Radiology and Pathology Correlation of Bone Tumors

A QUICK REFERENCE AND REVIEW

Radiology and Pathology Correlation of Bone Tumors

A QUICK REFERENCE AND REVIEW

Adam Greenspan, MD, FACR

Professor Emeritus of Radiology and Orthopedic Surgery
University of California, Davis School of Medicine
Former Director, Section of Musculoskeletal Imaging
Department of Radiology, University of California Davis Medical Center
Sacramento, California

Dariusz Borys, MD, FCAP

Associate Professor of Pathology and Orthopedic Surgery
Chief of Orthopaedic and Pediatric Pathology
Director of Digital Pathology
Loyola University Chicago
Chicago, Illinois

Foreword by

Lynne S. Steinbach, MD, FACR

Professor of Radiology and Orthopaedic Surgery
University of California San Francisco
San Francisco, California
President, International Skeletal Society
Schaumburg, Illinois

 Wolters Kluwer

Philadelphia · Baltimore · New York · London
Buenos Aires · Hong Kong · Sydney · Tokyo

Acquisitions Editor: Ryan Shaw
Product Development Editor: Lauren Pecarich
Senior Production Project Manager: Alicia Jackson
Senior Design Coordinator: Stephen Druding
Senior Manufacturing Coordinator: Beth Welsh
Marketing Manager: Dan Dressler
Prepress Vendor: SPi Global

Copyright © 2016 Wolters Kluwer

All rights reserved. This book is protected by copyright. No part of this book may be reproduced or transmitted in any form or by any means, including as photocopies or scanned-in or other electronic copies, or utilized by any information storage and retrieval system without written permission from the copyright owner, except for brief quotations embodied in critical articles and reviews. Materials appearing in this book prepared by individuals as part of their official duties as U.S. government employees are not covered by the above-mentioned copyright. To request permission, please contact Wolters Kluwer at Two Commerce Square, 2001 Market Street, Philadelphia, PA 19103, via email at permissions@lww.com, or via our website at lww.com (products and services).

9 8 7 6 5 4 3 2 1

Printed in China

Library of Congress Cataloging-in-Publication Data
Greenspan, Adam, author.
Radiology and pathology correlation of bone tumors : a quick reference and review / Adam Greenspan, Dariusz Borys.
    p. ; cm.
  Includes bibliographical references and index.
  ISBN 978-1-4698-9887-2 (alk. paper)
 I. Borys, Dariusz author. II. Title.
  [DNLM: 1. Bone Neoplasms—radiography. 2. Bone Neoplasms—physiopathology. WE 258]
  RC280.H47
  616.99'44107572—dc23
                                                                                       2015018485

This work is provided "as is," and the publisher disclaims any and all warranties, express or implied, including any warranties as to accuracy, comprehensiveness, or currency of the content of this work.

This work is no substitute for individual patient assessment based upon healthcare professionals' examination of each patient and consideration of, among other things, age, weight, gender, current or prior medical conditions, medication history, laboratory data and other factors unique to the patient. The publisher does not provide medical advice or guidance and this work is merely a reference tool. Healthcare professionals, and not the publisher, are solely responsible for the use of this work including all medical judgments and for any resulting diagnosis and treatments.

Given continuous, rapid advances in medical science and health information, independent professional verification of medical diagnoses, indications, appropriate pharmaceutical selections and dosages, and treatment options should be made and healthcare professionals should consult a variety of sources. When prescribing medication, healthcare professionals are advised to consult the product information sheet (the manufacturer's package insert) accompanying each drug to verify, among other things, conditions of use, warnings and side effects and identify any changes in dosage schedule or contraindications, particularly if the medication to be administered is new, infrequently used or has a narrow therapeutic range. To the maximum extent permitted under applicable law, no responsibility is assumed by the publisher for any injury and/or damage to persons or property, as a matter of products liability, negligence law or otherwise, or from any reference to or use by any person of this work.

LWW.com

To my wife Barbara, with all my love.

A.G.

To my wife Ewa and my children Adrianna and Francis, and to my parents Helena and Franciszek, and my brother Robert, for their love, encouragement and support.

D.B.

Foreword

It is a great honor and pleasure to introduce this much needed text: "*Outline of Bone Tumors Imaging and Pathology: A Quick Reference and Review,*" written by noted radiologist Adam Greeenspan, MD, FACR, and pathologist Dariusz Borys, MD, FCAP. Both authors are at the top of their subspecialties and have vast experience with imaging and pathology of bone tumors. They are also highly regarded members of the International Skeletal Society.

Dr. Greenspan is a Professor in the Department of Radiology and former Director of Musculoskeletal Imaging at the University of California, Davis Medical Center in Sacramento, California. He has authored over 140 peer-reviewed papers and edited 10 books including the highly acclaimed text, "*Orthopedic Imaging—A Practical Approach,*" which is in its sixth edition and has been translated into many foreign languages.

Dr. Borys is an Associate Professor of Pathology and Orthopedic Surgery at Loyola University Medical Center in Chicago where he is currently the Chief of Orthopedic and Pediatric Pathology and Director of the Digital Pathology Laboratory. Dr. Borys has coauthored more than 30 peer-reviewed manuscripts and is the editor and founder of an Orthopedic and Podiatric Pathology Web site which can be found at www.pedorthopath.com.

What makes this book special? It provides timely information that is helpful to all those who are involved in diagnosing and treating bone tumors. This includes the current classification systems, newly revised in 2013. The organization is comprehensive yet concise, with the information presented in optically pleasing color displays with short bullet points. These make it easy to master the major concepts of the material that one is reviewing. A variety of imaging modalities (including radiography, scintigraphy, CT, MRI, PET, and PET-CT) are used to depict the various tumors with high-quality figures. Learning is enhanced with professional color diagrams, charts, and tables. Pathologic discussions include the latest in histopathology, genetics, staining, and immunohistochemistry with classic examples that are easy to recall. The references are up to date and carefully chosen. Board-style questions are an additional useful feature that make this book relevant to all who are studying this field, as testing has become universal for physicians in all stages of practice.

This book is intended for radiologists, pathologists, and orthopedic surgeons who deal with bone tumors. Trainees, seasoned practitioners, and academicians will also benefit from the material presented in this text. Whether one reads this book from cover-to-cover, uses it as a reference for cases that come into the office daily or monthly, or studies for an examination, there is satisfaction in knowing that this is an effective, efficient, and valuable way to get this type of information. The reader will be rewarded with a satisfying learning experience from a book that is likely to become a classic, as have many of Dr. Greenspan's previous texts.

Lynne S. Steinbach, MD, FACR
Professor of Radiology and Orthopaedic Surgery
University of California San Francisco
San Francisco, California
President, International Skeletal Society
Schaumburg, Illinois

Preface

Musculoskeletal tumors are one of the most challenging subjects not only to physicians in training, but probably also to some board-certified radiologists and pathologists as well. In conversation with the radiology, pathology, and orthopedic surgery residents and fellows taking the specialty boards, invariably we have heard a great deal of anxiety and frustration on their part when it comes to choose a correct answer to the questions concerning musculoskeletal neoplasms, mainly because of rarity of these abnormalities in the clinical practice when compared, for example, to those related to traumatic conditions, arthritic diseases, or infections. Although bone tumors are rare, nevertheless their imaging and histopathologic evaluation is crucial from the teaching and practical point of view. In order to facilitate the complex and commonly difficult process of diagnostic investigation in bone tumors, we have assembled a large amount of information into a single, easy-to-use book for fast review for those individuals who prepare for the specialty board examinations, as well as for physicians who may encounter the musculoskeletal neoplasm in their daily clinical practice. The past decade have brought significant modifications to the imaging of musculoskeletal lesions, as well as changes in the understanding the pathology of many tumors. Under discussion, there are varieties of osseous lesions, benign and malignant, their radiologic imaging appearances (including radiography, scintigraphy, CT, MRI, PET, and PET-CT), and pathologic (including gross specimens, histopathology, immunohistochemistry, and genetics) findings. We illustrated typical and some atypical presentations, including pertinent differential diagnosis. We based the discussion of several bone tumors on the revised histopathologic classification issued by World Health Organization (WHO) in 2013. For each lesion, we provided the crucial information, such as its definition, epidemiology, sites of involvement, clinical findings, imaging characteristics, histopathology, immunohistochemistry, genetics, complications, prognosis, and differential diagnosis. The pertinent references are cited at the end of each chapter. We also created a number of questions very similar to the actual specialty boards examinations questions. In the answers to these questions, we provided not only the correct choice but also elaborated why the particular answer is correct or wrong.

We hope the practical aspect of this text will be effective as a teaching tool to resolve the diagnostic problems that arise in musculoskeletal pathology, as well as to be a helpful compendium for those individuals who train in radiology, anatomic pathology, and orthopedic surgery as they prepare for specialty boards examinations. The practicing physicians, particularly radiologists, pathologists, and orthopedic oncologists may also find this book useful in their everyday practice.

Adam Greenspan, MD, FACR
Dariusz Borys, MD, FCAP

Acknowledgments

We would like to express our appreciation to many individuals from Wolters Kluwer Health who closely supervised the production of this work, but particularly to Ryan Shaw, the Acquisition Editor, for his vision and confidence that this text will be beneficial for the targeted audience. Special thanks go to Nicole Dernoski and Lauren Pecarich, Product Development Editors, and Alicia Jackson, Senior Production Project Manager, for their attentive review of the manuscript, editorial advice, and purposeful suggestions during revisions of the text. We also would like to acknowledge Steve Druding, Design Coordinator, for his beautiful design of the cover and interior of the book. A special note of acknowledgment goes to Julie Ostoich-Prather, a Senior Photographer at the Department of Radiology, University of California, Davis Medical Center in Sacramento, California, for creating some of the digital images, and to Michael Greenspan and Samantha Greenspan for their help in solving some encountered technical problems.

We are indebted to Gernot Jundt, MD, Professor of Pathology and Head of Swiss Bone Tumor Reference Center, Institute of Pathology at the University of Basel, Switzerland, Michael J. Klein, MD, Professor of Pathology and Laboratory Medicine, Pathologist in Chief and Director, Department of Pathology at the Hospital for Special Surgery, New York, New York, Peter G. Bullough, MB, ChB, Professor of Pathology, Former Director of Pathology and Laboratory Medicine at the Hospital for Special Surgery, New York, New York, and Javier Beltran, MD, FACR, Professor and Chairman of Radiology at Maimonides Medical Center, Brooklyn, New York, for permission to use some of the pathology and radiology images from their files. We are grateful to Lynne S. Steinbach, MD, FACR, Professor of Radiology and Orthopaedic Surgery, Department of Radiology at University of California, San Francisco, for writing a Foreword for this book. Finally, many thanks to Leslie Jebaraj, Project Manager at SPi, for supervision and help during final composition of this text. It is our belief that without the dutiful and diligent efforts of the many individuals acknowledged here, this project could not have been successfully completed.

Contents

Foreword vii
Preface ix
Acknowledgments xi

1. DIAGNOSIS OF BONE TUMORS: RADIOLOGIC AND PATHOLOGIC APPROACH   1

Radiology   1
  Conventional Radiography   2
    Site of the Lesion   2
    Borders of the Lesion   3
    Type of Bone Destruction   6
    Periosteal Reaction   7
    Soft-Tissue Mass   8
    Composition of Tumor Tissue (Type of Lesion Matrix)   11
    Benign versus Malignant Nature   12
  Computed Tomography and Magnetic Resonance Imaging   12
  Scintigraphy (Radionuclide Bone Scan)   17
  Positron Emission Tomography, PET-CT, and PET-MRI   18
Pathology   20
  Basic Techniques and Decalcification   20
  Special Stains   21
  Immunohistochemistry   23
    Antibodies against Intermediate Filaments   23
    Antibodies against Hematopoietic and Lymphoid Cells, and Vascular Antigens   25
    Antibodies against Muscle and Neuroectodermal Antigens   25
    Other Useful Antibodies in Bone Tumor Pathology   26
  Electron Microscopy   27
  Genetics of Bone Tumors   27
    Cytogenetics   27
    Molecular Cytogenetics   28
References   29

2. BONE-FORMING (OSTEOGENIC) LESIONS   32

A. Benign Bone-Forming Lesions   32
  Osteoma   32
  Osteoid Osteoma   35
  Osteoblastoma   40
B. Malignant Bone-Forming Tumors   47
  Osteosarcomas   47
    Conventional Osteosarcoma   47
    Telangiectatic Osteosarcoma   61
    Small Cell Osteosarcoma   64
    Low-Grade Central Osteosarcoma   66
    Giant Cell–Rich Osteosarcoma   68
    Multifocal (Multicentric) Osteosarcoma   68
    Surface Osteosarcomas   69
  Secondary Osteosarcomas   78
    Postradiation Osteosarcoma   78
    Paget Osteosarcoma   79
    Osteosarcoma Associated with Fibrous Dysplasia   79
  Soft-Tissue (Extraskeletal) Osteosarcoma   81
References   86

3. CARTILAGE-FORMING (CHONDROGENIC) LESIONS   90

A. Benign Cartilage-Forming Lesions   90
  Enchondroma   90
  Enchondromatosis, Ollier Disease, and Maffucci Syndrome   97
  Periosteal (Juxtacortical) Chondroma   99
  Soft-Tissue Chondroma   104
  Synovial (Osteo) Chondromatosis   107
  Osteochondroma (Osteocartilaginous Exostosis)   114
  Multiple Hereditary Osteochondromata (Diaphyseal Aclasis)   121
  Chondroblastoma   124
  Chondromyxoid Fibroma   134
B. Malignant Cartilage-Forming Tumors   138
  Chondrosarcomas   138
    Conventional Chondrosarcoma (Central or Medullary Chondrosarcoma)   139
    Clear Cell Chondrosarcoma   145
    Mesenchymal Chondrosarcoma   152
    Myxoid Chondrosarcoma (Chordoid Sarcoma)   157
    Dedifferentiated Chondrosarcoma   157
    Periosteal (Juxtacortical) Chondrosarcoma   164
    Soft-Tissue (Extraskeletal) Chondrosarcomas   169
  Secondary Chondrosarcomas   171
    Malignant Transformation of Osteochondroma   171
    Malignant Transformation of Enchondroma   171
    Chondrosarcoma Arising in Primary (Osteo) Chondromatosis   175
    Chondrosarcoma Arising in Pagetic Bone   175
References   175

4. FIBROGENIC, FIBRO-OSSEOUS, AND FIBROHISTIOCYTIC LESIONS   180

A. Benign Fibrous Lesions   181
  Fibrous Cortical Defect/Nonossifying Fibroma   181
  Benign Fibrous Histiocytoma   189
  Periosteal Desmoid (Cortical Desmoid)   192
  Fibrous Dysplasia   194
  Fibrocartilaginous Dysplasia   197
  Osteofibrous Dysplasia (Kempson-Campanacci Lesion)   206
  Desmoplastic Fibroma (Desmoid Tumor of Bone)   210
B. Malignant Fibrohistiocytic Tumors   218
  Fibrosarcoma   218
  Malignant Fibrous Histiocytoma (Pleomorphic Undifferentiated Sarcoma)   221
  Angiomatoid Fibrous Histiocytoma of Bone   223
References   226

5. ROUND CELL LESIONS   230

A. Benign Round Cell Lesions   231
  Langerhans Cell Histiocytosis (LCH, Eosinophilic Granuloma)   231
  Rosai-Dorfman Disease   241
  Erdheim-Chester Disease (Lipogranulomatosis)   242

B. Malignant Round Cell Tumors 244
  Ewing Sarcoma/Primitive Neuroectodermal Tumor
    (PNET) 244
  Malignant Lymphoma of Bone 254
  Multiple Myeloma (Plasma Cell Myeloma,
    Plasmacytoma) 263
References 269

6. VASCULAR LESIONS 272
A. Benign Vascular Lesions 273
  Intraosseous Hemangioma 273
  Epithelioid Hemangioma (Angiolymphoid Hyperplasia
    with Eosinophilia) 282
  Cystic Angiomatosis 282
  Gorham Disease (Disappearing Bone Disease, Massive
    Osteolysis) 284
  Synovial Hemangioma 285
  Lymphangioma, Lymphangiomatosis of Bone 285
  Glomus Tumor 289
    Variants of Glomus Tumor 290
B. Malignant Vascular Tumors 290
  Epithelioid Hemangioendothelioma 290
  Angiosarcoma 293
References 295

7. MISCELLANEOUS LESIONS 298
A. Benign Lesions 298
  Giant Cell Tumor (GCT) 298
  Simple Bone Cyst (SBC) 309
  Aneurysmal Bone Cyst (ABC) 311
  Giant Cell Reparative Granuloma (GCRG, Solid Variant
    of ABC) 323
  Intraosseous Lipoma 330

B. Malignant Tumors 334
  Adamantinoma of Long Bones 334
  Chordoma 339
  Leiomyosarcoma of Bone 344
  Liposarcoma of Bone 347
References 348

8. TUMORS AND TUMOR-LIKE LESIONS OF THE JOINTS 353
A. Benign Joint Lesions 353
  Synovial (Osteo)Chondromatosis 353
  Pigmented Villonodular Synovitis (PVNS, Diffuse-Type
    Tenosynovial Giant Cell Tumor) 353
  Localized Pigmented Nodular Tenosynovitis (Giant Cell
    Tumor of the Tendon Sheath, Localized Tenosynovial
    Giant Cell Tumor) 359
  Synovial Hemangioma 362
  Lipoma Arborescens 364
  Juxta-Articular Myxoma 366
B. Malignant Joint Tumors 369
  Synovial Sarcoma 369
  Synovial Chondrosarcoma 377
References 377

9. OSSEOUS METASTASES 381
Skeletal Metastases 382
References 397

10. MOCK-BOARD REVIEW QUESTIONS 399

Index 427

CHAPTER 1

Diagnosis of Bone Tumors: Radiologic and Pathologic Approach

An accurate diagnosis of bone tumors requires a high level of skill on the part of both radiologist and pathologist. It is true that imaging features correlate strongly with malignancy, with benignity, and even sometimes with a precise diagnosis based on histopathologic findings. It is also true that radiology offers the important advantage of being able to view the lesion in a three-dimensional fashion, thereby enhancing the pathologic assessment. It must be remembered, however, that a confident radiologic diagnosis may not override what the pathologist discovers from the microscopic appearance of the lesion. Both diagnostic components are necessary.

The following discussion centers first on the radiologic approach to osseous tumors and then on the pathologic approach.

Radiology
Conventional Radiography
Site of the Lesion
Borders of the Lesion
Type of Bone Destruction
Periosteal Reaction
Soft-Tissue Mass
Composition of Tumor Tissue (Type of Lesion Matrix)
Benign versus Malignant Nature
Computed Tomography and Magnetic Resonance Imaging
Scintigraphy (Radionuclide Bone Scan)
Positron Emission Tomography, PET-CT, and PET-MRI

Pathology
Basic Techniques and Decalcification
Special Stains
Immunohistochemistry
Antibodies against Intermediate Filaments
Antibodies against Hematopoietic and Lymphoid Cells, and Vascular Antigens
Antibodies against Muscle and Neuroectodermal Antigens
Other Useful Antibodies in Bone Tumor Pathology
Electron Microscopy
Genetics of Bone Tumors
Cytogenetics
Molecular Cytogenetics

RADIOLOGY

Musculoskeletal tumors are commonly suspected on the basis of the history and physical examination. They are most often revealed on conventional radiographic examination. The imaging of these tumors serves three purposes: (1) detection, (2) diagnosis and differential diagnosis, and (3) staging.

In spite of the spectacular advances in imaging technology that have taken place over the past few decades, *radiography* still figures most prominently in determining a diagnosis and in providing a basis for differential diagnosis. It offers the most useful data concerning location and morphology of a tumor, including information about zone of transition, periosteal reaction, ossifications, calcifications, and type of bone destruction (Fig. 1.1).

Some techniques have more limited, but still valuable, diagnostic functions. *Scintigraphy*, for instance, can distinguish multiple myeloma from metastases that are similar in appearance, or a bone island from a sclerotic tumor, but is only sometimes instrumental in making a precise diagnosis. *Ultrasonography* only seldom yields data that can be used to differentiate malignant from benign tumors. *Arteriography* sometimes can reveal abnormal tumor vessels and can help distinguish bone abscess from osteoid osteoma. Its main functions, though, are (1) to map out the lesion in the bone and determine the extent of disease and (2) to reveal the vascular supply of the tumor, localize vessels for preoperative intra-arterial chemotherapy, and pinpoint the area most suitable for open biopsy, as the most aggressive parts of a tumor lie within the most vascular sections of a tumor.

The most dramatic radiologic advances that have been made in the past couple of decades concern the staging

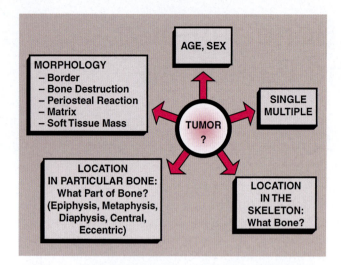

FIGURE 1.1 **Analytic approach to evaluation of the bone tumors.** Pragmatic analysis must include patient's age, multiplicity of the lesion, location in the skeleton and in the particular bone, and radiographic morphology.

has been of particular value in identifying primary, recurrent, and metastatic malignancies.

Conventional Radiography

Conventional radiographs provide abundant information about bone lesions:

- Location of the lesions in the skeleton and individual bone (topography of the lesion).
- Zone of transition (borders of the lesion).
- Type of bone destruction.
- Periosteal reaction (type of periosteal response to the lesion).
- Extent and quality of soft-tissue involvement.
- Composition of the tumor tissue (type of lesion matrix).

In the diagnosis of bone tumors, determining whether a lesion is solitary or multiple and the age of the patient are starting points.

Primary malignant tumors, including fibrosarcoma, malignant fibrous histiocytoma, Ewing sarcoma, chondrosarcoma, and osteosarcoma, do not often present as multiple lesions. Malignancies that are multifocal usually indicate multiple myeloma, metastatic disease, or lymphoma. Benign bone lesions with multifocal sites of involvement include, among others, polyostotic fibrous dysplasia, enchondromatosis, multiple cartilaginous exostoses (multiple hereditary osteochondromata), Langerhans cell histiocytosis (eosinophilic granuloma), hemangiomatosis, and osseous fibromatosis.

The patient's age is the most important item of clinical information that can be used along with the radiographic studies to reach a diagnosis. Certain bone tumors are found almost exclusively in certain age groups. For instance, metastatic lesions, conventional chondrosarcoma, and myeloma are usually seen in patients 40 years of age and older, and giant cell tumor of bone almost always arises after skeletal maturity (growth plate closure). In contrast, chondroblastoma, aneurysmal bone cyst, and chondromyxoid fibroma rarely are encountered in patients over 20 years old. When tumors do occur outside of their typical age group, they may not appear in the usual locations or may have a different radiographic appearance. This is the case with the simple bone cysts (so-called unicameral bone cysts). Before skeletal maturity, they usually arise in the proximal humerus or proximal femur. After skeletal maturity, however, they may be found in the calcaneus, scapula, or pelvis, among other places; with aging, they may look somewhat unconventional on radiography.

Site of the Lesion

A number of tumors have a predilection for specific bones or sites in bones, a fact that aids in diagnosis. The specific location is the result of developmental anatomy of the tumor-invaded bone and of the laws of field behavior. An example of such a tumor is chondroblastoma, which occurs mainly

(evaluation) of bone tumors. *Computed tomography (CT)* and *magnetic resonance imaging (MRI)* are indispensable in tumor staging for the following reasons: (1) their multiplanar capacities and outstanding soft-tissue contrast; (2) their ability to ascertain, with great accuracy, the tumor size, configuration, and location; (3) their capability in showing the intramedullary and extramedullary extension of tumors; and (4) their ability to reveal the relationship of tumors to nearby joints, as well as to muscles, muscle compartments, neurovascular bundles, and fascial planes. MRI, more than any other imaging modality, provides the most accurate anatomic staging. It should be noted that MRI, however, is not always successful in distinguishing benign from malignant tumors, even though attempts have been made to delineate the following markers: signal intensity patterns, the presence of edema, the appearance of tumor margins, and neurovascular bundle involvement.

Two techniques in particular are important in staging—*single photon emission computed tomography (SPECT)* and *scintigraphic techniques* using technetium-99m (^{99m}Tc), gallium-67 (^{67}Ga) citrate, and indium-111 (^{111}In)–labeled white blood cells. The radiopharmaceutical labeling enables these methods to yield information about the location and size of a tumor, as well as the pathophysiologic status of bone and the soft tissues surrounding it.

Positron emission tomography (PET), the most recent imaging modality to be applied to the diagnosis of musculoskeletal tumors alone or in combination with CT or MRI (PET-CT, PET-MRI), is able to correct for tissue attenuation signal loss and has relatively uniform spatial resolution. Because of these unique qualities, PET has gained wide acceptance. This technique has been able to supply information about the metabolism of musculoskeletal lesions, on the basis of high glycolysis rates in malignant tissues; whole-body ^{18}F-labeled 2-fluoro-2-deoxyglucose (^{18}FDG)-PET scanning

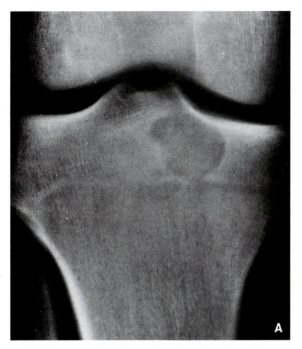
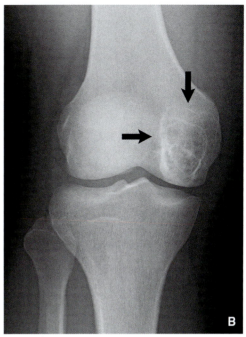

FIGURE 1.2 Predilection of the lesion for specific site within bone. Chondroblastoma has a predilection for the epiphysis of a long bone. **(A)** Anteroposterior radiograph of a knee of a 14-year-old boy shows a radiolucent lesion with thin sclerotic border in the proximal epiphysis of the right tibia. **(B)** Anteroposterior radiograph of the right knee of a 17-year-old girl shows a radiolucent lesion with chondroid calcifications in the medial femoral condyle (*arrows*).

in the epiphysis of the long bones before skeletal maturity has taken place (Fig. 1.2). Similarly, adamantinoma and osteofibrous dysplasia show a strong preference for the tibia (Fig. 1.3). Sometimes the location is so characteristic of the tumor that it alone can indicate the diagnosis, as in the case of parosteal osteosarcoma, which is found in most cases in the posterior aspect of the distal femur (Fig. 1.4). The site of the lesion can also be used in differential diagnosis. Because giant cell tumors are rarely found in another location than in the articular end of a bone, for instance, this diagnosis essentially should not be entertained if the lesion in question occurs in any other place (Fig. 1.5).

The relation of tumor to the central axis of the bone—especially a long tubular bone like the humerus, radius, tibia, and femur—is an equally significant component in assessing the site of the lesion. Some lesions appear centrally located; these include simple bone cyst (Fig. 1.6A), a focus or fibrous dysplasia (Fig. 1.6B), or enchondroma (Fig. 1.6C). An eccentric location is more typical of aneurysmal bone cyst (Fig. 1.7A), nonossifying fibroma (Fig. 1.7B), and chondromyxoid fibroma (Fig. 1.7C).

Borders of the Lesion

The lesion borders, or margins, can reveal much about how fast a lesion grows and thereby shed light on whether it is benign or malignant. A well-defined border indicates a slower growth rate and hence a greater likelihood of benignity (Fig. 1.8A). In contrast, an ill-defined border reflects a faster growth rate and thus a higher probability of malignancy (Fig. 1.8B).

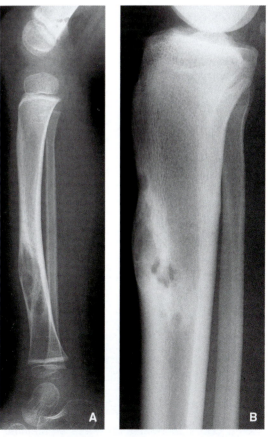

FIGURE 1.3 Predilection of the lesion for specific bone. The tibia is a common site for osteofibrous dysplasia **(A)** and adamantinoma **(B)**.

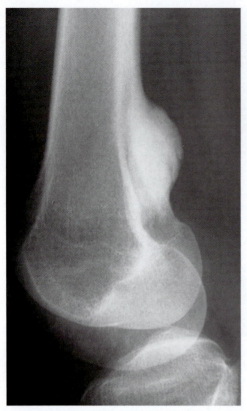

FIGURE 1.4 Predilection of the lesion for specific site within specific bone. Parosteal osteosarcoma has a strong predilection for the posterior aspect of the distal femur.

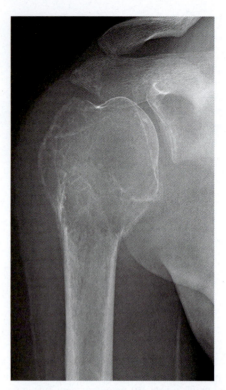

FIGURE 1.5 Predilection of the lesion for specific site within bone. One of the characteristic features of the giant cell tumor is its location in the articular end of a long bone, as seen in this 35-year-old woman who has a slightly expansive purely lytic lesion affecting right proximal humerus.

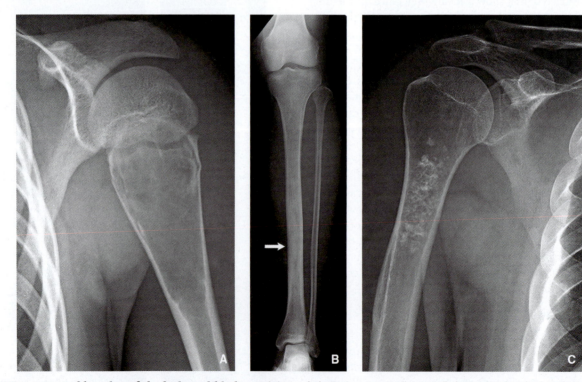

FIGURE 1.6 Central location of the lesion within bone. (A) Simple bone cyst is typically centrally located within the long bone, as seen in this 12-year-old boy who has a radiolucent lesion abutting the growth plate of the proximal humerus. **(B)** Majority of fibrous dysplasias are centrally located, as in this 28-year-old man with a sclerotic lesion affecting medullary portion of left tibia, exhibiting a "ground-glass" appearance (*arrow*). **(C)** Enchondroma is typically a central lesion, as demonstrated on this anteroposterior radiograph of the right humerus of the 52-year-old man.

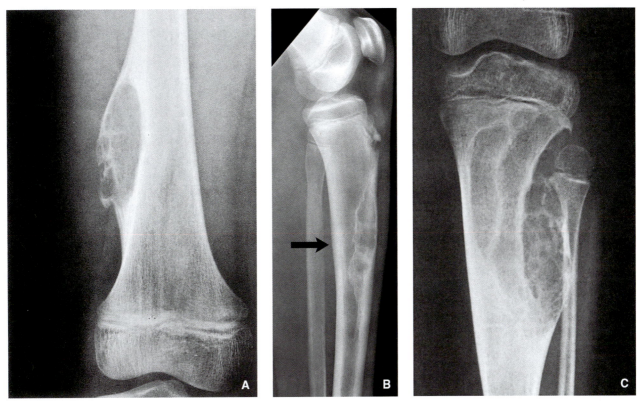

FIGURE 1.7 Eccentric location of the lesion within bone. (A) Aneurysmal bone cyst affecting the diaphysis of the right femur of an 8-year-old boy shows characteristic eccentric expansion. **(B)** Nonossifying fibroma seen here in the anterior aspect of the tibia of a 12-year-old girl exhibits a lobulated posterior margin and eccentric location within a bone (*arrow*). **(C)** Chondromyxoid fibroma, seen here affecting the metadiaphyseal portion of the left tibia of an 8-year-old girl, also displays characteristic eccentric location.

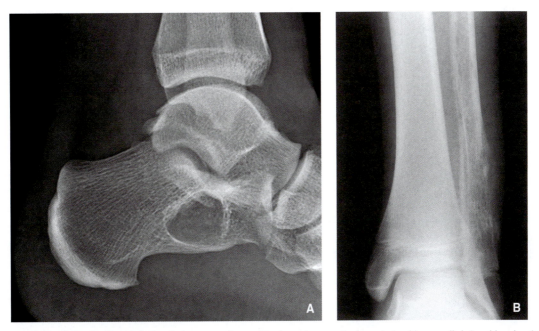

FIGURE 1.8 Borders of the lesion. (A) Simple bone cyst located in the calcaneus is characterized by a well-defined border. **(B)** Ewing sarcoma located in the fibula exhibits ill-defined border.

The margins can be divided into three types: (1) one sharply demarcated by sclerosis between the host bone and the peripheral aspect of the tumor (type IA margin); (2) one around the periphery of the lesion showing sharp demarcation but with no sclerosis (type IB margin); and (3) one with an ill-defined region where the lesion and host bone meet, involving either part of all of the circumference (type IC margin) (Fig. 1.9).

Benign tumors, such as aneurysmal bone cyst, chondromyxoid fibroma, simple bone cyst, and nonossifying fibroma, nearly always exhibit sharply defined borders (narrow zone of transition) with sclerosis at their margins (see Figs 1.7 and Fig. 1.8A). Conversely, malignant tumors, or those that are aggressive, instead are marked by indistinct borders (a wide zone of transition) (see Fig. 1.8B). Although radiotherapy or chemotherapy of malignant lesions can produce sclerosis, and thus a narrow zone of transition, in general, malignant or benign but aggressive tumors do not have sclerotic borders on radiographs. Such tumors include among others fibrosarcoma, malignant fibrous histiocytoma, multiple myeloma or solitary plasmacytoma, lymphoma, and metastases from primary tumors in the gastrointestinal tract, thyroid, and kidney.

Type of Bone Destruction

Destruction of bone may be caused by the tumor cells themselves. It may also result from the reaction of normal osteoclasts in the host bone to the growing pressure of the mass and to tumor-associated hyperemia. Although trabecular bone is destroyed at a faster rate than is cortical bone, cortical bone loss appears earlier on radiographs because its density is highly homogeneous compared with that of trabecular bone. About 70% of mineral content must be lost before trabecular bone loss shows on radiographs.

Three types of bone destruction can be defined, with the type of loss reflecting growth rate of the tumor. These types are (1) geographic (type I), marked by an area that is uniformly destroyed lying within sharply outlined borders; (2) moth-eaten (type II), characterized by small, multiple lytic areas, often clustered; and permeative (type III), showing as very small oval radiolucencies or lucent streaks that are ill defined (Fig. 1.10). These features alone do not define any specific tumors, but they are of help in differentiating benign from malignant lesions. Benign, slow-growing tumors, such as giant cell tumor, simple bone cyst, enchondroma, or chondromyxoid fibroma, show geographic bone destruction (Fig. 1.11A). In contrast, malignant tumors such as fibrosarcoma, Ewing sarcoma, myeloma, or lymphoma—all fast-growing and rapidly infiltrating tumors—have type II (Fig. 1.11C) or type III (Fig. 1.11B) destruction. It should be noted that some nonmalignant lesions may show this aggressive pattern. Examples include osteomyelitis, which may show both moth-eaten and permeative types of destruction, and hyperparathyroidism, which may produce a permeative pattern. Often, the same lesion may contain both types II and III, and distinguishing between them may present a challenge.

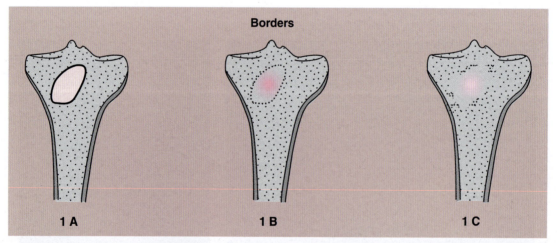

FIGURE 1.9 Types of the borders of the lesions. Borders of the lesion determine its growth rate. *1A*, sharp sclerotic; *1B*, sharp lytic; *1C*, ill defined. (Modified from Madewell JE, Ragsdale BD, Sweet DE. Radiologic and pathologic analysis of solitary bone lesions. Part I. Internal margin. *Radiol Clin North Am* 1981;19:715–748).

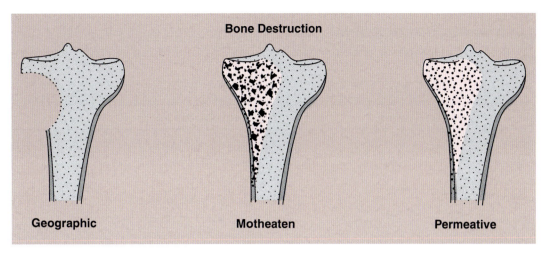

FIGURE 1.10 Patterns of bone destruction. Three types of bone destruction determine the lesion's growth rate. (Modified from Madewell JE, Ragsdale BD, Sweet DE. Radiologic and pathologic analysis of solitary bone lesions. Part I. Internal margin. *Radiol Clin North Am* 1981;19:715–748).

Periosteal Reaction

Like bone destruction, the periosteal reaction reveals the biologic activity of a lesion. It should be noted that no single periosteal response is unique to a particular lesion (Table 1.1). A periosteal process may manifest as any irregularity or broadening of the bone contour. Bone tumors produce periosteal reactions of two basic types: continuous (uninterrupted) and discontinuous (interrupted). The solid reaction, referred to as cortical thickening, can be a single solid layer or multiple closely apposed and fused layers of new bone that are joined to the cortex on its outer surface.

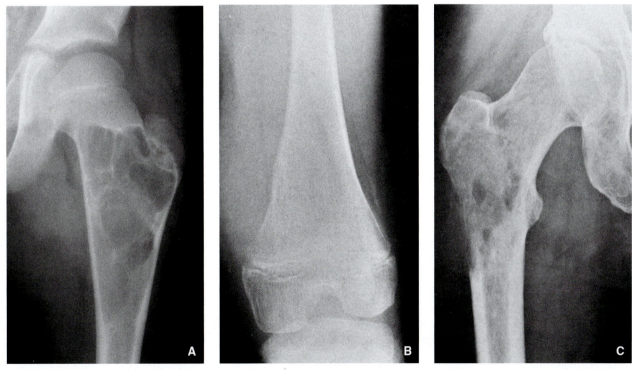

FIGURE 1.11 Patterns of bone destruction. (A) Simple bone cyst is typified by geographic type of bone destruction. **(B)** Ewing sarcoma exhibits a permeative pattern of bone destruction. **(C)** Myeloma characteristically shows moth-eaten type of bone destruction.

TABLE 1.1 Examples of Neoplastic and Nonneoplastic Processes Categorized by Type of Periosteal Reaction

Uninterrupted Periosteal Reaction

Benign tumors and tumor-like lesions	Nonneoplastic conditions
Osteoid osteoma	Osteomyelitis
Osteoblastoma	Langerhans cell histiocytosis
Aneurysmal bone cyst	Healing fracture
Chondromyxoid fibroma	Juxtacortical myositis ossificans
Periosteal chondroma	Hypertrophic pulmonary osteoarthropathy
Chondroblastoma	Hemophilia (subperiosteal bleeding)
Malignant tumors	Varicose veins and peripheral vascular insufficiency
Chondrosarcoma (rare)	Caffey disease
	Thyroid acropachy
	Treated scurvy
	Pachydermoperiostosis
	Gaucher disease

Interrupted Periosteal Reaction

Malignant tumors	Nonneoplastic conditions
Osteosarcoma	Osteomyelitis (occasionally)
Ewing sarcoma	Langerhans cell histiocytosis (occasionally)
Chondrosarcoma	Subperiosteal hemorrhage (occasionally)
Lymphoma (rare)	
Fibrosarcoma (rare)	
MFH (rare)	
Angiosarcoma	
Metastatic carcinoma	

From Greenspan A, Jundt G, Remagen W. Differential Diagnosis in Orthopaedic Oncology, 2nd ed. Philadelphia: Lippincott Williams & Wilkins; 2007.

Although the periosteal response is not a hallmark of any given lesion, as noted above, it has diagnostic value. A continuous reaction is likely to represent a benign lesion that is slow growing and usually indolent. The solid periosteal response may take many forms: (1) a single lamellar reaction, as seen with osteomyelitis, stress fracture, and Langerhans cell histiocytosis (Fig. 1.12A); (2) an undulating shape, seen in long-standing varicosities, chronic lymphedema, periostitis, pulmonary osteoarthropathy, and, rarely, with neoplasms (Fig. 1.12B); (3) a solid buttress, such as accompanying aneurysmal bone cyst and chondromyxoid fibroma (Fig. 1.12C); and (4) a solid elliptical or smooth layer, for example, present in osteoblastoma and osteoid osteoma (Fig. 1.12D).

In contrast, a discontinuous pattern most likely indicates primary malignant tumors and, less frequently, metastases and extremely aggressive nonmalignant lesions. The periosteal reaction in such tumors may have a characteristic sunburst (Fig. 1.13A) or onionskin arrangement (Fig. 1.13B and C). Another radiographic feature of note is the Codman triangle; this landmark is created when the tumor has invaded beyond the cortex and destroys newly lamellated bone, the remnants of which, on both ends of the breakthrough area, form this triangle (Fig. 1.13D).

Soft-Tissue Mass

The presence of a soft-tissue mass is a reliable indicator of an aggressive or malignant process. In contrast, benign bone neoplasms are not associated with soft-tissue mass, with certain exceptions, including among others desmoplastic fibroma, aneurysmal bone cyst, and giant cell tumor. Some nonneo-

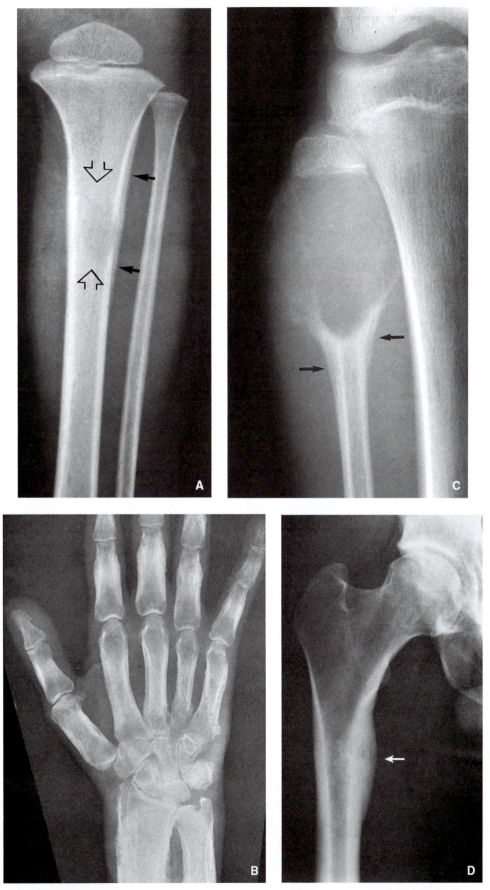

FIGURE 1.12 Types of periosteal reaction—uninterrupted. (A) Langerhans cell histiocytosis (*open arrows*) exhibits a single lamellar periosteal response (*arrows*). **(B)** Undulated type of periosteal reaction is seen in the distal radius and ulna, and metacarpals and phalanges in this patient with hypertrophic pulmonary osteoarthropathy due to lung carcinoma. **(C)** Solid buttress of periosteal reaction (*arrows*) accompanies the aneurysmal bone cyst. **(D)** Solid layer of periosteal reaction (*arrow*) is characteristic for cortical osteoid osteoma.

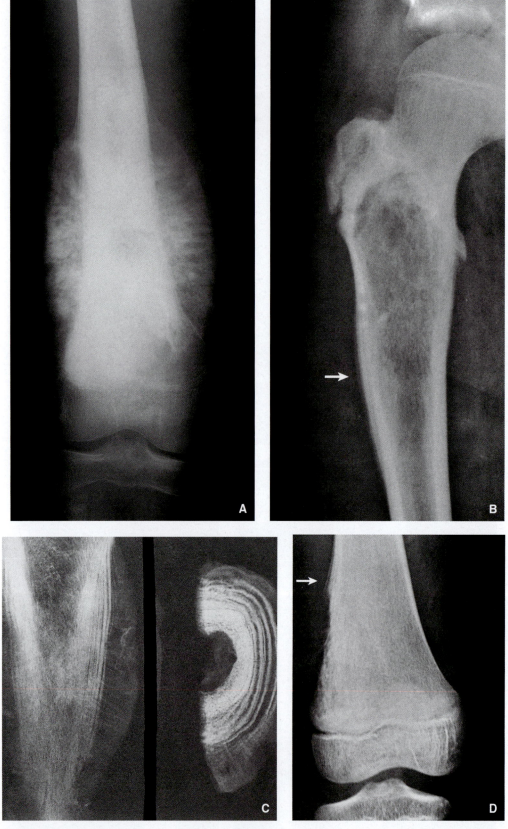

FIGURE 1.13 Types of periosteal reaction—interrupted. (A) Osteosarcoma exhibits characteristic sunburst type of periosteal reaction. **(B,C)** Ewing sarcoma is accompanied by onionskin type of periosteal reaction. **(D)** Typical Codman triangle (*arrow*) in a patient with osteosarcoma.

plastic processes can produce soft-tissue masses, as well; an example is osteomyelitis. In a condition such as this, the mass lacks sharp definition and the fatty tissue layers appear obliterated. Masses related to malignancy look quite different; they usually are well defined and extend through the damaged cortex, with tissue planes remaining intact (Fig. 1.14).

An important issue regarding soft-tissue masses is whether the mass is an extension of a primary bone tumor or is it a primary soft-tissue tumor invading bone. Making this determination often is challenging, as there are no hard-and-fast rules to follow. Careful observation may suggest answers. For example, if the bone lesion is small in relation to the soft-tissue mass, the bone lesion likely represents secondary bone involvement. Note, however, that in a small number of primary malignancies—notably, Ewing sarcoma—the bone lesion may be smaller than the accompanying soft-tissue mass. The periosteal response yields another clue. Primary malignant bone tumors usually elicit a periosteal response when they break through the cortex and invade neighboring soft tissues; conversely, primary soft-tissue tumors impinging on bone generally elicit no such response as they destroy the adjacent periosteum (Fig. 1.15).

Composition of Tumor Tissue (Type of Lesion Matrix)

Matrix, produced by mesenchymal cells, is intercellular material consisting of chondroid, myxoid, collagen, osteoid, and bone elements. A radiographic study of the matrix frequently can yield sufficient findings to differentiate between chondroblastic and osteoblastic processes and may help in distinguishing between lesions similar in appearance. Nonetheless, at times, it can be difficult to determine whether the matrix is osseous or cartilaginous. On the one hand, osseous matrix will appear fluffy, occasionally more organized, and trabecular. Conversely, cartilaginous matrix is more amorphous, typically with calcifications.

Osteosarcoma should be strongly considered if irregular, not fully mineralized bone matrix is identified on the radiograph as well as if cloud-like densities in the medullary cavity and neighboring soft tissues can be discerned (Fig. 1.16). It must be remembered, however, that tumor bone may bear a striking resemblance to reparative new bone generated after bone destruction by a process such as callus formation or reactive sclerosis.

In contrast to the cottony densities indicative of tumor bone, calcifications that lie within the tumor matrix suggest chondrogenic processes. They may take on any of three types of appearance: (1) stippled, or punctate; (2) flocculent, or irregularly shaped; or (3) annular or comma-shaped rings and arcs, producing a curvilinear look (Fig. 1.17). Calcifications occurring in a benign tumor or in a malignant tumor that is well differentiated may be the product of endochondral ossification. In making a differential diagnosis of the three types of calcifications, the following tumors may

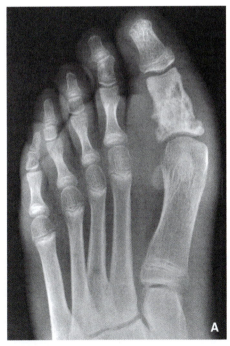
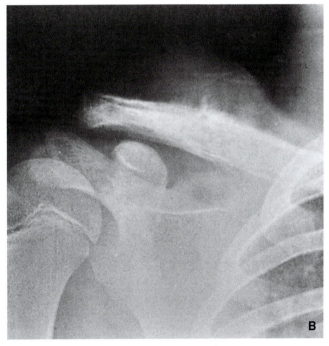

FIGURE 1.14 Soft-tissue mass. (A) Ill-defined soft-tissue mass in a patient with osteomyelitis of the proximal phalanx of the great toe. **(B)** Well-defined soft-tissue mass in a patient with osteosarcoma of the clavicle.

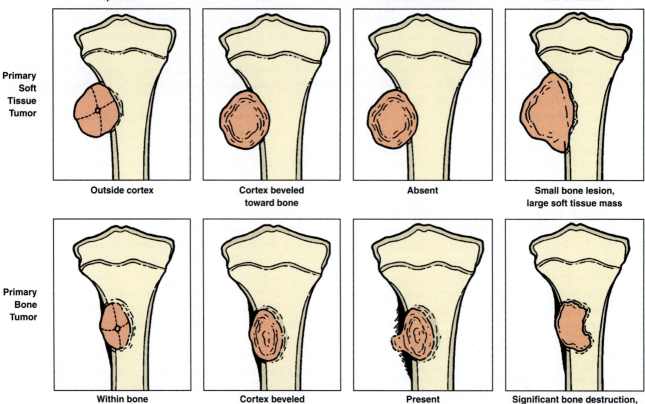

FIGURE 1.15 Soft-tissue mass—primary soft-tissue tumor versus primary tumor of bone with soft-tissue extension. Certain radiographic features may help in the differential diagnosis of these two possibilities.

be considered: chondrosarcoma, chondroblastoma, and enchondroma (Fig. 1.18 A,B).

If a lesion appears radiolucent, its origin could be either fibrous or cartilaginous. However, tumor-like lesions, such as an intraosseous ganglion or a simple bone cyst, that produce hollow structures may appear radiolucent, as well.

Benign versus Malignant Nature

Radiography alone is sometimes not sufficient for distinguishing between benign and malignant lesions. However, certain characteristics of the radiographic presentation can help the radiologist lean in one direction or the other. Malignant lesions show the following features:

- Borders that are poorly defined, with a wide zone of transition.
- A moth-eaten or permeative pattern to the bone destruction.
- A periosteal reaction with an interrupted, onionskin, or sunburst arrangement, with a neighboring soft-tissue mass.

On occasion, benign tumors may demonstrate aggressive characteristics such as those listed above. In general, however, benign lesions show the following features:

- Borders that are sharply defined and sclerotic.
- A geographic type of bone destruction.
- A periosteal reaction that is uninterrupted and solid, with no accompanying soft-tissue mass.

Computed Tomography and Magnetic Resonance Imaging

In determining whether tumor is present in the cortex, trabecular bone, or marrow cavity, CT and MRI have a high degree of accuracy. CT is not really of use in reaching a specific diagnosis, but it has great value because of the following capabilities: (1) it can clearly show a bone tumor that lies within an anatomically complex structure such as the pelvis, sacrum, or scapula; (2) it delineates with great precision how far a bone tumor extends and may reveal invasion of the cortex and surrounding soft tissues; (3) it shows surface lesions that occur on the bone, including juxtacortical chondrosarcoma, parosteal osteosarcoma, osteochondroma, and periosteal chondroma; and (4) three-dimensional CT images may offer a sharper and more complete view of the tumor.

The radiologist must decide when to use CT versus MRI. The choice is based on radiographic observations. If radiography does not reveal extension of the bone tumor into soft tissue, then CT is used because it can demonstrate, with

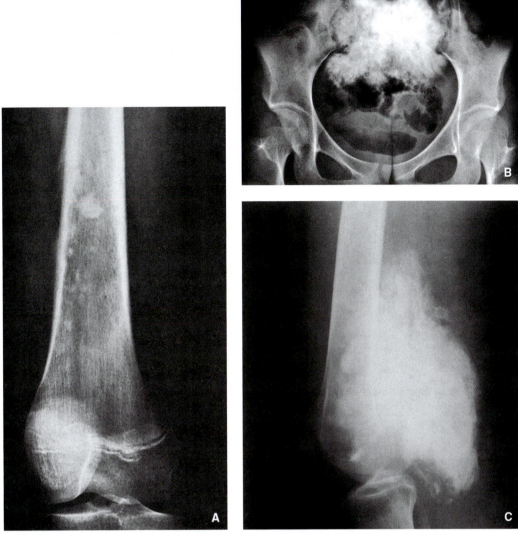

FIGURE 1.16 Composition of tumor tissue—osteoblastic matrix. The matrix of a typical osteoblastic tumor is characterized by the presence of fluffy, cotton-like densities within the medullary cavity such in this case of osteosarcoma of the distal femur **(A)**, by the presence of the wisps of tumor bone formation, like in this case of osteosarcoma of the sacrum **(B)**, or by the presence of a solid sclerotic mass, like in this case of parosteal osteosarcoma of the femur **(C)**.

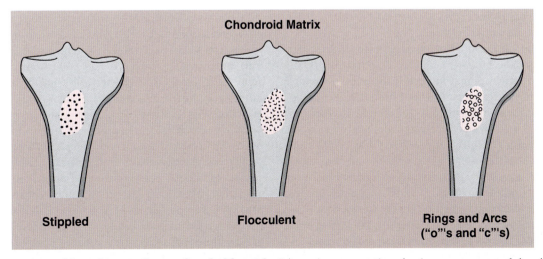

FIGURE 1.17 Composition of tumor tissue—chondroid matrix. Schematic representation of various appearances of chondroid matrix calcifications.

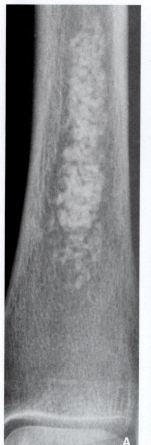
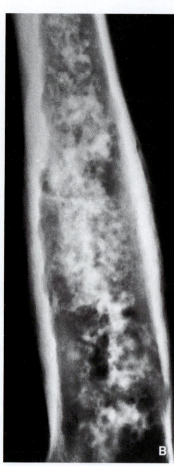

FIGURE 1.18 Composition of tumor tissue—chondroid matrix. Both enchondroma **(A)** and chondrosarcoma **(B)** display a typical chondroid matrix.

precision, cortical invasion and periosteal reaction, along with how far the tumor extends within the bone. If, however, radiography does show a soft-tissue mass together with cortical disruption or destruction, MRI would be the technique of choice because of its exceptional soft-tissue contrast and ability to reveal the extraosseous growth of the tumor. In fact, this attribute of providing superior soft-tissue contrast gives MRI a definite edge over CT. Furthermore, because of its ability to image on multiple planes (sagittal, coronal, axial, and oblique) and because it is not marked by beam-hardening artifacts from cortical bone, MRI is able to delineate intraosseous tumor extension, as well.

Spin echo (SE), short-time inversion recovery (STIR), gradient-recalled echo (GRE), and fast T2 or fat-suppressed T2-weighted sequences may be used to assess bone tumors. For identifying and staging most bone tumors, SE sequences are preferred, as the signal intensity for normal tissues is predictable. Bone marrow and fat display high signal intensity on T1 sequences; on T2 sequences, however, the signal intensity decreases to intermediate. Fluid shows intermediate signal intensity on T1-weighted images and high signal intensity on T2-weighted images. On both T1- and T2-weighted images, muscle has intermediate intensity. On both sequences, bone and fibrocartilage have low signal intensity. In imaging bone tumors (whose T1 and T2 relaxation times are increased relative to normal tissue), T1-weighted SE sequences show low or intermediate signal intensity, and T2-weighted sequences exhibit high signal intensity (Table 1.2). It should be noted that T1 and T2 images reveal different MRI characteristics of a bone tumor. On the one hand, contrast between tumor and bone, tumor and bone marrow, and tumor and fatty tissue is increased on T1-weighted SE sequences; on the other hand, contrast between tumor and muscle, as well as highlighting of peritumoral edema, is enhanced with T2-weighted SE, T2-weighted GRE, and other fluid-sensitive, such as STIR sequences (Fig. 1.19A–D).

Contrast-enhanced MRI with intravenous injection of gadopentetate dimeglumine (gadolinium diethylenetriamine-penta-acetic acid [Gd-DTPA]) offers further advantages. This enhancement reduces the T1 relaxation time on conventional T1-weighted sequences, allowing for higher signal intensity in the lesion and thus for enhanced delineation of the lesion (Figs. 1.20 and 1.21). This enhancement is especially notable in compressed tissue situated around the tumor, in heavily vascularized areas, and in muscle that is atrophic but greatly vascularized. Static and dynamic Gd-DTPA images are also of value in assessing musculoskeletal tumors. On T1 weighting, those areas showing contrast enhancement are usually more vascular; those not showing it generally consist of necrotic tissue. If a chemical shift (CHESS sequences) or fat suppression technique is used, an even greater advantage is conferred. In this technique, the fat signal is greatly

TABLE 1.2 Magnetic Resonance Imaging Signal Intensities of Various Tissues

Tissue	T1 Weighted	T2 Weighted
Hematoma, hemorrhage (acute, subacute)	High/intermediate	High
Hematoma, hemorrhage (chronic)	Low	Low
Fat, fatty marrow	High	Intermediate
Muscle, nerves, hyaline cartilage	Intermediate	Intermediate
Cortical bone, tendons, ligaments, fibrocartilage, scar tissue, air	Low	Low
Hyaline cartilage	Intermediate	Intermediate
Red (hematopoietic) marrow	Low	Intermediate
Fluid	Intermediate	High
Proteinaceous fluid	High	High
Tumors (generally)	Intermediate to low	High
Lipoma	High	Intermediate
Hemangioma	Intermediate (slightly higher than muscle)	High

From Greenspan A, Jundt G, Remagen W. *Differential Diagnosis in Orthopaedic Oncology.* 2nd ed. 27, Table 1-5.

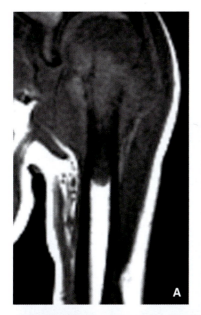
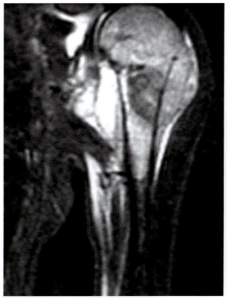
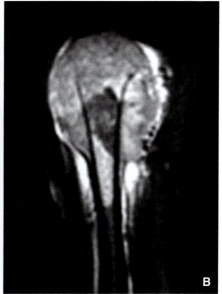
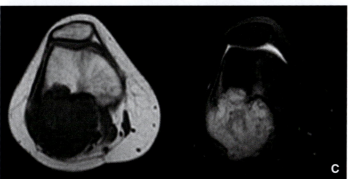

FIGURE 1.19 MRI of bone tumors, various sequences. **(A)** Coronal T1-weighted MR image of the left proximal humerus of a 14-year-old boy with conventional intramedullary osteosarcoma shows an intermediate-to-low signal intensity tumor destroying the cortex and extending into the soft tissues. **(B)** Coronal and sagittal T2-weighted fat-suppressed MR images show that the tumor exhibits heterogeneous but predominantly high signal. The areas of tumor bone formation are of low signal intensity. **(C)** In another patient, a 50-year-old woman with periosteal chondrosarcoma, axial T1- and T2-weighted fat-suppressed MR images demonstrate the tumor invading the lateral femoral condyle.

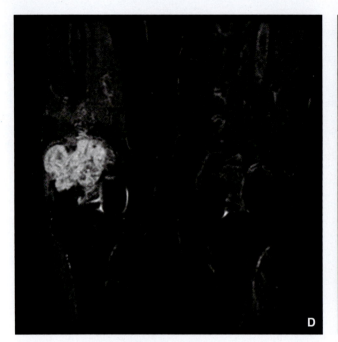
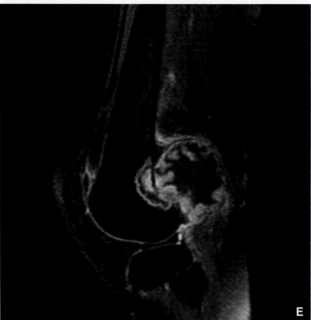

FIGURE 1.19 *(Continued)*. **(D)** Coronal inversion recovery (IR) MRI shows the tumor being of high signal intensity with internal foci of low signal, representing calcifications. **(E)** Sagittal T1-weighted fat-suppressed MR image obtained after intravenous administration of gadolinium demonstrates significant enhancement of the periphery of the tumor. Invasion of the medullary cavity of the femur is apparent.

suppressed, and the contrast-enhanced tumor shows a high signal intensity, resulting in an improved interface between tumor and reactive zone, tumor and peritumoral edema, and tumor and adjacent muscle.

The extent of extra- and intramedullary tumor within the context of surrounding structures is visualized much better with coronal-plane MRI than with axial CT, although the combination of coronal-plane MR images and CT scans does assist in evaluating important vascular structures next to tumors. Another way in which MRI surpasses CT is that it yields more defined images of tissue planes around a lesion and of neurovascular involvement, without the need for intravenous contrast. The superiority of MRI in differentiating normal from abnormal tissue, particularly in neoplasms

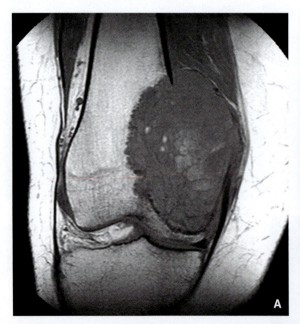
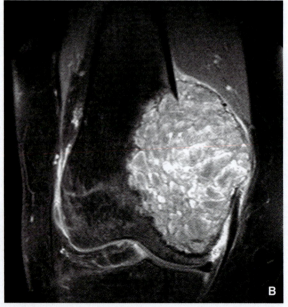

FIGURE 1.20 MRI enhanced with gadolinium of benign bone tumor. (A) Coronal T1-weighted MRI of the right knee of a 31-year-old woman demonstrates a large tumor destroying the cortex of the medial femoral condyle and extending into the soft tissues, exhibiting an intermediate but slightly heterogeneous signal intensity. **(B)** Coronal T1-weighted fat-suppressed MR image obtained after intravenous administration of gadolinium shows marked enhancement of the lesion, which on the histopathologic examination proved to be a benign giant cell tumor.

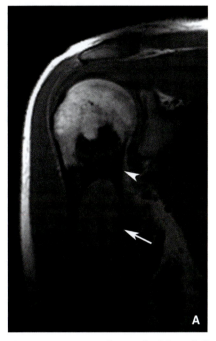 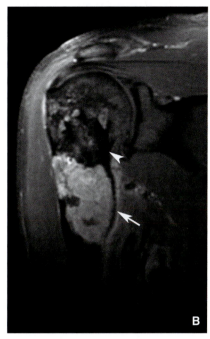 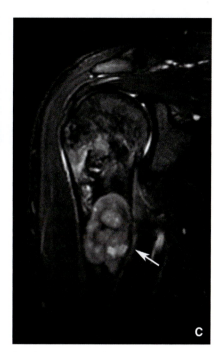

FIGURE 1.21 **MRI enhanced with gadolinium of malignant tumor. (A)** Coronal T1-weighted MR image of the right shoulder of a 22-year-old woman shows a lesion in the proximal humerus exhibiting low signal intensity in the proximal part of the tumor (*arrowhead*) and intermediate signal in the distal part (*arrow*). **(B)** Coronal T2-weighted MRI demonstrates that the proximal part is of mixed heterogeneous but predominantly of low signal intensity (*arrowhead*), whereas the distal part exhibits high signal intensity (*arrow*). **(C)** Coronal T1-weighted fat-suppressed MRI obtained after intravenous administration of gadolinium shows various degree of enhancement of the entire tumor, more prominent in the distal part (*arrow*). The excision biopsy revealed giant cell–rich osteosarcoma.

of the extremities, allows this technique to show, with a great measure of reliability, the following: extent of joint involvement, displacement and encasement of major neurovascular bundles, and tumor boundaries.

It must be noted that in certain respects, CT has the advantage over MRI. First, MRI is inferior to CT in depicting calcification in the tumor matrix, and when calcification is present in the image, it is not characterized as easily as on CT. Sometimes, small amounts of calcification have remained nearly undetected by MRI. Second, both CT and radiography have a greater capability than does MRI of showing cortical destruction and periosteal reaction.

Aside from the typical MRI characteristics of hemangioma and intraosseous lipoma, most of the time neither CT nor MRI is useful in defining the exact nature of a bone tumor. MRI in particular, however, has been touted as a reliable technique for differentiating benign from malignant lesions. Unfortunately, this has not been entirely borne out by the actual use of MRI. Several observations can be noted in this regard: (1) some malignant bone neoplasms can appear deceptively benign on MR scans, and, similarly, some benign bone lesions can appear deceptively malignant; (2) sometimes the classic features of malignancy and benignity overlap in MRI; (3) precise correlation between MRI findings and histologic diagnosis has not been achieved at this point; (4) the use of MRI signal intensities to characterize tissue is not yet reliable; and (5) because of the wide range of tumor composition and histologic patterns, signal intensity may be variable in histologically similar bone tumors, or the signal intensities of histologically dissimilar bone tumors may overlap. The bottom line is that MRI demonstrates high sensitivity in defining the extent of disease but remains somewhat nonspecific.

Scintigraphy (Radionuclide Bone Scan)

Bone-seeking radiopharmaceutical agents demonstrate enhanced deposition in bone that is undergoing change and repair; thus, a radionuclide bone scan, in reflecting mineral turnover, is helpful in localizing tumors and tumor-like lesions in the skeleton. For instance, it is instrumental in localizing small lesions not always detected by radiography, such as osteoid osteoma (Fig. 1.22). It is especially useful when more than one lesion is present, as in Langerhans cell histiocytosis, enchondromatosis, polyostotic fibrous dysplasia, and metastatic cancer. In determining whether a tumor is monostotic or polyostotic—hence in staging a tumor—technetium-99m methylene diphosphonate (MDP) scans are used. It should be kept in mind that the degree of abnormal uptake, which may reflect the aggressiveness of the lesion, does not show good correlation with histologic grade.

Skeletal scintigraphy has high sensitivity in detecting bone tumors, but its specificity is low. Because both benign and malignant conditions show increased blood flow with greater isotope deposition and increased osteoblastic activity, this technique cannot differentiate benign from malignant lesions. When, however, little or no radioactive isotope is absorbed, a distinction may be made. This may be the case with certain benign lesions. For example, scans using ^{67}Ga

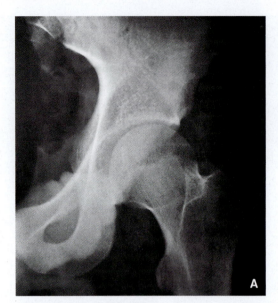 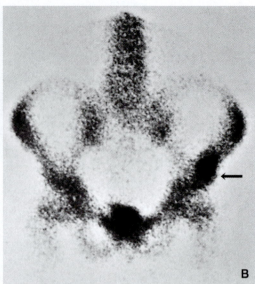

FIGURE 1.22 **Scintigraphy of osteoid osteoma. A:** Anteroposterior radiograph of the left hip of a 16-year-old boy with a typical history of osteoid osteoma is equivocal, although there is the suggestion of abnormal radiolucency in the supraacetabular portion of the ilium. **B:** Radionuclide bone scan shows an increased uptake of radiopharmaceutical agent *(arrow)* corresponding to questionable radiolucency seen on radiography. Osteoid osteoma was diagnosed on excision biopsy. (Reprinted with permission from Greenspan A. *Orthopedic imaging*, 4th ed. Philadelphia: Lippincott Williams & Wilkins, 2004.)

may reveal uptake in a soft-tissue sarcoma, which may help to distinguish it from a benign soft-tissue lesion. As another example, multiple myeloma usually does not exhibit much uptake of the radionuclide tracer and thereby may be differentiated from metastatic bone cancer, which usually does.

Thallium-201 (^{201}Tl) chloride has also been used in scintigraphy. In staging bone tumors and differentiating benign from malignant lesions, its use appears limited. However, it is useful in detection of some cartilaginous tumors and of primary and metastatic tumors, such as synovial sarcoma. In addition, ^{201}Tl in combination with pentavalent dimercaptosuccinic acid (DMSAV) may be of value in the differential diagnosis and grading of benign and malignant cartilage tumors.

In assessing a bone lesion, it is essential to determine intra- and extraosseous tumor extension and whether metastases are present. Scintigraphy is superior to radiography for evaluating the spread of a tumor beyond the site of origin. It also shows the degree of intramedullary involvement by tumor much better than does radiography. However, because the radionuclide tracer also localizes to hyperemic and edematous areas next to the tumor, a larger than actual area of extension is exhibited, and so bone scans cannot pinpoint the level of intramedullary invasion. That being said, with the single exception of MRI, scintigraphy is matchless in detecting skip lesions, which are remotely located skeletal lesions, and intraosseous metastases.

Scintigraphy and CT or MRI complement one another in the staging of bone tumors that require biopsy. Scintigraphy is of primary importance in evaluating the skeleton in general rather than in local staging. Its high sensitivity in this regard can suggest the presence of disseminated skeletal disease (Fig. 1.23). Although scintigraphy can yield information on the intraosseous extent of the disease, it falls short in giving a reliable representation of the local extent, for three reasons: (1) augmented uptake of the radionuclide, which has been described in osteosarcomas; (2) its relative lack of ability (compared with MRI) in distinguishing normal from abnormal marrow; and (3) its inability to reveal extracompartmental disease. Because any pathologic process that leads to new reactive or tumor bone formation, bone turnover, or increased blood flow will exhibit increased uptake of the radiopharmaceutical, scintigraphy is not specific enough to delineate a particular tumor type (except, sometimes, osteoid osteoma); nor is it sufficiently reliable in distinguishing between malignant and benign tumors. Nonetheless, this technique may yield valuable data on solitary bone tumors.

Scintigraphy should always be performed to assess whether skeletal involvement consists of solitary or multiple lesions. The most common malignant bone tumors are metastatic in nature. They can sometimes present as a solitary tumor in both pediatric and adult patients; for example, metastatic neuroblastoma and leukemia may be mistaken for solitary lesions like acute osteomyelitis, Langerhans cell histiocytosis, and Ewing sarcoma. Because synchronous and delayed skeletal metastases may occur in patients with Ewing sarcoma, scintigraphy is recommended at initial presentation as well as after excision of this tumor.

Positron Emission Tomography, PET-CT, and PET-MRI

In PET, biologic images are generated by detection of gamma rays emitted by a radioactive substance, such as 2-fluoro[fluorine-18]-2-deoxy-D-glucose (^{F18}FDG). This imaging technique makes possible the identification of physiologic and biochemical changes in the body, as well as evaluation of metabolic

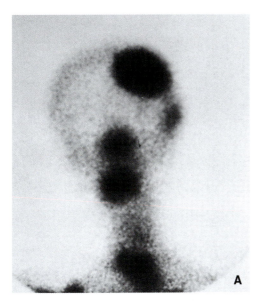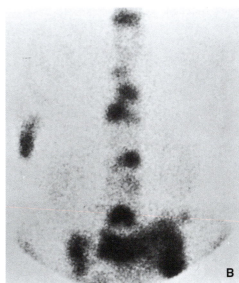

FIGURE 1.23 Scintigraphy of metastatic disease. A radionuclide bone scan was performed in a 68-year-old woman with breast carcinoma to determine the presence and distribution of metastases. After intravenous injection of 15 mCi (555 MBq) of ^{99m}Tc diphosphonate, an increased uptake of the radiopharmaceutical agent is seen in the skull and cervical spine **(A)** and lumbar spine and pelvis **(B)**, localizing the site of the multiple metastases.

activity and perfusion in organ systems. This technique has found significant application in oncology, in which it is used to determine the presence of primary and metastatic tumors (Fig. 1.24), as well as posttreatment recurrences. In this regard, PET appears to have greater sensitivity than does either CT or MRI. However, detection of bone marrow involvement is of uncertain reliability because physiologic bone marrow uptake of the radiopharmaceutical can be seen on ^{18}FDG PET images. Furthermore, despite a high degree of sensitivity, PET has low specificity because of accumulation of ^{18}FDG in benign aggressive lesions or those that are inflammatory. ^{11}C-methionine (MET) has been used in PET scanning of chordoma, with excellent results: an 80% sensitivity in the visualization of all tumors and a 100% sensitivity for recurrent tumors.

PET-CT combines in a single gantry system, a PET and a CT, allowing a sequential acquisition of images derived from both systems at the same time and thus combining them into a single superimposed image (Fig. 1.25). Two- and three-dimensional image reformation may be rendered as a function of a common software and control system. The simultaneous detection and precise localization of metabolic and biochemical activities by PET combined with anatomical details obtained by CT provides the radiologist with an unique opportunity not only to make a distinction between the normal and neoplastic processes but frequently between the various pathologic processes as well. The most common use of PET-CT is to improve the staging of bone tumors and evaluate their response to therapy and emergence of recurrences, as well as for detection and evaluation of metastatic disease.

PET-MRI is a newest hybrid technology with capabilities of instantaneous fusion of anatomic and functional data that allows an integrated scanning for simultaneous PET and MRI. This technique combines the strength of MRI, including lack of ionizing radiation and high resolution as well as

a high-contrast morphologic imaging of osseous structures and soft tissues with high sensitivity of PET and its ability to obtain functional images depicting metabolic and biochemical activity in the tissues, similar to PET-CT.

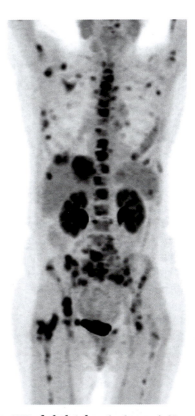

FIGURE 1.24 PET of skeletal metastases. A 65-year-old woman diagnosed with stage IV adenocarcinoma of the lungs developed widespread skeletal and internal organs metastases, as demonstrated on this whole-body PET scan.

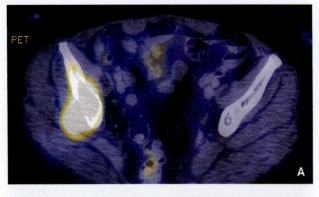
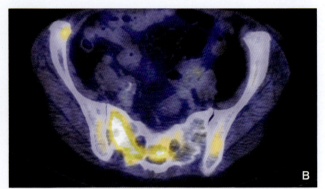
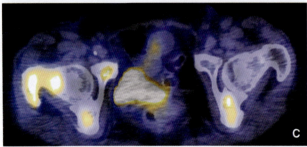

FIGURE 1.25 PET-CT. A 60-year-old woman with breast carcinoma underwent a PET-CT scanning. The axial fused PET-CT images generated several hypermetabolic foci of skeletal metastases including the right ilium **(A)**, sacrum **(B)**, right femur and both acetabula **(C)**, and thoracic vertebrae **(D)**.

PATHOLOGY

Diagnosis of osseous tumors, whether benign or malignant, is a complex and challenging process for both pathologists and radiologists. In bone tumor pathology, about 70 entities must be differentiated, many of which are rare.

In general, bone tumors are classified as primary or secondary lesions. Primary bone tumors account for only 1% of all malignancies, and about half of these represent multiple myeloma. They mainly occur (except for myeloma) in the first three decades of life, during the period of most active skeletal growth. Benign primary bone tumors are more common than malignant ones. According to some investigators, some of these lesions are not true neoplasms but, rather, are hamartomas (e.g., osteochondroma). The most common benign bone tumors are osteochondroma, enchondroma, and nonossifying fibroma. The most common primary malignant neoplasms are osteosarcoma and multiple myeloma, followed by chondrosarcoma and Ewing sarcoma. Secondary tumors can be further subdivided into metastatic tumors and malignant transformation of preexisting benign lesions (such as osteochondroma, enchondroma, Paget disease, bone infarct, or a chronic draining sinus tract of osteomyelitis). Metastatic carcinomas are the most frequently occurring malignant tumors of bone, found predominantly in adults over 40 years old or in children in the first decade of life. They are usually multifocal and are commonly seen in the axial skeleton (skull, vertebrae, ribs, and pelvis). In general, the location of the bone tumor and the patient's age correlate with bone tumor type (Tables 1.3 and 1.4).

The precise diagnosis of bone tumors is a formidable task, and if the diagnosis is in doubt, consultation with a specialized orthopedic pathologist is in order. The pathologist must review radiologic imaging studies to evaluate the size and growth pattern (behavior) of the tumor. Ordinarily, the pathologist receives a small, fragmented sample of bone biopsy tissue that may appear puzzling without radiologic correlation. Moreover, all tumor cases should also be discussed with an orthopedic surgical oncologist to relate all morphologic and imaging features to clinical information.

In summary, the correlation of morphologic, radiologic, and clinical findings is critical for making an accurate and definitive pathologic diagnosis.

Basic Techniques and Decalcification

For routine histologic diagnosis, hematoxylin and eosin (H&E) staining after decalcification is the gold standard for the orthopedic pathologist and should be sufficient for microscopic evaluation of tissue leading to the correct diagnosis (Figs. 1.26 and 1.27). In some cases, especially in small biopsy samples with tumor cells of unknown origin (metastases or primary sarcomas), histochemical and immunohistochemical stains may be needed but may be difficult to obtain after the decalcification process. Acidic decalcifiers such as formic acid (5% to 10% solutions) are commonly used. Formic acid

TABLE 1.3 Correlation Between Age Groups and Type of Bone Tumors

Age Group	Most Common Benign Lesions	Most Common Malignant Tumors
0–10	Simple bone cyst Langerhans cell histiocytosis (eosinophilic granuloma)	Ewing sarcoma Leukemic involvement Metastatic neuroblastoma
11–20	Nonossifying fibroma Fibrous dysplasia Simple bone cyst Aneurysmal bone cyst Osteochondroma (exostosis) Osteoid osteoma Osteoblastoma Chondroblastoma Chondromyxoid fibroma	Osteosarcoma Ewing sarcoma Adamantinoma
21–40	Enchondroma Giant cell tumor	Chondrosarcoma
41 and above	Osteoma	Metastatic tumors Myeloma Leukemic involvement Chondrosarcoma Osteosarcoma (Paget associated) MFH and fibrosarcoma Chordoma

is not as rapid a decalcifier as nitric acid, so tissue structure is well preserved and shows good staining for H&E. Most immunohistochemical stain protocols may also be applied. However, genetic studies may be affected owing to destruction of cell nuclear proteins. For genetic studies, decalcification with the chelating agent EDTA (ethylenediaminetetraacetic acid) is a better choice but is more time consuming. EDTA is effective for the rapid decalcification of small biopsy specimens.

Special Stains

Special stains are used when the H&E stain cannot provide answers to basic diagnostic, pathogenetic, and etiologic questions. Many special stains are available, but only a few can yield specific diagnostic information supporting an H&E diagnosis of skeletal tumor pathology. For instance, van Gieson stain, which is more commonly used in Europe, helps to identify the presence and amount of collagen in bone and other connective tissues by staining it intensively red (Fig. 1.28). Giemsa stain is occasionally used in the differentiation of small round cell tumors, particularly the lymphomas (Fig. 1.29). Reticulin fibers are usually stained with Gomori stain (Fig. 1.30) or Novotny stain (Fig. 1.31), which are helpful in differentiation against collagen fibers. Periodic acid–Schiff (PAS) stain coupled with diastase digestion is used to demonstrate intracytoplasmic glycogen. In bone tumor pathologic studies, PAS is often used to reveal glycogen in Ewing sarcoma and in clear cell chondrosarcoma (Fig. 1.32). Mucins stain can demonstrate metastatic adenocarcinoma whenever the tumor cells do not form glandular structures. Trichrome stain can reveal extracellular substances such as collagen, which may be useful in histomorphometric evaluation of mineralized versus nonmineralized osteoid in metabolic bone diseases. Several stains are used in the differential diagnosis to exclude bone tumors and to confirm another possibility. For example, certain stains document the presence of microorganisms. The Gram stain is used to classify bacterial organisms as gram positive or gram negative (Fig. 1.33); Grocott methenamine silver (GMS) stain identifies fungal organisms (Fig. 1.34); and Warthin-Starry stain is used to detect spirochetes and rickettsiae. The Congo red stain is used to highlight amyloid deposition, and green birefringence should be seen under polarized light. The von Kossa technique is used as a calcium stain, which proves useful in the histomorphometric assessment of metabolic bone disorders involving calcium.

TABLE 1.4 Most Common Skeletal Location of Bone Tumors

Lesions	Most Common Skeletal Sites
Ewing sarcoma Multiple myeloma Leukemia/lymphoma Metastatic cancers	Hematopoietic marrow sites in the axial skeleton (vertebrae, ribs, sternum, pelvis, cranium) and proximal long bones (femur, humerus)
Nonossifying fibroma	Femur and distal tibia
Simple bone cyst	Proximal humerus (50%), proximal femur (25%)
Chordoma	Base of the skull, C2, and sacrum (90%)
Adamantinoma	Mid-shaft of the tibia (90%), jaw bones
Chondroblastoma	75% long bones (distal and proximal femur, proximal tibia, and proximal humerus)
Giant cell tumor	Ends of long bones, the distal femur, proximal tibia, distal radius, and proximal humerus
Enchondroma	Most common in short tubular bones of the hand (~40% of cases)
Chondrosarcoma (primary and less commonly secondary)	About 75% occurs in the trunk, femur, and humerus, 25%–30% occurring in the pelvic bones
Fibrous dysplasia	Craniofacial bones and the femur are the most common sites for monostotic and polyostotic forms. In monostotic FD, most lesions are located in the femur, skull, and tibia
Osteochondroma	Most common in metaphyseal region of the distal femur, upper humerus, proximal tibia, and fibula
Osteoblastoma	Posterior elements of the spine and sacrum (40%–55%)
Aneurysmal bone cyst	Can affect any bone, but usually arises in the metaphysis of long bones: femur, tibia, and humerus
Chondromyxoid fibroma	Knee area (30%), pelvic bones, small bones of the feet
Hemangioma	Vertebral bodies are most common to be involved followed by craniofacial and long bones

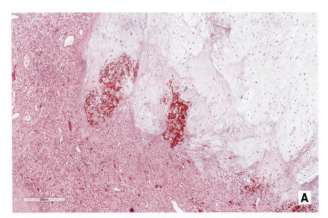 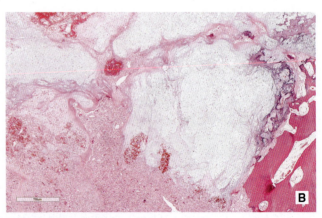

FIGURE 1.26 Hematoxylin and eosin (H&E) stain. *Dedifferentiated chondrosarcoma*. (A) There is sharp margin between two components of the tumor, consisting of a high-grade sarcoma that is stained pink (*lower left*) and low-grade cartilaginous tumor that is stained bluish (*upper right*). Note the malignant tumor invading the bone trabecula (*lower right*) (H&E, original magnification ×100). **(B)** Under higher magnification, markedly atypical sarcomatous cells and more benign looking cartilaginous cells are better appreciated (H&E, original magnification ×200).

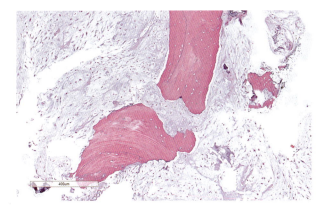

FIGURE 1.27 Hematoxylin and eosin (H&E) stain. *Conventional chondrosarcoma.* Cartilaginous tumor (*stained bluish*) permeates the bone trabecula (*stained pink*), the characteristic finding for this malignancy (H&E, original magnification ×200).

Immunohistochemistry

The immunohistochemistry (IHC) method is based on binding a specific cell antigen with a specific antibody on the cell surface or inner structures. Techniques using IHC are very helpful in distinguishing between tumors with similar histology but different origin. The best example is the use of this technique to differentiate among Ewing sarcoma/primitive neuroectodermal tumors (PNETs), lymphoma, metastatic neuroblastoma, and Wilms tumor in the differential diagnosis of small round cell tumors. Antigen retrieval methods rely on the use of enzyme-linked antibodies. The enzyme antibody converts a colorless substrate into a stained complex that is precipitated on the slide. The pathologist should be familiar with immunostaining patterns that may be diagnostically helpful but should also be aware of frequently occurring nonspecific staining patterns. Daily review of immunohistochemical results with external and internal positive and negative controls should be performed to avoid misinterpretation

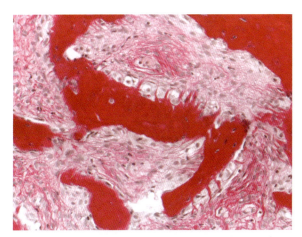

FIGURE 1.28 van Gieson stain. *Fibrous dysplasia.* Observe irregular woven bone trabeculae lacking osteoblastic activity, characteristic for this disorder. Collagenous fibers within the bone matrix are stained intensely red. Sharpey-like fibers in perpendicular arrangement to the trabecular surface extending into the adjacent stroma are conspicuous (van Gieson, original magnification ×200).

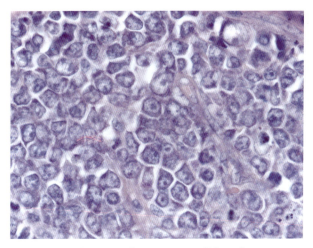

FIGURE 1.29 Giemsa stain. *Large B-cell lymphoma.* DNA, RNA, and basophilic cytoplasmic components are stained purple to gray-blue, helping to identify nuclear details of the lymphoma cells (Giemsa, original magnification ×630).

of ambiguous results. The pitfalls of IHC in general result in false-negative or false-positive diagnoses. The immunohistochemical technique is a powerful tool for providing diagnostically valuable information but should not be a substitute for the diagnostic approach to a specific bone tumor that incorporates additional clinical, radiologic, and histologic findings.

The most commonly used antibodies are briefly described in the following sections.

Antibodies against Intermediate Filaments

Intermediate filaments (IFs) are structural proteins with a diameter of 8 to 10 nm and a molecular weight of 40 to 110 KD. The most common antibodies used against IFs are as follows: **vimentin**, present in mesenchymal and some epithelial cells, and **cytokeratins (CKs)**, mostly found in epithelial cells. There are two groups of basic (CK 1–8) and acidic (CK 9–20) CKs. In practice, CKs are commonly divided into low molecular weight CKs (generally, CKs 8, 18, and 19) and

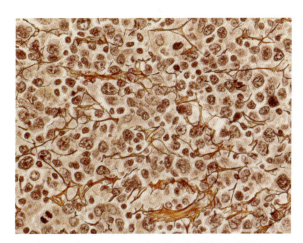

FIGURE 1.30 Gomori stain. *Large B-cell lymphoma.* Reticulin fibers appear as fine dark-brown to black network encircling lymphoma cells in a bone marrow biopsy specimen (Gomori, original magnification ×630).

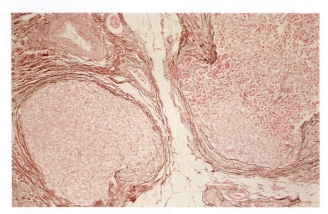

FIGURE 1.31 Novotny stain. *Ewing sarcoma*. Reticulin fibers that stain black are absent within tumor cell areas, thus excluding the diagnosis of malignant lymphoma and small cell osteosarcoma (Novotny, original magnification ×12).

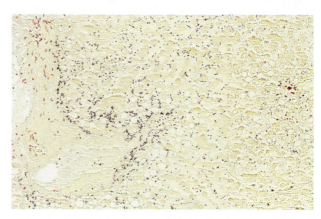

FIGURE 1.33 Gram stain. *Bacterial infection*. Gram stain highlights the chains of gram-positive bacteria, in this case *Staphylococcus aureus* (*brown organisms*).

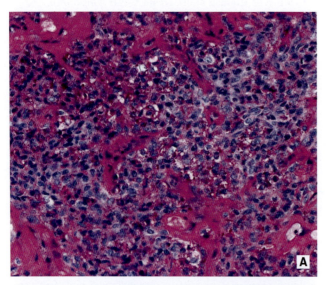

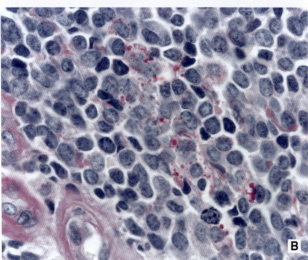

FIGURE 1.32 Periodic acid–Schiff (PAS) stain. *Ewing sarcoma*. **(A)** Glycogen droplets stain pink to red (PAS, original magnification ×100). **(B)** Under high magnification, glycogen droplets (*center*) and glycoprotein-containing basement membrane material of capillaries (*bottom left*) stain pink to red. Because glycogen is water soluble, it may be removed by formalin fixation (PAS, original magnification ×630).

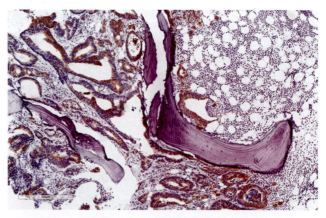

FIGURE 1.34 Grocott methenamine silver (GMS) stain. *Fungal infection*. This stain highlights the fungal organisms (*black*) in the infected tissue (GMS, original magnification ×100).

FIGURE 1.35 Immunohistochemistry. *Metastases*. Metastatic colonic adenocarcinoma to the bone is positive (*brown color*) for CK20 (CK20, original magnification ×100).

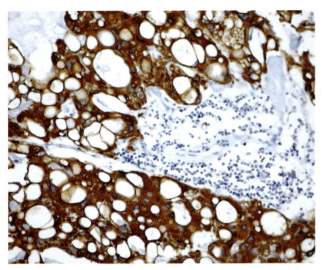

FIGURE 1.36 Immunohistochemistry. *Chordoma*. Tumor cells react positive with a cytokeratin antibody cocktail (CK22) directed against low molecular weight and high molecular weight cytokeratins. Lymphocytes (*center*) and cartilage cells (*upper left*) react negative (methylene blue counterstaining, original magnification ×400).

high molecular weight CKs (generally, CKs 1, 5, 10, and 14). CKs are highly sensitive markers for identification of metastatic carcinoma to bone (Fig. 1.35). Occasionally, they are effective in identification of Wilms tumor and chordoma (Fig. 1.36). From a practical point of view, we find it very useful to apply specific combinations of CK7 and CK20 for the preliminary differentiation of primary carcinoma origin, as follows: **CK7$^+$/CK20$^+$**—carcinoma of bile duct and primary mucous tumors of ovary, upper gastrointestinal tract, and endocervix; **CK7$^+$/CK20$^-$**—breast, endocervical, and endometrial carcinoma, carcinoma of esophagus, lung, salivary gland, thyroid, and mesothelioma; **CK7$^-$/CK20$^+$**—carcinoma of colon, primary carcinoma of adrenal cortex, and prostate carcinoma (Table 1.5).

Antibodies against Hematopoietic and Lymphoid Cells, and Vascular Antigens

Antibodies against hematopoietic and lymphoid cells are widely used in the diagnosis of lymphomas and hematologic malignancies. Most antibodies against these largely cell surface–based antigens have been categorized in workshops and statistically assigned to a so-called cluster of differentiation (CD) number that designates the respective antigens. These antigens are present not only on lymphatic or hematopoietic (as in Langerhans cell histiocytosis) cells (Fig. 1.37) but also in Ewing sarcoma and synovial sarcoma (CD99) (Fig. 1.38) and in endothelial and vascular tumors (CD31 and CD34).

Endothelial cells and endothelial cell–derived tumors are characterized by the expression of factor VIII–related antigen or von Willebrand factor (Fig. 1.39). This factor is a glucoprotein that is also synthesized in megakaryocytes. It is often used in combination with CD31 (platelet–endothelial cell adhesion molecule) and CD34 (hematopoietic progenitor cell antigen).

Antibodies against Muscle and Neuroectodermal Antigens

Desmin is a filamentous molecule expressed in smooth, skeletal, and cardiac muscles. In the pathologic study of bone, it is mainly used to detect metastatic sarcomas with muscle differentiation as leiomyosarcoma or a dedifferentiated rhabdomyoblastic component in dedifferentiated chondrosarcoma. Other markers used for muscle differentiation include **actin**, **myogenin**, and **MyoD**. Myogenin and MyoD are expressed in more than 90% of rhabdomyosarcomas and should be used in cases in which desmin is not strongly expressed but morphology is consistent with rhabdomyosarcoma.

Markers for nerve sheath differentiation include the **S100 protein**, which is expressed in a large number of tissues containing some neurons, glia, Schwann cells, melanocytes, and Langerhans cells. In the immunohistochemical diagnosis of bone tumors, it is of most value in Langerhans cell histiocytosis and clear cell sarcoma. Neuroectodermal marker **CD99**, the product of the pseudoautosomal *MIC2* gene, is an important immunohistochemical marker for the diagnosis of the Ewing sarcoma/PNET family. Many studies have shown that over 90% of Ewing sarcoma/PNET expresses CD99 (see Fig. 1.38). Nevertheless, we have to recognize that significant subsets of small round cell tumors also stain positively for CD99. For example, CD99 is seen in more than 90% of lymphoblastic lymphomas, in 20% to 25% of

TABLE 1.5	CK7/CK20 Combination to Diagnose Primary Site of Metastatic Carcinoma
CK7$^+$/CK20$^+$:	Carcinomas of bile duct, also primary mucinous tumors of the ovary, upper GI tract, and endocervix
CK7$^+$/CK20$^-$:	Breast, endocervical and endometrial adenocarcinoma, esophagus, lung, salivary gland, thyroid; mesothelioma
CK7$^-$/CK20$^+$:	Carcinoma of colon, primary mucinous tumors of lower GI tract, primary bladder adenocarcinoma
CK7$^-$/CK20$^-$:	Carcinoma of adrenal cortex, prostate

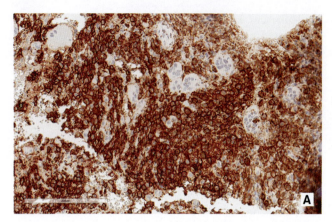
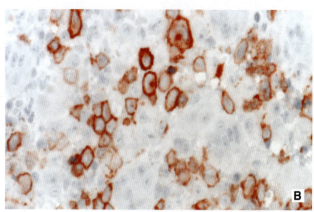

FIGURE 1.37 Immunohistochemistry. *Langerhans cell histiocytosis*. (A) Langerhans cells show strong membranous and cytoplasmic immunoreactivity for CD1a (CD1a, original magnification ×200). **(B)** Under higher magnification, observe that accompanying lymphocytes, macrophages, and giant cells are negative for this marker (methylene blue counterstaining, original magnification ×400).

primitive rhabdomyosarcomas, in more than 75% of poorly differentiated synovial sarcomas (primary synovial sarcomas of bone have been described in the literature, occurring mainly in older patients), and in approximately 50% of mesenchymal chondrosarcomas (small round cell component).

Other Useful Antibodies in Bone Tumor Pathology

Markers of *melanocytic differentiation* include **HMB45** and **Melan A**, mostly useful in detecting metastatic melanoma to bone and primary clear cell sarcoma. Markers of *endothelial differentiation* include CD34, CD31, and factor VIII. From a practical viewpoint, all three immunostains should be used to make a diagnosis of vascular tumors. CD34 (human hematopoietic progenitor cell antigen) is expressed on hematopoietic stem cells, endothelium, the interstitial cells of Cajal, and dendritic cells. However, CD34 is not limited to vascular tumors only and can be expressed in dermatofibrosarcoma protuberans (DFSP), solitary fibrous tumor (SFT), and malignant peripheral nerve sheath tumor (MPNST). CD31 (platelet–endothelial cell adhesion molecule-1) is expressed in 90% of angiosarcomas, hemangioendotheliomas, and hemangiomas. CD31 may also be expressed on macrophages and platelets. We have seen cases of the diffuse type of pigmented villonodular synovitis with prominent reactive atypia positive for CD31, resembling angiosarcoma.

Other useful markers in bone tumor pathology include the CD68 marker for histiocytes; β-catenin, positive in fibromas; CD1a, positive in Langerhans cells (see Fig. 1.37); MDM2, positive in low-grade osteosarcomas and liposarcomas; bcl-2, positive in follicular lymphomas; and p16, positive in most osteosarcomas (Fig. 1.40). Our recent study has shown clinical prognostic application in the adjuvant therapy of these tumors; for example, osteosarcomas positive for p16 had a better response to therapy than did p16-negative tumors.

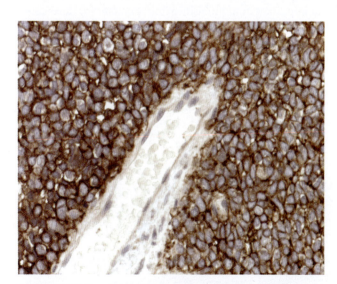

FIGURE 1.38 Immunohistochemistry. *Ewing sarcoma*. Tumor cells show a positive membrane-bound reaction for CD99. Nuclei are contrastained with methylene blue. Centrally located capillary with endothelial cells serve as a negative control (CD99, original magnification ×400).

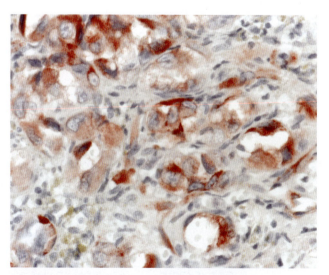

FIGURE 1.39 Immunohistochemistry. *Epithelioid angiosarcoma*. Observe strong intracytoplasmic immunoreactivity for factor VIII–related antigen (methylene blue counterstaining, original magnification ×400).

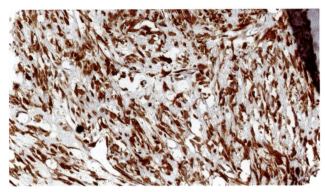

FIGURE 1.40 Immunohistochemistry. *Osteosarcoma.* p16 shows strong nuclear immunoreactivity in osteosarcoma cells (p16, original magnification ×100).

Electron Microscopy

Electron microscopy (EM) does not have a prominent role in the study of bone tumor pathology. Ultrastructural investigations, however, are still of help in the evaluation of small cell neoplasms (e.g., PNET may show neurosecretory granules), or in Langerhans cell histiocytosis, demonstrating characteristic Birbeck granules (Fig. 1.41).

Genetics of Bone Tumors

Genetic studies of bone tumors may demonstrate specific chromosomal changes in cancer cells, which may act as diagnostic, prognostic, and targeted therapy markers. To detect these changes, new diagnostic methods such as flow cytometry (FCM), digital cytogenetics, and molecular cytogenetics were developed.

Flow cytometry (FCM) is a quantitative automated method used to analyze the DNA content and proliferation rate of isolated cells. To determine DNA content, the DNA is stained with specific fluorescent dyes, and the emitted

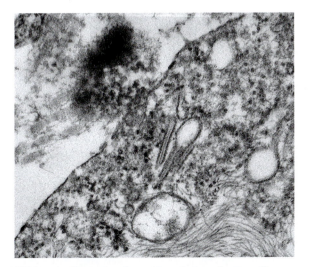

FIGURE 1.41 Electron microscopy. *Langerhans cell histiocytosis.* Rod-like and tennis racquet–shaped cytoplasmic structures (Birbeck granules) are characteristic for this lesion (EM, original magnification ×64,000).

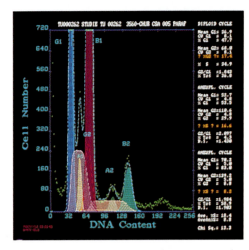

FIGURE 1.42 Flow cytometry. *Chondrosarcoma.* Flow cytometry histogram of chondrocytes of grade 2 tumor presents multiploid DNA pattern.

fluorescent signal is measured as the nuclei pass one by one through a nozzle-equipped chamber (flow cell). The intensity of the signal is proportional to the amount of DNA in the isolated nuclei. DNA distribution and the respective number of cells are calculated, compared with a standard (usually lymphocytes) and then assigned to each phase of the cell cycle. In FCM, the total amount of DNA is assessed without considering the distribution of single chromosomes. The prefix DNA, along with the ploidy terms, is used to determine FCM. Normal or tumor cells with the same amount of DNA as normal control cells (e.g., lymphocytes) are called DNA diploid, whereas cells with less or more DNA content are called DNA aneuploid. In the G0 phase of the cell cycle, cells are DNA diploid. Then, they enter the predivision period, the G1 phase, which is followed by the phase of DNA synthesis, the S phase. The number of cells in the S phase of the cell cycle represents the proliferating cell fraction (S-phase fraction, SPF). The amount of DNA gradually doubles until the cells are DNA tetraploid. Then, the cells enter the premitotic G2 phase, after which mitotic division is performed during the M phase. It is well known that DNA aneuploidy and often increased SPF are found in most carcinomas. DNA aneuploidy and increased SPF have been described in cartilaginous tumors (Fig. 1.42).

Cytogenetics

Cytogenetics is a branch of genetics that is concerned with studying the structure and function of the cell, especially the chromosomes. The karyotyping and identification of numerical and structural chromosomal abnormalities have an important role in diagnosing bone tumors—for example, in recurrent chromosomal translocations involving chromosomes 11 and 22 [t (11;22) (q24;q12)] or chromosomes 21 and 22 [t (21;22) (q22;q12)] in Ewing sarcoma. To evaluate tumor cells for growth, tissue has to be sent fresh, delivered immediately to the laboratory, and cultured in appropriate media. Mitoses of the tumor cells are interrupted during metaphase, and spread chromosomes are stained with special dyes (e.g., Giemsa). A metaphase chromosome is divided into two arms by a central region, the centromere (the constricted site on the chromosome to which the fibers of the mitotic spindle attach). The short arm is labeled with the letter p (petite) and the long arm with the letter q. The chromosomal ends (ter) are called telomeres (tel). Analysis of banded chromosomes is done microscopically by a clinical laboratory specialist in cytogenetics, who analyzes chromosomes and is able to recognize deletions, translocations, and other chromosomal aberrations. Generally, 20 cells are analyzed, which is enough to rule out mosaicism to an acceptable level.

Molecular Cytogenetics

With the development of **fluorescent in situ hybridization (FISH)**, genetic analyses of interphase nuclei became possible, even in fixed and paraffin-embedded material, by application of differentially labeled centromere-specific and sequence-specific probes to nuclear material. Multicolor labeling techniques made it possible to identify more than one DNA sequence simultaneously. Break-apart probes, with differentially labeled DNA fragments flanking—for example, the EWS breakpoint region on chromosome 22q12 in Ewing sarcomas—indicate translocations by the splitting of the normally paired green and red (or fused yellow) signal (Fig. 1.43). These results can be generated in 48 hours

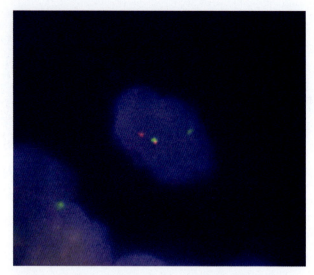

FIGURE 1.43 Fluorescence in situ hybridization (FISH). Ewing sarcoma. FISH using commercially available break-apart probe involving the *EWSR1* (Ewing sarcoma breakpoint region 1) gene on chromosome 22q12. Two probes, labeled in red and green, are applied flanking the breakpoint region from both sides. If no translocation is present, both colors should be in close contact. However, when translocation is present, the green and red signals are separated. The cell in center shows one fusion and one rearrangement (FISH, original magnification ×1,000).

TABLE 1.6 Most Common Translocation and Fusion Protein in Sarcomas

Type of sarcoma	Translocation	Fusion Protein
Alveolar rhabdomyosarcoma	t(2;13)(q35;q14)	PAX3-FKHR
	t(1;13)(p36;q14)	PAX7-FKHR
Alveolar soft part sarcoma	t(X;17)(p11.2;q25)	ASPL-TFE3
Clear cell sarcoma (malignant melanoma of soft parts)	t(12;22)(q13;q12)	ATF1-EWS
Congenital fibrosarcoma and mesoblastic nephroma	t(12;15)(p13;q25)	ETV6-NTRK3
Dermatofibrosarcoma protuberans (giant cell fibroblastoma)	t(17;22)(q22;q13)	COL1A1-PDGFB
Desmoplastic round cell tumor	t(11;22)(p13;q12)	WT1-EWS
Ewing sarcoma/primitive neuroectodermal tumors	t(11;22)(q24;q12)	EWS-FLI1
	t(21;22)(q22;q12)	EWS-ERG
	t(7;22)(p22;q12)	EWS-ETV1
	t(17;22)(q12;q12)	EWS-E1AF
	t(2;22)(q33;q12)	FEV-EWS
Inflammatory myofibroblastic tumor	t(2;19)(p23;p13.1)	ALK-TPM4
	t(1;2)(q22-23;p23)	TPM3-ALK
Myxoid chondrosarcoma, extraskeletal	t(9;22)(q22;q12)	EWS-CHN(TEC)
	t(9;17)(q22;q11.)	RBP56-CHN(TEC)
	t(9;15)(q22;q21)	TEC/TCF12
Myxoid liposarcoma	t(12;16)(q13;p11)	TLS(FUS)-CHOP
	t(12;22)(q13;q12)	EWS-CHOP
Synovial sarcoma	t(X;18)(p11;q11)	SYT-SSX1
		SYT-SSX2

with FISH. Comparative genomic hybridization (CGH) also uses DNA hybridization procedures. Tumor DNA and differentially labeled reference DNA are hybridized to normal metaphase chromosomes. Changes in the ratio of the two fluorochromes (i.e., red for tumor DNA, green for normal DNA) reflect losses or gains of tumor DNA that may be caused by amplifications, deletions, or duplications along the respective chromosomes. CGH is therefore a very useful tool to detect changes in DNA copy number.

The **polymerase chain reaction (PCR)** is a revolutionary method developed by Kary B. Mullis in the 1980s. PCR is based on the ability of DNA polymerase to synthesize new strands of DNA complementary to the offered template strand. Because DNA polymerase can add a nucleotide only to a preexisting 3′-OH group, it needs a primer to which it can add the first nucleotide. This requirement makes it possible to delineate a specific region of template sequence that the researcher wants to amplify. At the end of the PCR, the specific sequence will be accumulated in billions of copies (amplicons). This method enables detection of chromosomal translocation t(11;22) in Ewing sarcoma from even a very small sample of biopsy tissue. Table 1.6 shows most common translocation in sarcomas important for diagnosis and prognosis.

To summarize, the pathologist must diagnose a bone tumor on the basis of imaging correlation and evaluation of small amounts of biopsy material. Sometimes, this may be a very difficult assignment. In most cases, the morphologic features of tumor, such as pleomorphism, hyperchromatism, atypical mitotic figures, and the presence of necrosis, will help to distinguish between malignant and benign tumors. However, in some malignancies, like Ewing sarcoma, which belongs to the group of small round cell tumors, the features described above (particularly pleomorphism and atypical mitoses) are not present, which makes it rather difficult in most cases to differentiate this malignancy from lymphoma, metastatic neuroblastoma, small round cell sarcoma or embryonal rhabdomyosarcoma. In these instances, additional advanced molecular genetic studies can help to establish the correct diagnosis.

In the end, close cooperation between the radiologist, the pathologist, and the orthopedic surgeon in the review of clinical history, imaging studies, and biopsy material will lead to an accurate diagnosis of bone lesions. For the most part, careful analysis of all above-discussed elements enables identification of various benign and malignant tumors and tumor-like conditions of bones.

REFERENCES

Alho A, Connor JF, Mankin HJ, Schiller AL, Campbell CJ. Assesment of malignancy of cartilage tumors using flow cytometry. *J Bone Jont Surg Am.* 1983;65:779–785.

Alho A, Skjeldal S, Pettersen EO, Melvik JE, Larsen TE. Aneuploidy in benign tumors and nonneoplastic lesions of musculoskeletal tissues. *Cancer.* 1994;73:1200–1205.

An Y, Martin K, eds. *Handbook of Histological Methods for Bone and Cartilage.* Totowa, NJ: Humana Press; 2003.

Aoki J, Wanatabe H, Shinozaki T, et al. FDG PET of primary benign and malignant bone tumors: standardized uptake value in 52 lesions. *Radiology.* 2001;219:774–777.

Berquist TH. Magnetic resonance imaging of primary skeletal neoplasms. *Radiol Clin North Am.* 1993;31:411–424.

Bisseret D, Kaci R, Lafage-Proust M-H, et al. Periosteum: characteristic imaging findings with emphasis on radiologic-pathologic comparisons. *Skeletal Radiol.* 2015;44:321–338.

Bloem JL, Reiser MF, Vanel D. Magnetic resonance contrast agents in evaluation of the musculoskeletal system. *Magn Res Q.* 1990;6:136–163.

Bloem JL, Taminiau AHM, Eulderink F, Hermans J, Pauwels EK. Radiologic staging of primary bone sarcoma: MR imaging, scintigraphy, angiography, and CT correlated with pathologic examination. *Radiology.* 1988;169:805–810.

Bloem JL. *Radiological Staging of Primary Malignant Musculoskeletal Tumors. A Correlative Study of CT, MRI, ^{99m}Tc Scintigraphy and Angiography.* The Hague, the Netherlands: A. Jongbloed; 1988.

Bodner G, Schocke MFH, Rachbauer F, et al. Differentiation of malignant and benign musculoskeletal tumors: combined color and power Doppler US and spectral wave analysis. *Radiology.* 2002;223:410–416.

Borys D, Cantor R, Horvai A, et al. P16 expression predicts necrotic response among patients with osteosarcoma receiving neoadjuvant chemotherapy. *Hum Pathol.* 2012;43:1948–1954.

Bridge JA, Sndberg AA. Cytogenetic and molecular genetic techniques as adjunctive approaches in the diagnosis of bone and soft tissue tumor. *Skeletal Radiol.* 2000;29:249–258.

Bridge RS, Rajaram V, Dehner LP, Pfeifer JD, Perry A. Molecular diagnosis of Ewing sarcoma/primitive neuroectodermal tumor in routinely processed tissue: a comparison of two FISH strategies and RT-PCR in malignant round cell tumors. *Mol Pathol.* 2005;19:1–8.

Brown KT, Kattapuram SV, Rosenthal DI. Computed tomography analysis of bone tumors: patterns of cortical destruction and soft tissue extension. *Skeletal Radiol.* 1986;15:448–451.

Cindre JM. Immunohistochemistry in the diagnosis of soft tissue tumors. *Histopathology.* 2003;43:1–16.

Dahlin DC, Unni KK. *Bone Tumors: General Aspects and Data on 8542 Cases.* 4th ed. Springfield, MA: Charles C. Thomas; 1986.

Davies MA, Wellings RM. Imaging of bone tumors. *Curr Opin Radiol.* 1992;4:32–38.

Dilhon AP, Rhode J, Leathem M. Neurone specific enolase: an aid to the diagnosis of melanoma and neuroblastoma. *Histopathology.* 1982;6:81–92.

Dinauer PA, Brixey CJ, Moncur JT, Fanburg-Smith JC, Murphey MD. Pathologic and MR imaging features of benign fibrous soft-tissue tumors in adults. *Radiographics.* 2007;27:173–187.

Dorfman DH, Czerniak B. *Bone Tumors.* 1st ed. C.V. Mosby; 1998.

Dorfman HD, Czerniak B. *Bone Tumors.* St. Louis, MO: Mosby; 1998:1–33.

Dwek JR. The periosteum: what is it, where is it, and what mimics it in its absence? *Skeletal Radiol.* 2010;39:319–323.

Edeiken J, Hodes PJ, Caplan LH. New bone production and periosteal reaction. *Am J Roentgenol.* 1966;97:708–718.

Elias DA, White LM, Simpson DJ, et al. Osseous invasion by soft-tissue sarcoma: assessment with MR imaging. *Radiology.* 2003;229:145–152.

Enneking WF, Spanier SS, Goodman MA. A system for the surgical staging of musculoskeletal sarcoma. *Clin Orthop.* 1980;153:106–120.

Enneking WF. Staging of musculoskeletal neoplasms. *Skeletal Radiol.* 1985;13:183–194.

Erlemann R, Reiser MF, Peters PE, et al. Musculoskeletal neoplasms: static and dynamic Gd-DPTA-enhanced MR imaging. *Radiology.* 1989;171:767–773.

Ewing J. A review and classification of bone sarcomas. *Arch Surg.* 1922;4:485–533.

Fayad LM, Bluemke DA, Weber KL, Fishman EK. Characterization of pediatric skeletal tumors and tumor-like conditions: specific cross-sectional imaging signs. *Skeletal Radiol.* 2006;35:259–268.

Fechner RE, Mills SE. *Tumors of the Bones and Joints.* Washington DC: Armed Forces Institute of Pathology; 1993:1–16.

Fletcher DM, Unni KK, Mertens F, eds. *World Health Organization Classification of Tumors: Pathology and Genetics of Tumors of Soft Tissue and Bones*. Lyon, France: IARC Press; 2013.

Fletcher, CDM, Bridge JA, Hogendoorn P, Mertens F. *WHO Classification of Tumors of Soft Tissue and Bone*. 4th ed. Lyon, France; 2013.

Frank JA, Ling A, Patronas NJ, et al. Detection of malignant bone tumors: MR imaging vs. scintigraphy. *Am J Roentgenol*. 1990;155:1043–1048.

Franke WW, Schiller DL, Moll R, et al. Diversity of cytokeratins. Differentiation specific expression of cytokeratin polypeptides in epithelial cells and tissues. *J Mol. Biol.* 1981;153:933–959.

Galasko CS. The pathological basis for skeletal scintigraphy. *J Bone Joint Surg Br.* 1975;57:353–359.

Gao Z, Kahn LB. The application of immunohistochemistry in the diagnosis of bone tumors and tumor-like lesions. *Skeletal Radiol*. 2005;34: 755–769.

Gatenby RA, Mulhern CB, Moldofsky PJ. Computed tomography guided thin needle biopsy of small lytic bone lesions. *Skeletal Radiol*. 1984;11: 289–291.

Gillespy T III, Manfrini M, Ruggieri P, Spanier SS, Pettersson H, Springfield DS. Staging of intraosseous extent of osteosarcoma: correlation of preoperative CT and MR imaging with pathologic macroslides. *Radiology*. 1988;167:765–767.

Gold RH, Bassett LW. Radionuclide evaluation of skeletal metastases: practical considerations. *Skeletal Radiol*. 1986;15:1–9.

Golfieri R, Baddeley H, Pringle JS, et al. Primary bone tumors. MR morphologic appearance correlated with pathologic examinations. *Acta Radiol*. 1991;32:290–298.

Greenfield GB, Warren DL, Clark RA. MR imaging of periosteal and cortical changes of bone. *Radiographics*. 1991;11:611–623.

Greenspan A, Jundt G, Remagen W. *Differential Diagnosis in Orthopaedic Oncology*. 2nd ed. Philadelphia, PA: Lippincott Williams & Wilkins; 2007.

Greenspan A, Jundt G, Remagen W. *Differential Diagnosis in Orthopaedic Oncology*. 2nd ed. Lippincott Williams & Wilkins; 2007:1–35.

Greenspan A, Klein MJ. Radiology and pathology of bone tumors. In: Lewis MM, ed. *Musculoskeletal Oncology. A Multidisciplinary Approach*. Philadelphia, PA: WB Saunders; 1992:13–72.

Greenspan A, Stadalnik RC. Central versus eccentric lesions of long tubular bones. *Semin Nucl Med*. 1996;26:201–206.

Greenspan A. Pragmatic approach to bone tumors. *Semin Orthop*. 1991;6:125–133.

Hamada K, Ueda T, Tomita Y, et al. False positive 18F-FDG PET in an ischial chondroblastoma; an analysis of glucose transporter 1 and hexokinase II expression. *Skeletal Radiol*. 2006;35:306–310.

Hanna SL, Langston JW, Gronemeyer SA, Fletcher BD. Subtraction technique for contrast-enhanced MR images of musculoskeletal tumors. *Magn Reson Imaging*. 1990;8:213–215.

Hayes CW, Conway WF, Sundaram M. Misleading aggressive MR imaging appearance of some benign musculoskeletal lesions. *Radiographics*. 1992;12:1119–1134.

Helms C, Munk P. Pseudopermeative skeletal lesions. *Br J Radiol*. 1990;63:461–467.

Helms CA. Skeletal "don't touch" lesions. In: Brant WE, Helms CA, eds. *Fundamentals of Diagnostic Radiology*. Baltimore, MD: Lippincott Williams & Wilkins; 1994:963–975.

Hiddeman W, Schumman J, Andreef M, et al. Convention on nomenclature for DNA cytometry. Committee on Nomenclature, Society for Analytical Cytology. *Cancer Genet Cytogenet*. 1984;13:181–183.

Hudson TM. *Radiologic-pathologic Correlation of Musculoskeletal Lesions*. Baltimore, MD: Williams & Wilkins; 1987.

Huvos AG. *Bone Tumors. Diagnosis, Treatment and Prognosis*. Philadelphia, PA: WB Saunders; 1979.

Jaffe E, Harris N, Stein et al. *Tumours of Hematopoietic and Lymphoid Tissues*. Lyon, France: IARC Press; 2001.

Jaffe HL. *Tumors and Tumorous Conditions of the Bones and Joints*. Philadelphia, PA: Lea & Febiger; 1968.

Jelinek JS, Murphey MD, Welker JA, et al. Diagnosis of primary bone tumors with image-guided percutaneous biopsy: experience with 110 tumors. *Radiology*. 2002;223:731–737.

Johnson LC. A general theory of bone tumors. *Bull N Y Acad Med*. 1953;29:164–171.

Kallioniemi A, Kallioniemi OP, Sudar D, et al. Comparative genomic hybridization for molecular cytogenetic analysis of solid tumors. *Science*. 1992;258:818–821.

Kastan MB, Bartek J. Cell-cycle check points and cancer. *Nature*. 2004;432:316–323.

Kloiber R: Scintigraphy of bone tumors. In: *Current Concepts of Diagnosis and Treatment of Bone and Soft Tissue Tumors*. Berlin, Germany: Springer-Verlag; 1984:55–60.

Kransdorf M, Jelinek J, Moser RP Jr, et al. Soft-tissue masses. Diagnosis using MR imaging. *Am J Roentgenol*. 1989;153:541–547.

Kransdorf MJ, Murphey MD, Sweet DE. Liposclerosing myxofibrous tumor: a radiologic-pathologic-distinct fibro-osseous lesion of bone with a marked predilection for the intertrochanteric region of the femur. *Radiology*. 1999;212:693–698.

Kransdorf MJ. Magnetic resonance imaging of musculoskeletal tumors. *Orthopedics*. 1994;17:1003–1016.

Kransdorf MJ. Malignant soft-tissue tumors in a large referral population: distribution of diagnoses by age, sex, and location. *Am J Roentgenol*. 1995;164:129–134.

Kreisbergs A. DNA cytometry of musculoskeletal tumors. *Acta Orthop Scand*. 1990;61:282–297.

Kricun ME. Radiographic evaluation of solitary bone lesions. *Orthop Clin North Am*. 1983;14:39–64.

Lang P, Honda G, Roberts T, et al. Musculoskeletal neoplasm: perineoplastic edema versus tumor on dynamic postcontrast MR images with spatial mapping of instantaneous enhancement rates. *Radiology*. 1995;197:831–839.

Larson SE, Lorentzon R. The incidence of malignant primary bone tumors in relation to age, sex and site. A study of osteogenic sarcoma, chondrosarcoma, and Ewing's sarcoma diagnosed in Sweden from 1958-1968. *J Bone Joint Surg Br*. 1974;56B:534–540.

Larsson SE, Lorentzon R. The incidence of malignant primary bone tumors in relation to age, sex and site. A study of osteogenic sarcoma, chondrosarcoma, and Ewing's sarcoma diagnosed in Sweden from 1958–1968. *J Bone Joint Surg Br*. 1974;56B:534–540.

Lewis MM, Sissons HA, Norman A, Greenspan A. Benign and malignant cartilage tumors. In: Griffin PP, ed. *Instructional Course Lectures*. Chicago, IL: American Academy of Orthopaedic Surgeons; 1987:87–114.

Lichtenstein L. *Bone Tumors*. 5th ed. St. Louis, MO: Mosby; 1977.

Lodwick GS, Wilson AJ, Farrell C, Virtama P, Dittrich F. Determining growth rates of focal lesions of bone from radiographs. *Radiology*. 1980;134:577–583.

Lodwick GS, Wilson AJ, Farrell C, Virtama P, Smeltzer FM, Dittrich F. Estimating rate of growth in bone lesions. Observer performance and error. *Radiology*. 1980;134: 585–590.

Lodwick GS. A systematic approach to the roentgen diagnosis of bone tumors. In: *M.D. Anderson Hospital and Tumor Institute—Clinical Conference on Cancer: Tumors of Bone and Soft Tissue*. Chicago, IL: Year Book; 1965:49–68.

Lodwick GS. Solitary malignant tumors of bone: the application of predictor variables in diagnosis. *Semin Roentgenol*. 1966;1:293–313.

Ma LD, Frassica FJ, McCarthy EF, Bluenke DA, Zerhouni EA. Benign and malignant musculoskeletal masses: MR imaging differentiation with rim-to-center differential enhancement ratios. *Radiology*. 1997;202:739–744.

Ma LD, Frassica FJ, Scott WW Jr, Fishman EK, Zerhouni EA. Differentiation of benign and malignant musculoskeletal tumors: potential pitfalls with MR imaging. *Radiographics*. 1995;15:349–366.

Mackay B, Ordonez NG. Pathological evaluation of neoplasms with unknown primary tumor site. *Semin Oncol*. 1993;20:206–228.

Madewell JE, Ragsdale BD, Sweet DE. Radiologic and pathologic analysis of solitary bone lesions. Part I: Internal margins. *Radiol Clin North Am*. 1981;19:715–748.

Magid D. Two-dimensional and three-dimensional computed tomographic imaging in musculoskeletal tumors. *Radiol Clin North Am*. 1993;31:425–447.

McCarthy EF. CT-guided needle biopsies of bone and soft tissue tumors: a pathologist's perspective. *Skeletal Radiol.* 2007;36:181–182.

McCarthy EF. Histological grading of primary bone tumors. *Skeletal Radiol.* 2009;38:947–948.

McCarville B. The role of positron emission tomography in pediatric musculoskeletal oncology. *Skeletal Radiol.* 2006;35:553–554.

McNeil BJ. Value of bone scanning in neoplastic disease. *Semin Nucl Med.* 1984;14:277–286.

McNeil N, Ried TN. Novel molecular cytogenetic techniques for identifying complex chromosomal rearrangements: technology and applications in molecular medicine. *Expert Rev Mol Med.* 2000;2000:1–14.

Miller TT. Bone tumors and tumorlike conditions: analysis with conventional radiography. *Radiology.* 2008;246:662–674.

Mirowitz SA. Fast scanning and fat-suppression MR imaging of musculoskeletal disorders. *Am J Roentgenol.* 1993;161:1147–1157.

Mirra JM, Picci P, Gold RH. *Bone Tumors: Clinical, Radiologic and Pathologic Correlations*. Philadelphia, PA: Lea & Febiger; 1989.

Mittinen M. Antibody specific to muscle actin in the diagnosis and classification of soft tissue tumors. *Am J Pathol.* 1988;130:205–215.

Moll R., Franke WW, Schiller DL. The catalog of human cytokeratins: patterns of expression in normal epithelia, tumors and cultured cells. *Cell.* 1982;31:11–24.

Moore SG, Bisset GS, Siegel MJ, Donaldson JS. Pediatric musculoskeletal MR imaging. *Radiology.* 1991;179:345–360.

Moser RP, Madewell JE. An approach to primary bone tumors. *Radiol Clin North Am.* 1987;25:1049–1093.

Moser RP. Cartilaginous tumors of the skeleton. In: *AFIP Atlas of Radiologic-Pathologic Correlations*. Fasicle II. St. Louis, MO: Mosby-Year Book; 1990.

Mulder JD, Kroon HM, Schütte HE, Taconis WK. *Radiologic Atlas of Bone Tumors*. Amsterdam, the Netherlands: Elsevier; 1993:9–46.

Mulligan ME, Badros AZ. PET/CT and MR imaging in myeloma. *Skeletal Radiol.* 2007;36:5–16.

Munk PL, Lee MJ, Janzen DL, et al. Lipoma and liposarcoma: evaluation using CT and MR imaging. *Am J Roentgenol.* 1997;169:589–594.

Murray RO, Jacobson HG. *The Radiology of Bone Diseases*. 2nd ed. New York, NY: Churchill Livingstone; 1977.

Negendank WG, Crowley MG, Ryan JR, Keller NA, Evelhoch JL. Bone and soft-tissue lesions: diagnosis with combined H-1 MR imaging and P-31 MR spectroscopy. *Radiology.* 1989;173:181–188.

Nelson SW. Some fundamentals in the radiologic differential diagnosis of solitary bone lesions. *Semin Roentgenol.* 1966;1:244–267.

Nkajima T, Wantanabe S, Sato Y, Kameya T, Hirota T, Shimosato Y. An immunoperoxidase study of S-100 protein distribution in normal neoplastic tissues. *Am J Surg Pathol.* 1982;6:715–727.

Norman A, Schiffman M. Simple bone cyst: factors of age dependency. *Radiology.* 1977;124:779–782.

Nuovo MA, Norman A, Chumas J, Ackerman LV. Myositis ossificans with atypical clinical, radiographic, or pathologic findings: a review of 23 cases. *Skeletal Radiol.* 1992;27:87–101.

Olson P, Everson LI, Griffith HJ. Staging of musculoskeletal tumors. *Radiol Clin North Am.* 1994;32:151–162.

Ordonez NG, Mackay B. Electron microscopy in tumor diagnosis: indications for its use in the immunohistochemical era. *Hum Pathol.* 1998;29:1403–1411.

Panicek DM, Gatsonis C, Rosenthal DI, et al. CT and MR imaging in the local staging of primary malignant musculoskeletal neoplasms: report of the Radiology Diagnostic Oncology Group. *Radiology.* 1997;202:237–246.

Peterson JJ, Kransdorf MJ, Bancroft LW, O'Connor MI. Malignant fatty tumors: classification, clinical course, imaging appearance and treatment. *Skeletal Radiol.* 2003;32:493–503.

Peydro-Olaya A, Llombart-Bosch A, Carda-Battala C, pez-Guerrero JA. Electron microscopy and other ancillary techniques in the diagnosis of small round cell tumors. *Semin Diagn Pathol.* 2003;20;25–45.

Prophet E, Mills B, Arrington J, et al. *Laboratory Methods in Histotechnology*. Washington, DC: Armed Force Institute of Pathology; 1992.

Ragsdale BD, Madewell JE, Sweet DE. Radiologic and pathologic analysis of solitary bone lesions. *Part II: Periosteal reactions. Radiol Clin North Am.* 1981;19:749–783.

Rana RS, Wu JS, Eisenberg RL. Periosteal reaction. *Am J Roentgenol.* 2009;193:W259–W272.

Reinus WR, Wilson AJ. Quantitative analysis of solitary lesions of bone. *Invest Radiol.* 1995;30:427–432.

Rgazzini P, Gamberi G, Benassi MS, et al. Analysis of SAS gene and CDK4 and MDM2 proteins in low grade osteosarcoma. *Cancer Detect Prev.* 1999;23:129–136.

Schaffer L, Tommerup N, eds. *An International System for Human Cytogenetic Nomenclature*. Basel, Switzerland: Karger; 2005.

Schajowicz F. *Tumors and Tumorlike Lesions of Bone. Pathology, Radiology, and Treatment*. 2nd ed. Berlin, Germany: Springer-Verlag; 1994:1–21.

Seeger LL, Widoff BE, Bassett LW, Rosen G, Eckardt JJ. Preoperative evaluation of osteosarcoma: value of gadopentetate dimeglumine-enhanced MR imaging. *Am J Roentgenol.* 1991;157:347–351.

Selby S. Metaphyseal cortical defects in the tubular bones of growing children. *J Bone Joint Surg.* 1961;43:395–400.

Shibata Y, Fujita S, Yamaguchi A, Koji T. Assessment of decalcifying protocols for detection of specific RNA by non-radioactive in situ hybridization in calcified tissues. *Histochem Cell Biol.* 2000:113:153–159.

Shin DS, Shon OJ, Han DS, Choi JH, Chun KA, Cho IH. The clinical efficacy of 18F-FDG-PET/CT in benign and malignant musculoskeletal tumors. *Ann Nucl Med.* 2008;22:603–609.

Shuman WP, Patten RM, Baron RL, Liddell RM, Conrad EU, Richardson ML. Comparison of STIR and spin-echo MR imaging at 1.5T in 45 suspected extremity tumors: lesion conspicuity and extent. *Radiology.* 1991;179:247–252.

Skinner R. Decalcification of bone tissue. In: An Y. Martin K, eds, *Handbook of Histological Methods for Bone and Cartilage*. Totowa NJ; Humana Press; 2003:167–184.

Sostman HD, Charles HC, Rockwell S, et al. Soft-tissue sarcomas: detection of metabolic heterogeneity with P-31 MR spectroscopy. *Radiology.* 1990;176:837–843.

Speicher MR, Gwyn Ballard S, Ward DC. Karyotyping human chromosomes by combinatorial multi-flour FISH. *Nat Genet.* 1996;12:368–375.

Spjut HJ, Dorfman HD, Fechner RE, Ackerman LV. Tumors of bone and cartilage. In: *Atlas of Tumor Pathology*. Fasicle 5. Washington, DC: Armed Forces Institute of Pathology; 1971.

Sundaram M, McLeod R. MR imaging of tumor and tumorlike lesions of bone and soft tissue. *Am J Roentgenol.* 1990;155:817–824.

Sweet DE, Madewell JE, Ragsdale BD. Radiologic and pathologic analysis of solitary bone lesions. *Part III: Matrix patterns. Radiol Clin North Am.* 1981;19:785–814.

Tateishi U, Yamaguchi U, Seki K, Terauchi T, Arai Y, Kim EE. Bone and soft-tissue sarcoma: preoperative staging with Fluorine 18 fluorodeoxyglucose PET/CT and conventional imaging. *Radiology.* 2007;245:839–847.

Thomas C. *Histopathology. Textbook and Color Atlas*. 8th ed. Toronto, BC: Decker; 1989:305–309.

Trian R, Su M, Trian Y, et al. Dual-time point PET/CT with F-18 FDG for differentiation of malignant and benign bone lesions. *Skeletal Radiol.* 2009;38:451–458.

Unni KK, ed. *Bone Tumors*. New York, NY: Churchill Livingstone; 1988.

Vanel D, Verstraete KL, Shapeero LG. Primary tumors of the musculoskeletal system. *Radiol Clin North Am.* 1997;35:213–237.

Verstraete KL, De Deene Y, Roels H, Dierick A, Uyttendaele D, Kunnen M. Benign and malignant musculoskeletal lesions: dynamic contrast-enhanced MR imaging—parametric "first-pass" images depict tissue vascularization and perfusion. *Radiology.* 1994;192:835–843.

Volberg FM Jr, Whalen JP, Krook L, Winchester P. Lamellated periosteal reactions: a radiologic and histologic investigation. *Am J Roentgenol.* 1977;128:85–87.

Widmann G, Riedl QA, Schoepf D, et al. State-of-the-art HR-US imaging findings of the most frequent musculoskeletal soft-tissue tumors. *Skeletal Radiol.* 2009; 38:637–649.

CHAPTER 2

Bone-Forming (Osteogenic) Lesions

Disregarding, whether benign or malignant, the most characteristic feature of bone-forming neoplasms is the formation of osteoid tissue or mature bone directly by the tumor cells.

A. Benign Bone-Forming Lesions
Osteoma
Osteoid Osteoma
Osteoblastoma

B. Malignant Bone-Forming Tumors
Osteosarcomas
Conventional Osteosarcoma
  Osteoblastic
  Chondroblastic
  Fibroblastic
Telangiectatic Osteosarcoma
Small Cell Osteosarcoma
Low-Grade Central Osteosarcoma
Giant Cell–Rich Osteosarcoma
Multifocal (Multicentric) Osteosarcoma
Surface Osteosarcomas
  Parosteal Osteosarcoma
  Periosteal Osteosarcoma
  High-Grade Surface Osteosarcoma
Secondary Osteosarcomas
Postradiation Osteosarcoma
Paget Osteosarcoma
Osteosarcoma Associated with Fibrous Dysplasia
Soft-Tissue (Extraskeletal) Osteosarcoma

A. BENIGN BONE-FORMING LESIONS

Osteoma

Although not regarded as a neoplastic lesion by the World Health Organization, osteoma is included in this chapter because traditionally it has been regarded as a bone-forming lesion and because of its importance in differential diagnosis of osteoblastic tumors.

Definition:
- Slow-growing osteoblastic surface lesion.

Epidemiology:
- Fourth and fifth decades of life; men and women equally affected.

Sites of Involvement:
- Occurs most commonly in skull and facial bones, including mandible, maxilla, frontal sinuses, ethmoid sinuses, paranasal sinuses, orbital bones, and calvarium; rarely involves the clavicles and long bones.

Clinical Findings:
- On surface of bone—asymptomatic. If located in the paranasal sinuses, may cause mucocele, sinusitis, nasal discharge, and headache.
- Orbital tumors may produce diplopia, exophthalmos, and blindness.
- Presence of osteoma of long bones or multiple osteomas may be associated with Gardner syndrome (osteomas, colonic polyposis, skin fibromatoses, desmoids tumors, and epidermal and sebaceous cysts of skin).

Imaging:
- Radiography shows a homogenously dense, ivory-like sclerotic mass with sharply demarcated smooth borders, occasionally lobulated, attached to the cortex (Fig. 2.1A,B).
- Computed tomography (CT) demonstrates a surface lesion without cortical invasion (Fig. 2.1C,D).
- Magnetic resonance imaging (MRI) shows a lesion exhibiting low-signal intensity on all imaging sequences.

Pathology:
Gross (Macroscopy):
- Nodular or dome-shaped mass, containing dense cortical bone (Fig. 2.2A).

Histopathology:
Three types:
- *Cancellous* (cancellous trabecular architecture with fatty marrow in the intertrabecular spaces; woven bone with plait of collagen fibers; roundish spindle-shaped osteocyte lacunae) (Fig. 2.2B,C).

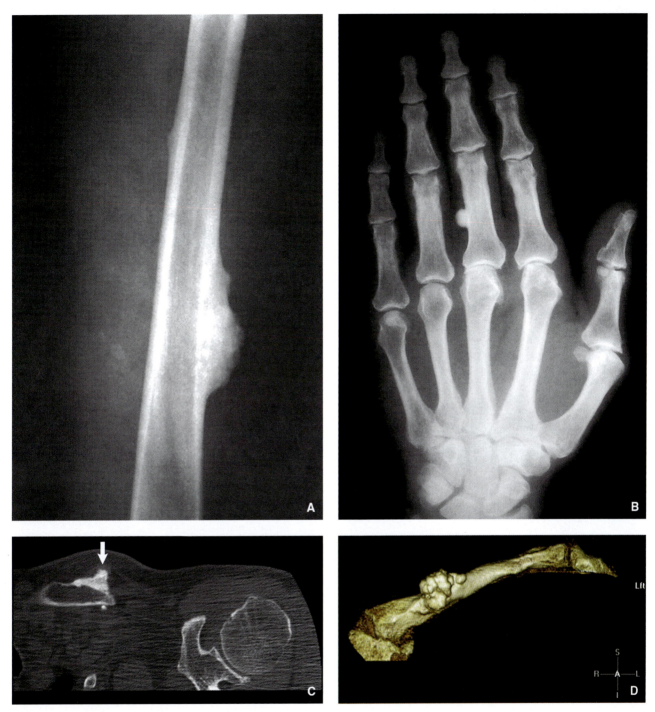

FIGURE 2.1 Osteoma. (A) Anteroposterior radiograph of the femur shows a sclerotic, ivory-like homogenous mass attached to the medial cortex. **(B)** Dorsovolar radiograph of the right hand shows a small homogenously sclerotic mass attached to the medial cortex of the proximal phalanx of the middle finger. **(C)** Coronal CT image of the left shoulder shows a sclerotic mass attached to the clavicle (*arrow*). Note lack of cortical invasion. **(D)** Three-dimensional CT image of the same patient as in **(C)** shows slightly lobulated mass on the surface of the clavicle.

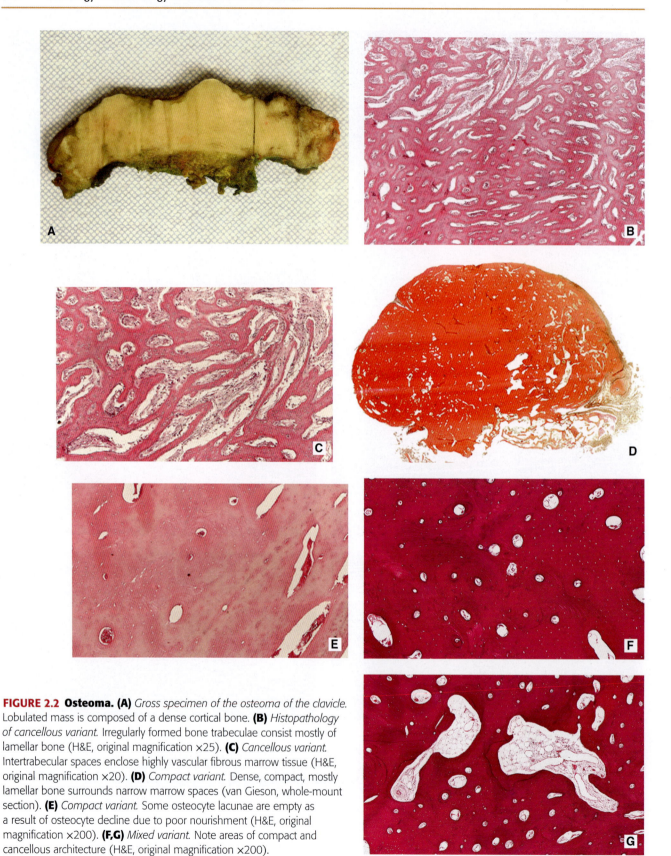

FIGURE 2.2 **Osteoma.** (A) *Gross specimen of the osteoma of the clavicle.* Lobulated mass is composed of a dense cortical bone. (B) *Histopathology of cancellous variant.* Irregularly formed bone trabeculae consist mostly of lamellar bone (H&E, original magnification ×25). (C) *Cancellous variant.* Intertrabecular spaces enclose highly vascular fibrous marrow tissue (H&E, original magnification ×20). (D) *Compact variant.* Dense, compact, mostly lamellar bone surrounds narrow marrow spaces (van Gieson, whole-mount section). (E) *Compact variant.* Some osteocyte lacunae are empty as a result of osteocyte decline due to poor nourishment (H&E, original magnification ×200). (F,G) *Mixed variant.* Note areas of compact and cancellous architecture (H&E, original magnification ×200).

- *Compact* (dense, compact, mature lamellar bone; no Haversian systems) (Fig. 2.2D,E).
- *Mixed* (admixed areas of compact and cancellous architecture) (Fig. 2.2F,G).

Prognosis:
- No recurrence after surgical excision.

Differential Diagnosis:
- **Parosteal osteosarcoma**
  Irregular outer contour.
  Commonly lack of homogeneity, periphery of the tumor may be less dense than the center.
  Occasionally invasion of the cortex by tumor.
  Incomplete cleft between the tumor and adjacent cortex commonly present.
  Histopathology shows streamers of woven to woven–lamellar bone with heavy collagenized stroma. Moderately cellular foci with nuclei exhibiting slight pleomorphism.
- **Sessile osteochondroma**
  Cortex of the host bone merges without interruption with cortex of the lesion, and respective cancellous portions of adjacent bone and osteochondroma communicate.
  Histopathology shows cartilaginous cap composed of hyaline cartilage arranged similarly to growth plate. Beneath it, zone of endochondral ossification with vascular invasion and replacement of calcified cartilage by newly formed bone.
- **Well-matured focus of parosteal myositis ossificans**
  Zonal phenomenon (periphery of the lesion more mature than the center).
  Radiolucent cleft separates the lesion from adjacent cortex.
  Regression of the lesion with time.
  Histopathology shows trabecular bone and fibrous marrow. Histologic zonal phenomenon consists of immature bone in the center with proliferating osteoblasts, fibroblasts, and areas of hemorrhage and necrosis; mature bone on periphery.
- **Monostotic form of melorheostosis (forme fruste)**
  Wavy outline of cortical thickening resembling wax dripping down one side of a candle.
  Occasionally, lesion extends into the medullary portion of bone.
  Histopathology shows thickened cortical bone containing irregularly arranged Haversian canals surrounded by cellular fibrous tissue. Osteoblastic activity usually present.

Osteoid Osteoma

Osteoid osteoma is a benign osteoblastic lesion characterized by a nidus of osteoid tissue, which may be purely radiolucent or have a sclerotic center. The nidus has a limited growth potential and usually measures less than 2 cm in diameter. It is often surrounded by a zone of reactive bone formation. Very rarely, an osteoid osteoma may have more than one nidus, in which instant it is called a multicentric or multifocal osteoid osteoma. Depending upon its location in a particular part of the bone, the lesion is classified as cortical, medullary (cancellous), or subperiosteal. Osteoid osteoma can be further subclassified as extracapsular or intracapsular (intra-articular).

Definition:
- Benign bone-forming tumor.
- Similar to osteoblastoma but smaller in size (nidus 1.5 to 2.0 cm).

Epidemiology:
- Usually occurs in second or third decade.
- Male-to-female ratio of 3:1.

Sites of Involvement:
- Most common in long bones—femur/tibia (cortex of metaphysis).
- May be found in any bone.
- Rare cases in ethmoid bone have been reported.

Clinical Findings:
- Intense localized pain particularly at night.
- Pain relieved by aspirin, nonsteroidal anti-inflammatory drugs (NSAIDs), surgery, or radiofrequency ablation.
- When osteoid osteoma is present in the small bones of the hands and feet, patients are typically misdiagnosed and treated for an inflammatory process (such as osteomyelitis, arthritis).

Imaging:
Radiography:
- Small, round radiolucency, surrounded by zone of sclerosis (particularly in cortical location) (Fig. 2.3A,B).
- Small, round radiolucency without zone of sclerosis (particularly in cancellous bone) (Fig. 2.3C).
- Small sclerotic or radiolucent lesion without zone of sclerosis, but with minimal periosteal response (in subperiosteal location) (Fig. 2.3D).
- If lesion localized within the joint (intracapsular)—periarticular osteoporosis and precocious osteoarthritis (Fig. 2.3E).
- Periosteal reaction (in intracortical location) (see Fig. 2.3B).

Scintigraphy:
- Increased activity of the radiopharmaceutical agent on both immediate and delayed images (Fig. 2.5).
- Characteristic "double-density" sign (Fig. 2.6).

Computed Tomography:
- Better characterization of the lesion (Fig. 2.7).
- Measurements of the nidus can be obtained.
- Vascular groove sign.

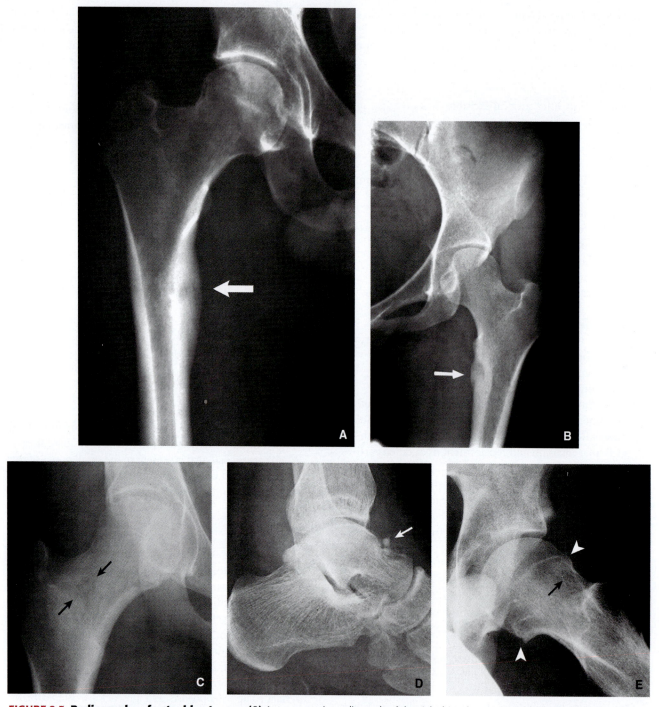

FIGURE 2.3 Radiography of osteoid osteoma. (A) Anteroposterior radiograph of the right hip of a 27-year-old man shows a radiolucent lesion within the medial femoral cortex associated with peripheral sclerosis (*arrow*). **(B)** Anteroposterior radiograph of the left hip of a 22-year-old woman shows similar radiolucent nidus surrounded by sclerotic reaction in the medial femoral cortex (*arrow*). **(C)** Intramedullary nidus within the femoral neck (*arrow*) shows no evidence of reactive sclerosis. **(D)** Subperiosteal lesion on the surface of the talus (*arrow*) show minimal periosteal reaction and no evidence of reactive sclerosis. **(E)** Intracapsular lesion is present in the left femoral neck (*arrow*) without evident perilesional sclerosis in a 14-year-old boy. Observe periarticular osteoporosis and early osteoarthritic changes in form of osteophytes (*arrowheads*).

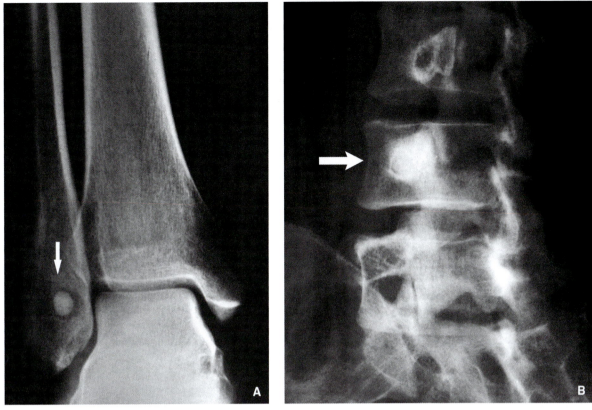

FIGURE 2.4 Radiography of osteoid osteoma. (A) Anteroposterior radiograph of the ankle shows a radiolucent lesion within the distal fibula with sclerotic center (*arrow*). **(B)** Oblique radiograph of the lumbar spine shows purely sclerotic nidus of osteoid osteoma affecting the pedicle of L4 (*arrow*).

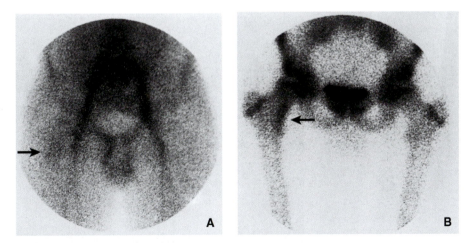

FIGURE 2.5 Scintigraphy of osteoid osteoma. (A) In the *first phase* of a three-phase radionuclide bone scan, 1 minute after intravenous injection of 15 mCi (555 MBq) technetium-99m–labeled MDP, there is increased activity in the iliac and femoral vessels. Discrete activity in the area of the medial left femoral neck (*arrow*) is related to the nidus of osteoid osteoma. **(B)** In the *third phase*, 2 hours after injection, there is accumulation of a bone-seeking tracer in the femoral neck lesion (*arrow*). (Reprinted from Greenspan A. Benign bone-forming lesions: osteoma, osteoid osteoma, and osteoblastoma. *Skeletal Radiol.* 1993;22:490–500, with permission.)

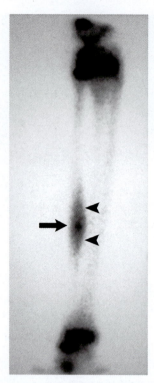

FIGURE 2.6 Scintigraphy of osteoid osteoma. Radionuclide bone scan shows a classic "double density" sign of osteoid osteoma located in the tibia: markedly increased radioactivity in the center (*arrow*) is related to the nidus, less active areas (*arrowheads*) represent reactive sclerosis.

Ultrasound:
- Focal cortical irregularity and adjacent hypoechoic synovitis at the site of intra-articular lesion.

Magnetic Resonance Imaging:
- High-signal intensity of the nidus on T2-weighted and inversion recovery (IR) sequences (Fig. 2.8).
- Occasionally confusing pattern, may be mistaken for inflammation or malignancy.

Pathology:
Gross (Macroscopy):
- Small, cortically based, red, gritty round lesion (Fig. 2.9).

Histopathology:
- Limited growth pattern (1.5 to 2.0 cm).
- Sharp circumscription of the nidus near cortical surface (Fig. 2.10A).
- Nidus composed of anastomosing bone trabeculae with variable mineralization (Fig. 2.10B).
- Bone trabeculae lined by plump osteoblasts (Fig. 2.10C).
- Osteoblastic and osteoclastic activities often prominent.
- Vascularized connective tissue, surrounded by sclerotic bone displaying a variety of maturation patterns.
- Benign giant cells may be present.

Genetics:
- Described loss of 17q.
- Structural alterations of chromosome 22 – [del(22)(q13.1)].

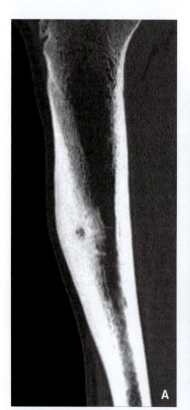
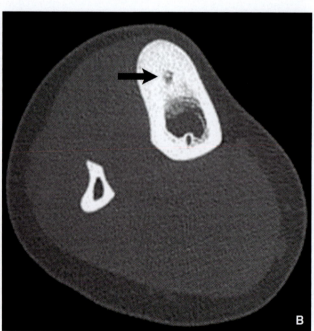

FIGURE 2.7 Computed tomography of osteoid osteoma. (A) Coronal reformatted CT image of the tibia and **(B)** axial CT of the same patient show a well-defined low-attenuation nidus with sclerotic center located in the anterior cortex (*arrow*).

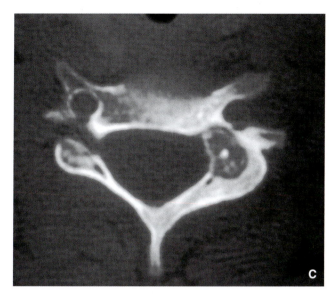

FIGURE 2.7 *(Continued).* **(C)** Axial CT image of the cervical vertebra C6 of another patient shows a low-attenuation nidus with a sclerotic center, located in the left pedicle and extending to the lamina. (**C**—Reprinted with permission from Greenspan A. Benign bone-forming lesions: osteoma, osteoid osteoma, and osteoblastoma. *Skeletal Radiol.* 1993;22:490–500).

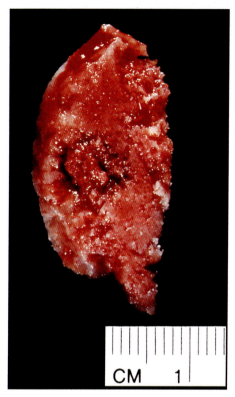

FIGURE 2.9 Osteoid osteoma, gross specimen. Note well-circumscribed nidus exhibiting hypervascular zone with surrounding sclerotic rim.

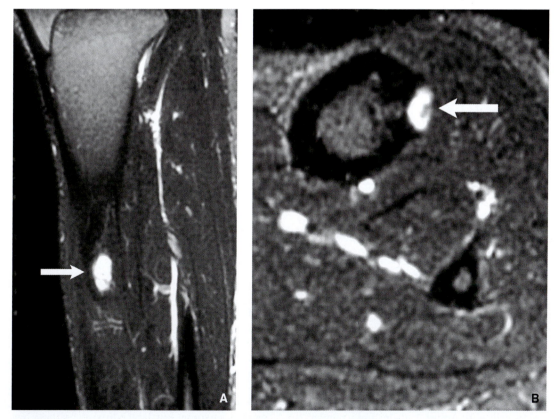

FIGURE 2.8 Magnetic resonance imaging of osteoid osteoma. (A) Sagittal and **(B)** axial T2-weighted MR images show a high-signal-intensity nidus in posterolateral cortex of tibia (*arrows*).

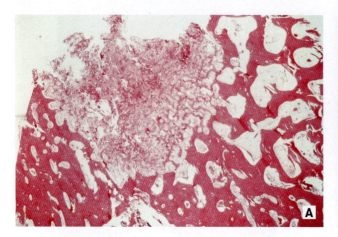
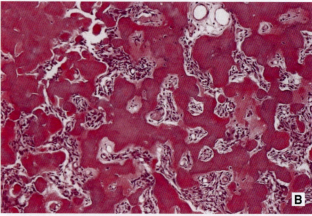
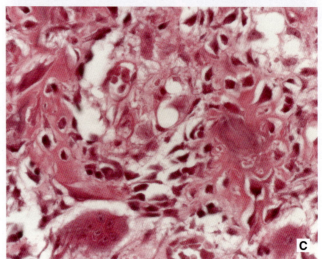

FIGURE 2.10 Osteoid osteoma, histopathology. (A) Low-power magnification shows a well-demarcated nidus composed of trabeculae and immature woven bone (*center*), surrounded by sclerotic bone (H&E, original magnification ×6). **(B)** Higher magnification of the center of the nidus shows interconnected, ossified bone trabeculae within areas of vascularized connective tissue, and osteoblastic activity (H&E, original magnification ×100). **(C)** High-power photomicrograph of the nidus shows bone trabeculae rimmed by osteoblasts (H&E, original magnification ×400).

Complications:
- Accelerated bone growth if nidus located near the growth plate.
- Painful scoliosis if nidus located within the vertebra (particularly within the neural arch).
- Precocious arthritis if lesion located within the joint (intracapsular).
- Recurrence if lesion not completely excised.

Prognosis:
- Excellent, after total surgical excision or radiofrequency thermal ablation (RFTA).

Differential Diagnosis:
- ***Osteoblastoma***
  Larger nidus (more than 2 cm).
  Less reactive sclerosis, but more prominent periosteal reaction.
  Histopathology is similar to osteoid osteoma, but less organized pattern of osteoid and reticular bone distribution; occasionally, spindle-shaped hyperchromatic cells with uniform nuclei and irregular eosinophilic cytoplasm interdispersed between immature bone trabeculae.
- ***Bone abscess***
  Serpentine radiolucent track extending from the lesion. May cross the growth plate.
  Histopathology shows inflammatory cells and areas of necrosis.
- ***Bone island (enostosis)***
  "Thorny radiations" (pseudopodia) at periphery of the lesion (brush borders) that blend with trabeculae of the host bone.
  Usually no significant activity on scintigraphy.
  Histopathology shows focus of mature compact bone; wide bands of parallel or concentric lamellae; marrow spaces resemble haversian canals.
- ***Stress fracture***
  More linear radiolucency with perpendicular or oblique orientation.

Osteoblastoma

Osteoblastoma is a benign bone-forming tumor, similar to osteoid osteoma, but larger in size. Natural history differs from that of osteoid osteoma: whereas the latter lesion tends toward regression, osteoblastoma tends toward progression, and even malignant transformation, although this possibility remains controversial. Toxic osteoblastoma, a rare variant of this tumor, has also been reported. It is associated with systemic manifestations, including diffuse periostitis of multiple bones, fever, and weight loss. Although the long bones are commonly affected by osteoblastoma, the lesion has a predilection for the vertebral column.

Definition:
- Benign bone-forming neoplasm producing woven bone spicules bordered by prominent osteoblasts (measuring more than 2.0 cm).

Epidemiology:
- About 1% of all primary bone tumors, and 3% of all benign bone tumors.
- Age: 10 to 30 years (but predominantly teenagers).
- Male-to-female ratio of 2.5:1.

Sites of Involvement:
- Predilection for the spine (40% to 55% of cases).
- Other common sites—femur and proximal tibia.
- Cementoblastoma of the jaw is considered osteoblastoma and is attached to the root of tooth.

Clinical Findings:
- Dull, localized pain, rarely interfered with sleep.
- Tenderness on palpation at the tumor site.
- Lesion in the spine may cause back pain, scoliosis, and nerve root compression.
- Jaw lesion may produce tooth pain.
- Aspirin does not relieve pain.
- Tendency to progression (question of malignant transformation, a controversial issue).

Imaging:
Distinctive four types of the lesion:
- Giant osteoid osteoma (Fig. 2.11A–C).
- Lytic expansive lesion, similar to aneurysmal bone cyst (ABC), with central mineralization (usually spine lesions) (Fig. 2.11D,E).
- Aggressive lesion simulating a malignant tumor (Fig. 2.11F–H).
- Juxtacortical (periosteal) in location (Fig. 2.11I–L).

General imaging features:
- Radiolucent well-circumscribed oval or round lesion.
- May or may not exhibit perilesional sclerosis.
- Prominent periosteal reaction.
- Scintigraphy invariably demonstrates intense focal accumulation of radiopharmaceutical.

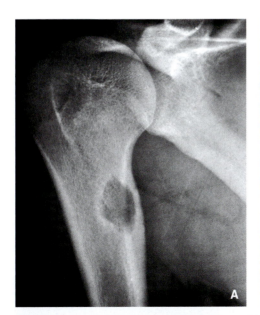 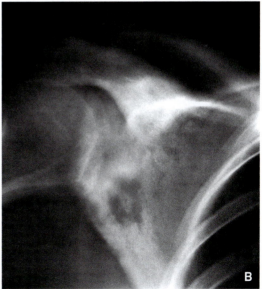

FIGURE 2.11 Radiography of osteoblastoma. *"Giant" osteoid osteoma-like lesions.* Note that all three lesions are very similar to osteoid osteoma, but much larger, and periosteal reaction is more prominent **(A–C)**. *Aneurysmal-like expansion with central radiodensities.* This type of presentation is usually seen in the spine lesions.

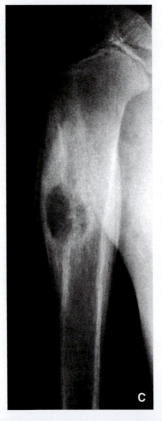
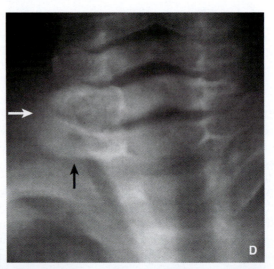
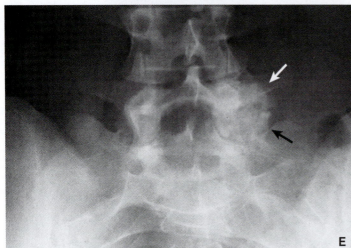
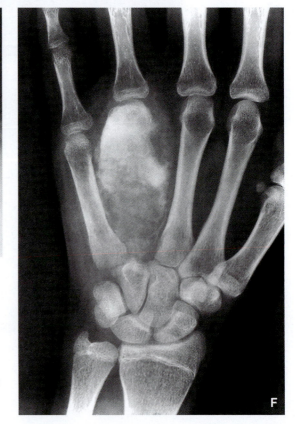

FIGURE 2.11 *(Continued).* **(D)** Expansive blow-out lesion with central opacities is seen in the lamina of C6 (*arrows*) and **(E)** in the lamina, pedicle, and transverse process of L5 (*arrows*). *Aggressive lesion mimicking malignant tumors.* **(F)** The lesion affecting the forth metacarpal bone completely destroyed the bone, having an appearance of osteosarcoma.

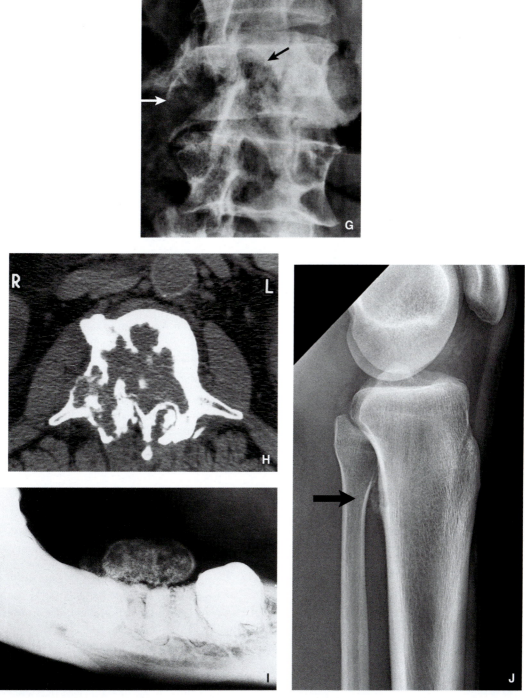

FIGURE 2.11 *(Continued).* (G,H) Aggressive osteoblastoma destroyed part of the vertebral body of L3 (*arrows*). *Periosteal location.* **(I)** Juxtacortical lesion of the mandible.

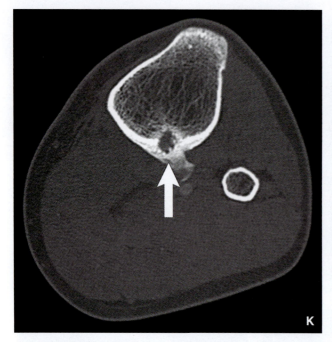
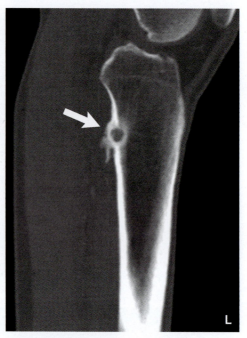

FIGURE 2.11 *(Continued).* **(J–L)** Juxtacortical location in the posterior cortex of proximal tibia, invading the endocortex and evoking periosteal reaction (*arrows*). (**D,E,G,H**—Reprinted with permission from Greenspan A. Benign bone-forming lesions: osteoma, osteoid osteoma, and osteoblastoma. *Skeletal Radiol.* 1993;22:494–500).

- CT better characterizes the lesion and allows to obtain measurements (Fig. 2.12).
- MRI shows extensive peritumoral bone marrow edema, and low signal intensity on all sequences when lesion is heavily mineralized (exhibiting predominantly osteoblastic matrix) (Fig. 2.13), but high signal intensity on T2-weighted and IR sequences in less mineralized (radiolucent) lesions.

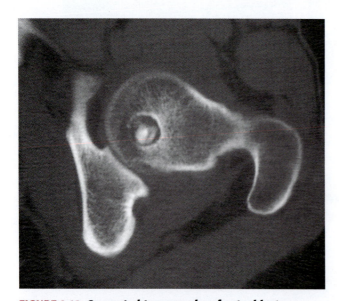

FIGURE 2.12 Computed tomography of osteoblastoma. Axial CT image of the left hip of a 20-year-old man shows a low-attenuation lesion with sclerotic center within the femoral head, measuring 2.75 cm.

Pathology:
Gross (Macroscopy):

- Central nidus is red, soft, and friable (vascular).
- Often with gritty or sandpaper consistency, if calcified may be yellow and gritty.
- Cortical bone may be thin-out or destroyed, occasionally with cyst formation representing formation of secondary ABC.

Histopathology:

- Nidus appears well circumscribed, with tumor osteoid merging with adjacent uninvolved bone.
- Composed of woven bone spicules or trabeculae lined by a single layer of osteoblasts (Fig. 2.14A).
- Irregular interlacing network of osteoid with prominent osteoblastic rimming and features of woven bone (Fig. 2.14B,D).
- Osteoblasts exhibit benign cytologic features, although increased mitotic activity without atypical forms may be present.
- Osteoid may be fine and lace-like with variable mineralization, separated by fibrovascular stroma containing multinucleated osteoclast-like giant cells (Fig. 2.14C).
- Rich vascularity of stroma (see Fig. 2.14A).
- Large blood lakes representing secondary aneurysmal cystic changes may be seen (Fig. 2.14E).
- Scattered osteoclast-type multinucleated giant cells are often present (see Fig. 2.14C).
- Focal blood-filled spaces mimicking ABC may be present (Fig. 2.14E).

Chapter 2 • Bone-Forming (Osteogenic) Lesions   45

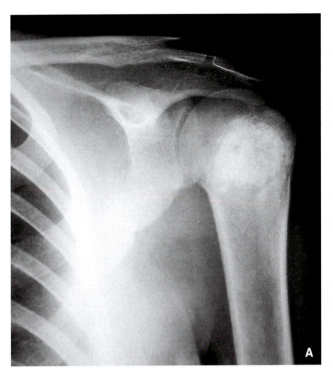
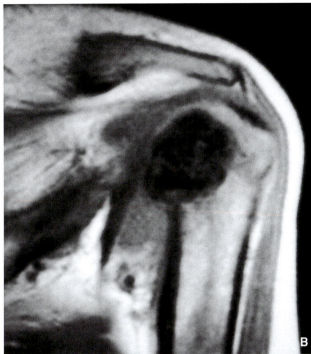
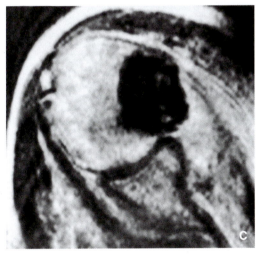

FIGURE 2.13 Magnetic resonance imaging of osteoblastoma.
(A) Anteroposterior radiograph of the left shoulder shows a large sclerotic lesion within the humeral head. **(B)** Coronal T1-weighted MR image shows the lesion to be of low-signal intensity. **(C)** Axial spin-echo T2-weighted MRI shows that the lesion remains of low-signal intensity, indicating osteoblastic matrix.

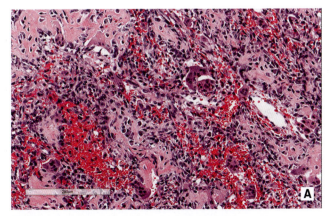
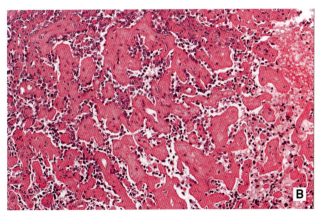

FIGURE 2.14 Histopathology of osteoblastoma. (A) Low-power photomicrograph shows irregular trabeculae of woven bone (osteoid) surrounded by densely arranged osteoblasts and some giant cells. Note also several ectatic blood vessels (H&E, original magnification ×50). **(B)** At higher magnification, the osteoblastic rimming of the trabeculae is conspicuous (H&E, original magnification ×100).

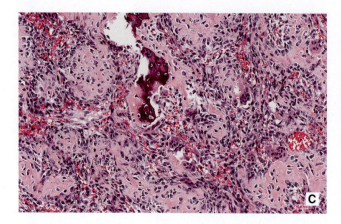
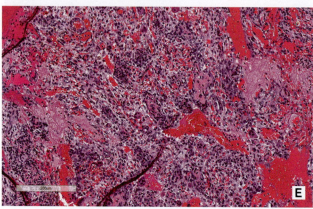

FIGURE 2.14 *(Continued).* **(C)** Densely arranged small trabeculae made up of woven bone are surrounded by osteoblasts. In the narrow marrow spaces, some capillaries and giant cells of the osteoclast type are seen (H&E, original magnification ×200). **(D)** High-power photomicrograph reveals osteoblasts and osteoclasts on the surface of the immature bone trabeculae (H&E, original magnification ×400). **(E)** Trabeculae of woven bone rimmed with osteoblasts and large blood lakes representing secondary aneurysmal cystic changes are present (H&E, original magnification ×100).

- Osteoblastomas do not infiltrate and isolate preexisting lamellar bone structures as does osteosarcoma.
- Cartilage usually not present.
- Epithelioid features may be seen represented by large cells with abundant eosinophilic cytoplasm and enlarged nuclei containing large nucleoli.
- Rare cytologically atypical multinucleated giant cells without mitotic activity may be seen (tumors with these features may be designated bizarre osteoblastoma or pseudomalignant osteoblastoma).

Prognosis:
- Excellent.
- Recurrences unusual if totally excised.

Differential Diagnosis:
- *Osteoid osteoma*
  Smaller nidus (less than 2 cm).
  More reactive sclerosis.
  Vascular groove sign on CT.
  Different clinical presentation (pain relief by salicylates).
  Histopathology similar to osteoblastoma, but at the periphery of the nidus, a fibrovascular rim is present, and nidus itself exhibits a distinct zonal pattern with central maturation to more mineralized woven bone.
- *Bone abscess (Brodie abscess)*
  Serpentine radiolucent track extending from the lesion.
  May cross the growth plate.
  Histopathology shows inflammatory cells and areas of necrosis.
- *Aneurysmal bone cyst*
  More prominent expansion and ballooning.
  Buttress of periosteal reaction.
  Histopathology shows multiple blood-filled sinusoid spaces separated by fibrous septae displaying lamellae of primitive woven bone; may contain hemosiderin and reactive foam cells; solid areas composed of fibrous elements contain irregular bone trabeculae and giant cells.
- *Enchondroma* (in short tubular bone)
  Central chondroid calcifications.
  Lack of periosteal reaction (unless pathologic fracture).
  Histopathology shows lobules of hyaline cartilage of variable cellularity with evidence of endochondral ossification at the periphery of the lobules; the tissue is sparsely cellular, and the cells containing small dark-staining nuclei are located in the lacunae; intercellular matrix has a uniform translucent appearance and contains relative little collagen; matrix calcifications may be present.

- *Osteosarcoma*
  More aggressive presentation.
  Interrupted periosteal reaction (sunburst, lamellated, Codman triangle).
  Make look very similar to aggressive osteoblastoma.
  Histopathology shows permeation of cortical bone; attenuation and "trapping" of lamellar bone; atypical mitoses and anaplasia of cells; hyperchromatism and pleomorphism of cells and nuclei; tumor bone and tumor cartilage formed by malignant cells.

B. MALIGNANT BONE-FORMING TUMORS

Osteosarcomas

Osteosarcomas, the most common primary malignant tumors of bone, comprise a family of connective tissue tumors with various degrees of malignant potential. There are several types of osteosarcoma (Fig. 2.15), each having distinctive clinical, imaging, and histopathologic characteristics. The common feature of all types is that the osteoid and bone matrix are formed directly by the malignant cells of connective tissue. The majority of osteosarcomas are of unknown cause and therefore are referred to as *primary* or *idiopathic*. A smaller number of tumors are related to known factors predisposing to malignancy, such as Paget disease, fibrous dysplasia, external ionizing irradiation, or ingestion of radioactive substances. These lesions are referred as to as *secondary* osteosarcomas. All types of osteosarcomas may further be subdivided by anatomic sites into tumors of appendicular skeleton and axial skeleton, as well as may be classified on the basis of their location in the bone as central (intramedullary), intracortical, and juxtacortical. A separate group consists of primary osteosarcomas originating in soft tissues (extraskeletal or soft-tissue osteosarcomas). Finally, yet another group comprises metastatic lesions (in the lungs, bones, and soft tissues).

It is important to mention here that there are numerous genetic disorders, marked by chromosome instability, associated with the development of various tumors, including osteosarcomas. Among these rare conditions are Rothmund-Thomson syndrome, Werner syndrome, Li-Fraumeni syndrome, retinoblastoma syndrome, and Bloom syndrome.

Histopathologically, osteosarcomas are graded on the basis of their cellularity, nuclear pleomorphism, and degree of mitotic activity (Table 2.1). The grading has clinical, therapeutic, and prognostic values.

Conventional Osteosarcoma

Definition:
- Primary intramedullary high-grade malignant sarcoma in which neoplastic cells produce osteoid or bone.

Epidemiology:
- Most common primary nonhematopoietic malignancy of bone.
- Incidence in the United States is 4 to 5 per million individuals with 1,000 to 1,500 new cases diagnosed annually, which accounts for approximately 20% of all primary malignant tumors.
- Most common in second decade of life with 60% of tumors in patients younger than 25 years.
- About 30% occur in patients over 40 years of age (predisposing conditions include radiation therapy and Paget disease of bone).
- Male-to-female ratio of 3:2.
- Osteosarcoma in children 5 years and younger is very uncommon, accounting for less than 2% of osteosarcomas in the pediatric population.

Sites of Involvement:
- Osteosarcoma most commonly involves long bones of the appendicular skeleton with preference to the distal femur, proximal tibia, and proximal humerus.
- Most of the tumors are centered in metaphysis of long bones (90%), followed by diaphysis (9%), and rarely epiphysis.
- Involvement of other sites than long bones (i.e., jaws, pelvis, spine, and skull) tends to increase with age.

Clinical Presentation:
- Typically presents as progressively enlarging mass.
- Pain is deeply seated and boring in nature, commonly noted months prior to the diagnosis, and usually increases in intensity over time.
- Skin overlying the tumor may be warm, erythematous, edematous, with prominent engorged veins.
- Large tumors near the joints may restrict the range of motion and produce joint effusion.
- Advanced cases result in weight loss and cachexia.
- Pathologic fracture through the destructive mass may be seen.

Imaging:
Radiography:
- Variable radiographic appearances, reflecting histopathology; conventional tumors usually present as a large, destructive, poorly defined, mixed lytic and blastic lesions exhibiting wide zone of transition and moth-eaten bone destruction, accompanied by cortical invasion and extension into the soft tissues (Figs. 2.16 and 2.17). Purely sclerotic (osteoblastic) (Fig. 2.18A,B) and purely lytic (chondroblastic or fibroblastic) (Fig. 2.18C) lesions may also be encountered.
- Tumor/periosteal interaction leads to variety of manifestations secondary to periosteal reaction (periosteal reactive bone formation), such as fine triangular structures (Codman triangle) (Fig. 2.19A), fine, ill-defined perpendicular spiculations (velvet type) (see Fig. 2.16A,B), perpendicular or radiating coarse striations ("hair-on-end"

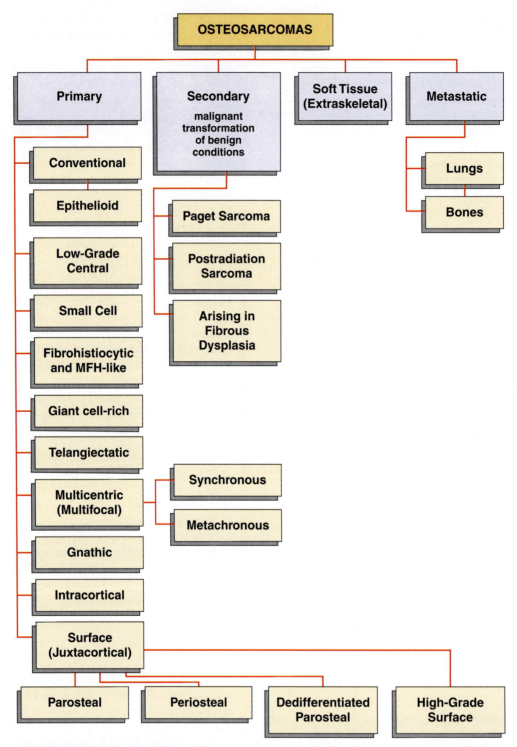

FIGURE 2.15 Classification of osteosarcomas.

or "sunburst" periosteal reaction) (Fig. 2.19B, see also Fig. 2.16A,B), or less common lamellated periosteal layers ("onion skin" type of periosteal reaction) (Fig. 2.19C).

Scintigraphy:

- Invariably increased uptake of radiopharmaceutical agent (Figs. 2.20 and 2.21); may show "skipped" lesions (Fig. 2.22).

Computed Tomography:

- Demonstrates intramedullary and extracortical extension of the tumor and periosteal reaction (Fig. 2.23).
- Accurately demonstrates cortical destruction.
- Using Hounsfield values, one can distinguish between tumor tissue, peritumoral edema, and normal bone marrow.

TABLE 2.1 Histologic Grading of Osteosarcoma[a]

Grade	Histologic Features
1	Cellularity: slightly increased Cytologic atypia: minimal to slight Mitotic activity: low Osteoid matrix: regular
2	Cellularity: moderate Cytologic atypia: mild to moderate Mitotic activity: low to moderate Osteoid matrix: regular
3	Cellularity: increased Cytologic atypia: moderate to marked Mitotic activity: moderate to high Osteoid matrix: irregular
4	Cellularity: markedly increased Cytologic atypia: markedly pleomorphic cells Mitotic activity: high Osteoid matrix: irregular, abundant

[a]According to Unni KK, Dahlin DC. Grading of bone tumors. *Semin Diagn Pathol.* 1984;1:165–172.

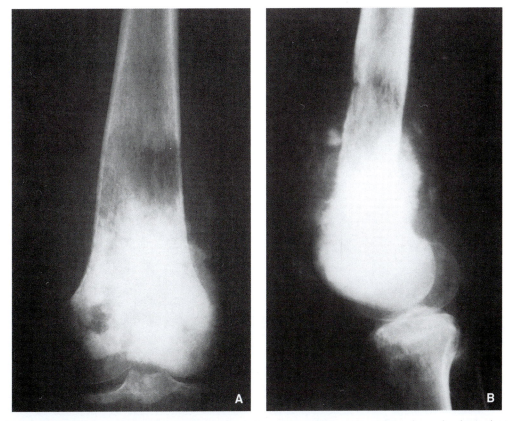

FIGURE 2.16 Radiography of conventional osteosarcoma. Anteroposterior **(A)** and lateral **(B)** radiographs shows the typical features of this tumor in the distal femur of a 19-year-old woman. Medullary and cortical destruction is present, associated with aggressive periosteal reaction of the velvet and sunburst types. A soft-tissue mass is present containing foci of tumor bone.

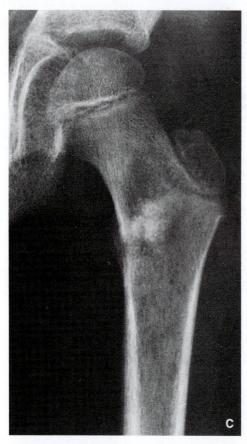

Magnetic Resonance Imaging:

- Similarly to CT shows intramedullary extension of the tumor and well characterizes soft-tissue mass (Figs. 2.24 to 2.27).
- Usually heterogenous low signal intensity on T1-weighted and heterogenous high signal on T2-weighted and other water-sensitive sequences (Fig. 2.28).
- Allows distinction between the tumor and peritumoral edema (postcontrast studies using gadolinium).
- Allows evaluation of involvement of neurovascular structures by the tumor.

Pathology:

Gross (Macroscopy):

- Heterogeneous large fleshy mass with ossified and non-ossified components and occasionally foci of cartilage (Fig. 2.29).
- Commonly the tumor breaks through the cortex and is invading the adjacent soft tissues, where foci of tumor bone formation and hemorrhage may be seen (Fig. 2.30).
- The tumor may invade the nearby joint (Fig. 2.31).
- New bone formation (periosteal reaction) at periphery of the tumor.

Histopathology:

- Tumor cells show prominent atypia and pleomorphism and may exhibit epithelioid, plasmacytoid, fusiform, ovoid, small round, or spindled appearances (Fig. 2.32).

FIGRE 2.16 *(Continued).* **(C)** In another patient, a 12-year-old boy, anteroposterior radiograph of the left femur demonstrates a mixed, lytic, and sclerotic tumor in the intertrochanteric region.

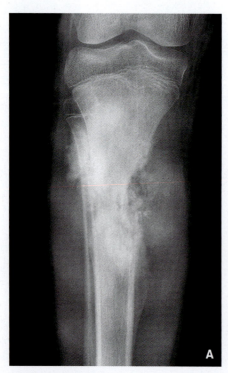
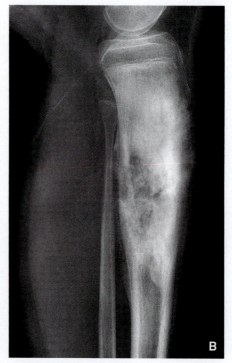

FIGURE 2.17 Radiography of conventional osteosarcoma. (A) Anteroposterior and **(B)** lateral radiographs of the right proximal leg of a 12-year-old boy show a sclerotic lesion affecting diaphysis of the tibia, associated with destruction of the medial cortex, aggressive periosteal reaction, and a soft-tissue mass.

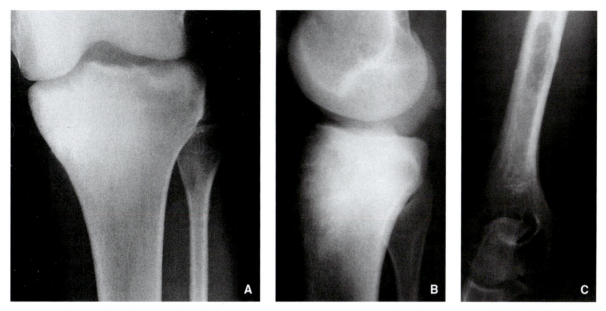

FIGURE 2.18 Radiography of conventional osteosarcoma. Anteroposterior **(A)** and lateral **(B)** radiographs demonstrate sclerotic variant of this tumor affecting proximal tibia. **(C)** Anteroposterior radiograph shows a destructive purely lytic lesion in the distal humerus, proven on histopathologic examination to represent fibroblastic osteosarcoma.

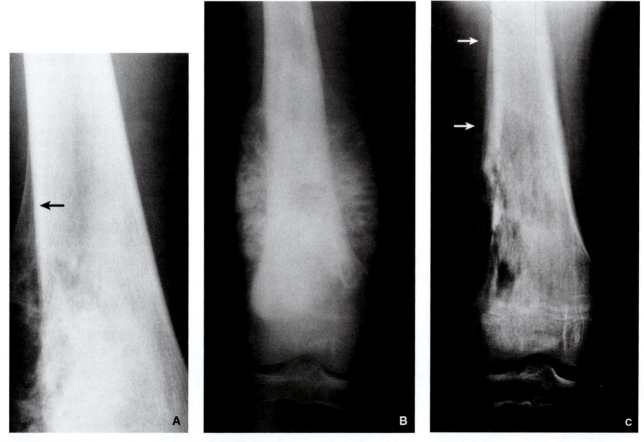

FIGURE 2.19 Radiography of periosteal reaction in osteosarcoma. (A) Typical Codman triangle (*arrow*). **(B)** Typical sunburst pattern. **(C)** Typical lamellated (onion skin) pattern (*arrows*).

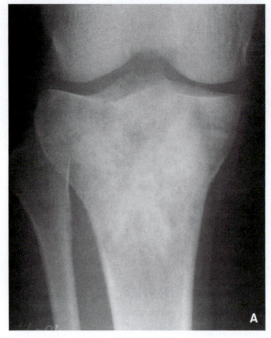
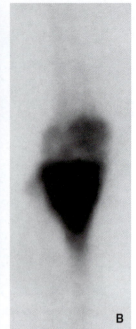

FIGURE 2.20 Scintigraphy of conventional osteosarcoma. (A) Anteroposterior radiograph of the right knee shows a sclerotic variant in the proximal tibia. **(B)** After intravenous injection of 15 mCi (555 MBq) of technetium-99m–labeled methylene diphosphonate, there is significant uptake of the radiopharmaceutical agent by the tumor.

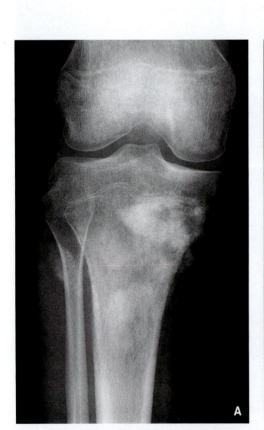
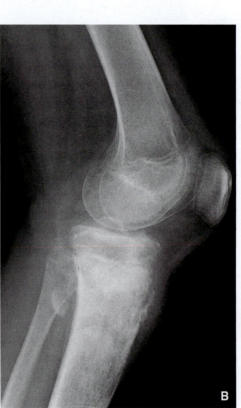
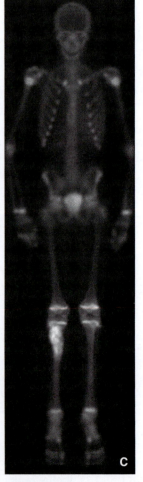

FIGURE 2.21 Scintigraphy of conventional osteosarcoma. (A) Anteroposterior and **(B)** lateral radiographs of the right knee of a 13-year-old girl show a sclerotic lesion affecting the metaphysis and diaphysis of the tibia. **(C)** A total body radionuclide bone scan and

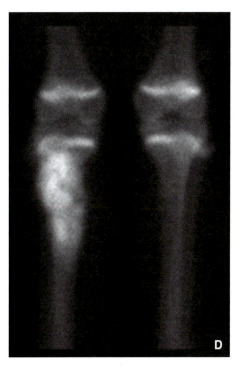

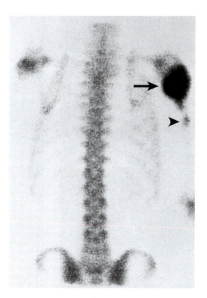

FIGURE 2.22 Scintigraphy of conventional osteosarcoma. In a 7-year-old-boy with a lesion in the proximal left humerus, radionuclide bone scan shows increased uptake of the tracer by the tumor (*arrow*). In addition, a small focus of activity (*arrowhead*) represents a skip lesion.

FIGURE 2.21 *(Continued).* **(D)** coned-down scintigraphic images of the knees show significantly increased uptake of the radiopharmaceutical agent by a tumor in the proximal right tibia.

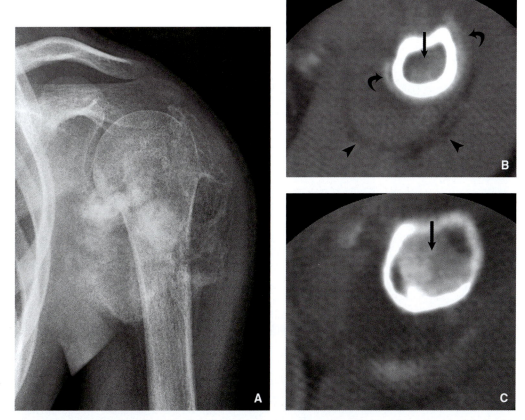

FIGURE 2.23 Computed tomography of conventional osteosarcoma. (A) Anteroposterior radiograph of the left shoulder shows a bone-forming tumor affecting proximal humerus associated with aggressive periosteal reaction and soft-tissue mass. **(B,C)** Two CT axial sections show high-attenuation tumor replacing the bone marrow (*arrows*), periosteal reaction (*curved arrows*), and soft-tissue mass (*arrow heads*).

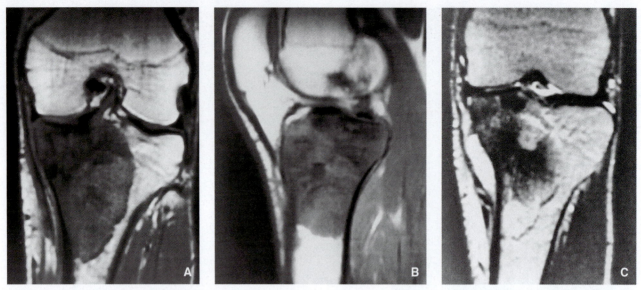

FIGURE 2.24 Magnetic resonance imaging of conventional osteosarcoma. (A) Coronal and **(B)** sagittal T1-weighted MR images of the knee of a 17-year-old boy show a heterogenous but predominantly low signal intensity appearance of the tumor affecting proximal tibia. **(C)** On T2-weighted MR image, the sclerotic parts of the tumor remain of low signal intensity, whereas the more distal, nonmineralized tissue and soft-tissue mass exhibit high signal intensity.

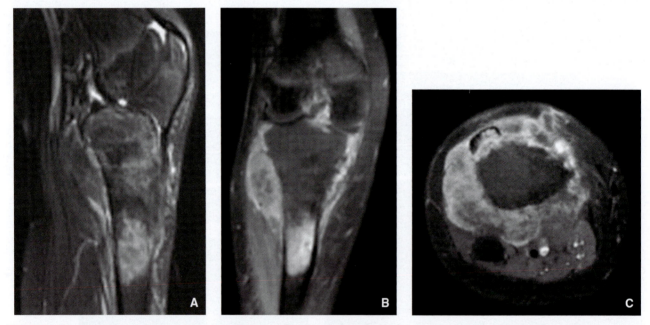

FIGURE 2.25 Magnetic resonance imaging of conventional osteosarcoma. (A) Sagittal T2-weighted MR image of the knee shows a tumor affecting proximal tibia, exhibiting heterogenous mixed high and low signal intensities. Soft tissue extension of the tumor is not well depicted. Coronal **(B)** and axial **(C)** T1-weighted MR images obtained after intravenous injection of gadolinium show lack of enhancement of the sclerotic part of the tumor, but significant enhancement of the lytic part proximally. Note also enhancement of a soft-tissue mass containing tumor-bone imaged as low signal intensity foci.

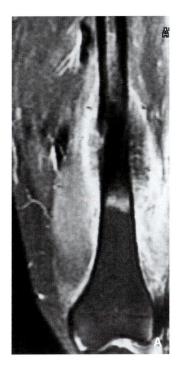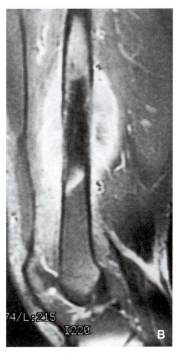

FIGURE 2.26 Magnetic resonance imaging of conventional osteosarcoma. Coronal **(A)** and sagittal **(B)** T1-weighted fat-suppressed MR images of a 29-year-old man obtained after intravenous injection of gadolinium show tumor enhancement in the medullary portion of the femur and in the soft-tissue mass. Heavy mineralized portion of the tumor does not enhance and remains of low signal intensity.

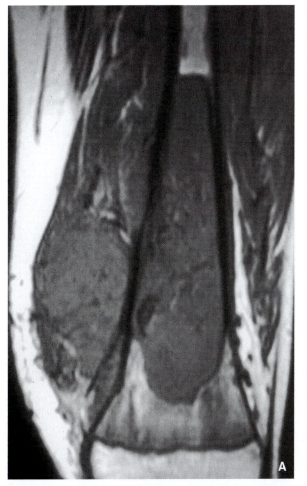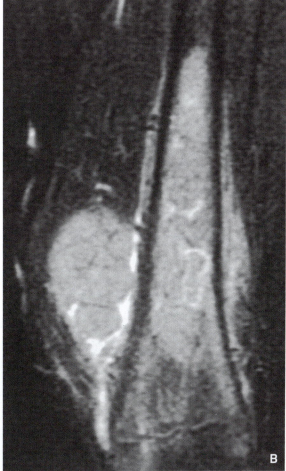

FIGURE 2.27 Magnetic resonance imaging of chondroblastic osteosarcoma. (A) Coronal T1-weighted MR image of the distal femur of a 14-year-old boy with chondroblastic osteosarcoma shows a large low-signal-intensity tumor in the bone marrow associated with a soft-tissue mass. **(B)** After intravenous administration of gadolinium, there is diffuse enhancement of both intramedullary tumor and soft-tissue mass.

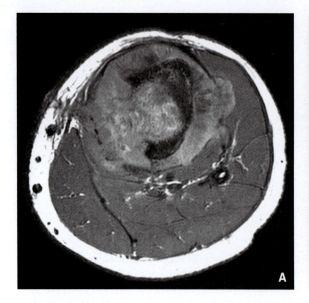
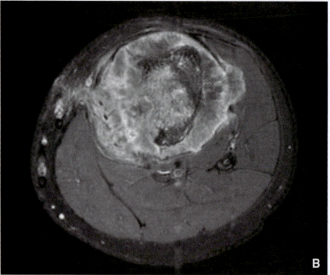
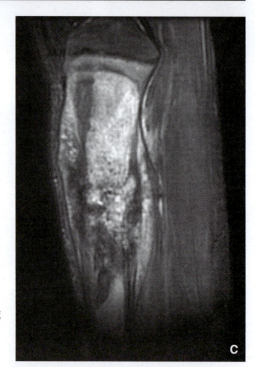

FIGURE 2.28 Magnetic resonance imaging of chondroblastic osteosarcoma. (A) Axial T1-weighted MRI shows a tumor within tibia, breaking into the soft tissues, exhibiting heterogenous signal. Axial **(B)** and sagittal **(C)** inversion recovery (IR) MR images demonstrate mixed although predominantly high-signal intensity of the lesion.

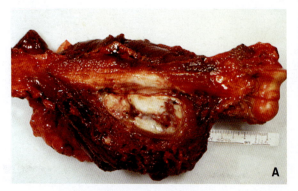
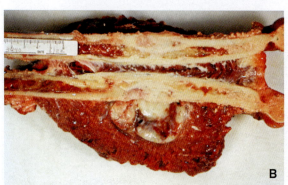

FIGURE 2.29 Gross specimen of conventional osteosarcoma. (A) Surgical specimen shows a hard tumor breaking through the cortex of the distal femur and forming a large soft-tissue mass. **(B)** Coronal section shows the neoplasm involving the medullary cavity, destroying the cortex, and forming tumor bone within the soft tissue extension.

Chapter 2 • Bone-Forming (Osteogenic) Lesions   **57**

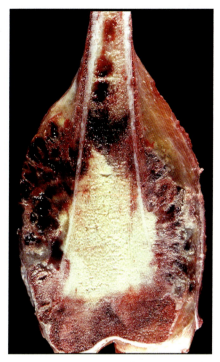

FIGURE 2.30 Gross specimen of conventional osteosarcoma. Predominantly osteoblastic tumor breaking through the cortex of the distal femur and producing tumor bone matrix in the soft-tissue mass. Areas of hemorrhage are present in the medullary cavity and in the soft-tissue mass.

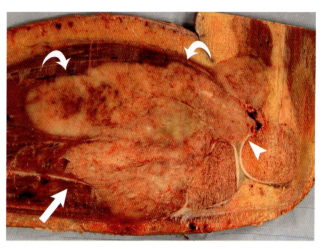

FIGURE 2.31 Gross specimen of conventional osteosarcoma. Tumor arising in the medullary portion of the proximal tibia (*arrow*) is breaking through the cortex and invading fibula, adjacent soft tissues (*curved arrows*), and knee joint space (*arrowhead*).

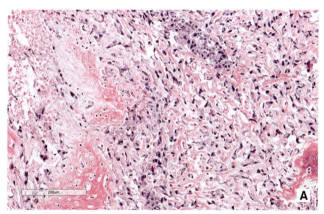

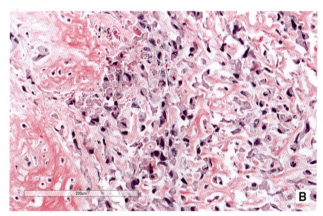

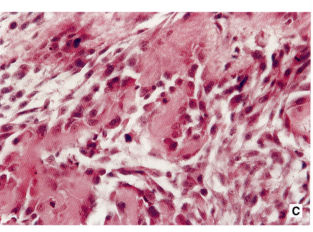

FIGURE 2.32 Histopathology of conventional osteoblastic osteosarcoma. (A) A pleomorphic malignant cells are producing osteoid (H&E, original magnification ×100). **(B)** Spindle to epithelioid tumor cells are producing osteoid (H&E, original magnification ×200). **(C)** On a high magnification note irregular woven bone trabeculae rimmed by pleomorphic tumor osteoblasts with hyperchromatic nuclei (H&E, original magnification ×400).

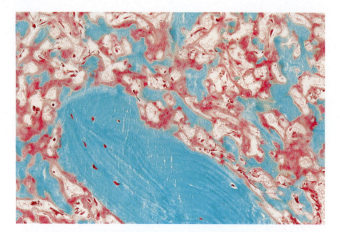

FIGURE 2.33 Histopathology of conventional osteoblastic osteosarcoma. In the marrow spaces around a normal bone trabecula (*lower center*), there are newly formed, fully mineralized irregular, smaller tumor trabeculae, surrounded by tumor cells (nondecalcified preparation, Goldner trichrome, original magnification ×50).

- The cytoplasm is most often eosinophilic but may be clear.
- May produce varying amounts of osteoid, bone, cartilage, and fibrous tissue.
- Amount of various components allows classification of conventional osteosarcoma into three subtypes: osteoblastic (50%), chondroblastic (25%), and fibroblastic (25%).
- In osteoblastic subtype, bone and/or osteoid is the predominant matrix; the extremes of matrix production are thin arborizing osteoid to dense, compact osteoid and bone (sclerotic) (Fig. 2.33).
- In chondroblastic subtype, chondroid matrix is predominant (Figs. 2.34 and 2.35); it tends to be high-grade hyaline cartilage, which is intimately associated and randomly mixed, with nonchondroid elements without sharp margin between two components (also known as tumor chondrosteoid) (Fig. 2.36).
- In fibroblastic subtype, high-grade spindle cell malignancy with sometimes minimal amount of osseous matrix with or without cartilage is present (Figs. 2.37 and 2.38); the overall histologic appearance is similar to fibrosarcoma or pleomorphic undifferentiated sarcoma (malignant fibrous histiocytoma [MFH]), which may be difficult to diagnose on small biopsy samples.

Genetics and Immunohistochemistry:
- Loss of heterozygosis of chromosome arm 3q, 6q, 9, 10, 13q, 17p, and 18q is most common. Gains of portions of chromosomes 1p, 1q, 6p, 8q, and 17p have also been reported. Deregulations of *TP53* is also thought to be significant in the development of osteosarcoma and occurs due to mutations of the gene or gross changes to the gene locus at chromosome band 17p13.1. Aberrations of the gene *RECQL4* located at chromosome band 8q24.4 are also associated with the development of this tumor.
- Amplification of the cyclin-dependent kinase gene (*CDK4*) located at chromosome band 12q13-14 has been detected in approximately 10% of the tumors.
- Deletion of 9p21 and the CDKN2A gene was reported in approximately 15% of the tumors. Loss of CDKN2A (p16) is associated with reduced survival. Recent study showed p16 loss as negative prognostic marker in osteosarcomas.
- Amplification at 1q21-23 and 17p are frequent findings in conventional osteosarcoma.

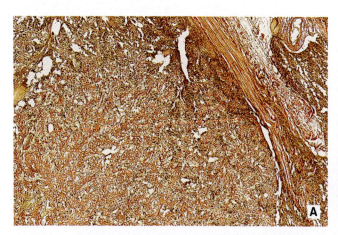
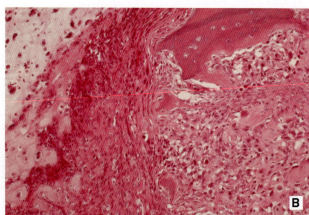

FIGURE 2.34 Histopathology of chondroblastic osteosarcoma. (A) Osteoblastic tumor tissue with moderate osteoid formation extending into the periosteum (*right upper corner*) (van Gieson, original magnification ×25). **(B)** In another field of view, the tumor is composed of chondroblastic tissue invading the adjacent trabecula (*right upper corner*). Osteoid-producing malignant cells (*bottom right*) are also visible (H&E, original magnification ×100).

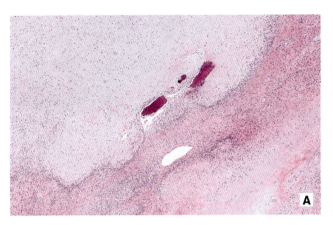
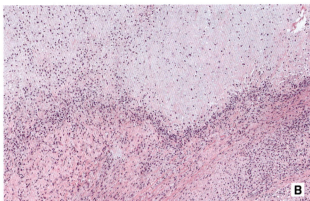
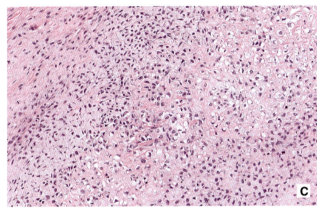

FIGURE 2.35 Histopathology of chondroblastic osteosarcoma. (A) Cartilaginous component consists mainly of high-grade hyaline cartilage mixed with nonchondroid component (H&E, original magnification ×50). **(B)** The tumor is composed mainly of cartilaginous tissue (chondroid matrix) with only scanty amount of tumor osteoid (H&E, original magnification ×100). **(C)** In another field of view, malignant cells are producing tumor osteoid (H&E, original magnification ×200).

Differential Diagnosis:

- *Ewing sarcoma*
  Location usually in diaphysis.
  Permeative type of bone destruction more common than "moth-eaten".
  "Saucerization" of the cortex.
  Lack of mineralization of the matrix.
  "Onion skin" (lamellated) type of periosteal reaction more common than sunburst.
  Occasionally soft-tissue mass disproportionally larger in comparison to the osseous involvement.
  Histopathology shows small, uniform-sized cells exhibiting indistinct borders, with round, slightly hyperchromatic nuclei and scant eosinophilic cytoplasm.
- *Malignant fibrous histiocytoma*
  Location usually at the articular end of bone.
  May look like a giant cell tumor.

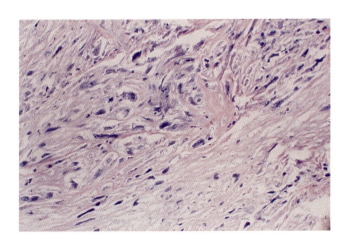

FIGURE 2.36 Histopathology of chondroblastic osteosarcoma. Marrow space with two bone trabeculae (*upper right and lower middle*) that are destroyed by tumor consisting of chondrosteoid (osteoid and cartilage matrix merging into one another without clear separation) is typical for many osteosarcomas (H&E, original magnification ×50).

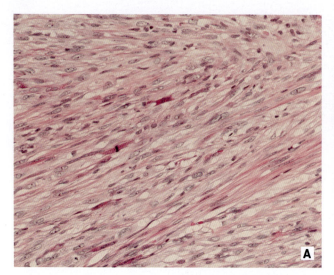
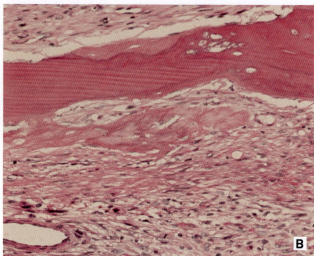

FIGURE 2.37 Histopathology of fibroblastic osteosarcoma. (A) Predominantly spindle fibroblast-like tumor cells with deeply stained nuclei are arranged in sheaths (H&E, original magnification ×200). **(B)** In another field, malignant cells adjacent to the remnants of destroyed trabecula produce osteoid (H&E, original magnification ×200).

Histopathology shows bundles of fibers and spindle-shaped, fibroblast-like cells arranged in a cartwheel or storiform pattern, exhibiting mitotic activity and features of atypia; rounded and foam cells with histiocytic features and well-defined cytoplasmic borders, exhibiting often grooved or indented nuclei.

- *Fibrosarcoma*
  Purely lytic lesion, commonly exhibiting a moth-eaten or permeative pattern of bone destruction, with no evidence of reactive sclerosis and without matrix mineralization, eccentric in location, closed to or in the articular end of bone.
  Small sequester-like fragments of bone within the lesion.
  Aggressive periosteal reaction may be seen.
  Histopathology shows formation of interlacing bundles of collagen fibers by spindle-shaped tumor cells, exhibiting a herringbone pattern, and lack of tumor bone or cartilage formation.
- *Chondrosarcoma*
  Occurs in the older population.
  Exhibits characteristic chondroid matrix.
  Less aggressive type of periosteal reaction.
  Histopathology shows lack of osteoid or tumor bone formation, but production of malignant cartilage by the tumor cells accompanied by infiltration of the marrow cavity and entrapment of preexisting bone trabeculae; destruction of bone and infiltration of Haversian systems; myxoid changes of the stroma.

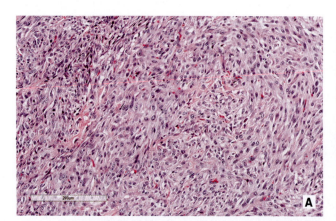
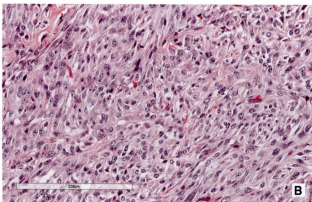

FIGURE 2.38 Histopathology of fibroblastic osteosarcoma. (A) High-grade spindle cell malignancy with minimal amount of tumor osteoid (H&E, original magnification ×100). **(B)** Spindle cell proliferation with prominent pleomorphism and atypical mitotic figures, and scant osteoid production by malignant cells (H&E, original magnification ×200).

- *Malignant lymphoma*
  Generally, older age.
  Diaphyseal rather than metaphyseal location.
  Periosteal reaction and soft-tissue mass are present in less than 50% of cases.
  Histopathology shows aggregates of malignant lymphoid cells that are usually rounded, ovoid, or pleomorphic. The cytoplasm is basophilic and exhibits well-defined outline. Large nuclei, containing rather scanty chromatin, are sometimes indented (cleaved) or horseshoe shaped with prominent nucleoli.

Complications:
- Pathologic fractures.
- Metastases (lungs, bones, soft tissues).

Prognosis:
- Depends on type of the tumor, size, location, stage, resectability, and presence of metastases.
- Untreated, conventional osteosarcoma is fatal.
- Aggressive local growth, rapid hematogenous systemic dissemination, and pulmonary metastases are bad prognostic features.
- Treatment of conventional osteosarcoma is tailored to the location, size, and stage of the tumor.
- Chemotherapy is usually employed in the preoperative setting and continued after surgical resection.
- Survival is directly related to response to preoperative therapy. In those patients whose tumors have greater than 90% tumor necrosis, long-term survival is generally 80% to 90%.
- In patients with less than 90% response to therapy, the survival is poor, usually less than 15%.
- P16 negativity in osteosarcoma shows correlation with worse response to therapy.

Telangiectatic Osteosarcoma

Definition:
- Malignant bone-forming tumor characterized by large spaces with or without septa, filled with blood.

Epidemiology:
- Accounts for less than 4% of all cases of osteosarcomas.
- Most common in the second decade of life but was described in younger patients.
- Male-to-female ratio of 1.5:1.

Sites of Involvement:
- Most common location is distal femoral metaphysis followed by the upper tibia, proximal humerus, and proximal femur.

Clinical Presentation:
- Similar to conventional osteosarcoma.
- Common pathologic fracture (1/4 of the cases), because of massive bone destruction.

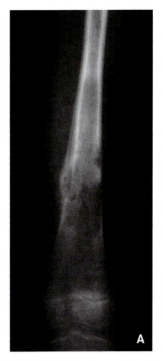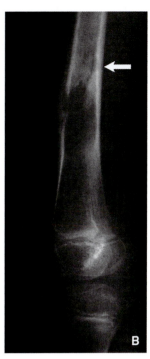

FIGURE 2.39 Radiography of telangiectatic osteosarcoma.
(A) Predominantly osteolytic tumor associated with periosteal reaction is seen in the distal femoral diaphysis of this 6-year-old girl. **(B)** On the lateral radiograph, the pathologic fracture is well demonstrated (*arrow*). (Courtesy of Dr. K.K. Unni, Rochester, Minnesota.)

Imaging:
- Purely osteolytic, large bone destruction without distinct surrounding bony sclerosis (Figs. 2.39 and 2.40).
- Most lesions are located in metaphysis and usually extend into the epiphysis.
- Tumor often expands and disrupts the cortex, extending into the soft tissues.
- Periosteal reaction including Codman triangle, velvet type, and "onion skin" is common.
- MRI, T1-weighted images may show increased signal intensity due to the presence of methemoglobin, and T2-weighted images show high signal intensity with several cystic areas and fluid–fluid levels, associated with an extraskeletal extension of the tumor, similar to the ABC (Fig. 2.41).

Pathology:
Gross (Macroscopy):
- Dominant cystic architecture in the medullary space (Fig. 2.42).
- Cystic portions of the tumor are filled incompletely with blood clots, described as "a bag of blood."
- Lack of sclerotic tumor bone formation.

Histopathology:
- Tumor contains solid areas mixed with blood-filled or empty spaces separated by thin septa simulating ABC (Fig. 2.43).

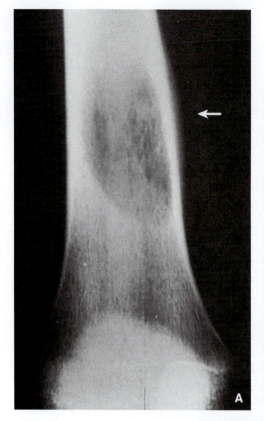
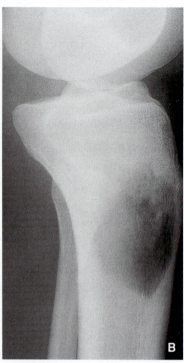

FIGURE 2.40 Radiography of telangiectatic osteosarcoma. **(A)** Purely destructive lesion in the femoral diaphysis of a 17-year-old girl. Note the velvet type of periosteal reaction (*arrow*). **(B)** Lateral radiograph of the proximal tibia of a 21-year-old man shows a purely lytic lesion with relatively narrow zone of transition.

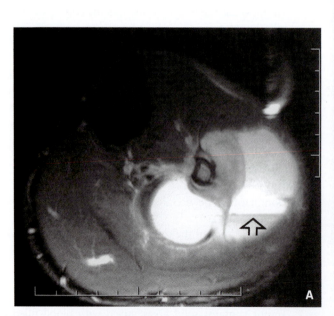
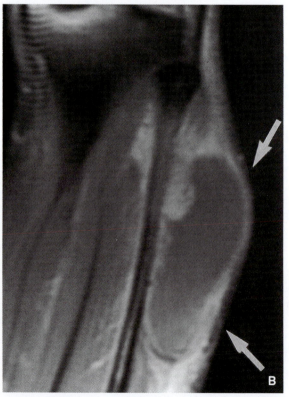

FIGURE 2.41 Magnetic resonance imaging of telangiectatic osteosarcoma. (A) Axial fat-suppressed T2-weighted image of the proximal leg of an 18-year-old woman shows a large tumor affecting the fibula and extending into the soft tissues. Note fluid–fluid level (*open arrow*), characteristic for this neoplasm. **(B)** Coronal fat-suppressed T1-weighted MR image obtained after intravenous administration of gadolinium shows enhancement of both intramedullary portion of the tumor and the periphery of the large soft-tissue mass (*arrows*). The cystic part of the mass does not enhance.

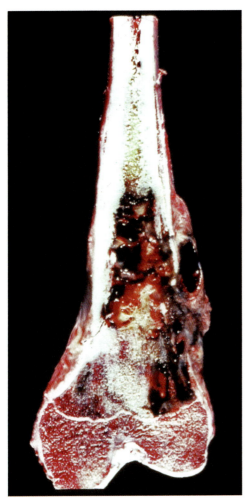

FIGURE 2.42 Gross specimen of telangiectatic osteosarcoma. Areas of solid tumor and dominant cystic architecture partially filled with blood clots are typical for this neoplasm. Note that the tumor did not invade the growth plate.

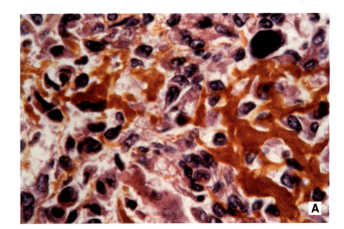

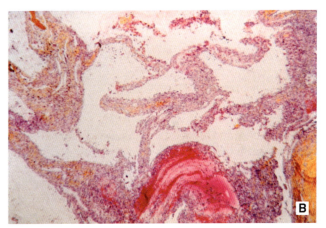

FIGURE 2.43 Histopathology of telangiectatic osteosarcoma. (A) Solid areas of the tumor show pleomorphic malignant cells with hyperchromatic nuclei, forming tumor bone (H&E, original magnification ×400). **(B)** In another section, there is almost no evidence of the cells, but large vascular spaces separated by thin septae are present characteristic for this tumor (H&E, original magnification ×100).

- Some tumors may be more solid with less cystic spaces (Fig. 2.44).
- The septa are cellular, containing atypical mononuclear tumor cells.
- Tumor cells are hyperchromatic and pleomorphic with high mitotic activity including atypical mitoses (Fig. 2.45).
- Amount of osteoid may vary, but usually fine, lace-like osteoid is observed in minimal amount.
- Cellular septae contain many benign-looking multinucleated giant cells, which may be difficult to differentiate from giant cell tumor.

Genetics:
- Mutations in the *TP53* and *RAS* genes, LOH at *TP53*, *CDKN2A*, and *RB1*.
- Amplifications of *MDM2* and *MYC* are rare.

Differential Diagnosis:
- **Aneurysmal bone cyst**
  Usually less aggressive presentation, but not infrequently very similar to the telangiectatic osteosarcoma, with fluid–fluid levels seen on MRI.
  Commonly solid buttress of periosteal reaction.
  Histopathology shows multiple blood-filled spaces lined by a single layer of flat undifferentiated cells, alternating with more solid areas composed of fibrous, richly vascular connective tissue. The fibrous lining contains many giant cells, usually in clusters. Lamellae of primitive woven bone may be present. Deposit of an iron pigment is a common finding.
- **Giant cell tumor**
  Invariably in the mature skeleton (after the closure of the physis), at the articular end of bone.

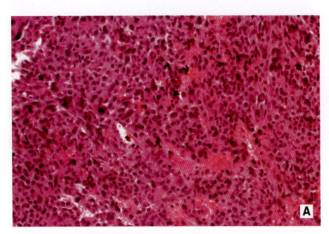 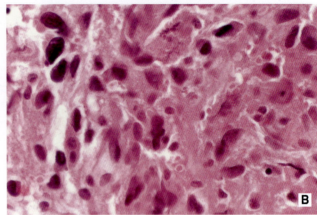

FIGURE 2.44 **Histopathology of telangiectatic osteosarcoma. (A)** Marked polymorphism and pleomorphism of the tumor with malignant cells forming osteoid (H&E, original magnification ×100). **(B)** On higher magnification, observe the pleomorphic tumor cells forming osteoid (H&E, original magnification ×400).

Lack of matrix mineralization.
Periosteal reaction rarely present.
Histopathology shows dual population of spindle fibrocytic and monocytic mononuclear stromal cells and giant cells that are usually uniformly distributed throughout the tumor. Giant cells never exhibit mitotic activity. Areas of hemorrhage, and occasionally groups of foam cells and hemosiderin-laden macrophages, are commonly present.

Prognosis:
- Similar to conventional osteosarcoma.
- Sensitive to chemotherapy.

Small Cell Osteosarcoma

Definition:
- Osteosarcoma composed of small cells with variable degree of osteoid production.

Epidemiology:
- About 1.5% of all osteosarcomas.
- Age range from 5 to 80 years old, although most common in the second decade of life.
- Slight predilection for females.

Sites of Involvement:
- Metaphysis of long bones (distal femur, proximal tibia, proximal humerus).
- Multiple sites may be affected.

Clinical Presentation:
- Pain and swelling of involved site.

Imaging:
- Aggressive process with destruction of the medullary cavity and cortex.
- Aggressive type of periosteal reaction.

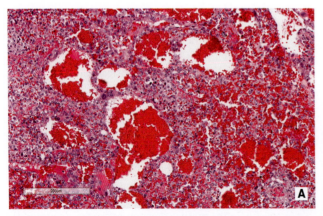 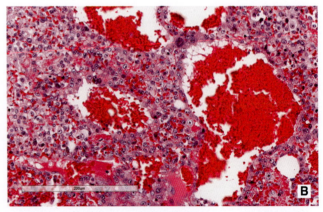

FIGURE 2.45 **Histopathology of telangiectatic osteosarcoma. (A)** Several blood-filled and empty cystic spaces are separated by thin septa (H&E, original magnification ×100). **(B)** Surrounding the cystic spaces are pleomorphic malignant cells exhibiting high mitotic activity and forming tumor osteoid (H&E, original magnification ×200).

- There is always a lytic component exhibiting permeative pattern of bone destruction, usually combined with radiodense areas.
- Mineralized tissue is seen, either intramedullary or in soft-tissue tumor extension.

Pathology:

Histopathology:

- Small blue cell proliferation exhibiting round-to-oval nuclei with fine-to-coarse chromatin (Fig. 2.46A,B).
- Nuclear diameter of round cells can range in size from very small to medium; the smaller ones are comparable to those of Ewing sarcoma or lymphoma.
- Cells show scant eosinophilic cytoplasm.
- Mitoses range from 3 to 5 per HPF.
- Less common spindle cell type show short, oval-to-spindle nuclei with a granular chromatin, inconspicuous nucleoli, and scanty amounts of cytoplasm.
- Lace-like osteoid is always present (Fig. 2.46C).
- Biopsy from small cell osteosarcoma may resemble Ewing sarcoma. In these cases, cytogenetic study for t(11,22) is the best diagnostic tool, which is negative in small cell osteosarcoma.

Immunohistochemistry:

- Positive for CD99, vimentin, osteocalcin, and osteonectin.

Genetics:

- Negative for t(11,22) in comparison to Ewing sarcoma, which is the best marker for differentiation of these two very similar morphologically tumors.

Differential Diagnosis:

- ***Ewing sarcoma***
  Diaphyseal location.
  Saucerization of the cortex.
  Lack of mineralization of the matrix.
  Occasionally soft tissue component disproportionally larger in comparison to osseous involvement.

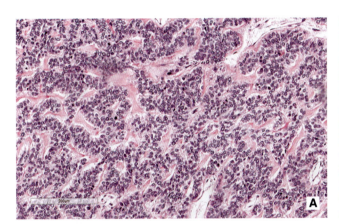
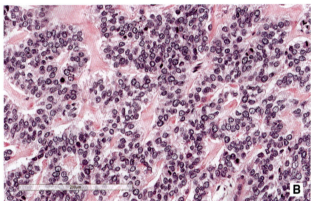
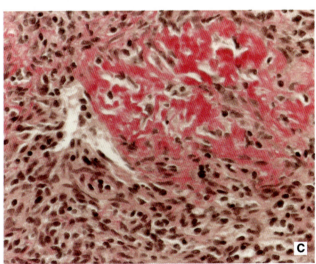

FIGURE 2.46 Histopathology of small cell osteosarcoma. (A) Small round blue cells are forming tumor osteoid (H&E, original magnification ×100). **(B)** The nuclei of the cells are round to oval with fine or coarse chromatin (H&E, original magnification ×200). **(C)** Tumor tissue consists of medium-sized round and oval cells with indistinct cytoplasm and pleomorphic and hyperchromatic nuclei resembling those of Ewing sarcoma. In contrast to Ewing sarcoma, however, there is osteoid formation (*red areas*) by malignant cells (H&E, original magnification ×400).

Histopathology shows small, uniform-sized cells exhibiting indistinct borders, with round, slightly hyperchromatic nuclei and almost clear cytoplasm.
Translocation t(11,22).
- **Malignant lymphoma**
Usually localized in the shafts of long bones.
Geographic or moth-eaten types of lytic bone destruction with prominent endosteal reaction.
When affecting the flat bones or vertebral bodies, sclerotic changes predominate.
Periosteal reaction and soft-tissue mass are present in less than 50% of cases.
Histopathology shows aggregates of malignant lymphoid cells that are usually rounded, ovoid, and pleomorphic. The cytoplasm is basophilic and exhibits well-defined outline. Large nuclei, containing rather scanty chromatin, are sometimes indented (cleaved) or horseshoe shaped with prominent nucleoli.

Prognosis:
- Poor.

Low-Grade Central Osteosarcoma

Definition:
- Low-grade tumor that arises from the medullary cavity of bone.

Epidemiology:
- 1% to 2% of all osteosarcomas.
- Males and females are equally affected.
- The peak incidence is in second to third decades of life.

Sites of Involvement:
- Most common in the long bones with predilection for the distal femur and proximal tibia.
- Flat bones are uncommonly affected.

Clinical Presentation:
- Pain and swelling are usual features.
- The duration of pain may be many months to even several years.

Imaging:
- Large metaphyseal or diaphyseal intramedullary tumors (Fig. 2.47).
- It is not uncommon to see extension into the end of the bone when the growth plate is closed.
- Majority of tumors are poorly marginated, up to 1/3 may show intermediate or well-defined margins suggestive of indolent or benign lesion.
- May mimic fibrous dysplasia (Fig. 2.48).
- Trabeculation and sclerosis are common findings that reflect indolent nature of this tumor.

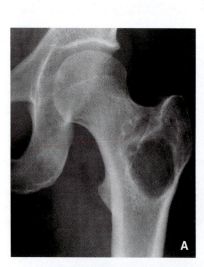 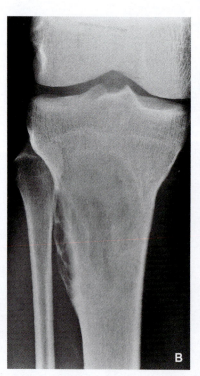 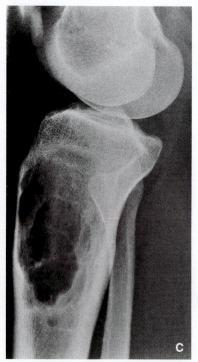

FIGURE 2.47 Radiography of low-grade central osteosarcoma. (A) Lytic lesion with narrow zone of transition and geographic type of bone destruction in the intertrochanteric region of left femur has a benign appearance. **(B)** Anteroposterior and **(C)** lateral radiographs of the right knee of another patient show a radiolucent lesion in the proximal tibial diaphysis slightly expanding the lateral cortex.

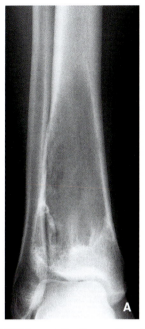
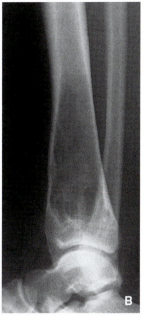

FIGURE 2.48 Radiography of low-grade central osteosarcoma. (A) Anteroposterior and **(B)** lateral radiographs of the distal leg of an 18-year-old woman show benign-appearing radiolucent lesion in the distal tibia exhibiting narrow zone of transition and geographic type of bone destruction, resembling fibrous dysplasia.

- Although rare, cortical destruction is the most convincing imaging feature to support malignant nature of the tumor.

Pathology:
Gross (Macroscopy):
- Grey-white tumor with a firm and gritty texture arising within the medullary cavity.

Histopathology:
Hypocellular-to-moderately cellular fibroblastic stroma with variable amounts of osteoid production (Fig. 2.49).
- Tumor cell shows some degree of cytologic atypia with nuclear enlargement and hyperchromasia.
- Occasional mitotic figures may be seen.
- Some tumors contain irregular anastomosing, branching, and curved trabeculae simulating the appearance of woven bone in fibrous dysplasia.
- Small scattered foci of atypical cartilage and multinucleated giant cells may occasionally be seen.

Genetics:
- Minor genetic alterations with gains at 12q13-14, 12p, and 6p21, resulting in overexpression of *CDK4* and *MDM2* and amplification of *SAS* (*s*arcoma-*a*mplified *s*equence).

Differential Diagnosis:
- ***Fibrous dysplasia***
  Monostotic form commonly exhibits "ground-glass" or smoky appearance and rind sign.
  Histopathology shows metaplastic immature woven bone trabeculae without osteoblastic activity (rimming), resembling Chinese characters, haphazardly arranged in loose fibrous stroma; no atypia in spindle cells.
- ***Desmoplastic fibroma***
  Usually expansive, radiolucent lesion, commonly trabeculated, yielding the honeycomb pattern of bone destruction, with sharply defined but nonsclerotic borders. No significant periosteal reaction.
  Histopathology shows very regular bundles of spindle-shaped or stellate fibroblasts with elongated or ovoid nuclei interspersed within a densely collagenized matrix. The cells show no evidence of mitotic activity.

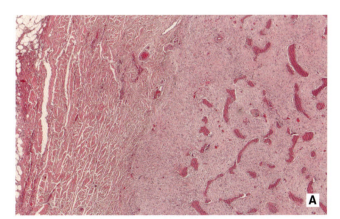
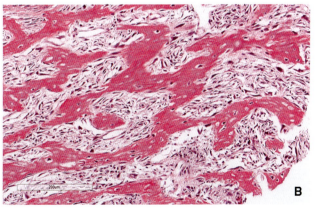

FIGURE 2.49 Histopathology of low-grade central osteosarcoma. (A) The cellular stroma contains irregularly formed woven bone trabeculae (*right*) resembling fibrous dysplasia (H&E, original magnification ×25). **(B)** Hypocellular-to-moderately cellular fibroblastic stroma with some degree of cellular atypia, and variable amount of osteoid production (H&E, original magnification ×100).

Prognosis:
- Low-grade central osteosarcoma behaves in a much more indolent fashion than conventional osteosarcoma.
- High incidence of local recurrence after inadequate excision.
- Recurrence may exhibit higher grade or differentiation with the potential for metastases.

Giant Cell–Rich Osteosarcoma

Definition:
- Osteosarcoma with giant cell component and a paucity of tumor osteoid and tumor bone.

Epidemiology:
- About 3% of all osteosarcomas.

Sites of Involvement:
- Metaphysis or diaphysis of long bones, usually femur and tibia.

Clinical Presentation:
- Similar to conventional osteosarcoma.

Imaging:
- Essentially similar to conventional osteosarcoma (Fig. 2.50).
- Periosteal reaction either absent or scant.
- Soft-tissue mass may be small or absent.

Pathology:
Gross (Macroscopy):
- Expansive solid mass with common involvement of and break through the cortex (Fig. 2.51).

Histopathology:
- Histologically related to telangiectatic and MFH-like osteosarcomas.
- Epithelioid or spindle osteosarcoma cells.
- Prominent nuclear atypia and hyperchromasia.
- Characteristic abundance of benign osteoclast-like giant cells.
- Paucity of tumor osteoid production.
- Resemble giant cell tumor (Fig. 2.52).

Multifocal (Multicentric) Osteosarcoma

Definition:
- Osteosarcoma developing simultaneously in several bones.

Epidemiology:
- Accounts for about 1.5% of all osteosarcomas, M > F.
- Most cases in children 5 to 10 years old.

Sites of Involvement:
- Distal end of femur, proximal end of tibia, but any bone can be affected, including small tubular bones.

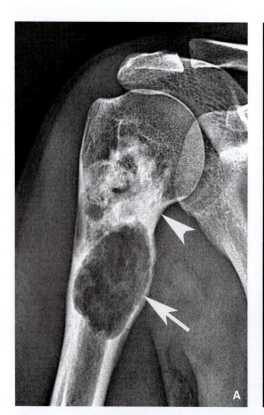 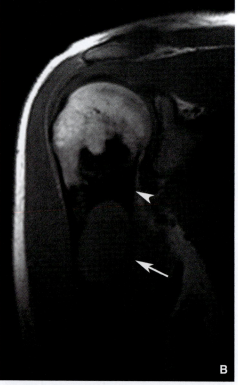

FIGURE 2.50 Radiography and magnetic resonance imaging of giant cell–rich osteosarcoma. (A) Anteroposterior radiograph of the right shoulder of a 22-year-old woman shows slightly expansive, mixed lytic (*arrow*) and sclerotic (*arrowhead*) lesion in the proximal humerus, exhibiting narrow zone of transition. **(B)** Coronal T1-weighted MR image shows the proximal sclerotic part of the tumor being of low-signal intensity (*arrowhead*), and the distal lytic part of intermediate signal (*arrow*).

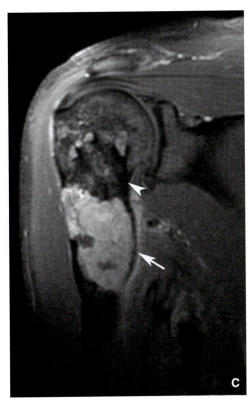 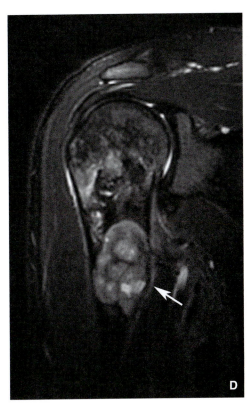

FIGURE 2.50 *(Continued).* **(C)** Coronal T2-weighted MR image demonstrates that the proximal part is of mixed heterogenous but predominantly of low signal intensity (*arrowhead*), whereas the distal part exhibits high signal (*arrow*). **(D)** Coronal T1-weighted fat-suppressed MR image obtained after intravenous administration of gadolinium shows various degree of enhancement of the entire tumor, more prominent in the distal part (*arrow*).

Clinical Presentation:
- Two variants have been described: synchronous (when several lesions appear simultaneously) and metachronous (when appearance of multiple lesions is separated by some lapse of time).

Imaging:
- Essentially very similar to conventional osteosarcoma, but affecting multiple bones (Fig. 2.53).
- Scintigraphy effective in localizing sites of involvement.

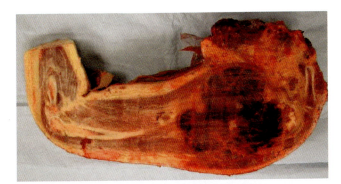

FIGURE 2.51 Gross specimen of giant cell–rich osteosarcoma. Solid tumor in the proximal humerus is breaking through the cortex invading soft tissues.

Pathology:
- Identical to conventional osteosarcoma.

Differential Diagnosis:
- **Skeletal metastases from primary osteosarcoma** (in which case lungs are usually affected as well).

Prognosis:
- Extremely poor.

Surface Osteosarcomas
Several types have been identified (Fig. 2.54).

Parosteal Osteosarcoma
Definition:
- Low-grade osteosarcoma which arises on the surface of bone.

Epidemiology:
- Accounts for about 4% of osteosarcomas.
- Most common surface osteosarcoma.
- Slight female predominance.
- Mostly young adults, about 1/3 of the cases occur in third decade of life.

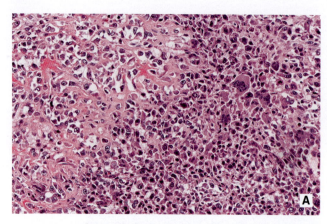
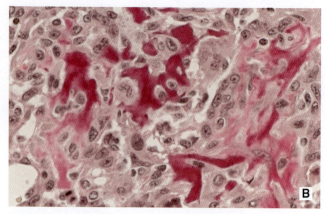

FIGURE 2.52 Histopathology of giant cell–rich osteosarcoma. (A) Proliferation of spindle-to-epithelioid cells with prominent atypia and pleomorphism producing osteoid. Note characteristic for this tumor abundance of benign osteoclast-like giant cells similar to giant cell tumor (H&E, original magnification ×200). **(B)** At high-power magnification, atypical cells with pleomorphic nuclei, irregular mitoses, and tumor osteoid formation are visible (van Gieson, original magnification ×400).

Sites of Involvement:
- Most of the cases involve the surface of the distal posterior femur, followed by proximal tibia and proximal humerus.

Clinical Presentation:
- Painless swelling; inability to flex the knee may be the initial symptom.
- Some patients may complain of a painful swelling.

Imaging:
- Heavily mineralized mass attached to the cortex with broad base (Fig. 2.55A).
- Incomplete cleft between the tumor and adjacent cortex (Fig. 2.55B).
- Tumor has tendency to wrap around the involved bone.
- CT and MRI are useful in evaluating the extent of cortical and medullary (rare) involvement (Figs. 2.56 and 2.57).

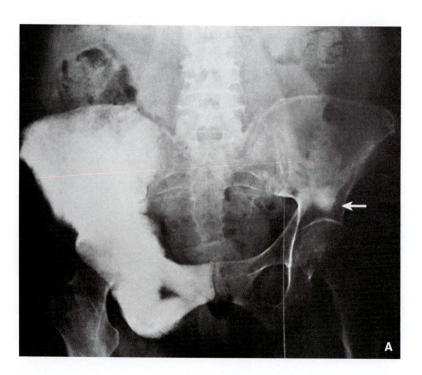

FIGURE 2.53 Radiography of multicentric osteosarcoma. (A) Anteroposterior radiograph of the pelvis shows sclerotic tumors affecting right ilium, ischium, and pubic bones. In addition, there is a sclerotic focus in the left ilium (*arrow*).

Chapter 2 • Bone-Forming (Osteogenic) Lesions 71

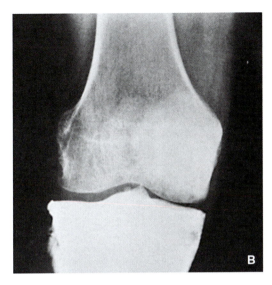

FIGURE 2.53 *(Continued).* **(B,C)** Distal femur, proximal and distal tibia, and several bones of the right foot are also affected in the same patient.

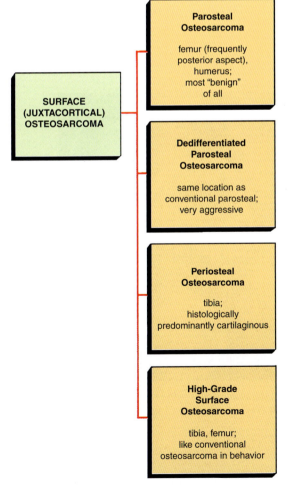

FIGURE 2.54 Variants of surface osteosarcomas.

Pathology:

Gross (Macroscopy):

- Hard lobulated mass attached to the underlying cortex with, occasionally present, incomplete cap-like cartilage covering the surface and thus suggesting a diagnosis of osteochondroma (Figs. 2.58 and 2.59).

Histopathology:

- Well-formed bone trabeculae in spindle cell stroma (Fig. 2.60).
- Spindle cells show minimal atypia, osteoid formation, and rare mitotic figures.
- Bone trabeculae are arranged in a parallel manner and simulate normal bone.
- The trabeculae may or may not show osteoblastic rimming.
- About 50% of the tumors will show cartilaginous differentiation.
- Cartilaginous component may form hypercellular nodules of cartilage within the tumor or cap on the surface.
- When cartilage cap is present it may be mildly hypercellular, and the cells may show mild atypia and lack of columnar arrangement seen in osteochondroma.
- About 15% will show high-grade spindle cell sarcoma (dedifferentiation).

Genetics:

- *SAS*, *CDK4*, and *MDM2* overexpression and coamplification were described in majority of cases.

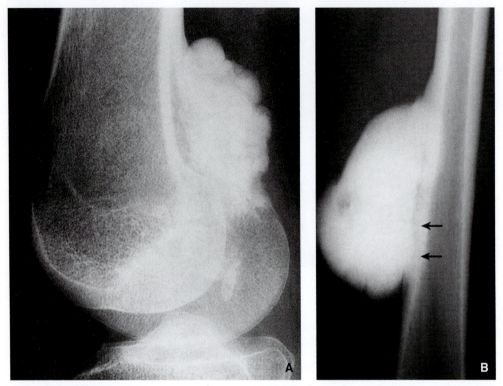

FIGURE 2.55 Radiography of parosteal osteosarcoma. (A) Sclerotic, lobulated mass is attached to the posterior cortex of distal femur. The periphery of the tumor is slightly less dense than the base. **(B)** Large sclerotic tumor is partially attached to the medial cortex of the femoral shaft displaying inferiorly a radiolucent cleft (*arrows*).

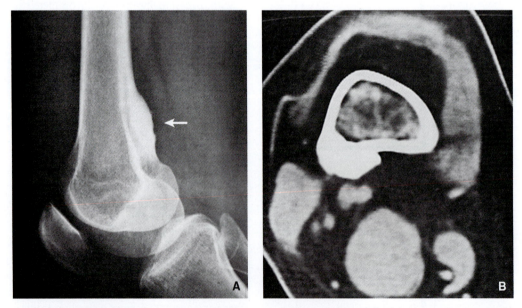

FIGURE 2.56 Computed tomography of parosteal osteosarcoma. (A) Lateral radiograph of the knee of a 37-year-old woman shows an ossific tumor attached to the posterior cortex of the distal femur (*arrow*). **(B)** Contrast-enhanced CT section shows that medullary cavity is not invaded.

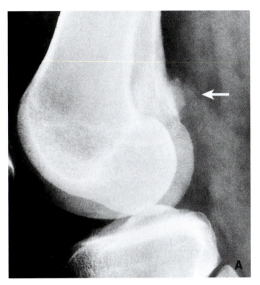
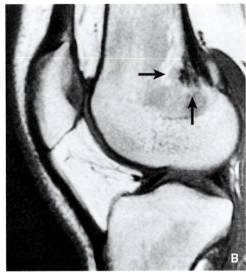

FIGURE 2.57 Magnetic resonance imaging of parosteal osteosarcoma. (A) Lateral radiograph of the knee of a 22-year-old woman shows a surface tumor involving the posterior aspect of the medial femoral condyle (*arrow*). The invasion of the cortex cannot be determined. **(B)** Sagittal MR image demonstrates the invasion of medullary cavity (*arrows*).

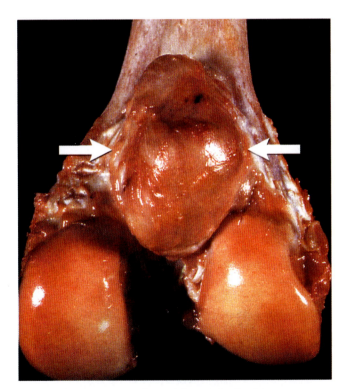

FIGURE 2.58 Gross specimen of parosteal osteosarcoma. Note a large surface lesion in the posterior aspect of the distal femur exhibiting glistening cartilaginous-like cap (*arrows*).

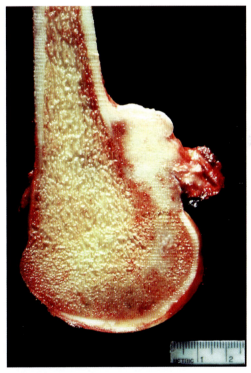

FIGURE 2.59 Gross specimen (sagittal section) of parosteal osteosarcoma. Although the entire tumor is on the surface of the bone, there is evidence of cortical invasion.

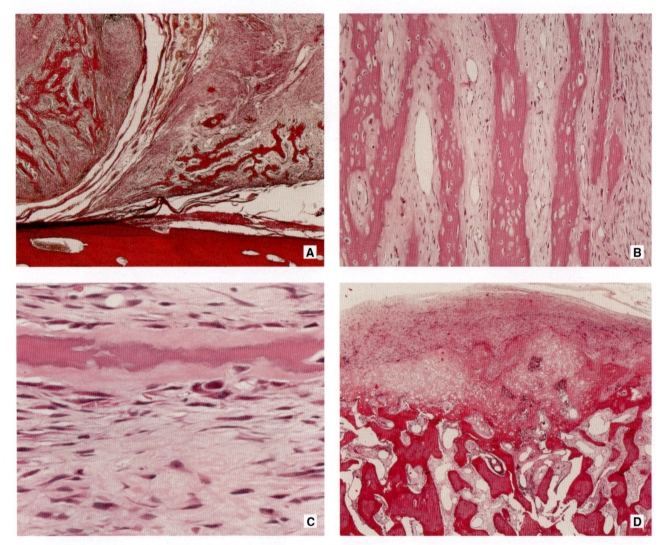

FIGURE 2.60 Histopathology of parosteal osteosarcoma. (A) The tumor originates at the surface of cortical bone (van Gieson, original magnification ×25). **(B)** At higher magnification, parallel arranged trabeculae of woven bone are separated by a fibrous stroma containing irregularly shaped spindle cells (H&E, original magnification ×100). **(C)** In some areas, spindle cells containing enlarged hyperchromatic nuclei are producing tumor bone (H&E, original magnification ×400). **(D)** On its surface, parosteal osteosarcoma may be covered by the cartilaginous cap resembling osteochondroma; however, subchondral areas contain spindle cells, and there is absence of hematopoietic or fatty marrow (H&E, original magnification ×25).

Differential Diagnosis:
- **Periosteal osteosarcoma**
  Heterogenous tumor matrix with calcified spiculations interspersed with areas of radiolucency representing uncalcified matrix.
  Endosteal surface of affected bone commonly spared.
  Extension of tumor into the soft tissues but medullary canal spared.
  Occasionally periosteal reaction in form of the Codman triangle.
  Histopathology shows low-grade to medium-grade malignancy with predominance of lobulated chondroid tissue exhibiting moderate cellularity.

- **Parosteal osteoma**
  Homogenously dense, ivory-like sclerotic mass attached to the cortex, with sharply demarcated smooth borders, occasionally lobulated. No evidence of cortical invasion.
  Histopathology shows either cancellous trabecular architecture with fatty marrow in the intertrabecular spaces and woven bone with plait of collagen fibers and roundish spindle-shaped osteocyte lacunae, or dense, compact mature lamellar bone without Haversian systems.

- **Juxtacortical myositis ossificans**
  Zonal phenomenon (periphery of the lesion more mature than the center). Radiolucent cleft separates

the lesion from adjacent cortex. Regression of the lesion with time.

Histopathology shows trabecular bone and fibrous marrow. Immature bone in the center of the lesion with proliferating osteoblasts, fibroblasts, and areas of hemorrhage and necrosis, but mature bone on the periphery.

- **Sessile osteochondroma**

  Cortex of the host bone merges without interruption with cortex of the lesion, and respective cancellous portions of osteochondroma and adjacent bone communicate.

  Histopathology shows cartilaginous cap composed of hyaline cartilage arranged similarly to the growth plate. Beneath it, there is zone of endochondral ossification with vascular invasion and replacement of calcified cartilage by newly formed bone.

- **Parosteal lipoma with ossifications**

  Lobulated mass containing irregular ossifications and radiolucent areas of fat; hyperostosis of adjacent cortex occasionally present.

  Histopathology shows formation of mature bone with adipose tissue; occasionally foci of necrosis and calcifications.

Prognosis:
- Excellent, with overall 91% survival rate at 5 years.

Periosteal Osteosarcoma
Definition:
- Intermediate-grade chondroblastic osteosarcoma arising on the surface of the bone.

Epidemiology:
- Less than 2% of all osteosarcomas.
- It is more common than surface high-grade osteosarcoma, but about 1/3 as common as parosteal osteosarcoma.
- The peak incidence is the second and third decades of life.
- Slight male predominance.

Sites of Involvement:
- Diaphysis or diaphyseal–metaphyseal area of long bones, with the tibia and femur most commonly affected.

Clinical Presentation:
- Painless mass or limb swelling is the most common initial finding with pain and tenderness later developing in the affected area.

Imaging:
- Arising on the surface of a bone, displays heterogeneous, calcified spiculations that are oriented perpendicular to the cortex and give the overall sunburst appearance (Fig. 2.61).
- The lesion decreases in density from the cortical base to the surface, where the tumor has a relatively well-demarcated margin.
- Commonly, the cortex appears thickened as a result of the production of ossified matrix.
- Occasionally, Codman triangle is present.
- Medullary cavity of the affected bone is usually spared.
- CT and MRI important in the evaluation of tumor size, integrity of the cortex, and soft tissue extension (Figs. 2.62 and 2.63).

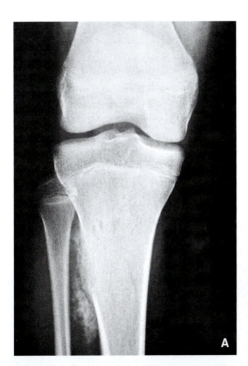 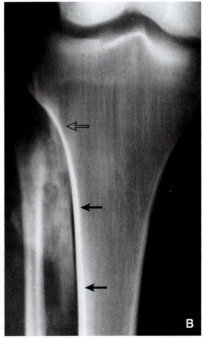

FIGURE 2.61 Radiography of periosteal osteosarcoma. (A) Frontal radiograph of the right knee of a 12-year-old girl with discomfort in the upper leg for 2 months shows poorly defined calcifications and ossifications in a mass attached to the surface of the lateral tibial cortex. **(B)** Anteroposterior tomography shows the ossified mass. Although attached to the tibia proximally (*open arrow*), it is partially separated from the lateral cortex by a narrow radiolucent cleft (*arrows*), very similar to that seen in the juxtacortical myositis ossificans.

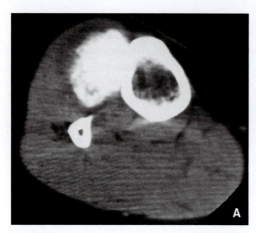 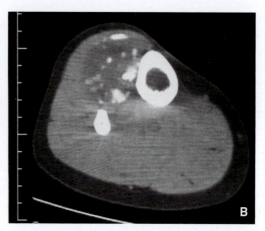

FIGURE 2.62 Computed tomography of periosteal osteosarcoma (same patient as depicted in Fig. 2.61). (A) CT section obtained through the proximal part of the tumor of the same patient as in Figure 2.61 clearly demonstrates the attachment of the lesion to the tibial cortex. The medullary cavity is not affected. **(B)** CT section through the distal part of the tumor shows the extent of the soft-tissue mass. Note low attenuation of the mass with high-attenuation ossifications.

Pathology:
Gross (Macroscopy):

- Tumor arises from the bone surface and may involve part of the bone or the entire circumference.

Histopathology:

- The tumor has the appearance of a moderately differentiated chondroblastic osteosarcoma (Fig. 2.64).
- Ossified mass is generally found arising from the cortex and is made up of relatively mature bone.
- Cartilaginous component predominates, but elements of intermediate-grade osteosarcoma are invariably present.
- Cartilaginous component may show varying degrees of cytologic atypia, and matrix may be myxoid.
- Periphery most of the time is not calcified and made up of fascicles of spindle cells.

Genetics:

- Rare +17 chromosome was described in a few cases.

Differential Diagnosis:

- *Periosteal chondrosarcoma*
  Sometimes difficult to differentiate, but no evidence of osteoid formation.
- *Parosteal osteosarcoma*
  Homogenously dense mass exhibiting more mature appearance on imaging studies, sharply demarcated from the soft tissues.
  Occasionally present an incomplete radiolucent cleft, partially separating the tumor from the cortex of the affected bone.
  Histopathology shows well-formed bone trabeculae within spindle cell stroma, arranged in a parallel manner that simulate normal bone. Minimal atypia, osteoid formation, and rare mitotic figures. About 50% of tumors show cartilaginous differentiation in form of hypercellular nodules, cartilage in tumor stroma, or cartilaginous cap on the tumor surface.
- *Juxtacortical myositis ossificans*
  Classic zonal phenomenon (see previous text).
  Cleft separating the lesion from the adjacent cortex.
  Histopathology shows lack of tumor osteoid or tumor bone formation.
- *Nora lesion (bizarre parosteal osteochondromatous proliferation, BPOP)*
  Hands and feet most commonly affected.

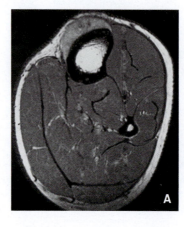 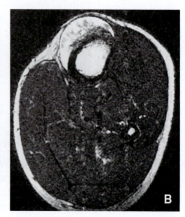

FIGURE 2.63 Magnetic resonance imaging of periosteal osteosarcoma. (A) Axial T1-weighted MR image shows a tumor adjacent to the anterior cortex of the tibia displays slightly higher signal than muscles. **(B)** On T2-weighted MRI, the mass becomes bright except for the central areas at which bone formation displays low signal.

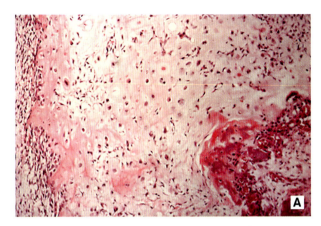
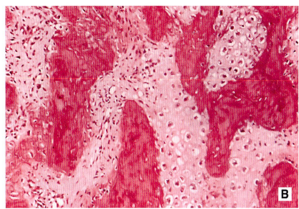
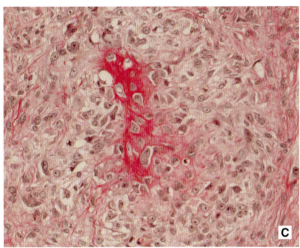

FIGURE 2.64 Histopathology of periosteal osteosarcoma. (A) Note predominantly cartilaginous component of the tumor with pseudotrabeculae of tumor bone formed by the malignant cells (H&E, original magnification ×100). **(B)** In another section, the cartilaginous tissue predominates, but there are areas of tumor osteoid and tumor bone formation as well (*left lower corner*) (H&E, original magnification ×100). **(C)** At high magnification, note scanty osteoid formation by malignant cells (H&E, original magnification ×200).

Heavy calcified or ossified mass with a broad base attached to the adjacent cortex.

Histopathology shows bizarre hypercellular cartilage formation and irregular short bone trabeculae, without invasion of soft tissue; spindle cells within the intertrabecular spaces.

- *Florid reactive periostitis*

  Aggressive periosteal reaction usually affecting small tubular bones of the hand and feet.

  Soft tissue swelling may be present.

  Histopathology shows woven bone and areas of osteoblastic activity, as well as hypercellular spindle cell stroma without pleomorphism or cellular atypia.

Prognosis:
- Better prognosis than conventional osteosarcoma, but still have tendency to recur and metastasize.
- Medullary involvement of the bone may have poorer prognosis.
- About 70% recurrence rate after excision.
- Rate of metastasis has been reported to be about 15%.

High-Grade Surface Osteosarcoma
Definition:
- High-grade bone-forming malignancy that arises on the surface of the bone.

Epidemiology:
- Less than 1% of all osteosarcomas.
- Peak incidence in second decade of life.
- Slight male predilection.

Sites of Involvement:
- Femur is most commonly affected followed by the humerus and tibia.

Clinical Presentation:
- Patients commonly present with the mass or pain at the site of the tumor.

Imaging:
- Surface mass, partially mineralized, extending to soft tissue (Fig. 2.65).
- The underlying cortex is partially destroyed, and periosteal new bone formation is commonly present at the periphery of the tumor.
- Cross-sectional imaging may show minimal medullary involvement, but for the most part, the tumor is relatively well circumscribed at its bone–soft tissue interface.

Pathology:
Gross (Macroscopy):
- Tumor is situated on the surface of the bone but may erode the underlying cortex.

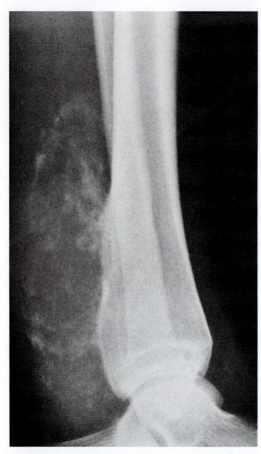

FIGURE 2.65 Radiography of high-grade surface osteosarcoma. Lateral radiograph of the distal leg of a 24-year-old man shows a tumor arising from the surface of the posterior tibial cortex. Note similarity of this tumor to the periosteal osteosarcoma depicted in Fig. 2.61.

Histopathology:
- Shows similar morphology to conventional osteosarcoma.
- Regions of predominantly osteoblastic, chondroblastic, or fibroblastic differentiation.
- All tumors show high-grade cytologic atypia and lace-like osteoid as seen in conventional osteosarcoma (Fig. 2.66).

Prognosis:
- As in conventional osteosarcoma, prognostic features depend upon positive response to chemotherapy.

Secondary Osteosarcomas

Definition:
- Bone-forming sarcomas occurring in bones affected by preexisting lesions, the most common being postirradiation therapy changes in the osseous structures, Paget disease, and rarely various other benign disorders such as fibrous dysplasia.

Postradiation Osteosarcoma

Definition:
- Osteosarcoma developing as a result of irradiation.

Epidemiology:
- Constitute 3.4% to 5.5% of all osteosarcomas and 50% to 60% of radiation-induced sarcomas.
- Estimated risk of developing osteosarcoma in irradiated bone is 0.03% to 0.8%.
- Children treated with high-dose radiotherapy and chemotherapy are at greatest risk.
- The prevalence of postirradiation osteosarcomas is increasing as children survive treatment of their malignant disease.

Criteria for the Diagnosis:
- The initial lesion and the postirradiation sarcoma must not be of the same histologic type.
- The site of the new tumor must be within field of irradiation.
- At least 3 years must have elapsed since the previous radiation therapy.

Sites of Involvement:
- Any irradiated bone, but the most common locations are the pelvis and the shoulder girdle.

Clinical Presentation:
- History of previous radiation therapy and tumor developing in the path of radiation beam.
- A symptom-free latent period may be long (4 to 40 years, median of 11 years) and inversely related to the radiation dose.
- Radiation doses are usually greater than 20 Gy.
- From experience, we have seen few osteosarcomas in young children with history of radiation therapy for synovial sarcoma.

Imaging:
- Tumors are densely sclerotic or lytic with a soft-tissue mass.
- Radiation osteitis is present in about 50% of cases (trabecular coarsening and lytic areas in cortex).

Pathology:
Histopathology:
- High-grade osteosarcoma predominates (see Conventional Osteosarcoma).

Differential Diagnosis:
- **Radiation-induced osteonecrosis** (MRI is helpful showing typical double-line signal intensity sign of bone infarction and lack of soft-tissue mass).

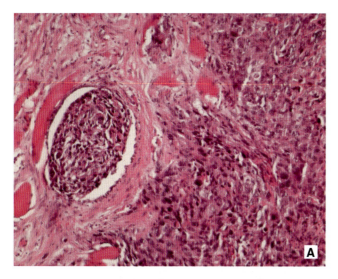
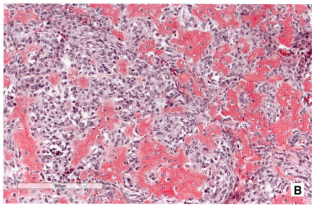
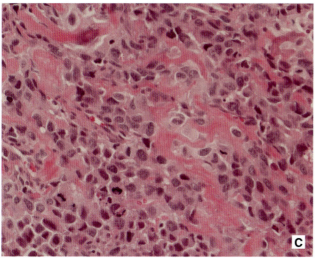

FIGURE 2.66 Histopathology of high-grade surface osteosarcoma. (A) High cellularity and marked pleomorphism of the stromal cells together with infiltration of the skeletal muscle and vascular invasion are characteristic features of this tumor (H&E, original magnification ×100). **(B)** Marked pleomorphism and cellular atypia with bone formation by malignant cells (H&E, original magnification ×100). **(C)** On higher magnification, high cellularity, numerous mitoses, and areas of tumor osteoid production indicate high-grade tumor (H&E, original magnification ×200).

Prognosis:
- The 5-year survival rate is of 68.2% for patients with extremity lesions, 27.3% for patients with axial lesions.

Paget Osteosarcoma
- Malignant transformation in Paget disease is very rare, estimated to be 0.7% to 0.95%, and osteosarcomas represent 50% to 60% of all Paget sarcomas.
- In most series, Paget osteosarcoma is more common in man (M:F 2:1), with an overall median age of 64 years.
- Most cases of malignant transformation occur in polyostotic form of disease.
- Pelvic bones and femur are preferential sites of this malignancy.
- It is osteosarcoma of older patients, not found in pediatric population.
- Imaging findings include typical pagetic bone with lytic destruction and soft-tissue mass (Figs. 2.67 and 2.68); periosteal reaction is rarely seen; pathologic fractures are not uncommon.
- Histopathology shows typical changes of high-grade osteosarcoma (with osteoblastic, fibroblastic, or chondroblastic differentiation) within mosaic pattern of Paget disease (Fig. 2.69).
- Genetic changes have been linked to multiple chromosomes. Mutations of *TNFRSF11A* (18q22.1) (critical receptor for osteoclastogenesis) were found in minority of patients with Paget disease. Somatic mutations in *SQSTM1* have been described in sporadic and familial cases of Paget disease and were linked to Paget osteosarcoma.
- Differential diagnosis should include metastases to pagetic bone from primary carcinomas (prostate, breast, kidney).
- Prognosis is poor.

Osteosarcoma Associated with Fibrous Dysplasia
- Most commonly associated with McCune-Albright syndrome (polyostotic fibrous dysplasia, skin pigmentation [café au lait spots exhibiting irregular, ragged borders—"coast of Maine"], precocious puberty, and other endocrine abnormalities).
- Rarely malignant transformation of monostotic fibrous dysplasia.

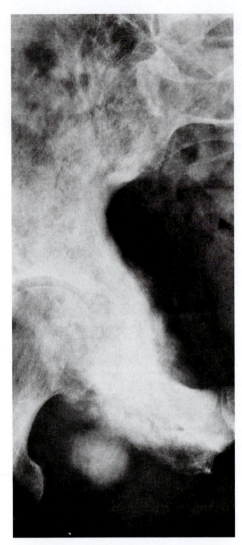

FIGURE 2.67 Radiography of Paget osteosarcoma. Anteroposterior radiograph of the right hip of a 66-year-old man with polyostotic Paget disease shows destruction of the cortex of the ischial bone associated with soft-tissue mass containing tumor bone.

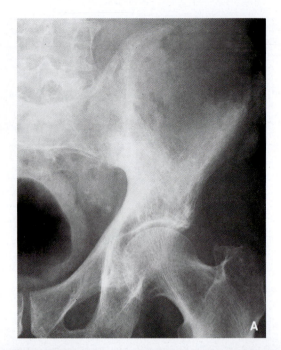
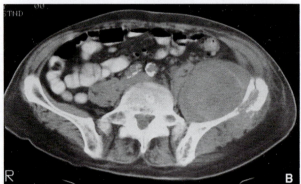

FIGURE 2.68 Computed tomography of Paget osteosarcoma. (A) Anteroposterior radiograph of the left hip of a 73-year-old man who had extensive skeletal involvement by Paget disease shows destructive lesion of the ilium. **(B)** Axial computed tomography section shows in addition the pathologic fracture and a large soft-tissue mass.

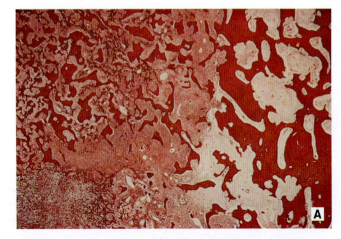
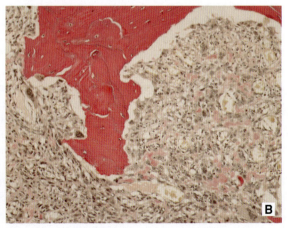

FIGURE 2.69 Histopathology of Paget osteosarcoma. (A) There is clear separation between the characteristic appearance of pagetic bone (*right*) and osteosarcoma (*left*) (H&E, original magnification ×15). **(B)** Pagetic bone exhibiting classic mosaic pattern (*upper left corner*) is invaded by pleomorphic osteosarcoma producing scant osteoid (H&E, original magnification ×100).

Soft-Tissue (Extraskeletal) Osteosarcoma

Definition:
- High-grade malignant mesenchymal tumor originating in the soft tissues, with the capacity to form neoplastic osteoid, bone, and cartilage.

Epidemiology:
- Constitute about 4% of all osteosarcomas.
- Most cases in middle and old age, mean age at presentation 54 years.

Sites of Involvement:
- Predilection for lower extremities and buttocks.

Clinical Presentation:
- Slowly enlarging mass with or without pain.

Imaging:
- Soft-tissue mass, various in size, with central amorphous calcifications and ossifications (Fig. 2.70).
- Reverse zonal phenomenon (Figs. 2.71 and 2.72).
- MRI shows similar presentation as in conventional osteosarcoma (Figs. 2.73 and 2.74).

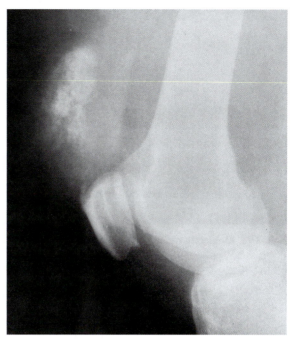

FIGURE 2.71 Radiography of soft-tissue osteosarcoma. Lateral radiograph of the knee of a 51-year-old woman shows a poorly defined soft-tissue mass situated above the patella, merging with the quadriceps muscle. Amorphous calcifications and ossifications are noted within the mass.

Pathology:

Gross (Macroscopy):
- Fleshy mass with areas of bone and cartilage (Fig. 2.75).

Histopathology:
- Indistinguishable from conventional osteosarcoma (Fig. 2.76) with the same spectrum of histologic morphology including osteoblastic, fibroblastic, or chondroblastic (in this order) differentiation.

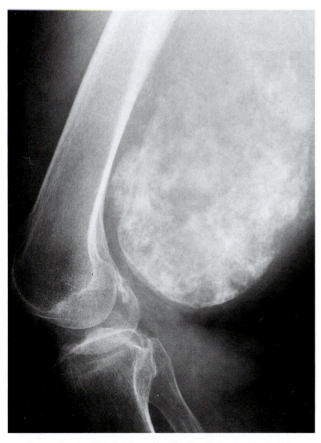

FIGURE 2.70 Radiography of soft-tissue osteosarcoma. A lateral radiograph of the knee of a 68-year-old woman shows a large soft-tissue mass sharply outlined in its distal extent but poorly demarcated proximally with calcifications and ossifications within the tumor.

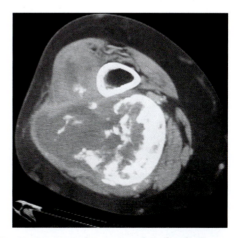

FIGURE 2.72 Computed tomography of soft-tissue osteosarcoma. Axial CT section of the tumor of the same patient as shown in Figure 2.70 shows reverse zoning phenomenon typical for this neoplasm.

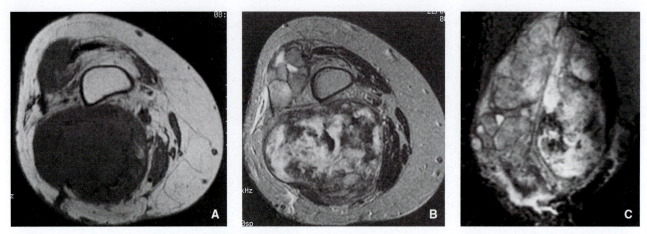

FIGURE 2.73 **Magnetic resonance imaging of soft-tissue osteosarcoma. (A)** Axial T1-weighted magnetic resonance image (same patient as shown in Fig. 2.70) shows a large soft-tissue mass displaying low-signal intensity. The bone is not affected. **(B)** Axial T2-weighted MRI reveals heterogeneity of the tumor. **(C)** Sagittal inversion recovery MR image shows internal septa and heterogenous character of the tumor.

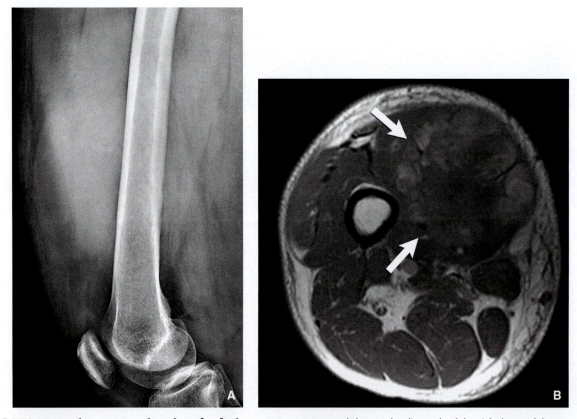

FIGURE 2.74 **Magnetic resonance imaging of soft-tissue osteosarcoma. (A)** Lateral radiograph of the right knee of the 70-year-old man shows a large soft-tissue mass projecting anteriorly to the distal femur with faint foci of ossifications in the center. **(B)** Axial T1-weighted MR image shows well-defined heterogeneous but predominantly of intermediate signal intensity mass (*arrows*).

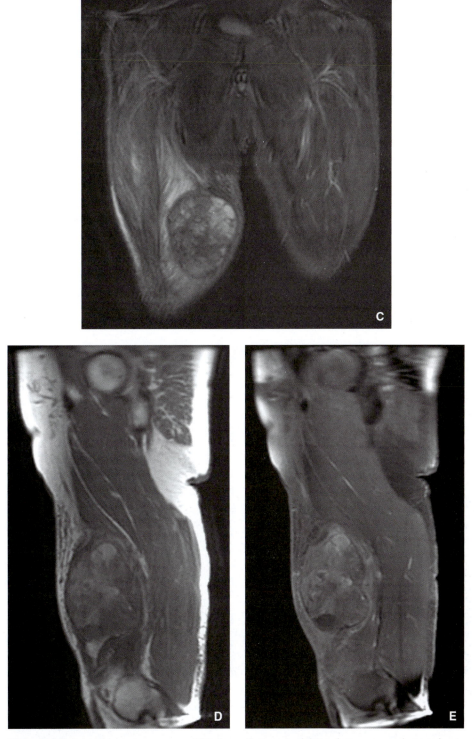

FIGURE 2.74 *(Continued).* **(C)** Coronal inversion recovery MRI shows the mass exhibiting heterogenous but predominantly high signal intensity. Sagittal T1-weighted **(D)** and sagittal T1-weighted postcontrast **(E)** image show mild enhancement of the tumor.

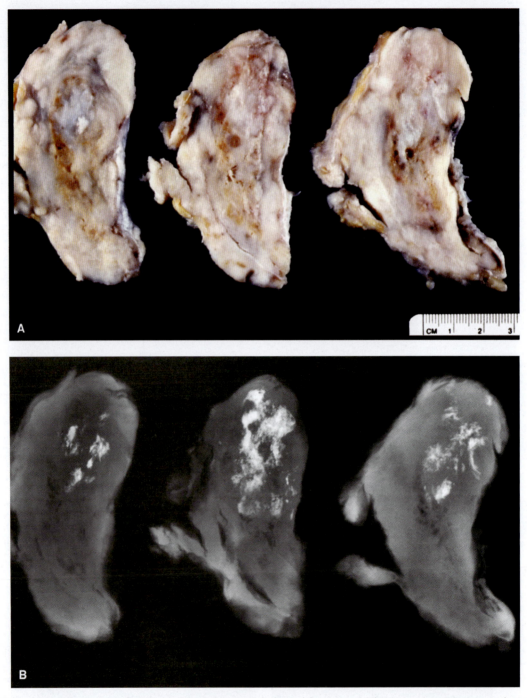

FIGURE 2.75 Gross specimen of soft-tissue osteosarcoma. (A) Three slab sections of the tumor (same patient as depicted in Fig. 2.70) show gritty, fleshy appearance of the mass with foci of bone. **(B)** Radiography of the specimen shows reverse zonal phenomenon.

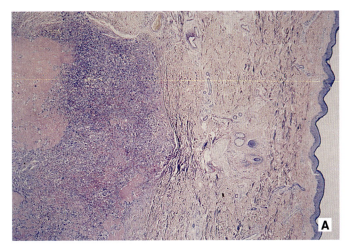
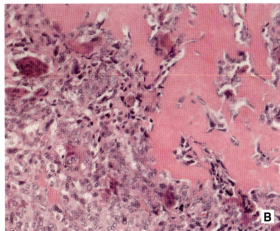
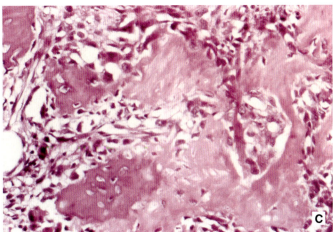

FIGURE 2.76 Histopathology of soft-tissue osteosarcoma. (A) Low-power magnification shows cellular tumor tissue containing tumor bone beneath the skin (*right*) (Giemsa, original magnification ×6). **(B)** At higher magnification, plate-like tumor osteoid is present adjacent to the cellular areas of the tumor containing some osteoclast-like giant cells (H&E, original magnification ×200). **(C)** High magnification shows malignant cells with hyperchromatic nuclei forming tumor bone (H&E, original magnification ×400).

Differential Diagnosis:

- ***Soft-tissue chondrosarcoma***
  Foci of chondroid calcifications within the mass.
  Histopathology shows malignant cartilage formation by the tumor cells, but lack of osteoid or tumor bone formation.
- ***Synovial sarcoma***
  Predominantly lower extremities, feet commonly affected.
  Close proximity to the joints.
  Foci of amorphous calcifications (but not tumor bone), commonly located at the periphery of tumor.
  Characteristic MRI feature consists of "triple signal intensity" sign, due to combination of cystic and solid elements, fibrous tissue, hemorrhage, and hemosiderin deposition.
  Histopathology, depending on the type of the tumor (biphasic, monophasic, or poorly differentiated), shows spindle cells and epithelial components arranged in glandular or nest-like patterns, or interdigitating fascicles and "ball-like" structures formed by the spindle cells.
- ***Myositis ossificans***
  Zonal phenomenon (more mature tissue at the periphery, less mature in the center of the lesion) in contrast to "reverse zonal" in soft-tissue osteosarcoma.
  Regression of the lesion with time.
  Histopathology shows trabecular bone and fibrous marrow, but lack of tumor bone formation.
- ***Any benign soft-tissue mass with calcifications or ossifications*** (e.g., *tumoral calcinosis*)

Prognosis:

- Poor.

REFERENCES

Abe K, Kumagai K, Hayashi T, et al. High-grade surface osteosarcoma of the hand. *Skeletal Radiol.* 2007;36:869–873.

Ackerman LV. Extra-osseous localized non-neoplastic bone and cartilage formation (so-called myositis ossificans). *J Bone Joint Surg Am.* 1958;40A:279–298.

Ahuja SC, Villacin AB, Smith J, et al. Juxtacortical (parosteal) osteosarcoma: histological grading and prognosis. *J Bone Joint Surg Am.* 1977;59A:632–647.

Aisen AM, Martel W, Braunstein EM, et al. MRI and CT evaluation of primary bone and soft-tissue tumors. *AJR Am J Roentgenol.* 1986;146:749–756.

Aizawa T, Okada K, Abe E, et al. Multicentric osteosarcoma with long-term survival. *Skeletal Radiol.* 2004;33:41–45.

Alpert LI, Abaci IF, Werthamer S. Radiation-induced extraskeletal osteosarcoma. *Cancer.* 1973;31:1359–1363.

Amanatullah DF, Mallon ZO, Mak WH, Borys D, Tamurian RM. Pelvic osteoid osteoma in a skeletally mature female. *Am J Orthop.* 2011;40:476–478.

Amstutz HC. Multiple osteogenic sarcomata—metastatic or multicentric? *Cancer.* 1969;24:923–931.

Anderson RB, McAlister JA Jr, Wrenn RN. Case report 585. Intracortical osteosarcoma. *Skeletal Radiol.* 1989;18:627–630.

Assoun J, Railhac JJ, Bonnevialle P, et al. Osteoid osteoma: percutaneous resection with CT guidance. *Radiology.* 1993;188:541–547.

Assoun J, Richardi G, Railhac JJ, et al. Osteoid osteoma: MR imaging versus CT. *Radiology.* 1994;191:217–223.

Atar D, Lehman WB, Grant AD. Tips of the trade: computerized tomography—guided excision of osteoid osteoma. *Orthop Rev.* 1992;21:1457–1458.

Ayala AG, Ro JY, Raymond AK, et al. Small cell osteosarcoma. A clinicopathologic study of 27 cases. *Cancer.* 1989;64:2162–2173.

Azura M, Vanel D, Alberghini M, Picci P, Staals E, Mercuri M. Parosteal osteosarcoma dedifferentiating into telangiectatic osteosarcoma: importance of lytic changes and fluid cavities at imaging. *Skeletal Radiol.* 2009;38:685–690.

Ballance WA Jr, Mendelsohn G, Carter JR, Abdul-Karim FW, Jacobs G, Makley JT. Osteogenic sarcoma. Malignant fibrous histiocytoma subtype. *Cancer.* 1988;62:763–771.

Bane BL, Evans HL, Ro JY, et al. Extraskeletal osteosarcoma. A clinicopathologic review of 26 cases. *Cancer.* 1990;65:2762–2770.

Baruffi MR, Volpon JB, Net JB, Casartelli C. Osteoid osteoma with chromosome alteration involving 22q. *Cancer Genet Cytogenet.* 2001;124:127–131.

Bathurst N, Sanerkin N, Watt I. Osteoclast-rich osteosarcoma. *Br J Radiol.* 1986;59:667–673.

Bauer TW, Zehr RJ, Belhobek GH, Marks KE. Juxta-articular osteoid osteoma. *Am J Surg Pathol.* 1991;15:381–387.

Baum PA, Nelson MC, Lack EE, Bogumill GP. Case report 560. Parosteal osteoma of tibia. *Skeletal Radiol.* 1989;18:406–409.

Berquist TH. Magnetic resonance imaging of primary skeletal neoplasms. *Radiol Clin North Am.* 1993;31:411–424.

Bertoni F, Boriani S, Laus M, Campanacci M. Periosteal chondrosarcoma and periosteal osteosarcoma. Two distinct entities. *J Bone Joint Surg Br.* 1982;64B:370–376.

Bertoni F, Present DA, Enneking WF. Staging of bone tumors. In: Unni KK, ed. *Bone Tumors.* New York: Churchill Livingstone; 1988:47–83.

Bertoni F, Present D, Bacchini P, Pignatti G, Picci P, Campanacci M. The Instituto Rizzoli experience with small cell osteosarcoma. *Cancer.* 1989;64:2591–2599.

Bertoni F, Unni KK, Beabout JW, Sim FH. Parosteal osteoma of bones other than of the skull and face. *Cancer.* 1995;75:2466–2473.

Bettelli G, Tigani D, Picci P. Recurring osteoblastoma initially presenting as a typical osteoid osteoma. Report of two cases. *Skeletal Radiol.* 1991;20:1–4.

Biebuyck JC, Katz LD, McCauley T. Soft tissue edema in osteoid osteoma. *Skeletal Radiol.* 1993;22:37–41.

Blasius S, Link TM, Hillmann A, Rödl R, Edel G, Winkelmann W. Intracortical low grade osteosarcoma. A unique case and review of the literature on intracortical osteosarcoma. *Gen Diagn Pathol.* 1996;141:273–278.

Borys D, Cantor R, Horvai A, et al. P16 expression predicts necrotic response among patients with osteosarcoma receiving neoadjuvant chemotherapy. *Hum Pathol.* 2012;43:1948–1954.

Bridge JA, Nelson M, McComb E, et al. Cytogenetic findings in 73 osteosarcoma specimens and review of the literature. *Cancer Genet Cytogenet.* 1997;95:74–87.

Broders AC. The microscopic grading of cancer. In: Pack CT, Ariel IM, eds. *Treatment of Cancer and Allied Diseases, Vol 1.* 2nd ed. New York: Paul B. Hoeber; 1958:55–59.

Bronner MP. Gastrointestinal polyposis syndromes. *Am J Med Genet.* 2003;122:335–341.

Byun BH, Kong C-B, Lim I, et al. Comparison of (18)F-FDG PET/CT and (99m)Tc-MDP bone scintigraphy for detection of bone metastasis in osteosarcoma. *Skeletal Radiol.* 2013;42:1673–1681.

Campanacci M, Cervellati G. Osteosarcoma: a review of 345 cases. *Ital J Orthop Traumatol.* 1975;1:5–22.

Campanacci M, Pizzoferrato A. Osteosarcoma emorragico. *Chir Organi Mov.* 1971;60:409–421.

Campanacci M, Picci P, Gherlinzoni F, Guerra A, Bertoni F, Neff JR. Parosteal osteosarcoma. *J Bone Joint Surg Br.* 1984;66B:313–321.

Capanna R, Bertoni F, Bettelli G, et al. Dedifferentiated chondrosarcoma. *J Bone Joint Surg Am.* 1988;70A:60–69.

Carter TR. Osteoid osteoma of the hip: an alternate method of excision. *Orthop Rev.* 1990;19:903–905.

Cassar-Pullicino VN, McCall IW, Wan S. Intra-articular osteoid osteoma. *Clin Radiol.* 1992;45:153–160.

Cervilla V, Haghighi P, Resnick D, Sartoris DJ. Case report 596. Parosteal osteoma of the acetabulum. *Skeletal Radiol.* 1990;19:135–137.

Chang CH, Piatt ED, Thomas KE, Watne AL. Bone abnormalities in Gardner's syndrome. *AJR Am J Roentgenol.* 1968;103:645–652.

Chung EB, Enzinger FM. Extraskeletal osteosarcoma. *Cancer.* 1987;60:1132–1142.

Crim JR, Seeger LL. Diagnosis of low-grade chondrosarcoma. *Radiology.* 1993;189:503–504.

Crim JR, Mirra JM, Eckardt JJ, Seeger LL. Widespread inflammatory response to osteoblastoma: the flare phenomenon. *Radiology.* 1990;177:835–836.

Dahlin DC. Grading of bone tumors. In: Unni KK, ed. *Bone Tumors.* New York: Churchill Livingstone; 1988:35–45.

Dahlin DC, Coventry MB. Osteogenic sarcoma: a study of six hundred cases. *J Bone Joint Surg Am.* 1967;49A:101–110.

Dahlin DC, Johnson EW Jr. Giant osteoid osteoma. *J Bone Joint Surg Am.* 1954;36A:559–572.

Dahlin DC, Unni KK. Osteosarcoma of bone and its important recognizable varieties. *Am J Surg Pathol.* 1977;1:61–72.

Dahlin DC, Unni KK. Osteoma. In: *Bone Tumors. General Aspects on 8,542 Cases.* 4th ed. Springfield, IL: Charles C. Thomas; 1986:84–87, 308–321.

Dahlin DC, Unni KK. *Bone Tumors: General Aspects and Data on 8542 Cases.* 4th ed. Springfield, MA: Charles C. Thomas; 1986:227–259.

Dale S, Breidahl WH, Baker D, Robbins PD, Sundaram M. Severe toxic osteoblastoma of the humerus associated with diffuse periostitis of multiple bones. *Skeletal Radiol.* 2001;30:464–468.

Dardick I, Schatz JE, Colgan TJ. Osteogenic sarcoma with epithelial differentiation. *Ultrastruct Pathol.* 1992;16:463–474.

Della Rocca C, Huvos AG. Osteoblastoma: varied histological presentations with a benign clinical course, 55 cases. *Am J Surg Pathol.* 1996;20:841–850.

Denis F, Armstrong GW. Scoliogenic osteoblastoma of the posterior end of the rib: a case report. *Spine.* 1984;9:74–76.

deSantos LA, Murray JA, Finkelstein JB, Spjut HJ, Ayala AG. The radiographic spectrum of periosteal osteosarcoma. *Radiology*. 1978;127:123–129.

Dorfman HD, Weiss SW. Borderline osteoblastic tumors: problem in the differential diagnosis of aggressive osteoblastoma and low-grade osteosarcoma. *Semin Diagn Pathol*. 1984;1:215–234.

Ebrahim FS, Jacobson JA, Lin J, Housner JA, Hayes CW, Resnick D. Intraarticular osteoid osteomas: sonographic findings in three patients with radiographic, CT, and MR imaging correlation. *AJR Am J Roentgenol*. 2001;177:1391–1395.

Edeiken J, Raymond AK, Ayala AG, Benjamin RS, Murray JA, Carrasco HC. Small-cell osteosarcoma. *Skeletal Radiol*. 1987;16:621–628.

Ehara S, Rosenthal DI, Aoki J, et al. Peritumoral edema in osteoid osteoma on magnetic resonance imaging. *Skeletal Radiol*. 1999;28:265–270.

Ellis JH, Siegel CL, Martel W, Weatherbee L, Dorfman H. Radiologic features of well-differentiated osteosarcoma. *AJR Am J Roentgenol*. 1988;151:739–742.

Falappa P, Garganese MC, Crocoli A, et al. Particular imaging features and customized thermal ablation treatment for intramedullary osteoid osteoma in pediatric patients. *Skeletal Radiol*. 2011;40:1523–1530.

Farr GH, Huvos AG, Marcove RC, Higinbotham NL, Foote FW Jr. Telangiectatic osteogenic sarcoma: a review of twenty-eight cases. *Cancer*. 1974;34:1150–1158.

Fechner RE, Mills SE. Osseous lesions. In: Rosai J, Sobin L, eds. *Atlas of Tumor Pathology: Tumors of the Bones and Joints*. Washington, DC: Armed Forces Institute of Pathology; 1993:25–77.

Fine G, Stout AP. Osteogenic sarcoma of the extraskeletal soft tissues. *Cancer*. 1956;9:1027–1043.

Fletcher CDM, Unni KK, Mertens E, eds. *World Health Organisation Classification of Tumours of Soft Tissue and Bone*. Lyon, France: IARC Press; 2013:276.

Fletcher CDM, Unni KK, Mertens E, eds. *World Health Organisation Classification of Soft Tissue and Bone Tumours*. Lyon, France: IARC Press; 2013:277–278.

Fletcher CDM, Unni KK, Mertens E, eds. *World Health Organisation Classification of Soft Tissue and Bone Tumors*. Lyon, France: IARC Press; 2013:279–280.

Fletcher CDM, Unni KK, Mertens E, eds. *World Health Organisation Classification of Tumours of Soft Tissue and Bone*. Lyon, France: IARC Press; 2013:281–296.

Gentry JF, Schechter JJ, Mirra JM. Case report 574. Periosteal osteoblastoma of rib. *Skeletal Radiol*. 1989;18:551–555.

Geschickter CF, Copeland MM. Parosteal osteoma of bone: a new entity. *Ann Surg*. 1951;133:790–807.

Gherlinzoni F, Antoci B, Canale V. Multicentric osteosarcomata (osteosarcomatosis). *Skeletal Radiol*. 1983;10:281–285.

Gil S, Marco SF, Arenas J, et al. Doppler duplex color localization of osteoid osteoma. *Skeletal Radiol*. 1999;28:107–110.

Gitelis S, Schajowicz F. Osteoid osteoma and osteoblastoma. *Orthop Clin North Am*. 1989;20:313–325.

Glicksman AS, Toker C. Osteogenic sarcoma following radiotherapy for bursitis. *Mt Sinai J Med*. 1976;43:163–167.

Goldman AB. Myositis ossificans circumscripta: a benign lesion with a malignant differential diagnosis. *AJR Am J Roentgenol*. 1976;126:32–40.

Goldman AB, Schneider R, Pavlov H. Osteoid osteoma of the femoral neck: report of four cases evaluated with isotope bone scanning, CT, and MR imaging. *Radiology*. 1993;186:227–232.

Gomes H, Menanteau B, Gaillard D, Behar C. Telangiectatic osteosarcoma. *Pediatr Radiol*. 1986;16:140–143.

Good DA, Busfield F, Fletcher BH, et al. Linkage of Paget disease of bone to a novel region on human chromosome 18q23. *Am J Hum Genet*. 2002;70:517–525.

Greenspan A. Benign bone-forming lesions: osteoma, osteoid osteoma, and osteoblastoma. *Skeletal Radiol*. 1993;22:485–500.

Greenspan A. Bone island (enostosis): current concept. *Skeletal Radiol*. 1995;24:111–115.

Greenspan A, Klein MJ. Osteosarcoma: radiologic imaging, differential diagnosis, and pathological considerations. *Semin Orthop*. 1991;6:156–166.

Greenspan A, Elguezabel A, Bryk D. Multifocal osteoid osteoma. A case report and review of the literature. *AJR Am J Roentgenol*. 1974;121:103–106.

Greenspan A, Steiner G, Norman A, Lewis MM, Matlen J. Case report 436. Osteosarcoma of the soft tissues of the distal end of the thigh. *Skeletal Radiol*. 1987;16:489–492.

Greenspan A, Jundt G, Remagen W. *Differential Diagnosis in Orthopaedic Oncology*. 2nd ed. Philadelphia, PA: Lippincott Williams & Wilkins; 2007:40–51.

Greenspan A, Jundt G, Remagen W. *Differential Diagnosis in Orthopaedic Oncology*. 2nd ed. Philadelphia, PA: Lippincott Williams & Wilkins; 2007:51–74.

Greenspan A, Jundt G, Remagen W. *Differential Diagnosis in Orthopaedic Oncology*. 2nd ed. Philadelphia, PA: Lippincott Williams & Wilkins; 2007:84–148.

Griffith JF, Kumta SM, Chow LTC, Leung PC, Metreweli C. Intracortical osteosarcoma. *Skeletal Radiol*. 1998;27:228–232.

Haibach H, Farrell C, Gaines RW. Osteoid osteoma of the spine: surgically correctable case of painful scoliosis. *Can Med Assoc J*. 1986;135:895–899.

Hansen MF. Genetic and molecular aspects of osteosarcoma. *J Musculoskelet Neuronal Interact*. 2002;2:554–560.

Helms CA. Osteoid osteoma: the double density sign. *Clin Orthop*. 1987;222:167–173.

Hermann G, Abdelwahab IF, Kenan S, Lewis MM, Klein MJ. Case report 795. High-grade surface osteosarcoma of the radius. *Skeletal Radiol*. 1993;22:383–385.

Hermann G, Klein MJ, Springfield D, Abdelwahab IF, Dan SJ. Intracortical osteosarcoma; two-year delay in diagnosis. *Skeletal Radiol*. 2002;31:592–596.

Hopper KD, Moser RP Jr, Haseman DB, Sweet DE, Madewell JE, Kransdorf MJ. Osteosarcomatosis. *Radiology*. 1990;175:233–239.

Houghton MJ, Heiner JP, DeSmet AA. Osteoma of the innominate bone with intraosseous and parosteal involvement. *Skeletal Radiol*. 1995;24:445–457.

Hudson TM, Chew FS, Manaster BJ. Scintigraphy of benign exostoses and exostotic chondrosarcomas. *AJR Am J Roentgenol*. 1983;140:581–586.

Huvos AG, Rosen G, Bretsky SS, Butler A. Telangiectatic osteosarcoma: a clinicopathologic study of 124 patients. *Cancer*. 1982;49:1679–1689.

Jackson RP, Rockling FW, Mants FA. Osteoid osteoma and osteoblastoma. Similar histologic lesions with different natural histories. *Clin Orthop*. 1977;128:303–313.

Jaffe HL. Osteoid osteoma: a benign osteoblastic tumor composed of osteoid and atypical bone. *Arch Surg*. 1935;31:709–728.

Jaffe HL. Osteoid osteoma of bone. *Radiology*. 1945;45:319–334.

Jaffe HL. Benign osteoblastoma. *Bull Hosp Joint Dis*. 1956;17:141–151.

Jelinek JS, Murphey MD, Kransdorf MJ, Shmookler BM, Malawer MM, Hur RC. Parosteal osteosarcoma: value of MR imaging and CT in the prediction of histologic grade. *Radiology*. 1996;201:837–842.

Kaufman RA, Towbin RB. Telangiectatic osteosarcoma simulating the appearance of an aneurysmal bone cyst. *Pediatr Radiol*. 1981;11:102–104.

Keim HA, Reina EG. Osteoid osteoma as a cause of scoliosis. *J Bone Joint Surg Am*. 1975;57A:159–163.

Kenan S, Floman Y, Robin GC, Laufer A. Aggressive osteoblastoma. A case report and review of the literature. *Clin Orthop*. 1985;195:294–298.

Kenan S, Ginat DT, Steiner GC. Dedifferentiated high-grade osteosarcoma originating from low-grade central osteosarcoma of the fibula. *Skeletal Radiol*. 2007;36:347–351.

Klein MH, Shankman S. Osteoid osteoma: radiologic and pathologic correlation. *Skeletal Radiol*. 1992;21:23–31.

Klein MJ, Siegal GP. Osteosarcoma: anatomic and histologic variants. *Am J Clin Pathol*. 2006;125:555–581.

Kramer K, Hicks D, Palis J, et al. Epithelioid osteosarcoma of bone. Immunocytochemical evidence suggesting divergent epithelial and mesenchymal differentiation in a primary osseous neoplasm. *Cancer.* 1993;71:2977–2982.

Kransdorf MJ, Meis JM. Extraskeletal osseous and cartilaginous tumors of the extremities. *Radiographics.* 1993;13:853–884.

Kransdorf MJ, Stull MA, Gilkey FW, Moser RP Jr. Osteoid osteoma. *Radiographics.* 1991;11:671–696.

Kroon HM, Schurmans J. Osteoblastoma: clinical and radiologic findings in 98 new cases. *Radiology.* 1990;175:783–790.

Kyriakos M, Gilula LA, Besich MJ, Schoeneker PL. Intracortical small cell osteosarcoma. *Clin Orthop.* 1992;279:269–280.

Kyriakos M, El-Khoury GY, McDonald DJ, et al. A benign, multifocal osteoblastic lesion, distinct from osteoid osteoma and osteoblastoma, radiologically simulating a vascular tumor. *Skeletal Radiol.* 2007;36:237–247.

Landsman JC, Shall JF, Seitz WH Jr, Berner JJ. Pediatric update #15. Florid reactive periostitis of the digits. *Orthop Rev.* 1990;19:828–834.

Lichtenstein L. Benign osteoblastoma. A category of osteoid- and bone-forming tumors other than classical osteoid osteoma, which may be mistaken for giant-cell tumor or osteogenic sarcoma. *Cancer.* 1956;9:1044–1052.

Lichtenstein L, Sawyer WR. Benign osteoblastoma: further observations and report of twenty additional cases. *J Bone Joint Surg Am.* 1964;46A:755–765.

Lim C, Lee H, Schatz J, Alvaro F, Boyle R, Bonar SF. Case report: periosteal osteosarcoma of the clavicle. *Skeletal Radiol.* 2012;41:1011–1015.

Liu PT, Chivers FS, Roberts CC, Schultz CJ, Beauchamp CP. Imaging of osteoid osteoma with dynamic gadolinium-enhanced MR imaging. *Radiology.* 2003;227:691–700.

Liu TL, Kujak JL, Roberts CC, Chadaverian JP. The vascular groove sign: a new CT finding associated with osteoid osteoma. *AJR Am J Roentgenol.* 2012;96:168–173.

Logan PM, Mitchell MJ, Munk PL. Imaging of variant osteosarcomas with an emphasis on CT and MR imaging. *AJR Am J Roentgenol.* 1998;171:1531–1537.

Lopez BF, Rodriquez PJL, Gonzalez LJ, Sánchez-Herrera S, Sánchez-del-Charco M. Intracortical osteosarcoma. A case report. *Clin Orthop Relat Res.* 1991;268:218–222.

Lorigan JG, Lipshitz HI, Peuchot M. Radiation-induced sarcoma of bone: CT findings in 19 cases. *AJR Am J Roentgenol.* 1989;153:791–794.

Lucas DR, Unni KK, McLeod RA, O'Connor MI, Sim FH. Osteoblastoma: clinicopathologic study of 306 cases. *Hum Pathol.* 1994;25:117–134.

Maheshwari AV, Jelinek JS, Seibel NL, Meloni-Ehrig AM, Kumar D, Henshaw RM. Bilateral synchronous tibial periosteal osteosarcoma with familial incidence. *Skeletal Radiol.* 2012;41:1005–1009.

Matsuno T, Unni KK, McLeod RA, Dahlin DC. Telangiectatic osteogenic sarcoma. *Cancer.* 1976;38:2538–2547.

McKenna RJ, Schwinn CP, Soong KY, Higinbotham NL. Osteogenic sarcoma arising in Paget's disease. *Cancer.* 1964;17:42–66.

McLeod RA, Dahlin DC, Beabout JW. The spectrum of osteoblastoma. *AJR Am J Roentgenol.* 1976;126:321–325.

Meltzer CC, Scott WW Jr, McCarthy EF. Case report 698. Osteoma of the clavicle. *Skeletal Radiol.* 1991;20:555–557.

Miller CW, Aslo A, Won A, Tan M, Lampkin B, Koeffler HP. Alterations of the p53, Rb and MDM2 genes in osteosarcoma. *J Cancer Res Clin Oncol.* 1996;122:559–565.

Mindell ER, Shah NK, Webster JH. Postradiation sarcoma of bone and soft tissues. *Orthop Clin North Am.* 1977;8:821–834.

Moore TE, King AR, Kathol MH, el-Khoury GY, Palmer R, Downey PR. Sarcoma in Paget disease of bone: clinical, radiologic, and pathologic features in 22 cases. *AJR Am J Roentgenol.* 1991;156:1199–1203.

Mulder JD, Schütte HE, Kroon HM, Taconis WK. *Radiologic Atlas of Bone Tumors.* Amsterdam, the Netherlands: Elsevier; 1993:51–76.

Murphey MD, Robbin MR, McRae GA, Flemming DJ, Temple HT, Kransdorf MJ. The many faces of osteosarcoma. *Radiographics.* 1997;17:1205–1231.

Murphey MD, wan Joavisidha S, Temple HT, Gannon FH, Jelinek JS, Malawer MM. Telangiectatic osteosarcoma: radiologic-pathologic comparison. *Radiology.* 2003;229:545–553.

Nogues P, Marti-Bonmati L, Aparisi F, Saborido MC, Garci J, Dosdá R. MR imaging assessment of juxtacortical edema in osteoid osteoma in 28 patients. *Eur Radiol.* 1998;8:236–238.

Norman A. Persistence or recurrence of pain: a sign of surgical failure in osteoid osteoma. *Clin Orthop.* 1978;130:263–266.

Norman A, Dorfman H. Juxtacortical circumscribed myositis ossificans: evolution and radiographic features. *Radiology.* 1970;96:301–306.

Norman A, Abdelwahab IF, Buyon J, Matzkin E. Osteoid osteoma of the hip stimulating an early onset of osteoarthritis. *Radiology.* 1986;158:417–420.

Nuovo MA, Norman A, Chumas J, Ackerman LV. Myositis ossificans with atypical clinical, radiographic, or pathologic findings: a review of 23 cases. *Skeletal Radiol.* 1992;21:87–101.

O'Connel JX, Rosenthal DI, Mankin HJ, Rosenberg AE. Solitary osteoma of a long bone. *J Bone Joint Surg Am.* 1993;75A:1830–1834.

Okada K, Kubota H, Ebina T, Kobayashi T, Abe E, Sato K. High-grade surface osteosarcoma of the humerus. *Skeletal Radiol.* 1995;24:531–534.

Okada K, Unni KK, Swee RG, Sim FH. High grade surface osteosarcoma. A clinicopathologic study of 46 cases. *Cancer.* 1999;85:1044–1054.

Onikul E, Fletcher BD, Parham DM, Chen G. Accuracy of MR imaging for estimating intraosseous extent of osteosarcoma. *AJR Am J Roentgenol.* 1996;167:1211–1215.

Partovi S, Logan PM, Janzen DL, O'Connell JX, Connell DG. Low-grade parosteal osteosarcoma of the ulna with dedifferentiation into high-grade osteosarcoma. *Skeletal Radiol.* 1996;25:497–500.

Pasic I, Shlien AD, Durbin AD, et al. Recurrent focal copy-number changes and loss of heterozygosity implicate two noncoding RNAs and one tumor suppressor gene at chromosome 3q13.31 in osteosarcoma. *Cancer Res.* 2010;70:160–171.

Picci P, Gherlinzoni F, Guerra A. Intracortical osteosarcoma: rare entity or early manifestation of classical osteosarcoma? *Skeletal Radiol.* 1983;9:255–258.

Porcel Lopez MT, Fernandez GMA, Campos de Orellana A, Quiles GM. Florid reactive periostitis ossificans of the distal ulna. *Orthopedics.* 2008;31:286.

Price CHG, Goldie W. Paget's sarcoma of bone: a study of eighty cases from the Bristol and Leeds bone tumor registries. *J Bone Joint Surg Br.* 1969;51B:205–224.

Raymond AK, Ayala AG, Knuutila S. Conventional osteosarcoma. In: Fletcher CDM, Unni KK, Mertens F, eds. *Pathology and Genetics of Tumours of Soft Tissue and Bone.* Lyon, France: IARC Press; 2002:264–270.

Ritts GD, Pritchard DJ, Unni KK, Beabout JW, Eckardt JJ. Periosteal osteosarcoma. *Clin Orthop.* 1987;219:299–307.

Ruiter DJ, Cornelisse CJ, van Rijssel TG, van der Velde EA. Aneurysmal bone cyst and telangiectatic osteosarcoma. A histopathological and morphometric study. *Virchows Arch A Pathol Anat Histol.* 1977;373:311–325.

Saito T, Oda Y, Kawaguchi K, et al. Five-year evolution of a telangiectatic osteosarcoma initially managed as an aneurysmal bone cyst. *Skeletal Radiol.* 2005;34:290–294.

Sampath SC, Sampath SC, Rosenthal DI. Serially recurrent osteoid osteoma. *Skeletal Radiol.* 2015;44:875–881.

Sandberg AA, Bridge JA. Updates on the cytogenetics and molecular genetics of bone and soft tissue tumors: osteosarcoma and related tumors. *Cancer Genet Cytogenet.* 2003;145:1–30.

Sandry F, Hessler C, Garcia J. The potential aggressiveness of sinus osteomas. A report of two cases. *Skeletal Radiol.* 1988;17:427–430.

Schai P, Friederich NB, Kruger A, Jundt G, Herbe E, Buess P. Discrete synchronous multifocal osteoid osteoma of the humerus. *Skeletal Radiol.* 1996;25:667–670.

Schajowicz F, Lemos C. Malignant osteoblastoma. *J Bone Joint Surg Br.* 1976;58B:202–211.

Schajowicz F, Sissons HA, Sobin LH. The World Health Organization's histologic classification of bone tumors. A commentary on the second edition. *Cancer.* 1995;75:1208–1214.

Sciot R, Samson I, Dal Cin P, et al. Giant cell rich parosteal osteosarcoma. *Histopathology.* 1995;27:51–55.

Shaikh MI, Saiffudin A, Pringle J, Natali C, Sherazi Z. Spinal osteoblastoma: CT and MR imaging with pathologic correlation. *Skeletal Radiol.* 1999;28:33–40.

Sherazi Z, Saiffudin A, Shaikh MI, Natali C, Pringle JA. Unusual imaging findings in association with spinal osteoblastoma. *Clin Radiol.* 1966;51:644–648.

Sheth DS, Yasko AW, Raymond AK, et al. Conventional and dedifferentiated parosteal osteosarcoma: diagnosis, treatment and outcome. *Cancer.* 1996;78:2136–2145.

Shuhaibar H, Friedman L. Dedifferentiated parosteal osteosarcoma with high-grade osteoclast-rich osteogenic sarcoma at presentation. *Skeletal Radiol.* 1998;27:574–577.

Sim FH, Unni KK, Beabout JW, Dahlin DC. Osteosarcoma with small cells simulating Ewing's tumor. *J Bone Joint Surg Am.* 1979;61A:207–215.

Sordillo PP, Hajdu SI, Magill GB, Goldbey RB. Extraosseous osteogenic sarcoma. A review of 48 patients. *Cancer.* 1983;51:727–734.

Spjut HJ, Dorfman HD, Fechner RE, Ackerman LV. Tumors of bone and cartilage. In: Firminger HI, ed. *Atlas of Tumor Pathology*, 2nd Series, Fascicle 5. Washington, DC: Armed Forces Institute of Pathology; 1971.

Stern PJ, Lim EVA, Krieg JK. Giant metacarpal osteoma. A case report. *J Bone Joint Surg Am.* 1985;67A:487–489.

Stevens GM, Pugh DG, Dahlin DC. Roentgenographic recognition and differentiation of parosteal osteogenic sarcoma. *AJR Am J Roentgenol.* 1957;78:1–12.

Strong EB, Tate JR, Borys D. Osteoid osteoma of the ethmoid sinus: a rare diagnosis. *Ear Nose Throat J.* 2012;91:E19–E20.

Sundaram M, Falbo S, McDonald D, Janney C. Surface osteomas of the appendicular skeleton. *AJR Am J Roentgenol.* 1996;167: 1529–1533.

Takeushi K, Morii T, Yabe H, Morioka H, Mukai M, Toyama Y. Dedifferentiated parosteal osteosarcoma with well-differentiated metastases. *Skeletal Radiol.* 2006;35:778–782.

Thompson GH, Wong KM, Konsens RM, Vibhakars S. Magnetic resonance imaging of an osteoid osteoma of a proximal femur: a potentially confusing appearance. *J Pediatr Orthop.* 1990;10:800–804.

Torres FX, Kyriakos M. Bone infarct-associated osteosarcoma. *Cancer.* 1992;70:2418–2430.

Unni KK. Osteosarcoma of bone. In: Unni KK, ed. *Bone Tumors.* New York: Churchill Livingstone; 1988:107–133.

Unni KK. *Dahlin's Bone Tumors. General Aspects and Data on 11,087 Cases.* 5th ed. Philadelphia, PA: Lippincott-Raven; 1996:117–120.

Unni KK. *Dahlin's Bone Tumors: General Aspects and Data on 11,087 Cases.* 5th ed. Philadelphia, PA: Lippincott-Raven; 1996:185–196.

Unni KK, Dahlin DC. Premalignant tumors and conditions of bone. *Am J Surg Pathol.* 1979;3:47–60.

Unni KK, Dahlin DC. Grading of bone tumors. *Semin Diagn Pathol.* 1984;1:165–172.

Unni KK, Dahlin DC, Beabout JW. Periosteal osteogenic sarcoma. *Cancer.* 1976;37:2476–2485.

Unni KK, Dahlin DC, Beabout JW, Ivins JC. Parosteal osteogenic sarcoma. *Cancer.* 1976;37:2644–2675.

Unni KK, Dahlin DC, McLeod RA. Intraosseous well-differentiated osteosarcoma. *Cancer.* 1977;40:1337–1347.

van der Heul RO, von Ronnen JR. Juxtacortical osteosarcoma. Diagnosis, differential diagnosis, treatment, and an analysis of eighty cases. *J Bone Joint Surg Am.* 1967;49A:415–439.

Vanel D, Picci P, De Paolis M, Mercuri M. Radiological study of 12 high-grade surface osteosarcomas. *Skeletal Radiol.* 2001;30:667–671.

Wold LE, Unni KK, Beabout JW, Pritchard DJ. High-grade surface osteosarcomas. *Am J Surg Pathol.* 1984;8:181–186.

Wold LE, Unni KK, Beabout JW, Sim FH, Dahlin DC. Dedifferentiated parosteal osteosarcoma. *J Bone Joint Surg Am.* 1984;66A:53–59.

Yaniv G, Shabshin N, Sharon M, et al. Osteoid osteoma—the CT vessel sign. *Skeletal Radiol.* 2011;40:1311–1314.

Youssef BA, Haddad MC, Zahrani A, et al. Osteoid osteoma and osteoblastoma: MRI appearances and the significance of ring enhancement. *Eur Radiol.* 1996;6:291–296.

CHAPTER 3
Cartilage-Forming (Chondrogenic) Lesions

Diagnosis of a bone lesion as originating from cartilage is usually a simple task for the radiologist. The lesion's radiolucent matrix, scalloped margin, and punctate, annular, or comma-shaped calcifications usually suffice to establish its chondrogenic nature. Yet determination if a cartilage tumor is benign or malignant, often creates a problem for the radiologist and even for the pathologist. All cartilage tumors, regardless if benign or malignant, exhibit a positive reaction for S-100 protein, a helpful diagnostic hint. Histologically, cartilaginous lesions are usually recognized by the features of their intercellular matrix, which has a uniformly translucent appearance and contains less collagen than do the bone-forming tumors. The tumor cells are located in rounded spaces, called lacunae, as in normal cartilage. In benign cartilage tumors, like enchondroma, the tissue is sparsely cellular. The cells usually contain small darkly stained nuclei. The tumor tissue is avascular, and areas of calcified matrix are common. Because of their slow growth, enchondromas expand into the endocortex creating small erosions (scalloping). Conversely, chondrosarcomas exhibit pleomorphism, large nuclei, double nuclei, and mitoses. These tumors invade the endocortex, form deep scalloping, and are associated with cortical thickening, periosteal reaction, and not infrequently a soft-tissue mass.

A. Benign Cartilage-Forming Lesions
Enchondroma
Enchondromatosis, Ollier Disease, and Maffucci Syndrome
Periosteal (Juxtacortical) Chondroma
Soft-Tissue Chondroma
Synovial (Osteo) Chondromatosis
Osteochondroma (Osteocartilaginous Exostosis)
Multiple Hereditary Osteochondromata (Diaphyseal Aclasis)
Chondroblastoma
Chondromyxoid Fibroma

B. Malignant Cartilage-Forming Tumors
Chondrosarcomas
Conventional Chondrosarcoma (Central or Medullary Chondrosarcoma)
Clear Cell Chondrosarcoma
Mesenchymal Chondrosarcoma
Myxoid Chondrosarcoma (Chordoid Sarcoma)
Dedifferentiated Chondrosarcoma
Periosteal (Juxtacortical) Chondrosarcoma
Soft-Tissue (Extraskeletal) Chondrosarcomas
  Extraskeletal Myxoid Chondrosarcoma

Secondary Chondrosarcomas
Malignant Transformation of Osteochondroma
Malignant Transformation of Enchondroma
Chondrosarcoma Arising in Primary (Osteo) Chondromatosis
Chondrosarcoma Arising in Pagetic Bone

A. BENIGN CARTILAGE-FORMING LESIONS

Enchondroma

Definition:
- Benign hyaline cartilage neoplasm arising in the medullary portion of bone.

Epidemiology:
- Ten to twenty-five percent of all benign bone tumors.
- Age range from 5 to 80 years.
- Most common in the second through fourth decades of life.
- Solitary enchondromas are rare in young children, whereas multiple enchondromas are encountered more commonly.
- Both genders are equally affected.

Sites of Involvement:
- Any bone formed by endochondral ossification can be affected.

- Common in the short tubular bones (phalanges and metacarpals) of the hands, followed by bones of the feet, and the long bones, especially proximal humerus and proximal and distal femur.
- In the long bones, the tumors are usually centrally located within metaphysis or diaphysis.
- Epiphyseal involvement is rare.

Clinical Findings:
- In the small bones of the hands and feet typically presents as palpable swellings, with or without pain.
- Common expansion of small bones and attenuation of the cortex may cause pathologic fractures, which may resemble aggressive malignant behavior.
- In the long bone, tumors are more often asymptomatic and are detected incidentally in the imaging studies obtained for other reasons.

Imaging:
- Radiography shows well-marginated lesion that vary from radiolucent to heavily mineralized (calcified) (Figs. 3.1 and 3.2).
- Cortex is usually thinned out and expanded in symmetric fusiform fashion.
- Calcification pattern is characteristic, consisting of punctate (stippled), flocculent, or curvilinear (in form of ring, comma-shaped, and arc pattern) calcifications, exhibiting "popcorn"-like appearance (see Figs. 1.6C, 1.17, 1.18A, and 3.2).
- Lesions in the small tubular bones can be centrally or eccentrically located, and larger tumors may completely replace medullary cavity.
- Occasionally, intracortical lesions are present, resembling osteochondromas (see Fig. 3.12).
- Shallow endosteal scalloping is usually present (see Fig. 3.2C).
- There is no periosteal reaction, unless pathologic fracture has occurred.
- Cortical destruction and soft-tissue invasion should never be seen in enchondromas and would be most consistent with chondrosarcoma.
- Skeletal scintigraphy shows mildly increased uptake of radiopharmaceutical agent in uncomplicated lesions, whereas the presence of a pathologic fracture or malignant transformation is revealed by marked scintigraphic activity.
- Computed tomography further delineates the tumor and more precisely localizes it in the bone; it shows to better advantage the scalloped borders and matrix calcifications.
- Magnetic resonance imaging—T1-weighted sequences show the lesion to be of low-to-intermediate signal intensity, whereas on T2-weighted and other water-sensitive sequences, the lesions will exhibit high signal, with calcifications imaged as low signal intensity structures (Figs. 3.3 and 3.4). After intravenous administration of gadolinium, there is enhancement of the lesion (Figs. 3.5D and 3.6C).

Pathology:

Gross (Macroscopy):
- Most enchondromas measure less than 3 cm in length, and tumors larger than 5 cm are uncommon.
- Cartilaginous multinodular architecture is separated by bone marrow.
- Multinodular pattern is seen more often in long bones compared to confluent growth pattern in small tubular bones.

Histopathology:
- Cartilage nodules may cause shallow impressions on endocortex, but no invasion is present (Fig. 3.7).
- Cartilage nodules frequently undergo endochondral ossification (Fig. 3.8).
- Cartilage shows low-to-moderate cellularity and contains chondrocytes of variable size located in the lacunae, exhibiting small, round, and hyperchromatic nuclei (Figs. 3.9A,B and 3.10B).
- Occasionally, scattered binucleated cells are present (Fig. 3.9C).
- Nodules of hyaline cartilage are well demarcated by the surrounding bone and bone marrow (Fig. 3.10A).
- Calcifications may be present.

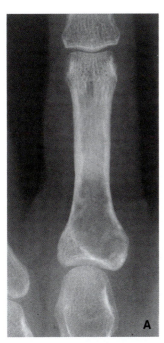 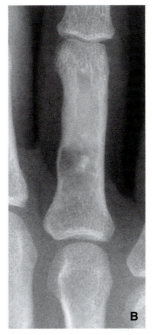

FIGURE 3.1 Radiography of enchondroma. (A) Radiolucent lesion in the proximal phalanx of the middle finger of a 40-year-old woman and **(B)** a similar lesion with central calcification in the proximal phalanx of the ring finger of a 42-year-old man are typical examples of enchondroma in the short tubular bones.

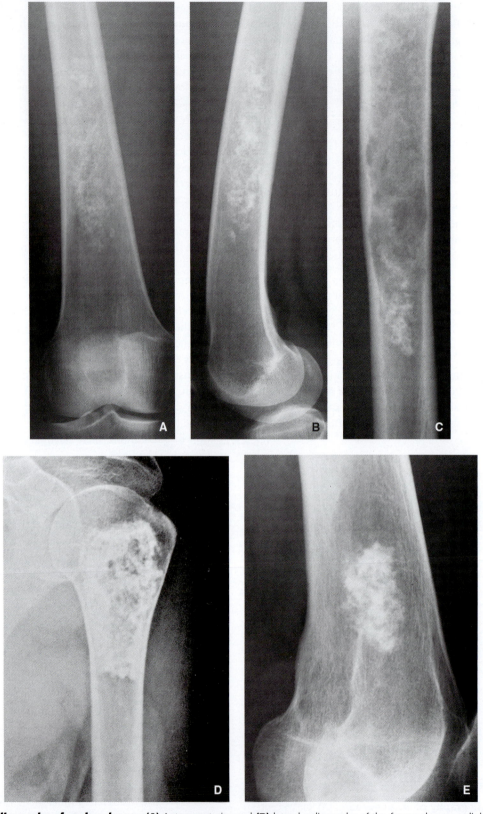

FIGURE 3.2 Radiography of enchondroma. (A) Anteroposterior and **(B)** lateral radiographs of the femur show a radiolucent lesion with "popcorn"-like calcifications. **(C)** In another patient, a radiolucent lesion in a long tubular bone exhibits central calcifications and shallow scalloping of the endocortex reflecting the lobular growth pattern of cartilage. At the site of the lesion, the cortex is thin-out. **(D)** A heavily calcified lesion (so-called calcifying enchondroma) is seen in the proximal humerus of a 58-year-old woman. Note that despite of the large size of the lesion, the cortex is not thickened. **(E)** Another lesion with typical stippled and annular calcification is present in the distal femur of a 30-year-old man.

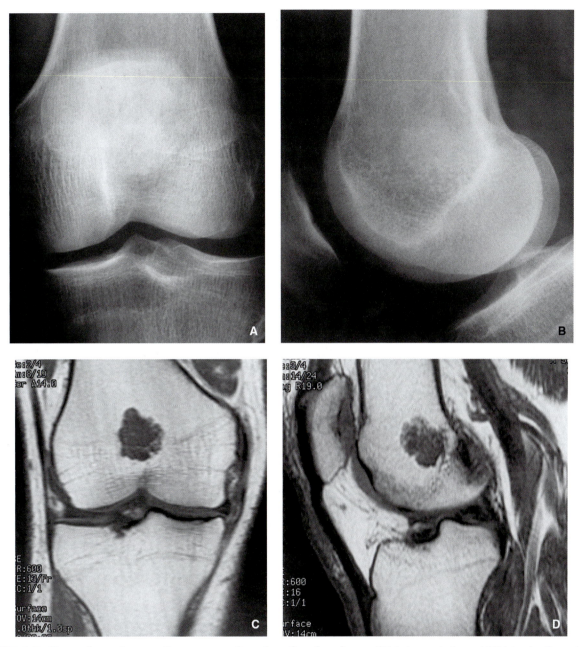

FIGURE 3.3 Radiography and magnetic resonance imaging of enchondroma. (A) Anteroposterior and **(B)** lateral radiographs of the left knee show an almost nondiscernible lesion in the distal femur. **(C)** Coronal and **(D)** sagittal T1-weighted MR images reveal the full extent of the tumor.

Genetics:
- Structural abnormalities involving chromosomes or chromosomal regions 4q, 7, 11, 14q, 16q22-q24, 20, and particularly rearrangement of chromosome 6 and 12q12-q15.

Complications:
- Pathologic fracture.
- Malignant transformation.

Prognosis:
- Solitary enchondromas are successfully treated by intralesional curettage in most cases, and local recurrences are uncommon.

Differential Diagnosis:
- *Medullary bone infarct*
  Well-defined, sclerotic, serpentine border.
  Lack of endosteal scalloping.

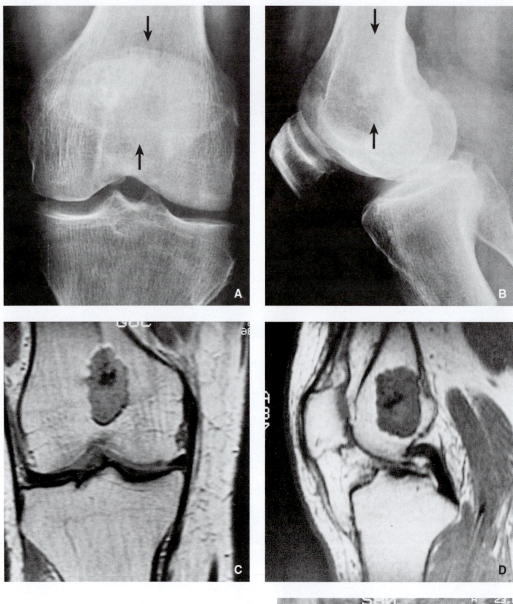
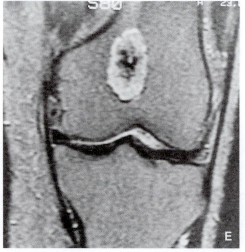

FIGURE 3.4 Radiography and magnetic resonance imaging of enchondroma. (A) Anteroposterior and (B) lateral radiographs of the knee of a 61-year-old man show a few calcifications in the distal femur (*arrows*). The nature and extent of the lesion cannot be adequately determined. (C) Coronal and (D) sagittal T1–weighted MR images demonstrate a well-circumscribed, lobulated lesion exhibiting intermediate signal intensity. The low signal intensity areas in the center represent calcifications. (E) Coronal T2–weighted MR image shows the lesion displaying a high intensity signal, with calcifications remaining of low signal.

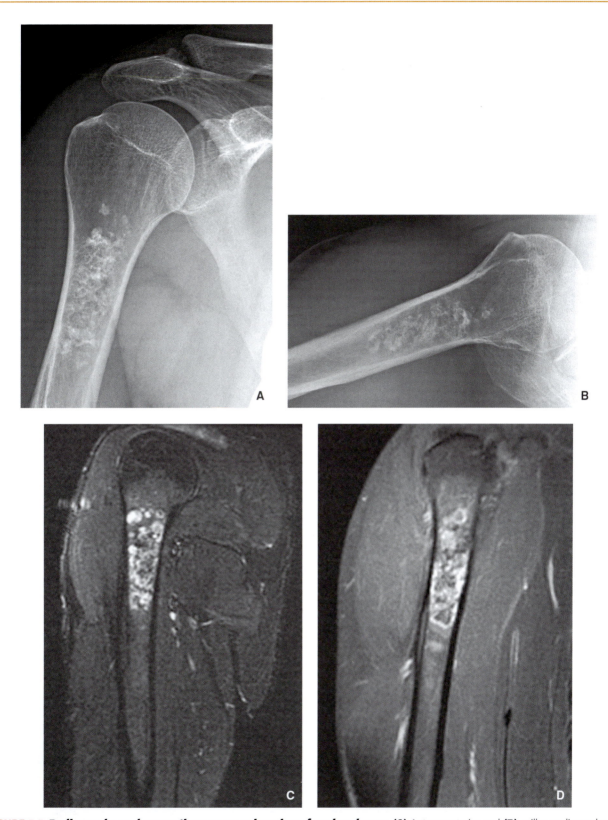

FIGURE 3.5 Radiography and magnetic resonance imaging of enchondroma. (A) Anteroposterior and **(B)** axillary radiographs of the right shoulder of a 52-year-old man show a radiolucent lesion in the proximal humerus with chondroid type of calcifications. Note that despite the size of the lesion that extends from the lateral to medial cortex, there is no endosteal scalloping and the cortex is not thickened, the typical signs of benignity. **(C)** Coronal inversion recovery MRI and **(D)** sagittal T1-weighted fat-suppressed contrast-enhanced MR image confirm that the lesion is entirely within the medullary portion of the bone. The cortex is intact, there is no periosteal reaction, and there is lack of soft-tissue extension.

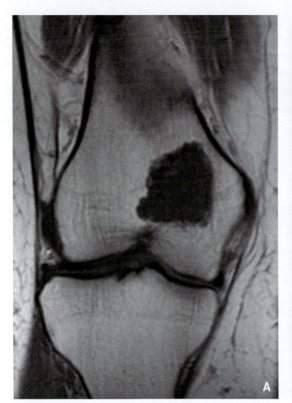
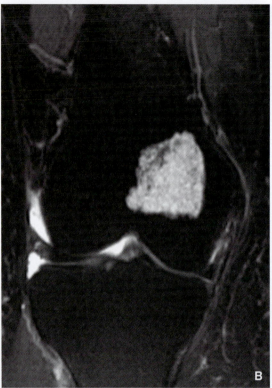
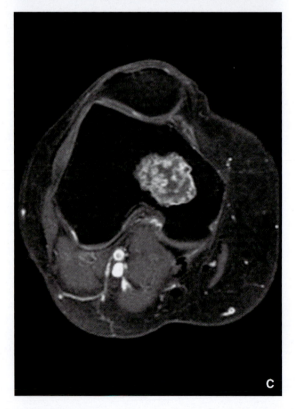

FIGURE 3.6 Magnetic resonance imaging of enchondroma. (A) Coronal T1–weighted MR image of the right knee of a 59-year-old woman shows a sharply demarcated lesion in the medial femoral condyle displaying low signal intensity. **(B)** Coronal T2–weighted MR image shows the lesion exhibiting high signal intensity with a few low signal foci, representing calcifications. **(C)** Axial T1–weighted fat-suppressed MRI obtained after intravenous administration of gadolinium shows significant enhancement of the tumor. Calcifications remain of low signal intensity.

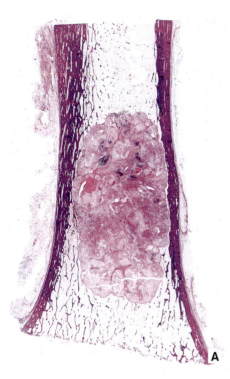
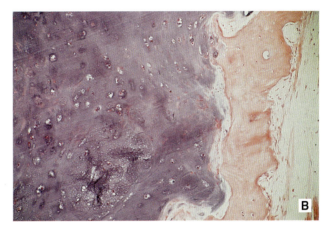

FIGURE 3.7 Histopathology of enchondroma. (A) Whole-mount section (H&E) shows the tumor consisting of cartilaginous lobules and extends from the medial to the lateral cortex of the femur causing shallow endosteal scalloping. **(B)** On the higher magnification, there is no evidence of invasion, only shallow pressure/erosion of the endocortex (H&E, original magnification ×183).

MRI (water-sensitive sequences) shows characteristic double-line signal intensity pattern.

- *Low-grade chondrosarcoma*
  Length of the lesion greater than 5 cm.
  Thickening of the cortex.
  Deep endosteal scalloping.
  Histopathology shows increased cellularity, cytologic atypia, hyperchromasia of the nuclei and binucleation, and occasionally stromal myxoid changes.
  Permeation and entrapment of bone trabeculae.

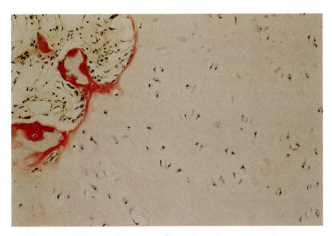

FIGURE 3.8 Histopathology of enchondroma. Cartilage lobules are surrounded by a narrow rim of bone, representing endochondral ossification (H&E, original magnification ×250).

Enchondromatosis, Ollier Disease, and Maffucci Syndrome

- Enchondromatosis—two or more enchondromas not associated with bone deformities or growth disturbance (Figs. 3.11 and 3.12).
- Ollier disease (nonhereditary disorder)—multiple enchondromas with strong preference for one side of the body (monomelic distribution), associated with bone growth disturbance (Figs. 3.13 to 3.16).
- Maffucci syndrome (nonhereditary disorder)—Ollier disease associated with hemangiomas of soft tissue (Figs. 3.17 and 3.18).
- Clinical features of both conditions are knobby swelling of the digits and gross disparity in the length of the forearms and legs.
- Clinical behavior of these conditions is unpredictable, and there is no specific treatment.
- Most serious complication is malignant transformation of an enchondroma in Ollier disease (25% to 30% of affected patients) and Maffucci syndrome (greater than 50%) (see Fig. 3.18).
- Patients with these conditions must have lifetime monitoring of their tumors.
- Histologically, the enchondromas of these entities are similar to those of sporadic solitary tumors; however, they frequently demonstrate a greater degree of cellularity, demonstrate cytologic atypia, and may contain myxoid stroma, which may suggest the diagnosis of chondrosarcoma.

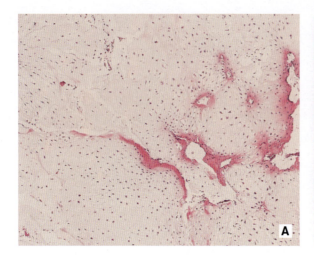
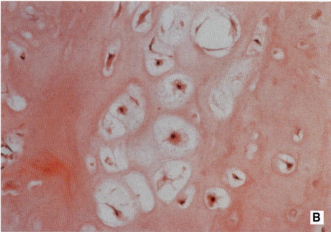
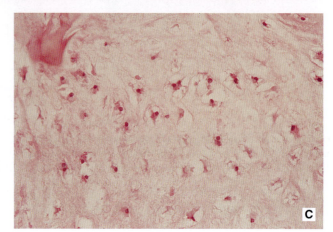

FIGURE 3.9 Histopathology of enchondroma. (A) Low-magnification photomicrograph shows that the lesion consists of hyaline cartilage exhibiting low-to-moderate cellularity (H&E, original magnification ×50). **(B)** At higher magnification, the chondrocytes with darkly stained nuclei are seen to be located in the lacunae (H&E, original magnification ×100). **(C)** Occasionally binucleated cells may be present (H&E, original magnification ×150).

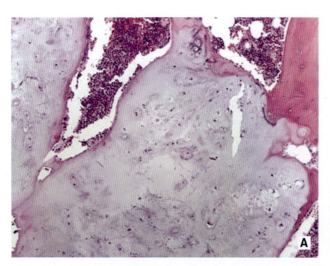
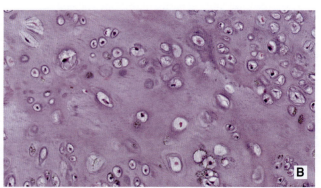

FIGURE 3.10 Histopathology of enchondroma. (A) Nodules of hyaline cartilage are well demarcated by the surrounding bone and bone marrow (H&E, original magnification ×50). **(B)** Higher-magnification photomicrograph shows low-to-moderate cellularity of the cartilage tissue containing chondrocytes of variable size located in the lacunae (H&E, original magnification ×200).

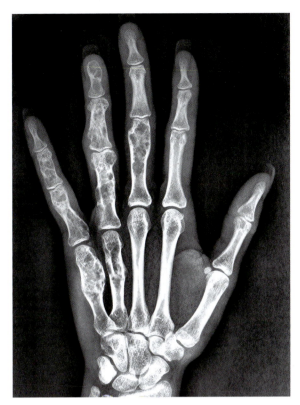

FIGURE 3.11 Radiography of enchondromatosis. Dorsovolar radiograph of the left hand of a 30-year-old woman shows several enchondromas affecting the fourth and fifth metacarpal bones, as well as the phalanges of the middle, ring, and small fingers. The remaining skeleton was not affected.

Periosteal (Juxtacortical) Chondroma

Definition:
- Benign cartilaginous lesion, almost identical to enchondroma, but growing on the surface of the bone in or beneath the periosteum.

Epidemiology:
- Less than 2% of all benign cartilaginous lesions.
- Most common in the second and third decades of life.
- Children and adults are equally affected.

Sites of Involvement:
- Long and short tubular bones with most common location in the proximal humerus.

Clinical Findings:
- Common presentation as palpable, often painful mass.

Imaging:
- Radiography shows cartilaginous lesion on the surface of the bone, with or without cortical erosion, that may contain calcifications, commonly associated with a buttress of periosteal reaction (Figs. 3.19 and 3.20); larger lesions resemble sessile osteochondromas (Fig. 3.21).

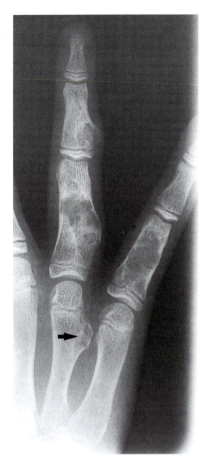

FIGURE 3.12 Radiography of enchondromatosis. In this 12-year-old boy, the intracortical lesion in the metaphysis of the forth metacarpal bone protrudes from the cortex (*arrow*), thus resembling an osteochondroma.

- CT and MRI demonstrate separation of the lesion from the medullary portion of host bone (Figs. 3.21 and 3.22).

Pathology:
Gross (Macroscopy):
- Well-marginated bone surface tumors.
- Cortex underlying the tumor is usually thickened and may be eroded.
- Most of the time, tumors are less than 6 cm in greatest diameter.

Histopathology:
- Can be more cellular than enchondroma, occasionally cellular atypia is present (Fig. 3.23).

Prognostic Factors:
- Recurrence rate is low after total excision.

Differential Diagnosis:
- ***Sessile osteochondroma***
  Continuity of the cortices of the lesion and host bone.
  Continuity of the cancellous portions of the lesion and host bone.

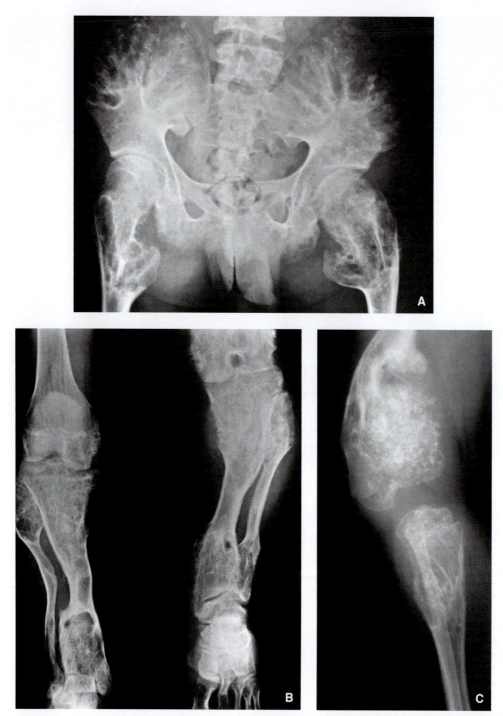

FIGURE 3.13 Radiography of Ollier disease. The classic features of this disorder in a 17-year-old boy are demonstrated in extensive involvement of multiple bones. **(A)** Anteroposterior radiograph of the pelvis shows crescent-shaped and ring-like calcifications in the tongues of cartilage extending from the iliac crests and proximal femora. **(B)** Anteroposterior radiograph of both legs shows growth stunting and deformities of the tibiae and fibulae. **(C)** In another patient, a 6-year-old boy, note extensive involvement of the distal femur and proximal tibia.

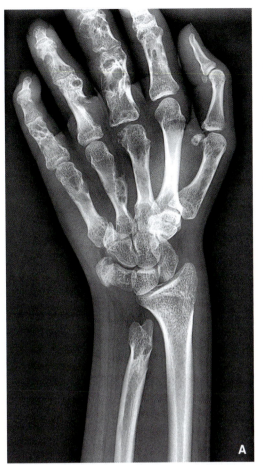
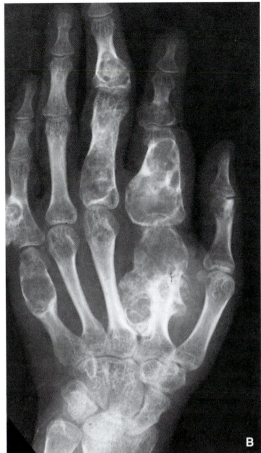
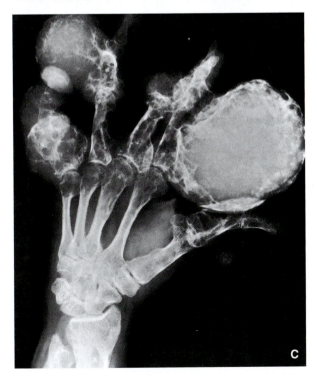

FIGURE 3.14 Radiography of Ollier disease. (A) Dorsovolar radiograph of the left hand of a 17-year-old girl shows extensive involvement of several metacarpals and phalanges by enchondromas. Note also involvement of the distal ulna, which in addition shows growth stunting, one of the features of this disorder. **(B)** Dorsovolar radiograph of the right hand of a 24-year-old woman shows extensive involvement of the metacarpals and phalanges by large expansive cartilaginous lesions. **(C)** Dorsovolar radiograph of the right hand of a 48-year-old man shows multiple enchondromas, some presenting as large lobulated cartilaginous masses of the phalanges.

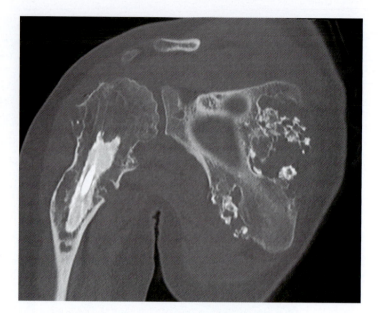

FIGURE 3.15 Computed tomography of Ollier disease. Coronal reformatted CT image of the right shoulder of a 23-year-old woman shows several enchondromas of different sizes affecting the proximal humerus and the scapula.

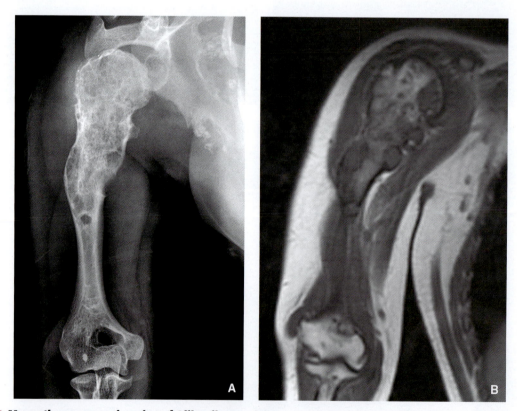

FIGURE 3.16 Magnetic resonance imaging of Ollier disease. (A) Anteroposterior radiograph of the right humerus of the same patient as depicted in Fig. 3.15 shows numerous enchondromas affecting proximal half of the bone. **(B)** Coronal T1–weighted MR image shows heterogeneous but predominantly low signal intensity of the lesions.

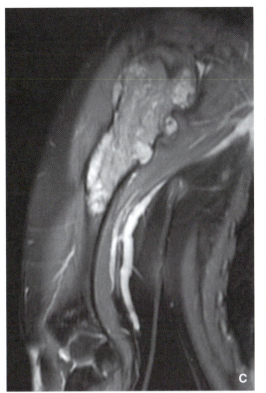
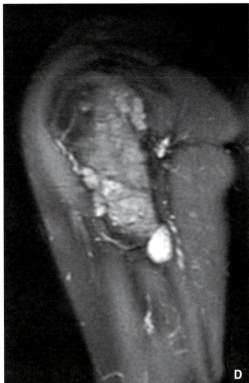
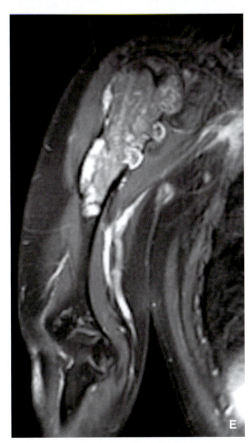

FIGURE 3.16 *(Continued).* **(C)** Coronal and **(D)** sagittal T2–weighted MR images show heterogeneous but predominantly high signal intensity of the lesions. **(E)** After intravenous administration of gadolinium, there is strong peripheral enhancement of multiple enchondromas.

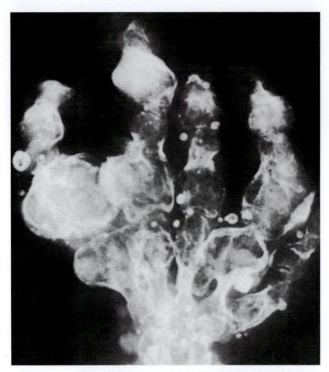

FIGURE 3.17 Radiography of Maffucci syndrome. Typical changes of this disorder consist of multiple enchondromas and soft-tissue hemangiomatosis, manifested by calcified phleboliths.

- *Periosteal osteoblastoma*
  Thin shell of newly formed periosteal bone usually covers the lesion.
  Bone formation within the lesion.
  Histopathology shows osteoid and immature bone trabeculae produced by osteoblasts.

Soft-Tissue Chondroma

Sites:
- Hands and feet.

Clinical Findings:
- Usually asymptomatic.

Imaging:
- Radiography shows small (2 to 4 cm) well-defined soft-tissue masses with chondroid type of calcifications.

Pathology:
Gross (Macroscopy):
- Well-circumscribed cartilaginous nodule.

Histopathology:
- Lesion composed of lobules of hyaline cartilage covered by fibrous tissue (Fig. 3.24).
- Sometimes partially myxoid, moderately cellular tissue with hyperchromatic nuclei.
- May contain focal areas of fibrosis, hemorrhage, necrosis, calcifications, and granuloma formation.

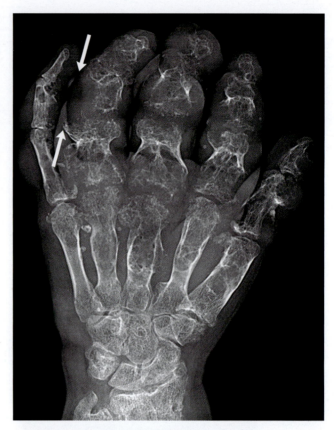

FIGURE 3.18 Radiography of Maffucci syndrome. Dorsovolar radiograph of the right hand of a 26-year-old woman shows multiple enchondromas affecting carpal bones, metacarpals, and phalanges. One of the lesions underwent malignant transformation to chondrosarcoma (*arrows*). Note numerous phleboliths within soft-tissue hemangiomas.

Differential Diagnosis:
- *Myositis ossificans*
  Imaging modalities and histopathology show lack of cartilage formation and classic zonal phenomenon (outer layer of mature bone formation and inner layer composed of reactive proliferation of spindle cells).
- *Synovial sarcoma*
  Lower extremities more commonly affected.
  May invade the adjacent bone.
  Periosteal reaction may be observed.
  MRI shows characteristic "triple-signal-intensity" pattern.
  Histopathology shows biphasic appearance with gland-like spaces and spindle cell sarcomatous areas; positivity for epithelial membrane antigen (EMA) and for bcl2 and CD99, but negative for S-100 protein.
- *Soft-tissue chondrosarcoma*
  Larger lesion.
  Histopathology shows undifferentiated mesenchymal cells with only rare islands of well-differentiated cartilage; frequent myxoid changes; and permeation and entrapment of bone trabeculae.

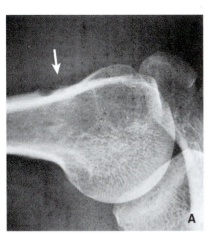
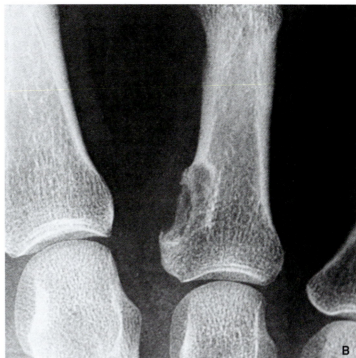
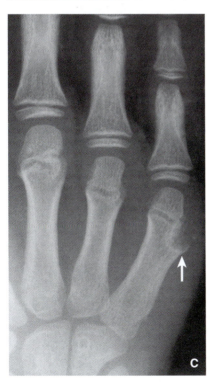

FIGURE 3.19 Radiography of periosteal chondroma. (A) Radiolucent lesion erodes the external surface of the cortex of proximal humerus (*arrow*) in this 24-year-old man. **(B)** Well-defined, saucer-like erosion of the cortex of the proximal phalanx is characteristic for this tumor. **(C)** Metaphyseal lesion erodes the cortex of the fifth metacarpal and evokes the buttress of periosteal reaction (*arrow*).

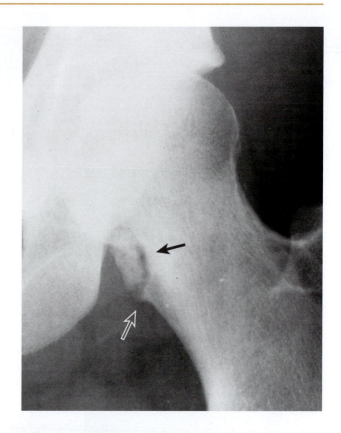

FIGURE 3.20 Radiography of periosteal chondroma.
A cartilaginous lesion is eroding the medial cortex of the neck of the femur (*arrow*) evoking a buttress of periosteal reaction (*open arrow*).

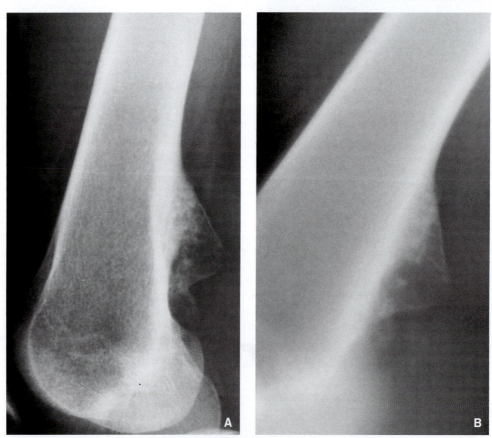

FIGURE 3.21 Radiography and computed tomography of periosteal chondroma. (A) Lateral radiograph of the distal femur shows a bony excrescence arising from the posterior cortex, resembling an osteochondroma. **(B)** Conventional tomography demonstrates calcifications at the base of the lesion and lack of communication of the medullary cavities of the lesion and a host bone, as invariably is seen in osteochondroma.

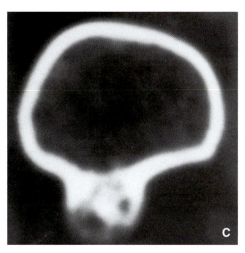

FIGURE 3.21 *(Continued).* **(C)** Computed tomography section demonstrates that the lesion is separated from the host bone by femoral cortex.

Synovial (Osteo) Chondromatosis

Definition:
- Benign metaplastic nodular cartilaginous proliferation arising in the synovial membrane of joints, bursae, or tendon sheaths.

Epidemiology:
- Uncommon condition.
- Mostly seen in adults.
- Male-to-female ratio of 2:1.

Sites of Involvement:
- Most of the time only one joint is involved.
- Most common involvement of the knee followed by the hip, elbow, wrist, ankle, and shoulder joint.

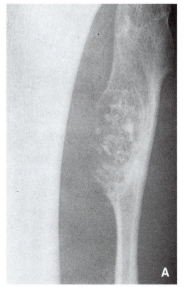
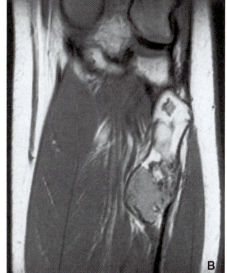
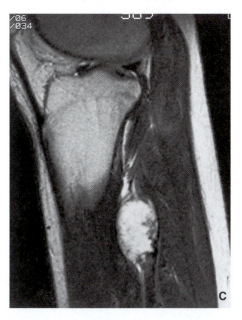

FIGURE 3.22 Radiography and magnetic resonance imaging of periosteal chondroma.
(A) Radiography shows a large lesion that blends imperceptibly with the medial cortex of the fibula, extending into the medullary portion of the bone. **(B)** Coronal proton density and **(C)** sagittal T2–weighted MR images show the lesion's extension into the medullary cavity.

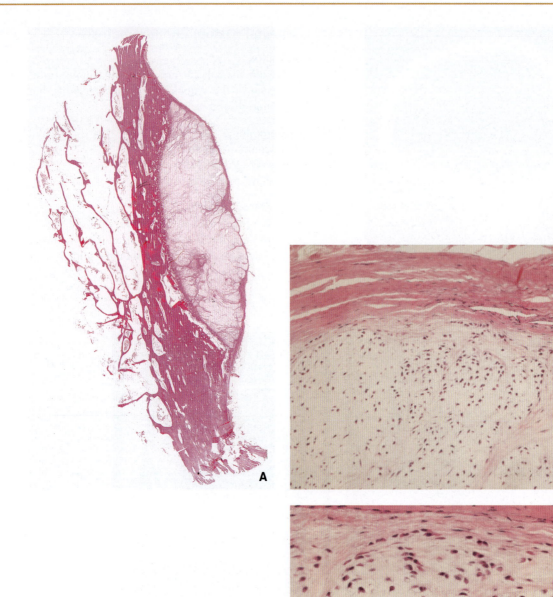

FIGURE 3.23 Histopathology of periosteal chondroma. (A) At the interface with the adjacent cortex, the cartilaginous tumor (*right*) erodes the bone (H&E, whole-mount section). **(B)** The higher magnification shows the tumor tissue more cellular than that of enchondroma, with some cells appearing atypical (H&E, original magnification ×100). **(C)** High magnification shows hyaline cartilage with rather dense cell population and slight cell enlargement, typical for this type of cartilage tumor (H&E, original magnification ×200).

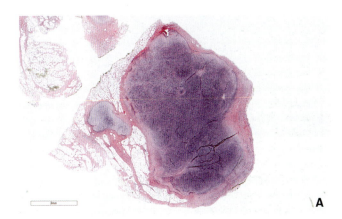
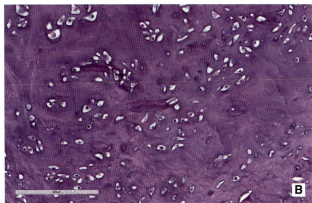

FIGURE 3.24 **Histopathology of soft-tissue chondroma.** **(A)** Lesion is composed of well-circumscribed hyaline cartilage covered by fibrous tissue (H&E, original magnification ×10). **(B)** Higher-magnification photomicrograph shows moderately cellular hyaline cartilage. Note benign chondrocytes with hyperchromatic nuclei (H&E, original magnification ×200).

Clinical Findings:
- Nonspecific symptoms with recurrent pain, swelling, joint effusion, and stiffness of joint.
- Sometimes lesion may present as painless soft-tissue mass adjacent to a joint.

Imaging:
- Radiographic findings depend upon the degree of calcification within the cartilaginous bodies, ranging from joint effusion only to visualization of many radiopaque joint bodies (Figs. 3.25 and 3.26). The bodies are small and uniform in size.
- CT and MRI demonstrate intra-articular loose bodies (even noncalcified), bone erosion, and (rare) extracapsular extension of the lesion (Figs. 3.27 to 3.29).

Pathology:
Gross (Macroscopy):
- Multiple blue/white ovoid bodies or nodules within synovial tissue (Fig. 3.30).
- Nodules may measure from a millimeters to several centimeters.

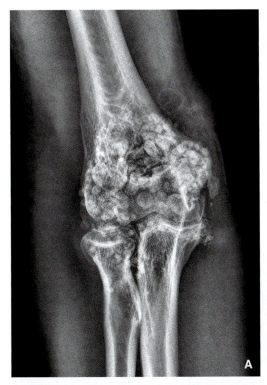
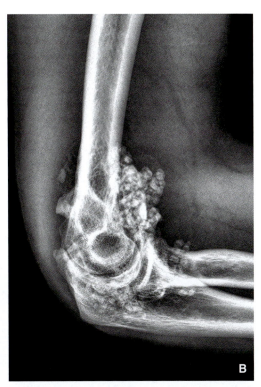

FIGURE 3.25 **Radiography of synovial (osteo)chondromatosis.** **(A)** Anteroposterior and **(B)** lateral radiographs of the elbow of a 27-year-old man show multiple osteochondral bodies within the joint, regularly shaped and uniform in size.

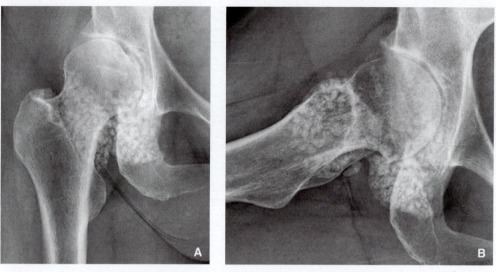

FIGURE 3.26 Radiography of synovial (osteo)chondromatosis. (A) Anteroposterior and **(B)** frog-lateral radiographs of the right hip of a 59-year-old woman demonstrate numerous uniform in size intra-articular osteochondral bodies.

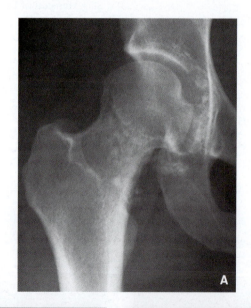

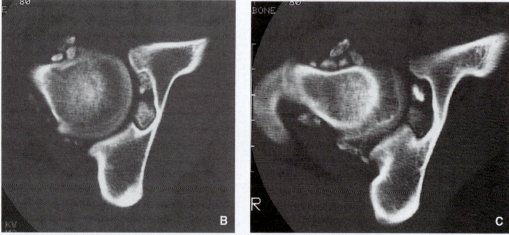

FIGURE 3.27 Radiography and computed tomography of synovial (osteo)chondromatosis. (A) Anteroposterior radiograph of the right hip of a 27-year-old woman shows multiple osteochondral bodies around the femoral head and neck. **(B,C)** Two axial CT sections, one through the femoral head and another through the femoral neck, demonstrate unquestionably the intra-articular location of multiple osteochondral bodies.

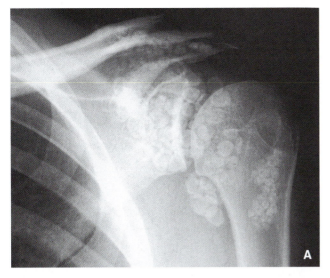
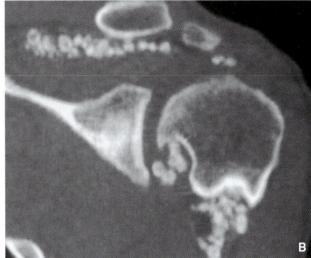
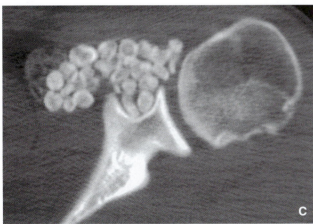

FIGURE 3.28 Radiography and computed tomography of synovial (osteo)chondromatosis. (A) Anteroposterior radiograph of the left shoulder of a 36-year-old man shows multiple osteochondral bodies around the glenohumeral joint. **(B)** Coronal CT section effectively shows location of the uniform in size calcified bodies in the glenohumeral joint and subacromial bursa. **(C)** Axial CT section confirms the intra-articular location of osteochondral bodies.

Histopathology:
- Variably cellular hyaline cartilage nodules covered by a fibrous tissue with synovial lining (Figs. 3.31 and 3.32A).
- Chondrocytes may form clusters with plump nuclei, and some of them may show moderate nuclear enlargement and binucleated cells (Fig. 3.32B).
- Uncommon mitotic figures.
- Ossifications and fatty marrow in intertrabecular spaces may be seen.

Genetics:
- Most cases show near-diploid or pseudodiploid karyotypes with some cases showing only simple numerical changes (−X, −Y, and +5, respectively).
- Some cases may display rearrangement of the bands 1p13-p22.

Prognostic Factors/Complications:
- Self-limiting process with potential local recurrence.
- Bone erosion has been described.
- Rare cases of chondrosarcoma arising in synovial chondromatosis were described.

Differential Diagnosis:
- ***Secondary osteochondromatosis (complication of osteoarthritis)***
  The osteochondral bodies are larger and not uniform in size. Affected joint shows degenerative changes (osteoarthritis).

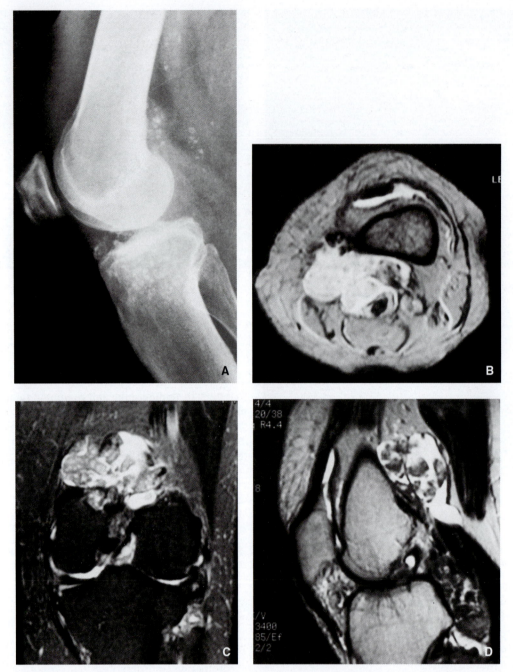

FIGURE 3.29 Radiography and magnetic resonance imaging of synovial (osteo)chondromatosis. (A) Lateral radiograph of the left knee of a 50-year-old man shows multiple osteochondral bodies in and around the joint. **(B)** Axial T2*–weighted (MPGR) MR image demonstrates high signal intensity joint effusion and multiple bodies of intermediate signal intensity, primarily located in a large popliteal cyst. **(C)** Coronal T2-weighted fat-suppressed and **(D)** sagittal fast spin echo MR images show to better advantage the distribution of numerous osteochondral bodies.

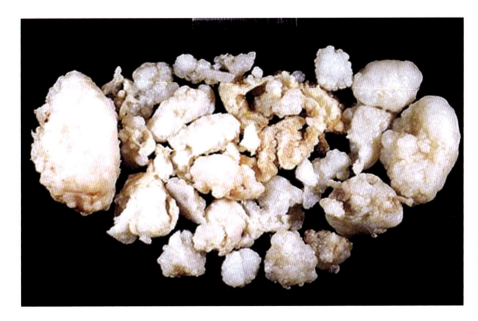

FIGURE 3.30 Gross specimen of synovial (osteo)chondromatosis. Multiple blue/white ovoid nodules of cartilage are scattered within the synovial tissue.

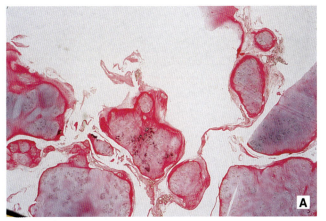
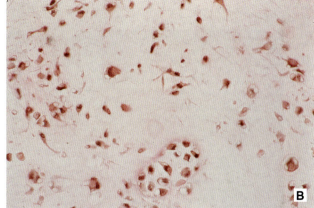

FIGURE 3.31 Histopathology of synovial (osteo)chondromatosis. (A) Photomicrograph of the synovium removed from the knee of a patient with primary synovial (osteo)chondromatosis shows nodules of irregular cellular cartilage covered by a thin layer of synovium (H&E, original magnification ×6). **(B)** High-power photomicrograph shows cells arranged in clusters with dark nuclei (H&E, original magnification ×100).

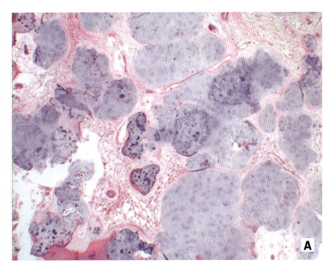
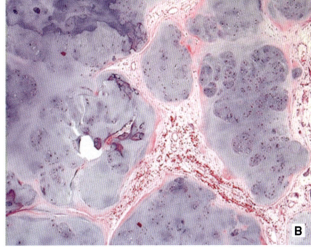

FIGURE 3.32 Histopathology of synovial (osteo)chondromatosis. (A) Variable cartilaginous nodules are covered by synovial tissue (H&E, original magnification ×100). **(B)** On higher magnification, note the clusters of chondrocytes with plump nuclei. Some of the cells show binucleation (H&E, original magnification ×200).

Osteochondroma (Osteocartilaginous Exostosis)

Definition:
- Cartilage-capped osseous projection (either sessile or pedunculated) arising on the external surface of a bone exhibiting an uninterrupted merging of the cortex of the host bone with the cortex of the lesion and communication of the medullary portions of the lesion and adjacent bone.

Epidemiology:
- Most common benign bone lesion (20% to 50% of all benign bone tumors).
- May be solitary or multiple, the latter occurring in the setting of hereditary multiple exostoses.
- Solitary lesions account for 80% of cases.
- Most common in the second decade of life.
- Male-to-female ratio of 1.5–2:1.

Sites:
- Most common sites: metaphyseal region of the distal femur, proximal humerus, and proximal tibia and fibula.

Clinical Findings:
- Most common presentation is that of a hard mass of long-standing duration.
- Majority of the lesions are asymptomatic and found incidentally.
- Symptoms are often related to the size and location of the lesion, pressure on the nerve or blood vessels, pathologic fracture, or bursitis exostotica.

Imaging:
- Radiography shows bulbous, cauliflower-like lesions (Fig. 3.33).
- The characteristic feature is continuation of the cortex of the lesion with that of a host bone and communication of the respected medullary portions (Figs. 3.34 to 3.36).

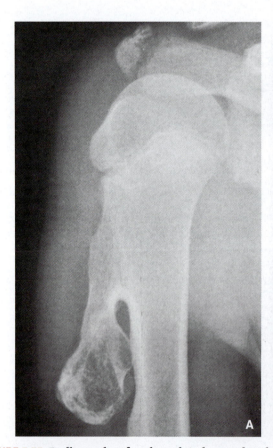 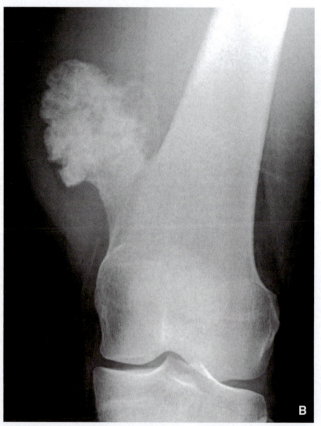

FIGURE 3.33 Radiography of pedunculated osteochondroma. (A) The typical pedunculated variant of this lesion is seen arising near the proximal growth plate of the right humerus of a 13-year-old boy. Note continuity of the cortex of the lesion with the cortex of a host bone and communication of their respective medullary cavities. **(B)** Pedunculated osteochondroma arising from the medial cortex of the distal left femur of a 22-year-old woman exhibits calcifications in the chondro-osseous zone of the stalk.

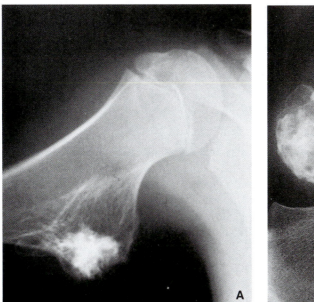
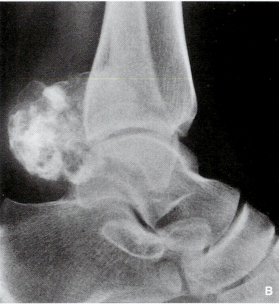

FIGURE 3.34 Radiography of sessile osteochondroma. (A) Broad-based lesion is seen arising from the medial cortex of the proximal diaphysis of the right humerus of a 14-year-old boy. Dense calcifications are present at the chondro-osseous junction of the lesion. **(B)** Lateral radiograph of the ankle of a 26-year-old woman shows a sessile osteochondroma arising from the posterior aspect of distal tibia.

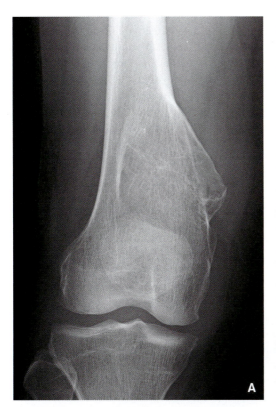
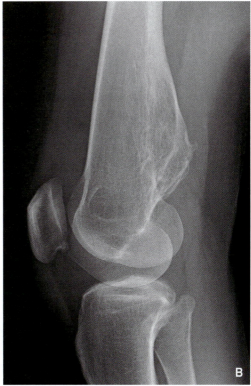

FIGURE 3.35 Radiography of sessile osteochondroma. (A) Anteroposterior and **(B)** lateral radiographs of the right knee of a 57-year-old woman show a sessile lesion arising from the posteromedial aspect of the distal femur, showing continuity of the cortex and medullary cavities of the lesion and host bone, and displaying no visible calcifications.

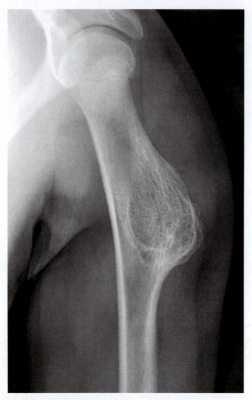

FIGURE 3.36 Radiography of sessile osteochondroma.
Anteroposterior radiograph shows a large sessile lesion arising from the lateral aspect of the proximal humeral diaphysis of an 11-year-old girl. Note that the cortex of the lesion and the host bone are in continuity, and the medullary portions are communicating.

- Calcifications in the chondro-osseous junction of the lesion (see Figs. 3.33B and 3.34A).
- Excessive cartilage-type flocculent calcifications, particularly dispersed calcifications into the cartilaginous cap, should raise the suspicion of malignant transformation (see Fig. 3.46 and Table 3.1).

- CT and MRI typically show unequivocally the lack of cortical interruption and the continuity of cancellous portions of the lesion and the host bone (Figs. 3.37 to 3.39). These modalities also demonstrate the thickness of the cartilaginous cap.

Pathology:

Gross (Macroscopy):

- May be sessile (Fig. 3.40) or pedunculated.
- The cortex and medullary cavity of the host bone extend into the lesion.
- The cartilage cap is usually thin.
- A thick cap (greater than 2 cm) may be indicative of malignant transformation.

Histopathology:

- The lesion has three layers—perichondrium (fibrous layer covering cartilage), cartilage, and bone (Figs. 3.41 and 3.42).
- The outer layer is a fibrous perichondrium that is continuous with the periosteum of the underlying bone.
- Underneath there is a cartilage cap that is usually less than 2 cm thick (thickness decreases with age).
- Within the cartilage cap, the superficial chondrocytes are clustered, whereas the ones close to bone resemble growth plate.
- Loss of the architecture of cartilage, wide fibrous bands, myxoid change, increased chondrocyte cellularity, mitotic activity, significant chondrocyte atypia, and necrosis are all features that may indicate secondary malignant transformation.

Genetics:

- Chromosomal aberrations involving *EXT1* gene 8q22-24.1 and *EXT2* 11p11-p12 defect.

TABLE 3.1 Clinical and Imaging Features Suggesting Malignant Transformation of Osteochondroma

Clinical Features	Radiologic Findings	Imaging Modality
Pain (in the absence of fracture, bursitis, or pressure on nearby nerves)	Enlargement of the lesion	Conventional radiography (comparison with earlier radiographs)
Growth spurt (after skeletal maturity)	Development of a bulky cartilaginous cap usually more than 2–3 cm thick	CT, MRI
	Dispersed calcifications in the cartilaginous cap	Radiography, CT, MRI
	Development of a soft-tissue mass with or without calcifications	
	Increased uptake of isotope after closure of growth place (not always reliable)	Scintigraphy

From Greenspan A, Beltran J. *Orthopedic Imaging.* 6th ed. Wolters Kluwer: Philadelphia 2015:745, Table 18.1.

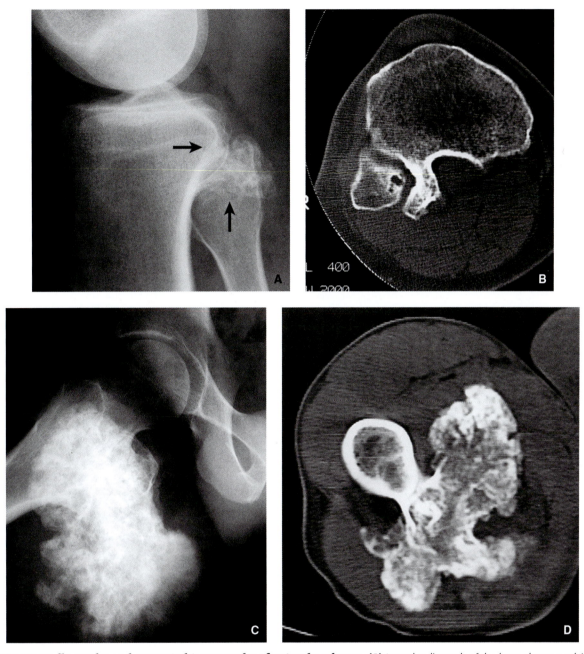

FIGURE 3.37 Radiography and computed tomography of osteochondroma. (A) Lateral radiograph of the knee shows a calcified lesion at the posterior aspect of the proximal tibia (*arrows*). The exact nature of the lesion cannot be ascertained. **(B)** CT section clearly establishes continuity of the cortex, which extends without interruption from osteochondroma into the tibia. Note also that the medullary portions of the lesion and the tibia communicate. **(C)** In another patient, a 26-year-old woman, a radiograph of the right hip shows a heavy calcified lesion arising from the intertrochanteric area of the femur. **(D)** CT section demonstrates a cauliflower-like mass exhibiting thin cartilaginous cap.

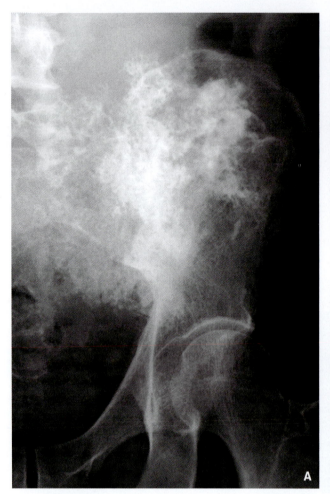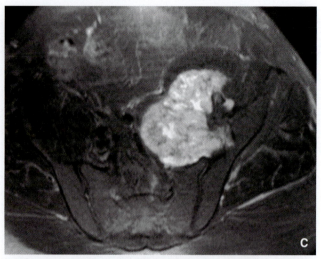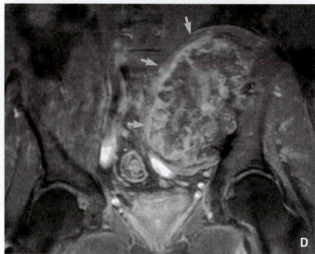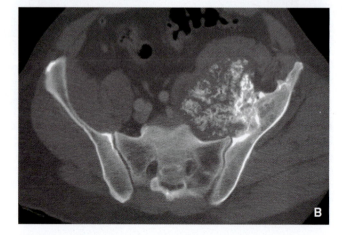

FIGURE 3.38 Radiography, computed tomography, and magnetic resonance imaging of sessile osteochondroma. **(A)** Anteroposterior radiograph of the left hemipelvis of a 29-year-old man shows a large cartilaginous lesion arising from the ilium. **(B)** Axial CT shows better the relationship between the lesion and the host bone. **(C)** Axial T2–weighted MR image demonstrates high signal intensity of the cartilaginous cap. **(D)** Coronal T1–weighted fat-suppressed MR image obtained after intravenous administration of gadolinium shows peripheral enhancement of the fibrovascular layer, which covers nonenhancing cartilaginous cap of the lesion (*arrows*).

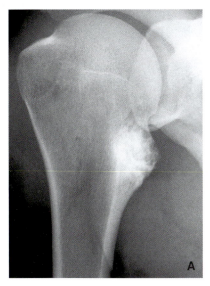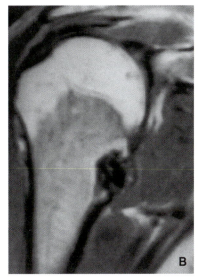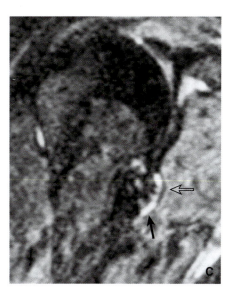

FIGURE 3.39 Radiography and magnetic resonance imaging of osteochondroma. (A) Radiograph of the right shoulder shows a sessile lesion at the medial aspect of the proximal humerus. **(B)** Coronal T1–weighted MR image reveals that the lesion exhibits low signal intensity due to heavy mineralization. **(C)** T2-weighted MRI shows a thin cartilaginous cap covering the lesion that exhibits high signal intensity (*arrow*), covered by linear strip of low signal intensity, representing perichondrium (*open arrow*).

Complications:
- Fracture of the lesion.
- Pressure/erosion and fracture of the adjacent bone (ulna, fibula) (Figs. 3.43 and 3.44).
- Bursitis (bursa exostotica) (Fig. 3.45).
- Pressure on nerves and blood vessels.
- Malignant transformation to chondrosarcoma (less than 1% in solitary lesions) (Fig. 3.46).

Prognosis:
- Excision is usually curative.
- Recurrence is seen with incomplete removal.

Differential Diagnosis:
- **Periosteal chondroma**
    Lesion separated from the host bone but may erode the cortex.
    Large lesion may mimic osteochondroma but lack cortical and medullary continuity.
    Value of attenuation coefficient of the lesion as determined by CT (Hounsfield values) is helpful in differential diagnosis: base of osteochondroma has higher values than does that of periosteal chondroma.
- **Trevor-Fairbanks disease (dysplasia epiphysealis hemimelica, intra-articular osteochondroma)**
    Asymmetric cartilaginous overgrowth of one or more epiphyses.
    Talus, distal femur, and distal tibia most commonly affected.
    Histopathologically almost identical with osteochondroma.
- **BPOP (Nora lesion, bizarre parosteal osteochondromatous proliferation)**
    Usually affects the metacarpals and phalanges of the hand.
    Mushroom-like-shaped osseous or cartilaginous mass attached to the cortex.
    Lack of communication with medullary cavity of the host bone.

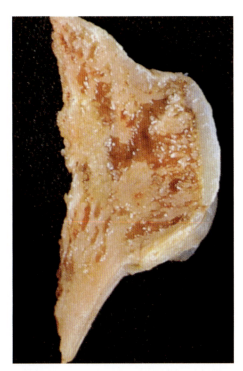

FIGURE 3.40 Gross specimen of sessile osteochondroma. Note continuity of the cortex and medullary cavities, and thin cartilaginous cap.

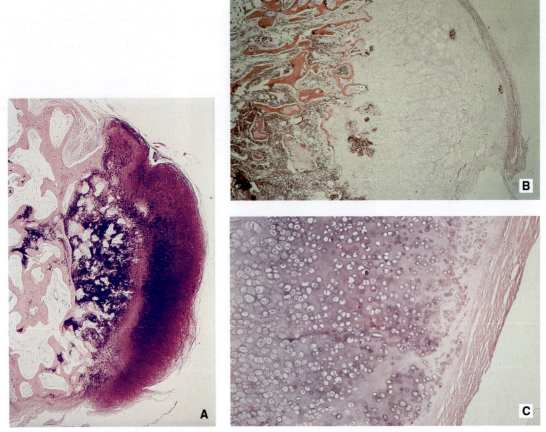

FIGURE 3.41 Histopathology of sessile osteochondroma. (A) The tumor consists of the hyaline cartilaginous cap with strong metachromasia of the matrix. A broad zone of endochondral ossification borders the cancellous bone containing the remnants of cartilaginous matrix (*center*) (Giemsa, original magnification ×6). **(B)** At higher magnification, foci of calcifications are seen at the chondro-osseous junction. These areas correspond to a zone of provisional calcification in the growth plate. Beneath the cap, there is evidence of transformation of the cartilage into bone by process of endochondral ossification (H&E, original magnification ×30). **(C)** Periphery of the lesion consists of a hyaline cartilaginous cap, which is covered by a thin fibrous membrane (perichondrium) (H&E, original magnification ×60).

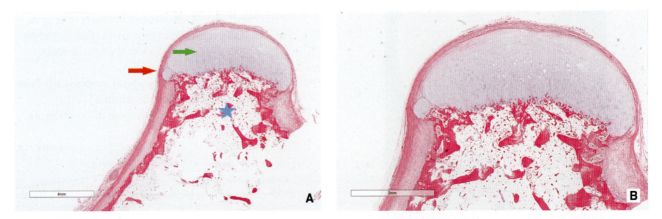

FIGURE 3.42 Histopathology of pedunculated osteochondroma. (A) The lesion consists of three layers: outer fibrous layer of perichondrium (*red arrow*), cartilaginous cap (*green arrow*), and osseous stalk (*star*) (H&E, original magnification ×5). **(B)** Higher magnification shows continuation of the perichondrium with the periosteum covering the stalk of the lesion (H&E, original magnification ×10).

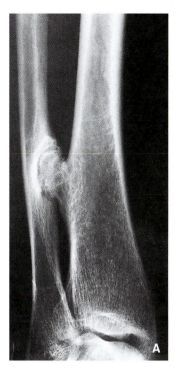 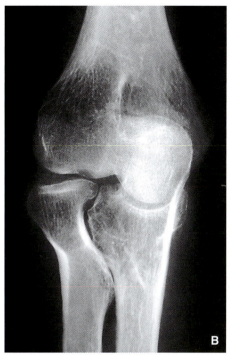 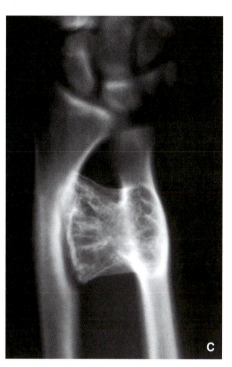

FIGURE 3.43 Complications of osteochondroma: pressure erosion of the adjacent bone. (A) Osteochondroma arising from the posterolateral aspect of the right distal tibia of a 24-year-old man has eroded the adjacent fibula. **(B)** In another patient, continued growth of the sessile osteochondroma of the proximal ulna resulted in pressure erosion of the head and neck of the radius. **(C)** Pedunculated lesion of the distal ulna has eroded medial aspect of the shaft of the radius.

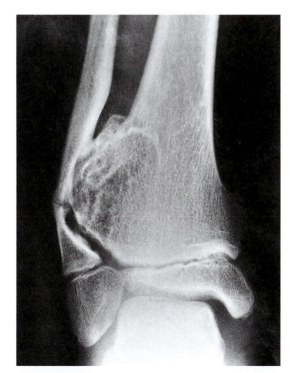

FIGURE 3.44 Complications of osteochondroma: fracture of the adjacent bone. The continued growth of a sessile osteochondroma of the distal tibial metaphysis of a 9-year-old boy has caused a fracture of the adjacent fibula.

- *Juxtacortical (parosteal) osteoma*
  Homogenously dense, sclerotic, ivory-like mass.
  No communication with the medullary portion of the host bone.
  Histopathology shows compact, dense, mature lamellar bone, or woven bone formation with transformation to lamellar bone, and osteocyte lacunae.

Multiple Hereditary Osteochondromata (Diaphyseal Aclasis)

- Autosomal dominant genetic disorder with incomplete penetrance in females.
- Male predominance 2:1.
- Most commonly affected sites are the knees, ankles, and shoulders.
- Imaging features similar to single osteochondromas, but lesions more commonly of sessile type (Figs. 3.47 to 3.52).
- Growth disturbance (dysplastic changes, retardation of longitudinal bone growth) (Figs. 3.48, 3.49, 3.50, and 3.53).
- Histopathologic features identical to those of solitary lesions.
- Genetic defect has recently been identified, a novel mutation in genes *EXT1* that maps to chromosome 8q24.1, *EXT2* that maps to chromosome 11p11-p12, and *EXT3* that maps to the short arm of chromosome 19.

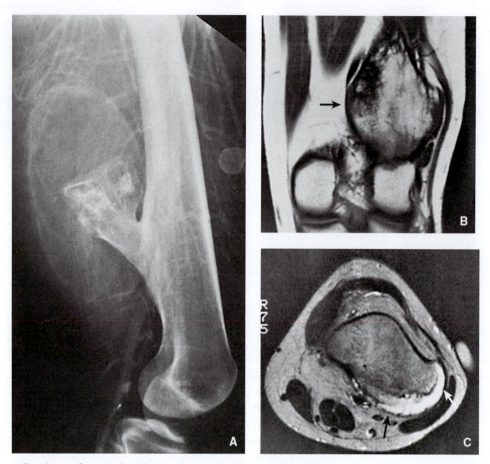

FIGURE 3.45 **Complications of osteochondroma: bursa exostotica. (A)** A 25-year-old man with a known solitary osteochondroma of the distal right femur presented with gradually increased pain. Malignancy was suspected, and arteriography was performed. The capillary phase of the arteriogram reveals a huge bursa exostotica, one of the complications of osteochondroma. **(B)** Coronal T1–weighted MR image of a 12-year-old girl who presented with pain in the popliteal fossa demonstrates a large osteochondroma arising from the posterolateral aspect of the distal femur (*arrow*). **(C)** Axial T2–weighted MRI shows a bursa exostotica distended with high-intensity fluid (*arrows*).

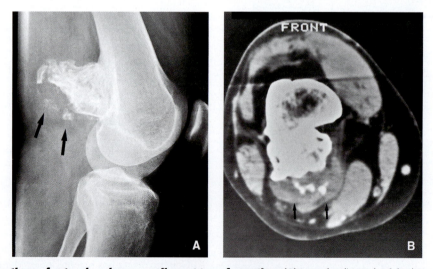

FIGURE 3.46 **Complications of osteochondroma: malignant transformation. (A)** Lateral radiograph of the knee of a 28-year-old man, who presented with pain in the popliteal region and increase in size of the mass he had been aware of for 15 years, shows a sessile osteochondroma arising from the posterior cortex of the distal femur. Note that calcifications not only are present at the chondro-osseous junction of the lesion but also are dispersed in the cartilaginous cap (*arrows*). **(B)** CT section confirms the increased thickness of the cartilaginous cap and dispersed calcifications within it (*arrows*), features of malignant transformation to chondrosarcoma, which was confirmed on histopathologic examination.

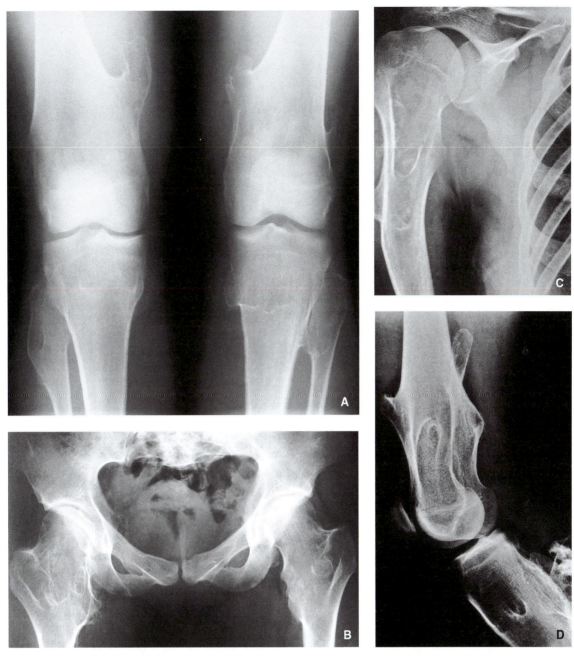

FIGURE 3.47 Radiography of multiple osteocartilaginous exostoses. (A) Anteroposterior radiograph of both knees of a 17-year-old boy shows numerous sessile and pedunculated osteochondromas. **(B)** Anteroposterior radiograph of the pelvis demonstrates numerous sessile osteochondromas affecting proximal femora. **(C)** Anteroposterior radiograph of the right shoulder of a 22-year-old man shows multiple sessile lesions involving the proximal humerus and scapula. **(D)** Lateral radiograph of the knee of the same patient shows involvement of the distal femur and proximal tibia.

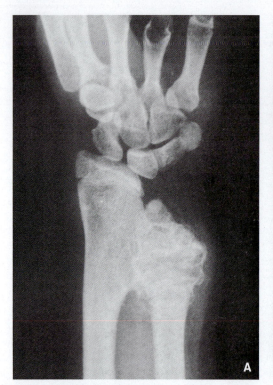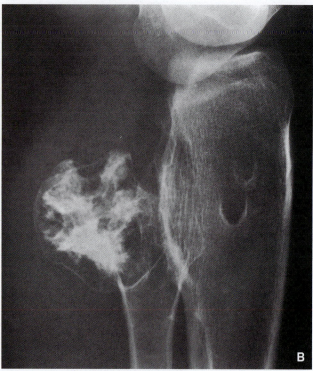

FIGURE 3.48 Radiography of multiple osteocartilaginous exostoses. (A) Radiograph of the distal forearm of an 8-year-old boy shows growth disturbance in the distal radius and ulna. **(B)** In another patient, a 21-year-old woman, observe growth disturbance of the proximal fibula.

Chondroblastoma

Definition:
- Benign, cartilage-producing neoplasm usually arising in the epiphyses of long bones of skeletally immature patients.

Epidemiology:
- Accounts for less than 1% of primary bone tumors.
- Most common between 10 and 25 years of age.
- Male predominance.
- Patients with skull and temporal bone involvement tend to present at an older age (40 to 50 years).

Sites of Involvement:
- Mostly involve epiphyses of the distal and proximal femur, followed by the proximal tibia and proximal humerus.
- Patients with tumors arising in the flat bones, vertebrae, and short tubular bones tend to be older and skeletally mature, although rare cases have been reported in children.

Clinical Findings:
- Majority of patients complain of localized pain, often mild, but sometimes of many years' duration.
- Soft-tissue swelling, joint stiffness and limitation, and limp are reported less commonly.
- Minority of patients may develop joint effusion, especially around the knee.

Imaging:
- Typically radiolucent, centrally or eccentrically located, relatively small lesion (3 to 6 cm), occupying less than one-half of the epiphysis (Fig. 3.54).
- Sharply demarcated, with or without a thin sclerotic border (Figs. 3.55 to 3.58).
- Matrix calcifications are only visible in about one-third of patients.
- Periosteal reaction remote from the tumor (see Figs. 3.56A and 3.57A).

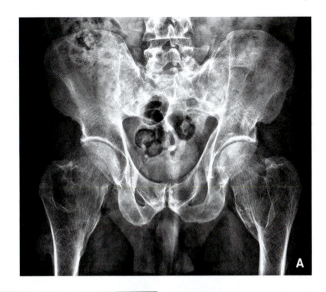
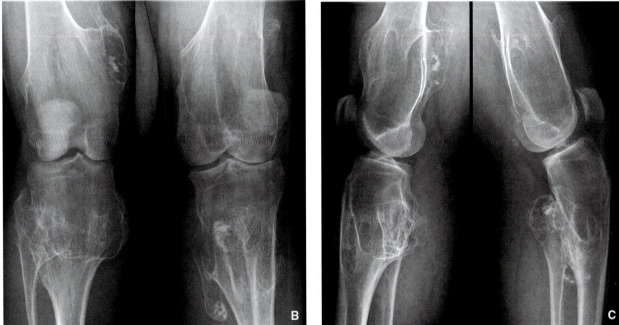

FIGURE 3.49 Radiography of multiple osteocartilaginous exostoses. (A) Anteroposterior radiograph of the pelvis of a 45-year-old man shows multiple lesions of the proximal femora. Note the broadening of the femoral necks. **(B)** Anteroposterior and **(C)** lateral radiographs of both knees of the same patient show classic appearance of this disorder: numerous sessile and pedunculated osteochondromas are seen arising from the distal femora and proximal tibiae and fibulae. Note also the growth disturbance due to defective metaphyseal remodeling commonly seen in this condition.

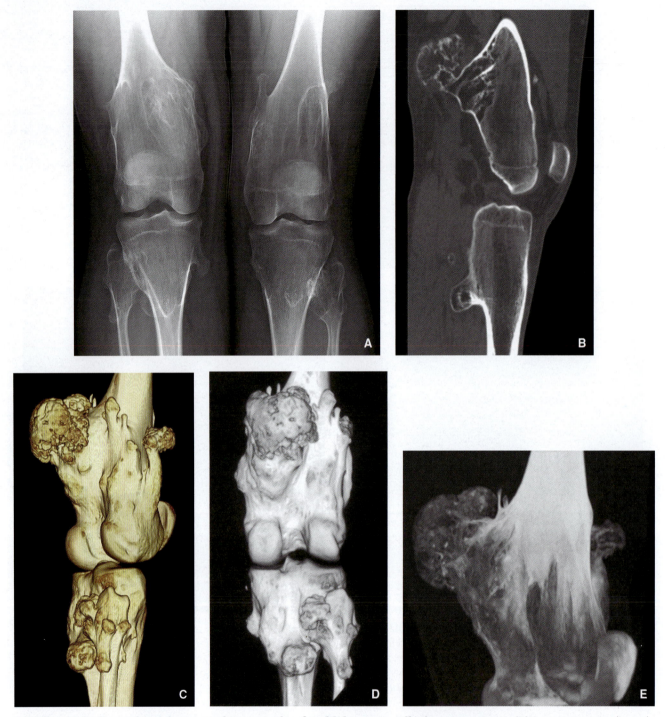

FIGURE 3.50 Radiography and computed tomography of multiple osteocartilaginous exostoses. (A) Anteroposterior radiograph of both knees of a 20-year-old man shows multiple osteochondromas arising from the distal femora and proximal tibiae and fibulae, associated with growth disturbance reflected by Erlenmeyer flask deformities. **(B)** Sagittal reformatted CT image shows osteochondromas arising from the posterior aspect of the distal femur and proximal tibia. Three-dimensional CT images with surface-rendering algorithm viewed from the lateral **(C)** and posterior **(D)** aspects of the knee show spatial distribution of numerous osteochondromas. **(E)** 3D CT image of the distal femur in maximum intensity projection (MIP) shows interior architecture of one of the sessile lesions.

Chapter 3 • Cartilage-Forming (Chondrogenic) Lesions

Pathology:

Gross (Macroscopy):

- Gritty and grayish white mass with areas of hemorrhage.

Histopathology:

- Densely cellular tissue composed of an admixture of mononuclear chondroblasts and multinucleated osteoclast-type giant cells (Fig. 3.59A).
- Chondroblasts grow in sheets, have eosinophilic cytoplasm, have well-defined cell borders, and have eccentrically placed reniform or coffee bean–shaped nuclei.
- Matrix generally consists of poorly formed matrix cartilage, which mineralization may form "chicken-wire" pattern around single cells (Figs. 3.59B and 3.60).
- Frequent mitotic activity but not atypical mitotic forms present.
- Osteoclast-type giant cells are scattered throughout the tumor but are most numerous in areas of matrix production and hemorrhage (Fig. 3.61).

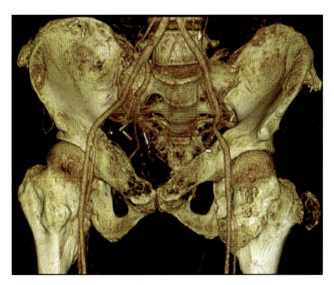

FIGURE 3.51 Computed tomography of multiple osteocartilaginous exostoses. Three-dimensional angio-CT image of the pelvis with surface-rendering algorithm of a 57-year-old woman shows multiple osteochondromas arising from the iliac wings, pubic bones, and proximal femora. The iliac and femoral arteries were not affected by the exostoses.

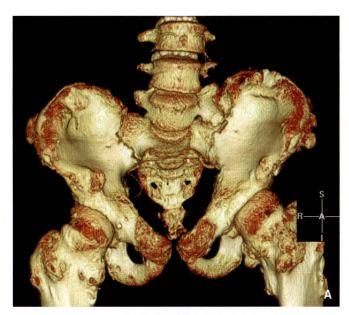
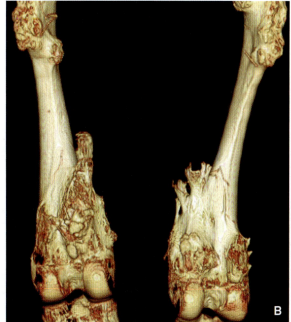

FIGURE 3.52 Computed tomography and magnetic resonance imaging of multiple osteocartilaginous exostoses. Three-dimensional CT images with surface-rendering algorithm of the pelvis **(A)** and femora **(B)** of a 16-year-old boy show multiple sessile and pedunculated osteochondromas typical for this disorder.

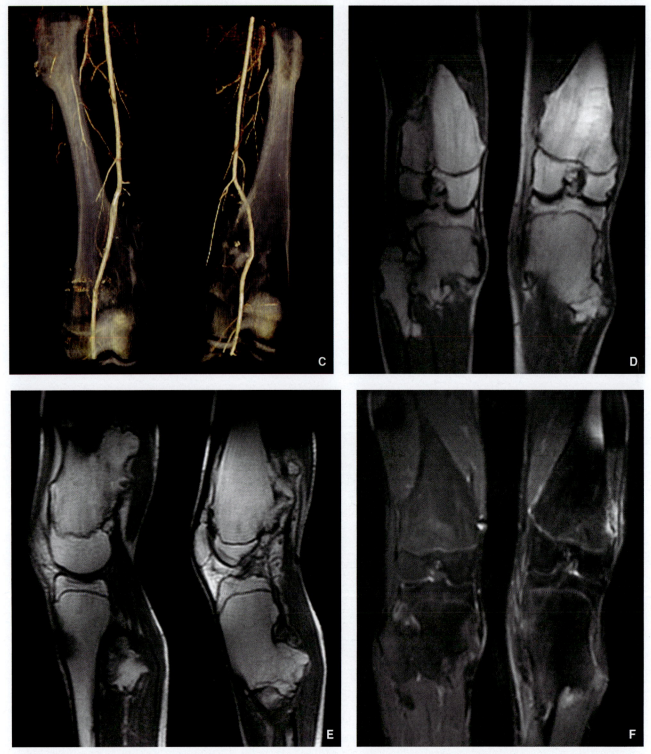

FIGURE 3.52 *(Continued).* **(C)** 3D CT angiogram was performed to rule out compression of the arteries of the lower extremities. The femoral and popliteal arteries were not affected by the lesions. **(D)** Coronal T1–weighted, **(E)** two sagittal T1–weighted, and **(F)** coronal T2–weighted fat-suppressed MR images show the lesions communicating with the medullary portions of the host bones.

Chapter 3 • Cartilage-Forming (Chondrogenic) Lesions   **129**

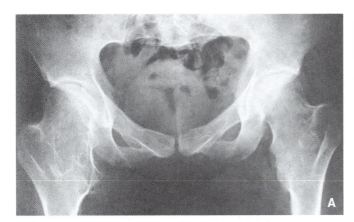

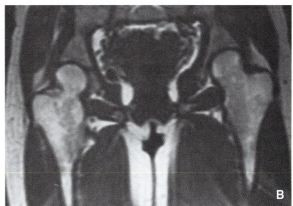

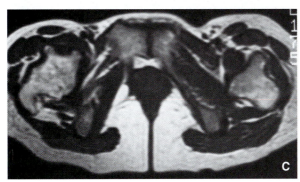

FIGURE 3.53 Radiography and magnetic resonance imaging of multiple osteocartilaginous exostoses. (A) Anteroposterior radiographs of the hips show multiple sessile osteochondromas affecting proximal femora. Some lesions are also present at the pubic bones. **(B)** Coronal and **(C)** axial T1–weighted MR images demonstrate continuity of the lesions with the medullary portion of the femora. Note also dysplastic changes expressed by abnormal tubulation of bones.

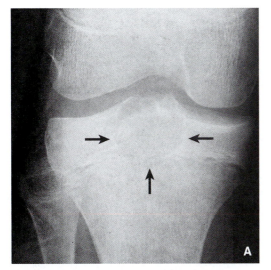

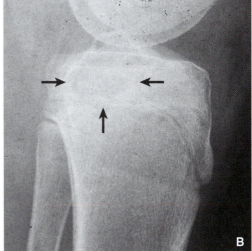

FIGURE 3.54 Radiography of chondroblastoma. (A) Anteroposterior and **(B)** lateral radiographs of the right knee of a 14-year-old boy show typical appearance of this tumor in the proximal epiphysis of tibia (*arrows*). The radiolucent, eccentrically located lesion exhibits a thin sclerotic margin.

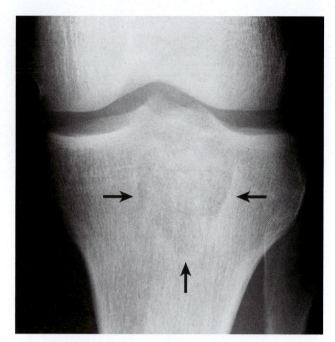

FIGURE 3.55 Radiography of chondroblastoma. Anteroposterior radiograph of the left knee of a 17-year-old boy shows a large radiolucent lesion with narrow zone of transition crossing the scarred growth plate of the proximal tibia and exhibiting matrix calcifications (*arrows*).

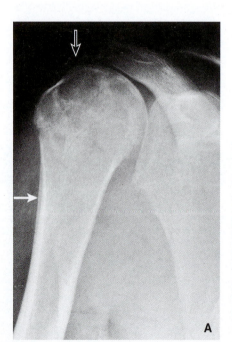
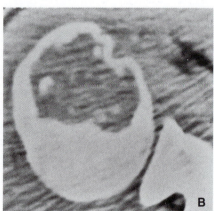

FIGURE 3.56 Radiography and computed tomography of chondroblastoma. (A) Anteroposterior radiograph of the right shoulder of a 16-year-old boy shows a lesion in the proximal humeral epiphysis (*open arrow*), but matrix calcifications are not well demonstrated. Note the well-organized layer of periosteal reaction at the lateral cortex, remote from the lesion (*arrow*). **(B)** CT section clearly demonstrates calcifications.

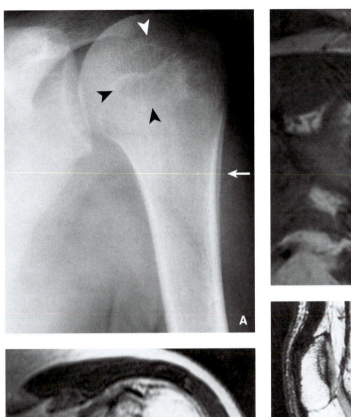
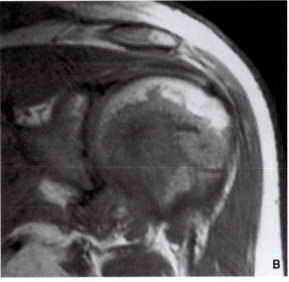
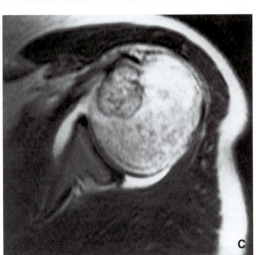
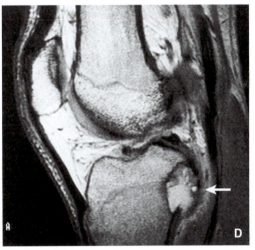
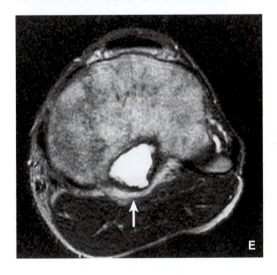

FIGURE 3.57 Radiography and magnetic resonance imaging of chondroblastoma. (A) Conventional radiograph shows a lesion (*arrowheads*) with a narrow zone of transition in the left humeral head of an 18-year-old man. Note benign type of periosteal reaction along the lateral cortex of the humeral diaphysis (*arrow*). **(B)** Coronal T1–weighted MR image shows the lesion displaying intermediate-to-low signal intensity. **(C)** Axial T2–weighted MR image shows sharp delineation of the lesion exhibiting a heterogeneous but mostly high signal. In another patient, a sagittal proton density–weighted **(D)** and axial T2–weighted **(E)** MR images show the lesion located in the posterior tibia exhibiting high signal and extending into the soft tissues (*arrows*).

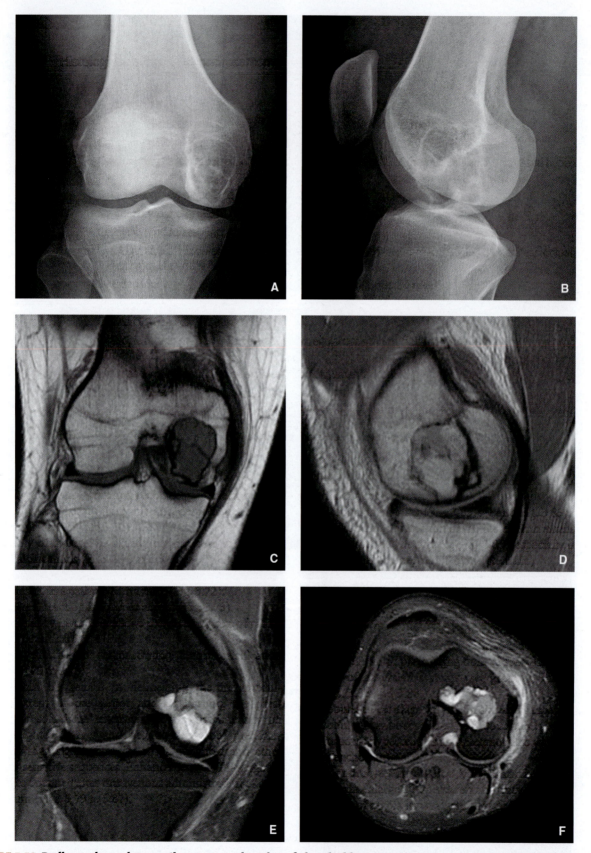

FIGURE 3.58 Radiography and magnetic resonance imaging of chondroblastoma. (A) Anteroposterior and **(B)** lateral radiographs of the right knee of a 22-year-old man show a radiolucent lesion with sclerotic border and central calcifications in the medial femoral condyle. **(C)** Coronal and **(D)** sagittal T1–weighted MR images show the tumor displaying intermediate signal intensity. The sclerotic margin is of low signal intensity. **(E)** Coronal and **(F)** axial fat-suppressed T2-weighted images demonstrate heterogeneous signal intensity of the lesion.

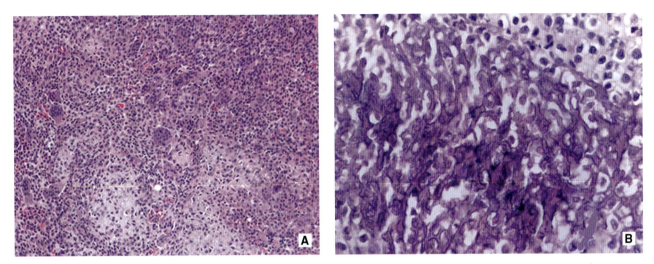

FIGURE 3.59 **Histopathology of chondroblastoma. (A)** Densely, cellular tissue is composed of an admixture of mononuclear chondroblasts and multinucleated osteoclast-type giant cells (H&E, original magnification ×100). **(B)** Higher magnification shows poorly formed primitive cartilaginous matrix with intercellular calcifications in form of chicken wire (H&E, original magnification ×200).

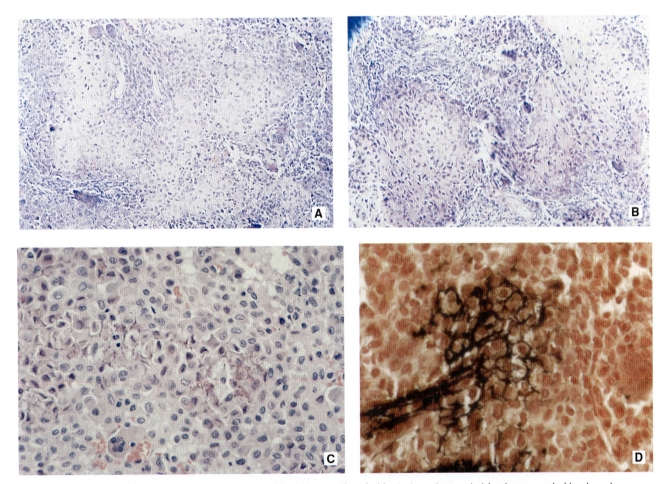

FIGURE 3.60 **Histopathology of chondroblastoma. (A)** Primitive chondroblastic tissue is seen in islands surrounded by densely arranged roundish cells. In addition, note the presence of numerous giant cells of osteo- and chondroblastic type (Giemsa, original magnification ×25). **(B)** At higher magnification, note the pleomorphism of chondrocytes within the cartilaginous matrix and some giant cells (Giemsa, original magnification ×50). **(C)** The chondrocytes, some with ovoid and some with elongated nuclei, are embedded in cartilaginous matrix. Surrounding the cells are fine, intercellular calcifications, forming a chicken-wire image (H&E, original magnification ×235). **(D)** High magnification shows to better advantage chicken-wire calcifications, characteristic for this tumor (von Kossa, original magnification ×400).

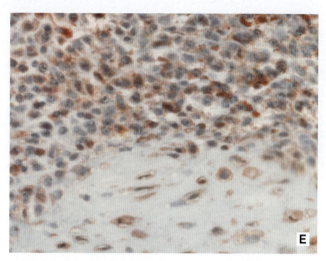

FIGURE 3.60 *(Continued).* (E) Tumor cells and adjacent hyaline cartilage are positive for S100 protein (biotin–streptavidin peroxidase, anti-S100, original magnification ×400).

Immunohistochemistry:

- Chondroblasts express positivity for S-100 protein and vimentin but may also stain for keratin and EMA (see Fig. 3.60E).

Genetics:

- Clonal anomalies including recurrent structural alterations in chromosomes 5 and 8 with rearrangements of band 8q21 and recurrent break points at 2q35, 3q21-q23, and 18q21.

Prognosis:

- Eighty to ninety percent of chondroblastomas are successfully treated by simple curettage with bone grafting.
- Local recurrence rates range between 14% and 18% and occur usually within 2 years.
- Rare development of pulmonary metastases in histologically benign chondroblastoma is well documented; however, these metastases are clinically nonprogressive and can often be satisfactorily treated by surgical resection and/or simple observation.

Differential Diagnosis:

- **Clear cell chondrosarcoma**
  MRI shows homogeneous intermediate signal intensity on T1-weighted images and heterogeneous but mostly increased signal on T2 weighting.
  Histopathology shows clusters of large chondrocytes with distinct cell boundaries, possessing small nuclei and abundant clear or eosinophilic cytoplasm. Osteoclasts-like giant cells and foci of reactive bone formation are also present.
- **Giant cell tumor**
  Skeletally mature patients (growth plate closed).
  Lack of sclerotic margin.
  Lack of matrix mineralization.
  Soft-tissue mass may be present.
  Histopathology shows dual population of fibrocytic or monocytic mononuclear stromal cells and uniformly distributed giant cells, which exhibit marked acid phosphatase activity.
- **Enchondroma**
  Extremely rare in epiphysis.
  Lack of periosteal reaction.
  Histopathology shows intercellular matrix of a uniformly translucent appearance containing relatively small amount of collagen. The tumor cells located in lacunae exhibit small darkly stained nuclei. Calcifications correspond to matrix calcifications or actual endochondral ossification at the periphery of the cartilaginous nodules, but there is lack of chicken-wire calcifications.
- **Intraosseous ganglion**
  Almost never seen before skeletal maturation.
  No intralesional matrix mineralization.
  Histopathology shows no presence of cartilage.
- **Geode (degenerative cyst)**
  Osteoarthritic changes of the joint invariably present.
  Cyst filled with fluid or gelatinous material.
- **Epiphyseal bone abscess**
  Rare in this location.
  Thicker sclerotic rim around the lesion.
  Serpentine tract extending toward the growth plate.
  Lack of calcifications within the lesion.
  Lack of periosteal reaction.
  Histopathology shows inflammatory changes.

Chondromyxoid Fibroma

Definition:

- Benign cartilage tumor characterized by lobules of spindle-shaped or stellate cells with abundant fibromyxoid or chondroid intercellular matrix.

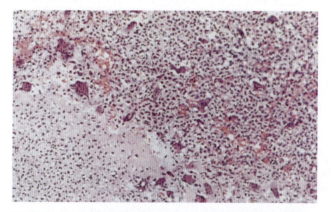

FIGURE 3.61 Histopathology of chondroblastoma. A highly cellular area of the tumor contains several giant cells (*upper right*). However, the juxtaposition of chondroid matrix (*lower left*) indicates the true nature of this tumor (H&E, original magnification ×100). (Reprinted with permission from Bullough PG. *Atlas of Orthopedic Pathology*. 2nd ed. New York: Gower; 1992:16.24).

Epidemiology:
- Uncommon tumor, constituting less than 1% of all primary bone tumors and less than 2% of benign bone tumors.
- More common in males than in females.
- Most common in the second and third decades of life.

Sites of Involvement:
- May occur in any bone but most common in long bones of lower extremity, especially in the proximal tibia (most common) and the distal femur.
- About 25% of cases occur in flat bones, mainly in the ilium.
- May be seen in bones of the feet especially in the metatarsals.
- Less common in ribs, vertebrae, and skull.

Clinical Findings:
- Chronic pain that may be present for several years.
- Swelling may be seen when the hands and feet are affected.

Imaging:
- Radiography shows characteristically round or ovoid radiolucent, eccentric, well-defined lesion exhibiting geographic type of bone destruction with buttress type of periosteal reaction; ballooning out of the cortex often seen; no visible calcifications (Figs. 3.62 to 3.64). MRI shows the lesion to be of low-to-intermediate signal intensity on T1-weighted images and of high signal on T2-weighted and water-sensitive sequences (Fig. 3.65).

Pathology:
Gross (Macroscopy):
- Expansive bluish, gray, or white tumor, without necrosis, cystic change, or liquefaction.
- In flat bones, the tumor is multilobulated and well demarcated from the surrounding normal bone.

Histopathology:
- May show variety of different morphologic features.
- Typically sharply demarcated from the normal bone.
- It is very rare to see entrapment of bone trabeculae, unless there was previous fracture.
- Classic morphology shows lobular pattern with stellate or spindle-shaped cells in fibromyxoid background and occasional giant cells (Figs. 3.66 and 3.67A).
- Lobules show hypocellular centers and cellular periphery (Fig. 3.67B).
- Tumor cells have oval to spindle nuclei and dense eosinophilic cytoplasm.
- Rare hyperchromatic and pleomorphic nuclei may be seen (these finding may be suspicious for malignancy, but usually, they are focal and show degenerative change).
- Microscopic cystic or liquefactive changes are rare and focal.
- Hyaline cartilage may be present.
- Focal hemosiderin deposition may be seen.
- Aneurysmal bone cyst–like changes may be seen in small percentage of cases.

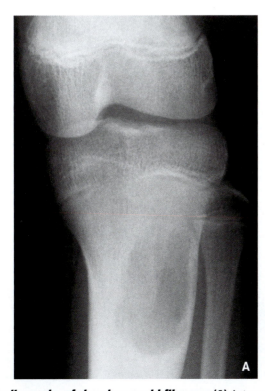 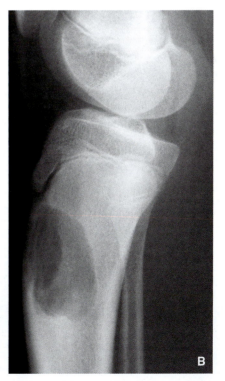

FIGURE 3.62 Radiography of chondromyxoid fibroma. (A) Anteroposterior and **(B)** lateral radiographs of the left knee of a 12-year-old girl show a radiolucent, slightly lobulated lesion with a thin sclerotic margin in the proximal tibial diaphysis, exhibiting geographic type of bone destruction.

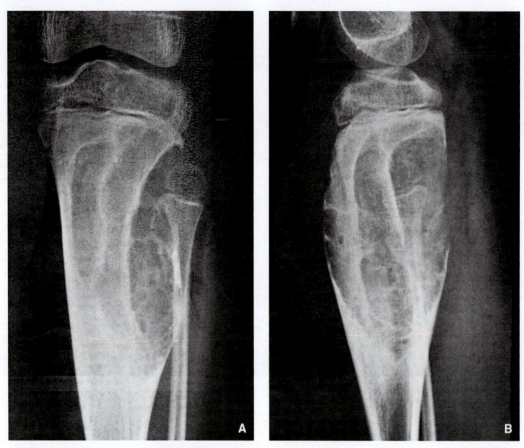

FIGURE 3.63 Radiography of chondromyxoid fibroma. (A) Anteroposterior and **(B)** lateral radiographs of the proximal left leg of an 8-year-old girl demonstrate a radiolucent lesion extending from the metaphysis into the diaphysis of the tibia, exhibiting a geographic type of bone destruction, internal septa, and a sclerotic scalloped border.

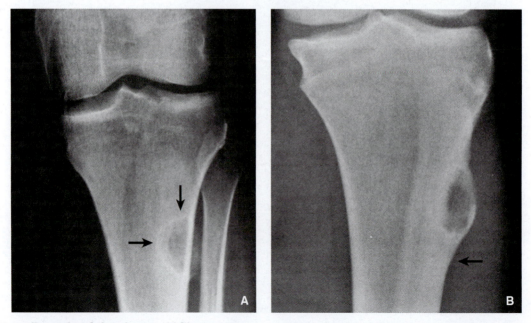

FIGURE 3.64 Radiography of chondromyxoid fibroma. (A) Anteroposterior radiograph of the left knee of an 18-year-old woman shows a radiolucent lesion located in the lateral aspect of proximal tibia (*arrows*). **(B)** An oblique radiograph shows that the lesion balloons out from the cortex and is supported by a solid buttress of periosteal reaction (*arrow*). This appearance closely resembles an aneurysmal bone cyst.

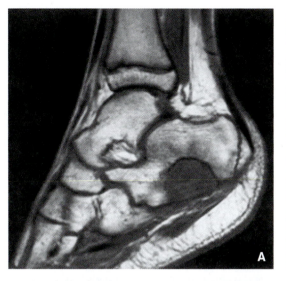
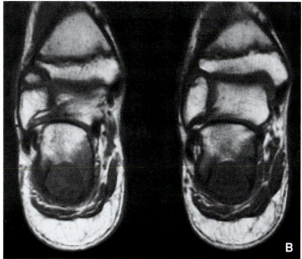
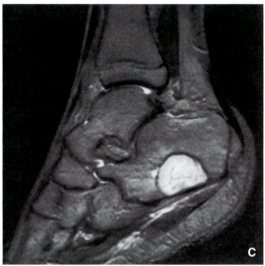

FIGURE 3.65 Magnetic resonance imaging of chondromyxoid fibroma. (A) Sagittal and **(B)** two coronal (short axis) T1–weighted MR images of the right ankle of a 10-year-old girl show a well-demarcated lesion in the plantar aspect of the calcaneus, displaying low signal intensity. **(C)** Sagittal T2–weighted MRI shows the lesion displaying homogenous high signal intensity. A sclerotic border is imaged as a rim of low signal intensity.

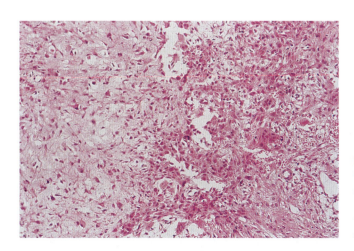

FIGURE 3.66 Histopathology of chondromyxoid fibroma. A photomicrograph shows the typical lobulated appearance of this tumor. Lobules of chondromyxoid tissue (*left and right*) are separated by the septum of cellular fibrous tissue (*center*), with occasional giant cells (H&E, original magnification ×50).

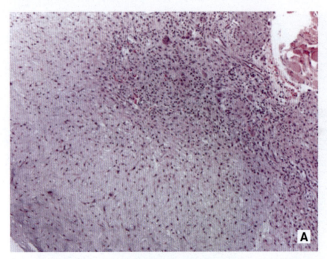 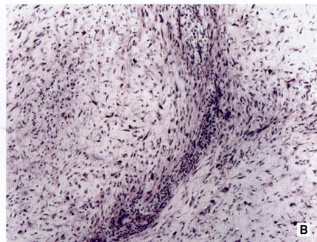

FIGURE 3.67 Histopathology of chondromyxoid fibroma. (A) Cartilaginous lesion shows lobular pattern with stellate and spindle-shaped cells in fibromyxoid background (H&E, original magnification ×100). **(B)** Higher-magnification photomicrograph demonstrates hypercellular areas at the periphery of the cartilaginous nodule and hypocellular areas in the center (H&E, original magnification ×200).

- Rare mitotic figures without atypia may be seen.
- Calcification may be seen in long-standing lesions.

Immunophenotype:
- S-100 may be positive in spindle cells.
- CD34 may be positive at the periphery.

Genetics:
- Clonal abnormalities of chromosome 6, most common rearrangement of the long arm chromosome 6 bands q13 and q25.

Prognostic Factors:
- Good prognosis.
- Recurrences are in the range of about 15%.

Differential Diagnosis:
- **Aneurysmal bone cyst**
  Cystic cavities.
  Fluid–fluid levels are characteristic.
  Scintigraphy may show characteristic increased uptake in a ring-like pattern around the periphery of the lesion.
  Histopathology shows multiple blood-filled spaces alternating with more solid areas; solid tissue is composed of fibrous, richly vascular connective tissue.
- **Nonossifying fibroma**
  No periosteal reaction.
  Lack of "ballooning."
  Histopathology shows bland monomorphous spindle cells admixed with histiocytic cells that often possess a clear or foamy cytoplasm and are arranged in storiform pattern.
- **Fibrous dysplasia**
  Usually central lesion.
  Rind sign.
  "Ground-glass" appearance.
  No periosteal reaction.
  Histopathology shows small trabeculae of woven bone of various shapes and sizes, resembling Chinese characters, scattered within the fibrous tissue without evidence of osteoblastic activity ("naked trabeculae").

B. MALIGNANT CARTILAGE-FORMING TUMORS

Chondrosarcomas

Chondrosarcoma is a malignant bone tumor characterized by the formation of a cartilage matrix by tumor cells, accompanied by infiltration of the marrow cavity and entrapment of preexisting bone trabeculae, destruction of normal bone, and infiltration of haversian systems. There are several types of this tumor (Fig. 3.68), each with characteristic clinical, imaging, and pathologic features. The degree of malignancy of chondrosarcoma is determined by several histologic criteria. These include structural characteristics (number of cells and appearance of matrix), cytologic findings (size of cells, pleomorphism, nuclear details, and presence or absence of bizarre cell forms), and replicate activity (mitotic figures, binucleated or multinucleated cells). There is a decided correlation between the histologic structure and the clinical behavior of these tumors. It is therefore important to differentiate between low-grade, intermediate-grade, and high-grade chondrosarcomas (grades 1, 2, and 3, respectively) (Table 3.2, also see Fig. 3.88). Such differentiation is based on several histologic characteristics, including the cellularity of the tumor tissue (e.g., hypocellular, hypercellular), the degree of pleomorphism observed in cells and nuclei (e.g., the presence of double and multinucleated cells, bizarre-shaped nuclei, large nuclei), and the degree of hyperchromasia of

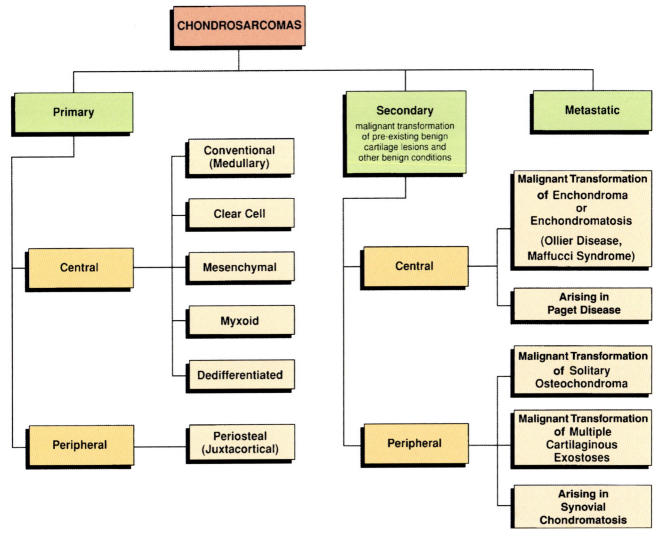

FIGURE 3.68 Classification of chondrosarcomas.

the nuclei (e.g., hyperchromatism). Certain other histologic signs are also indicative of degree of malignancy, such as invasion of trabeculae by tumor tissue, infiltration of bone marrow and haversian canals, and permeation through the cortex.

Conventional Chondrosarcoma (Central or Medullary Chondrosarcoma)

Definition:
- Malignant tumor with pure hyaline cartilage differentiation.
- Myxoid changes, calcifications, or ossifications may be present.

Epidemiology:
- Accounts for about 80% of all chondrosarcomas.
- Third most common primary malignancy of bone after myeloma and osteosarcoma.
- Tumor of adulthood and old age; the majority of patients are older than 50 years; the peak incidence is in the fifth to seventh decades of life.
- Slight preference for males.
- Very rare in younger patients (usually presents as high-grade malignancy).

Sites of Involvement:
- Most common skeletal sites are the bones of the pelvis (the ilium is the most frequently involved bone), followed by the proximal femur, proximal humerus, distal femur, and ribs.
- The small bones of the hands and feet are rarely involved.
- Extremely rare in the spine and craniofacial bones.

Clinical Findings:
- Local swelling and pain, alone or in combination.
- The symptoms are usually of long duration (several months or years).

TABLE 3.2 Histologic Grading of Chondrosarcoma

Grade	Histologic Features
0.5 (borderline)	Histologic features similar to enchondroma but imaging features more aggressive
1 (low grade)	Cellularity: slightly increased
	Cytologic atypia: slight increase in size and variation in shape of the nuclei; slightly increased hyperchromasia of the nuclei
	Binucleation: few binucleate cells are present
	Stromal myxoid change: may or may not be present
2 (intermediate)	Cellularity: moderately increased
	Cytologic atypia: moderate increase in size and variation in shape of the nuclei; moderately increased hyperchromasia of the nuclei
	Binucleation: large number of double-nucleated and trinucleated cells
	Stromal myxoid change: focally present
3 (high grade)	Cellularity: markedly increased
	Cytologic atypia: marked enlargement and irregularity of the nuclei; markedly increased hyperchromasia of the nuclei
	Binucleation: large number of double- and multinucleated cells
	Stromal myxoid change: commonly present
	Other: small foci of spindling at the periphery of the lobules of chondrocytes; foci of necrosis present

Modified from Dahlin DC. Grading of bone tumors. In: Unni KK, ed. *Bone Tumors*. New York: Churchill Livingstone; 1988:35–45.

Imaging:

- Radiography shows fusiform expansion of the medullary cavity with cortical thickening and deep endosteal scalloping (Figs. 3.69 and 3.70).
- Variably distributed punctate, comma-shaped, or ring-like calcifications (Figs. 3.70 and 3.71).
- Cortical erosion or destruction is usually present, which may result in a pathologic fracture (Fig. 3.72).
- Periosteal reaction is scant or absent (Fig. 3.73).
- Scintigraphy invariably shows increased uptake of radiopharmaceutical agent (Fig. 3.74).
- CT is effective in demonstrating matrix calcification (Figs. 3.75 to 3.78).
- MRI can be helpful in delineating the intramedullary extent of the tumor and establishing the presence of soft-tissue extension. Low signal intensity on T1-weighted images and heterogeneous but predominantly high signal intensity on T2-weighted and other water-sensitive sequences. Enhancement on T1-weighted images obtained after intravenous administration of gadolinium (Figs. 3.79 to 3.82).

Pathology:

Gross (Macroscopy):

- Translucent blue-gray or white in color mass, reflecting the presence of hyaline cartilage (Figs. 3.83 and 3.84).
- Lobular growth pattern is a consistent finding.
- There may be zones containing myxoid or mucoid material and cystic areas.
- Cortical thickening (Fig. 3.85, see also Fig. 3.83).
- Erosion and destruction of the cortex with extension into soft tissue may be present (Fig. 3.86), especially in the flat bones (pelvis, scapula, ribs, and sternum).

Histopathology:

- The histopathologic hallmark is production of malignant cartilage by the tumor cells accompanied by infiltration of the marrow cavity and entrapment and permeation of preexisting bone trabeculae and infiltration of haversian systems (see grading, Table 3.2, and Figs. 3.87 and 3.88).
- Lobules of cartilage varying in size and shape are present.
- Lobules may be separated by fibrous bands.
- Tumor is hypercellular and pleomorphic when compared to enchondroma.
- Chondrocytes are atypical, varying in size and shape, and contain enlarged, hyperchromatic nuclei.
- Extent of atypia is usually mild to moderate.
- Binucleation is commonly seen.
- Permeation of cortical and/or cancellous bone is an important characteristic that can be used to differentiate this tumor from enchondroma.
- Myxoid changes or chondroid matrix liquefaction is a common feature.

Chapter 3 • Cartilage-Forming (Chondrogenic) Lesions **141**

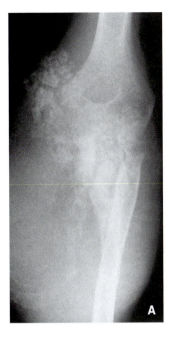
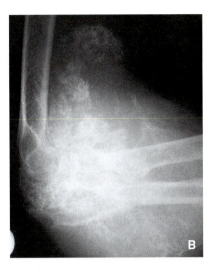

FIGURE 3.69 Radiography of conventional chondrosarcoma. (A) Anteroposterior and **(B)** lateral radiographs of the right elbow of a 55-year-old man show a tumor arising from the proximal ulna, associated with a large soft-tissue mass containing chondroid calcifications.

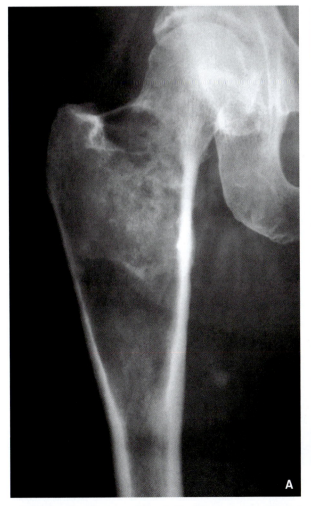
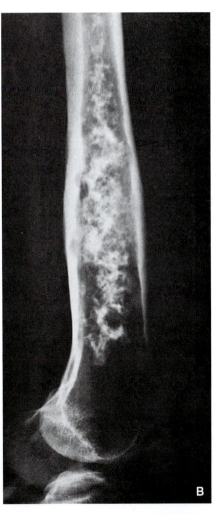

FIGURE 3.70 Radiography of conventional chondrosarcoma. (A) Anteroposterior radiograph of the proximal right femur of a 66-year-old woman shows a radiolucent lesion containing chondroid calcifications. Although the tumor did not penetrate the cortex, the medial cortex is thickened. **(B)** Lateral radiograph of the distal femur of a 46-year-old man shows the characteristic features of this tumor. Within the destructive lesion in the medullary portion of the bone, noted are annular and comma-shaped calcifications. The cortex is thickened due to periosteal new bone formation in response to tumor invasion. Also noted is typical deep scalloping of the endocortex.

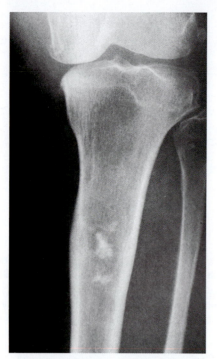

FIGURE 3.71 Radiography of conventional chondrosarcoma. Anteroposterior radiograph of the left proximal leg of a 48-year-old woman shows a radiolucent lesion in the tibia with wide zone of transition and chondroid calcifications. The bone is slightly focally expanded, and the cortex is thickened.

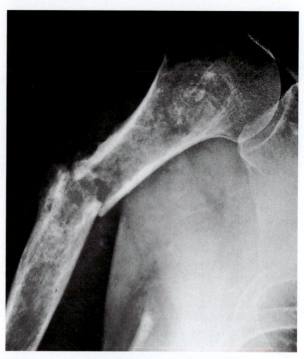

FIGURE 3.72 Radiography of complication of conventional chondrosarcoma. Note a pathologic fracture through a tumor affecting the right humerus of a 60-year-old man.

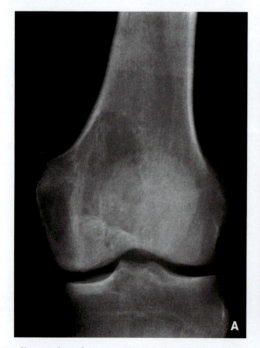
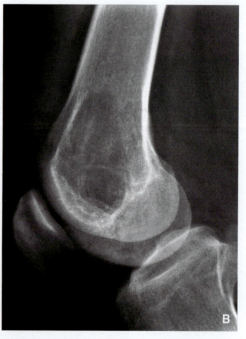

FIGURE 3.73 Radiography of conventional chondrosarcoma. (A) Anteroposterior and **(B)** lateral radiographs of the right knee of a 40-year-old man show a radiolucent lesion in the lateral femoral condyle, showing no visible calcifications nor periosteal reaction. The lesion resembles the giant cell tumor.

- Necrosis and mitoses can be present, particularly in high-grade tumors.
- The most significant histopathologic feature of tumor involving the small bones is permeation through the cortex into soft tissue and a permeative pattern in the cancellous bone.

Genetics:
- The most frequent numerical anomalies are loss of chromosomes 1, 6, 10, 13, 14, 15, and 22 and gain of chromosomes 2 and 20; also reported were rearrangements of chromosome bands 5q13, 1q21, 7p11, and 20q11.

Prognosis:
- Five-year survival is about 90% for patients with grade 1; the combined group of patients with grades 2 and 3 have a 5-year survival of 53%.
- Approximately 10% of tumors that recur have an increase in the degree of malignancy.

Differential Diagnosis:
- ***Osteosarcoma***
  Occurs in younger age.
  Metaphyseal involvement more common than diaphyseal.
  Tumor bone formation in form of fluffy densities within the lesion and in the soft-tissue mass.
  Aggressive sunburst or onionskin periosteal reaction.
  Histopathology shows tumor osteoid or tumor bone formation by malignant cells.

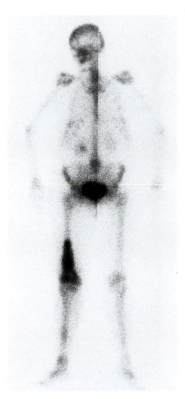

FIGURE 3.74 Scintigraphy of conventional chondrosarcoma. After intravenous administration of 15 mCi (555MBq) of technetium-labeled methylene diphosphonate (^{99m}Tc-MDP), radionuclide bone scan was obtained in a 61-year-old man with a tumor in the right femur. There is significantly increased uptake of the tracer localized to the site of the lesion.

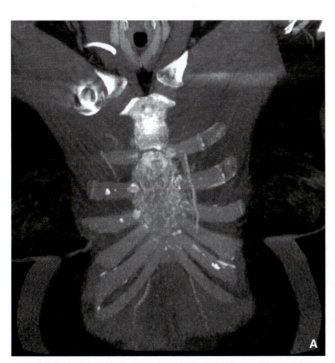
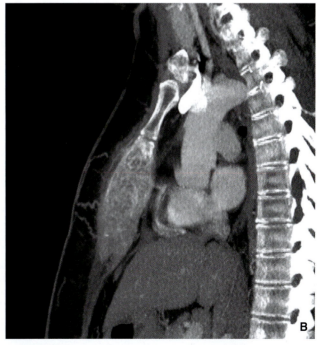

FIGURE 3.75 Computed tomography of conventional chondrosarcoma. (A) Coronal and **(B)** sagittal reformatted CT images of the chest of a 50-year-old man show an expansive osteolytic lesion within the body of the sternum containing chondroid calcifications.

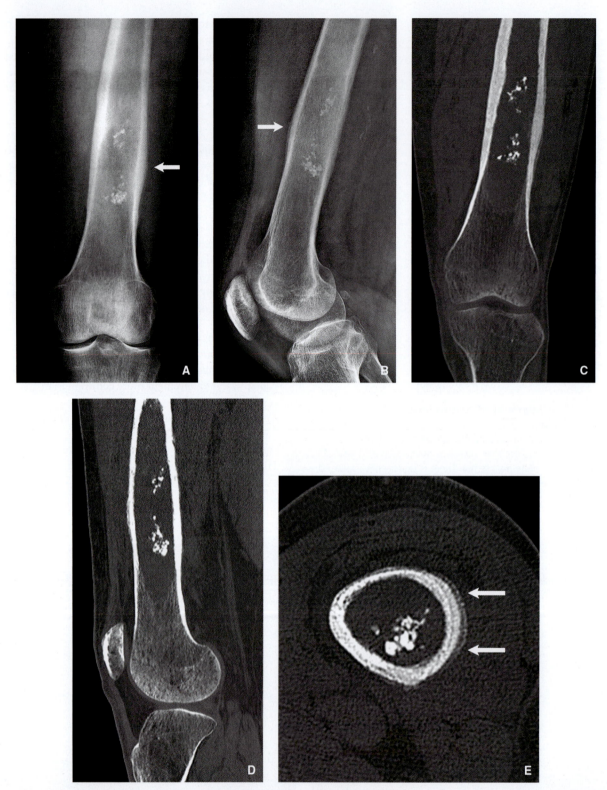

FIGURE 3.76 Radiography and computed tomography of conventional chondrosarcoma. (A) Anteroposterior and **(B)** lateral radiographs of the left distal femur show a radiolucent lesion with chondroid calcifications expanding the bone, associated with cortical thickening and periosteal reaction (*arrows*). **(C)** Coronal, **(D)** sagittal, and **(E)** axial CT images demonstrate cortical thickening and periosteal reaction to better advantage (*arrows*).

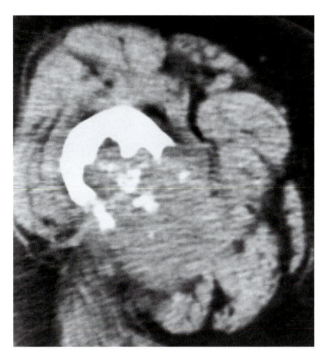

FIGURE 3.77 Computed tomography of conventional chondrosarcoma. CT section through the tumor located in the proximal right femur of a 69-year-old man shows thickening of the cortex, endosteal scalloping, chondroid calcifications, and a large soft-tissue mass.

- *Enchondroma*
  Lesion usually less than 5 cm in length.
  Lack of deep endosteal scalloping.
  Normal or thinned-out cortex.
  Lack of periosteal reaction.

Histopathology shows low-to-moderate cellularity; nodules of hyaline cartilage well demarcated by surrounding bone; lack of invasion and entrapment of trabeculae.

Clear Cell Chondrosarcoma

Definition:
- Rare, low-grade variant of chondrosarcoma, characterized histologically by bland clear cells in addition to hyaline cartilage.

Epidemiology:
- Represents about 2% of all chondrosarcomas and 0.2% of all primary bone tumors.
- Male-to-female ratio of 2:1.
- Patient age ranges between 25 and 50 years.

Sites of Involvement:
- Any bone can be involved; however, preferentially, the articular ends (epiphyses) of long tubular bones are most common locations, particularly humeral and femoral heads.

Imaging:
- Radiography shows predominantly lytic lesion with sclerotic border and central chondroid calcifications; occasionally endosteal scalloping is present; periosteal reaction is rare, as is soft-tissue mass. Frequently, the appearance of this tumor resembles chondroblastoma (Fig. 3.89A).
- Computed tomography shows calcification to better advantage (Fig. 3.89B).
- MRI shows homogeneous intermediate signal intensity on T1-weighted images and heterogeneous but mostly bright signal on T2 weighting and other water-sensitive sequences (Fig. 3.90).

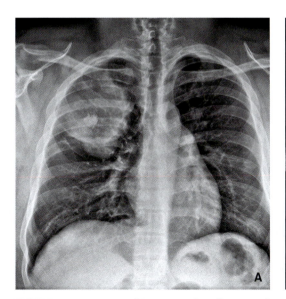
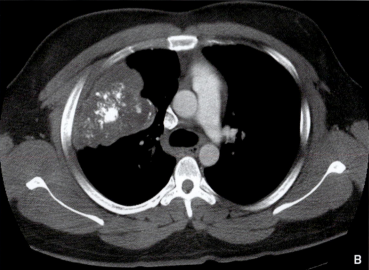

FIGURE 3.78 Computed tomography of conventional chondrosarcoma. (A) Posteroanterior radiograph of the chest of a 20-year-old man shows a large mass with central chondroid calcifications in the right upper lobe. **(B)** Axial CT image confirms the presence of a large lobulated mass containing chondroid calcifications arising from and destroying the right third rib and compressing the upper lobe of the right lung.

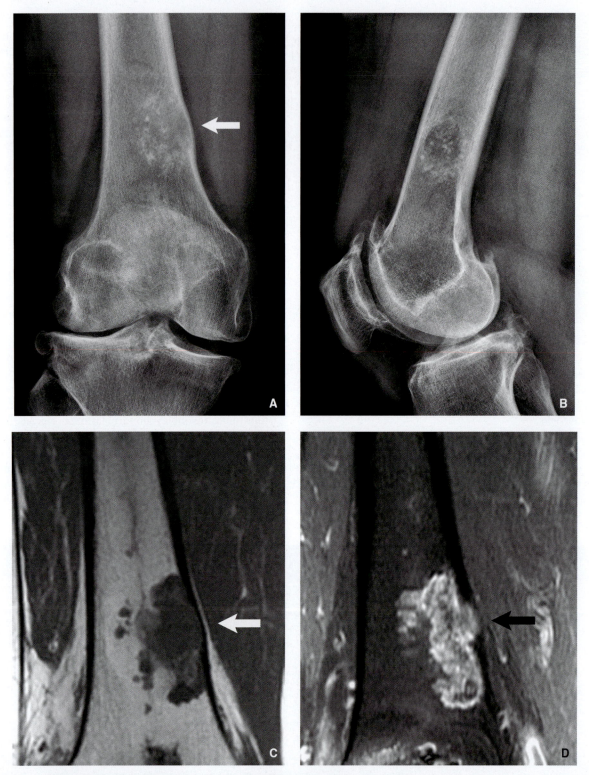

FIGURE 3.79 Radiography and magnetic resonance imaging of conventional chondrosarcoma. (A) Anteroposterior and **(B)** lateral radiographs of the right knee of a 58-year-old woman show a radiolucent lesion with chondroid calcifications in the medullary portion of the distal femur. Note deep endosteal scalloping of the posteromedial cortex (*arrow*). **(C)** Coronal T1–weighted and **(D)** T1-weighted fat-suppressed postcontrast MR images demonstrate the endosteal scalloping to better advantage (*arrows*). Observe heterogeneous signal of the tumor due to chondroid calcifications.

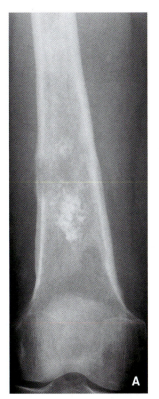
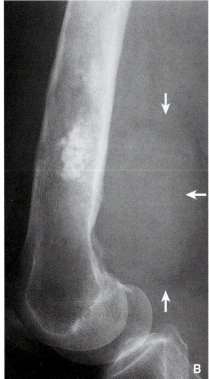
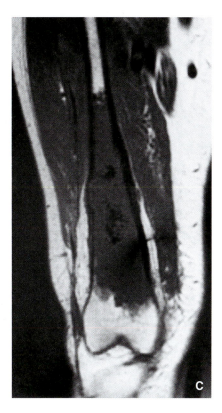
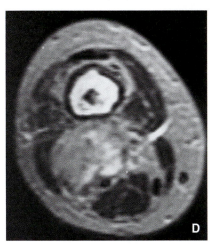

FIGURE 3.80 Radiography and magnetic resonance imaging of conventional chondrosarcoma. (A) Anteroposterior and **(B)** lateral radiographs of the distal femur show typical appearance of high-grade central medullary chondrosarcoma. The radiolucent tumor with chondroid calcifications destroys the cortex and forms a large soft-tissue mass (*arrows*). **(C)** Coronal T1–weighted MR image shows the tumor to be of low signal intensity. The central calcifications display signal void. **(D)** Axial T2–weighted MRI shows the tumor exhibiting high signal intensity with calcifications being of low signal. The soft-tissue extension of the tumor shows heterogeneous signal.

Pathology:

Gross (Macroscopy):

- Soft but gritty material with possible cystic changes.
- Size ranges between 2 and 13 cm.
- Cartilage may or may not be seen grossly.

Histopathology:

- Lobular groups of cells with round, small, or large centrally located nuclei and clear cytoplasm with distinct cytoplasmic membranes (Figs. 3.91 and 3.92).
- Some of the cells may have pink cytoplasm resembling the chondroblasts of chondroblastoma.
- Multinucleated osteoclast-like giant cells may be seen.
- Some lesions may show areas of conventional low-grade chondrosarcoma.
- Calcification, reactive woven bone, and areas of aneurysmal bone cyst may be seen in some cases.

Immunophenotype:

- Positive for S-100 protein and type II collagen.
- Immunoreactivity for type X collagen and osteonectin.

Genetics:

- *CDKN2A*/p16 alterations appear to be infrequent.
- Loss or structural aberrations of chromosome 9 and gain of chromosome 20.

Prognosis:

- *En bloc* excision with clear margins usually is curative.
- Marginal excision or curettage results in high recurrence (about 86%).

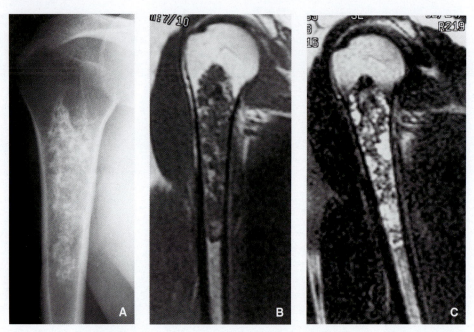

FIGURE 3.81 Radiography and magnetic resonance imaging of conventional chondrosarcoma. (A) Conventional radiograph of a 48-year-old man shows a cartilaginous lesion in the proximal right humerus. Although the cortex is not thickened, and there is no evidence of deep endosteal scalloping, the length of the lesion (15 cm) suggests malignancy. **(B)** Coronal T1–weighted and **(C)** T2-weighted MR images show heterogeneous signal intensity of the lesion and confirm lack of cortical thickening or endosteal scalloping. On biopsy, the tumor proved to be a low-grade chondrosarcoma.

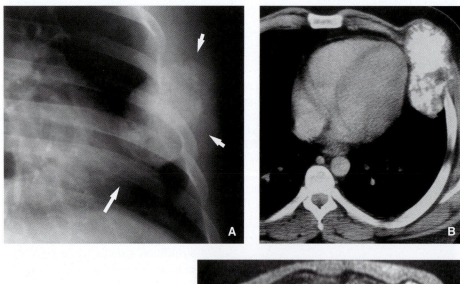
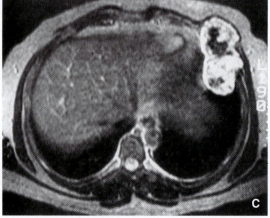

FIGURE 3.82 Computed tomography and magnetic resonance imaging of conventional chondrosarcoma.
(A) A large calcified mass arises from the left anterior sixth rib (*arrows*).
(B) Axial CT section reveals destruction of the rib and intrathoracic and extrathoracic extension of the tumor.
(C) Axial T2–weighted MR image demonstrates heterogeneity of the tumor. Areas of low-intensity signal represent calcified portion of the mass.

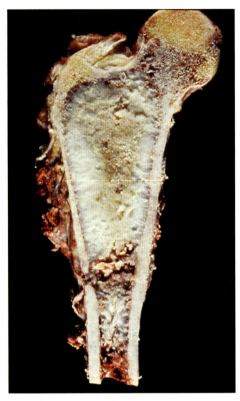

FIGURE 3.83 Gross specimen of conventional chondrosarcoma. Solid blue-gray cartilaginous tumor expands the proximal femoral shaft. The medial cortex is slightly thickened (same patient as shown in Fig. 3.70A).

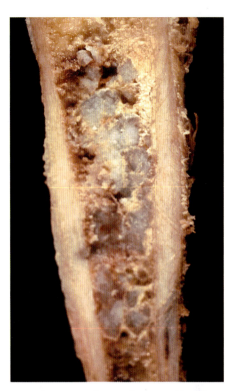

FIGURE 3.85 Gross specimen of conventional chondrosarcoma. Gray-blue lobules of malignant cartilage tissue expand the medullary portion of the tibia. The cortex is markedly thickened.

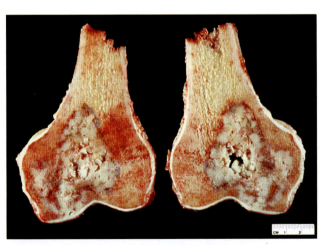

FIGURE 3.84 Gross specimen of conventional chondrosarcoma. Malignant cartilage tissue replaces cancellous bone in the distal femur. No visible calcifications are present. There is no obvious alteration of the cortex (same patient as depicted in Fig. 3.73).

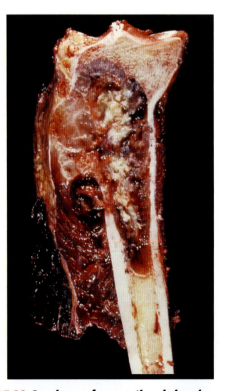

FIGURE 3.86 Specimen of conventional chondrosarcoma. A large cartilaginous tumor with calcifications is present in the medullary portion of the tibia, breaking through the cortex and forming a large soft-tissue mass.

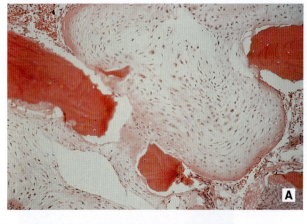
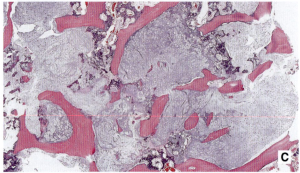
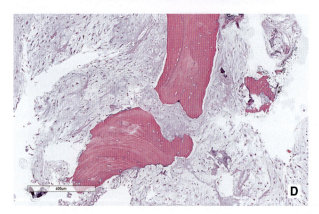
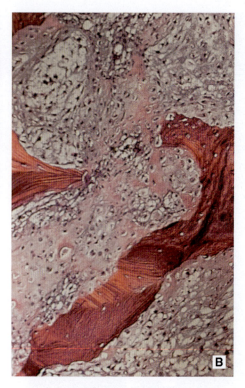

FIGURE 3.87 Histopathology of conventional chondrosarcoma. (A) Markedly cellular chondroid tissue invades the host bone trabeculae (H&E, original magnification ×25). **(B)** The cartilage lobules of the tumor showing pleomorphism and marked cellularity invades the preexisting bone trabeculae (H&E, original magnification ×100). **(C)** Entrapment and permeation of lamellar bone trabeculae and prominent myxoid changes are characteristic for this malignancy (H&E, original magnification ×100). **(D)** The higher magnification shows pleomorphism and hypercellularity of the tumor permeating the preexisting bone trabeculae (H&E, original magnification ×200).

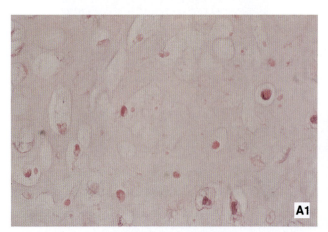
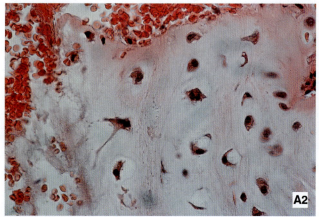

FIGURE 3.88 Histopathology of conventional chondrosarcoma. (A1) *Grade 1.* Low-cellularity tumor shows slightly abnormal nuclei (H&E, original magnification ×156). **(A2) *Grade 1.*** At higher magnification, note the variation in shape of the nuclei and hyperchromasia (H&E, original magnification ×400).

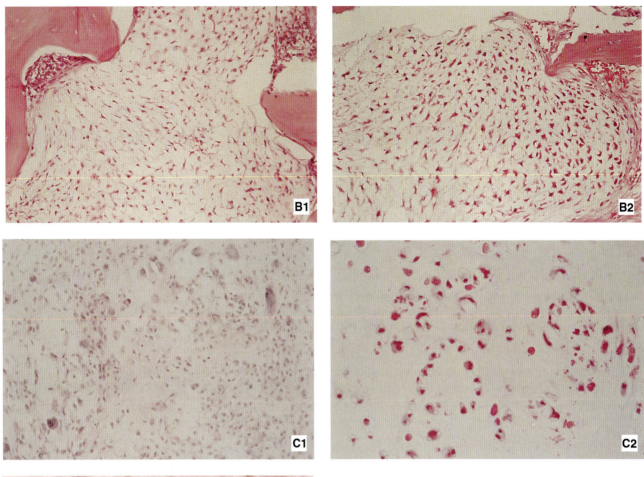
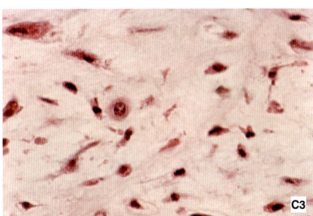

FIGURE 3.88 *(Continued).* **(B1)** *Grade 2.* The tumor exhibits moderately increased cellularity and several double-nucleated cells are present (H&E, original magnification ×25). **(B2)** *Grade 2.* At higher magnification, focal myxoid changes of the stroma are evident (H&E, original magnification ×50). **(C1)** *Grade 3.* The tumor is markedly cellular, showing pleomorphism and hyperchromatism of the nuclei. In addition to crowding of the cells, they are lying in a myxoid matrix (H&E, original magnification ×50). **(C2)** *Grade 3.* Note irregularly distributed cells with marked pleomorphism of nuclei. Numerous bi- and trinucleated cells are present (H&E, original magnification ×100). **(C3)** *Grade 3.* At high magnification, note markedly pleomorphic cells, some with double nuclei and some exhibiting mitosis (H&E, original magnification ×325).

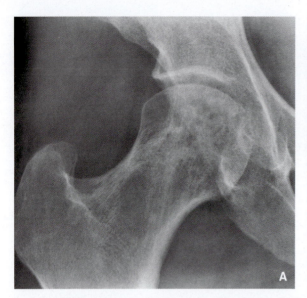
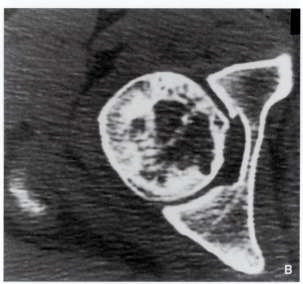

FIGURE 3.89 Radiography and computed tomography of clear cell chondrosarcoma. (A) Anteroposterior radiograph of the right hip shows a radiolucent lesion with chondroid calcifications within the femoral head. Note resemblance of the lesion to chondroblastoma. **(B)** Axial CT image shows the lytic character of the lesion and central calcifications to better advantage.

- In cases with incomplete excision, metastases to the other skeletal sites and lungs may develop.
- Dedifferentiation to high-grade sarcomas was reported.

Differential Diagnosis:

- ***Chondroblastoma***

    Imaging features very similar to clear cell chondrosarcoma.

    Histopathology shows nodules of fairly mature cartilage matrix surrounded by highly cellular, relatively undifferentiated tissue composed of round and polygonal chondroblast-like cells containing uniform shaped and moderate in size, usually indented nuclei. Characteristic are fine, lattice-like calcifications having a spatial arrangement that resemble hexagonal configuration of chicken wire.

Mesenchymal Chondrosarcoma

Definition:

- Rare malignant tumor characterized by a biomorphic pattern consisting of highly undifferentiated small round cells and islands of well-differentiated hyaline cartilage.

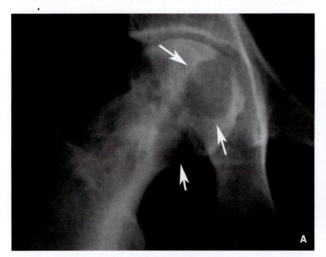
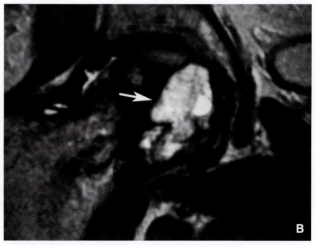

FIGURE 3.90 Radiography and magnetic resonance imaging of clear cell chondrosarcoma. (A) Anteroposterior radiograph of the right hip of a young man shows irregularly shaped lytic lesion with sclerotic margin in the femoral head and neck (*arrows*). **(B)** Coronal T2–weighted MR image demonstrates a hyperintense tumor, well demarcated from the normal bone (*arrow*).

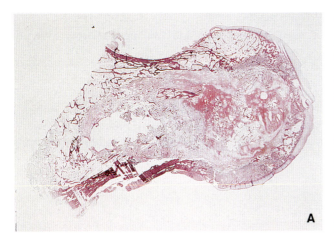
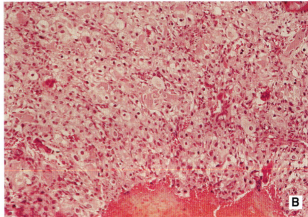
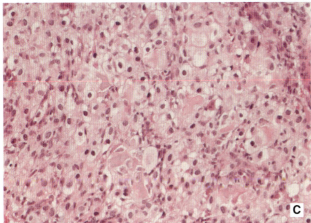

FIGURE 3.91 Histopathology of clear cell chondrosarcoma. **(A)** Coronal section of the resected femoral head and neck shows extension of the tumor from articular cartilage to the base of the neck (H&E, original magnification ×0.2). **(B)** There is solid arrangement of homogeneous area of large polygonal cells displaying a clear or slightly eosinophilic cytoplasm and small, dark, roundish nuclei. Some giant cells are also present. Note small areas of necrosis (*center and bottom*) (H&E, original magnification ×50). **(C)** Higher magnification shows large cells with clear or slightly eosinophilic cytoplasm and small nuclei, typical for this variant of chondrosarcoma. In addition, large eosinophilic deposits are present, resembling osteoid (H&E, original magnification ×200).

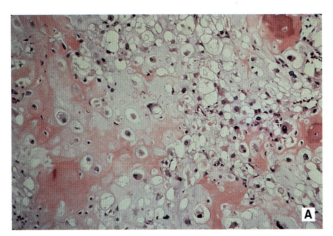
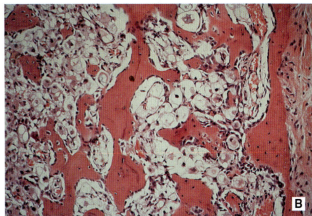

FIGURE 3.92 Histopathology of clear cell chondrosarcoma. **(A)** Large and vacuolated cells are dispersed in the intercellular cartilaginous matrix. Note small osteoid trabeculae (H&E, original magnification ×150). **(B)** In another area, vacuolated cells are seen in close proximity to reactive bone trabeculae (H&E, original magnification ×75).

Epidemiology:
- Represents less than 3% of all primary chondrosarcomas.
- May occur at any age, but the peak incidence is in the second and third decades of life.
- Equally affects men and women.

Sites of Involvement:
- Most common locations are craniofacial bones (mandible and maxilla), ribs, femur, fibula, ilium, and vertebrae.
- Multiple bones may be involved.
- About 30% of cases develop in extraskeletal site.

Clinical Findings:
- Long-standing pain and swelling associated with soft-tissue mass.
- Secondary osteogenic osteomalacia.

Imaging:
- This tumor exhibits no characteristic imaging pattern. It may resemble a conventional chondrosarcoma or present as a mixture of cartilage tumor and round cell tumor (Fig. 3.93).

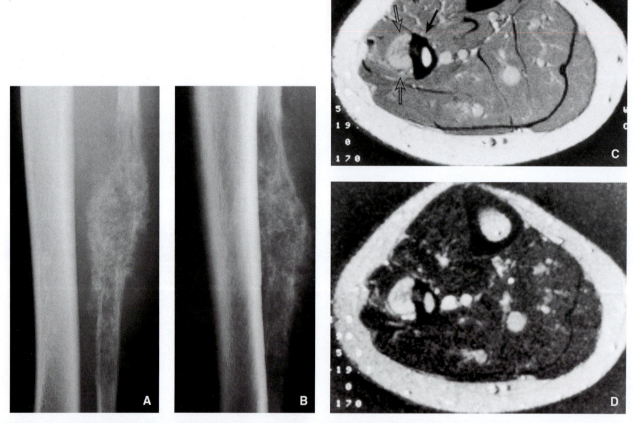

FIGURE 3.93 **Radiography and magnetic resonance imaging of mesenchymal chondrosarcoma.** (**A**) Anteroposterior and (**B**) lateral coned-down radiographs of the right leg of a 43-year-old woman show a destructive lesion of the midportion of the fibula. The central portion of the lesion exhibits comma-shaped and annular calcification typical of a cartilage tumor, but its periphery shows a permeative type of bone destruction, more characteristic of a round cell tumor. In another patient, axial T1–weighted MRI (**C**) shows a focus of intermediate signal intensity within the low signal intensity of the lateral cortex of the fibula (*arrow*). A soft-tissue mass displays a signal slightly higher than the muscles but lower than that of subcutaneous fat (*open arrows*). (**D**) Axial T2-weighted MR image shows the tumor displaying high signal intensity.

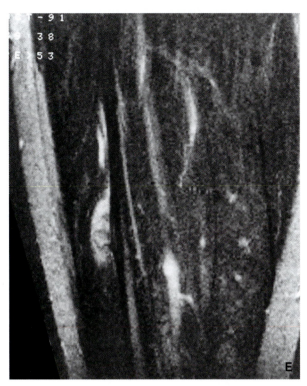
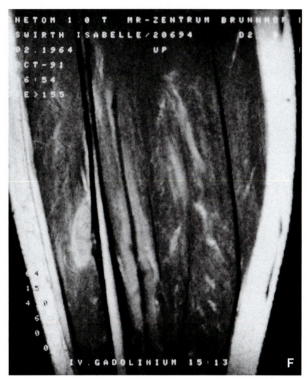

FIGURE 3.93 *(Continued).* **(E)** Coronal T2–weighted MR image better demonstrates the destruction of the fibular cortex. On these sequences, the soft-tissue mass becomes bright. **(F)** On coronal T1–weighted MR image obtained after intravenous administration of gadolinium, there is enhancement of the tumor.

Pathology:

Gross (Macroscopy):

- Solid gray-white to gray-pink, firm-to-soft, mostly well-defined, circumscribed mass, varying from 3 to 30 cm in diameter (Fig. 3.94).
- Rare lobulation.
- May show mineralization.
- Some tumors show clear cartilaginous component.
- Necrotic change and hemorrhage may be present.
- Common bone destruction and invasion of soft tissue.

Histopathology:

- Biphasic pattern consists of undifferentiated small round uniform-sized cells of mesenchymal tissue admixed with islands of well-differentiated hyaline cartilage, containing foci of calcifications and occasionally metaplastic bone encasement (Figs. 3.95 and 3.96).
- Cartilage may be well differentiated from the undifferentiated component or blend with it.
- Small round cell component may resemble Ewing sarcoma, which may be difficult to differentiate on biopsy tissue to distinguish these two different entities especially with lack of cartilaginous component.
- Small round cells may be spindle shaped to some extent.
- Rarely osteoclast-like giant cells and osteoid may be seen.
- Round cell component is positive for CD99 (Fig. 3.97A, see also Fig. 3.95E), and cartilaginous component is positive for S-100 protein (Fig. 3.97B).

Genetics:

- Negative for t(11,22), which is characteristic for Ewing sarcoma.
- Few cases showed t(13,21).
- Recurrent HEY1-NCOA2 fusion, representing fusion of HEY1 exon 4 to NCOA2 exon 13 at the mRNA level.

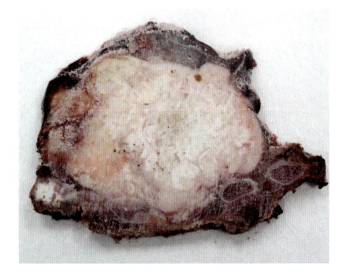

FIGURE 3.94 Gross specimen of mesenchymal chondrosarcoma. Solid cartilaginous tumor infiltrates the ribs and the soft tissues of the chest wall.

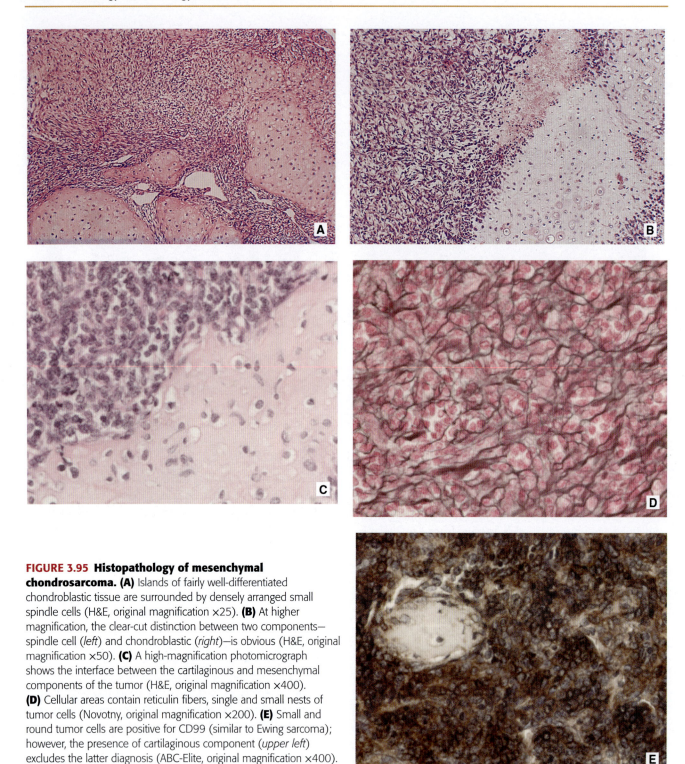

FIGURE 3.95 Histopathology of mesenchymal chondrosarcoma. (A) Islands of fairly well-differentiated chondroblastic tissue are surrounded by densely arranged small spindle cells (H&E, original magnification ×25). **(B)** At higher magnification, the clear-cut distinction between two components—spindle cell (*left*) and chondroblastic (*right*)—is obvious (H&E, original magnification ×50). **(C)** A high-magnification photomicrograph shows the interface between the cartilaginous and mesenchymal components of the tumor (H&E, original magnification ×400). **(D)** Cellular areas contain reticulin fibers, single and small nests of tumor cells (Novotny, original magnification ×200). **(E)** Small and round tumor cells are positive for CD99 (similar to Ewing sarcoma); however, the presence of cartilaginous component (*upper left*) excludes the latter diagnosis (ABC-Elite, original magnification ×400).

Chapter 3 • Cartilage-Forming (Chondrogenic) Lesions

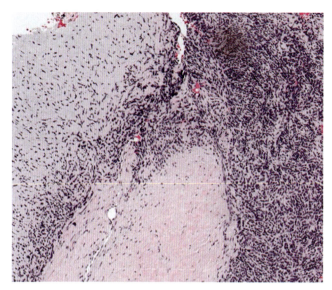

FIGURE 3.96 Histopathology of mesenchymal chondrosarcoma. Typical biphasic pattern consists of undifferentiated small round, uniform in size cells of mesenchymal tissue admixed with islands of well-differentiated hyaline cartilage (H&E, original magnification ×200).

Prognosis:
- Malignant tumor with a strong tendency toward local recurrence and distant metastases that are observed even after a delay of more than 20 years.

Myxoid Chondrosarcoma (Chordoid Sarcoma)
Definition:
- Very rare low-grade but locally aggressive malignant neoplasm showing chondroid differentiation.

Epidemiology:
- Represents approximately 12% of all chondrosarcomas of bone.
- Age range between 9 and 76 years, predominantly affecting males.

Sites of Involvement:
- Femur (50% of cases).

Imaging:
- Radiolucent, lobulated, sharply circumscribed lesion, commonly extending into the soft tissues (Fig. 3.98).

Pathology:
- Histopathology shows lobulated cartilaginous nodules with round stellate cells, some with acidophilic cytoplasm, and abundant myxoid matrix (Fig. 3.99). Occasionally, mitotic figures are present.

Differential Diagnosis:
- *Myxoid chondrosarcoma of soft tissues invading the bone* Very difficult to differentiate by imaging and histopathology.

Dedifferentiated Chondrosarcoma
Definition:
- Chondrosarcoma containing two clearly defined components, a well-differentiated cartilage tumor, either an enchondroma or a low-grade chondrosarcoma, with abrupt transition to a high-grade (not cartilaginous) sarcoma (most of the time malignant fibrous histiocytoma [MFH]).

Epidemiology:
- 10% of all chondrosarcomas.
- Average patient age between 50 and 60 years.

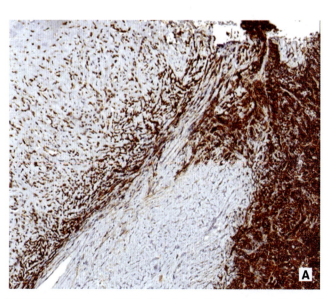 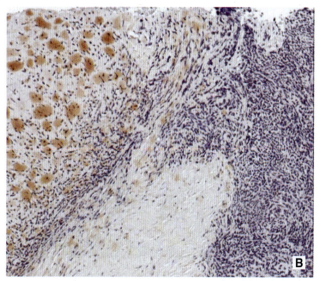

FIGURE 3.97 Immunohistochemistry of mesenchymal chondrosarcoma. (A) Cellular component of the tumor consisting of small round cells shows positivity for CD99 (brown stain) (original magnification ×200). **(B)** Well-differentiated hyaline cartilage is positive for S-100 protein (original magnification ×200).

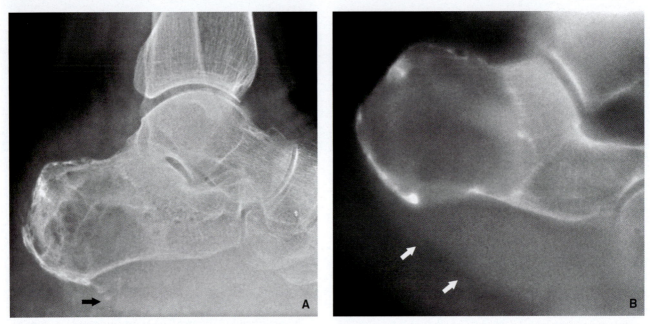

FIGURE 3.98 Radiography of myxoid chondrosarcoma. (A) Lateral radiograph of the hindfoot of a 65-year-old woman shows a large destructive lesion in the calcaneus. The tumor extends into the soft tissues (*arrow*). **(B)** Lateral conventional tomogram demonstrates the soft-tissue mass more effectively (*arrows*).

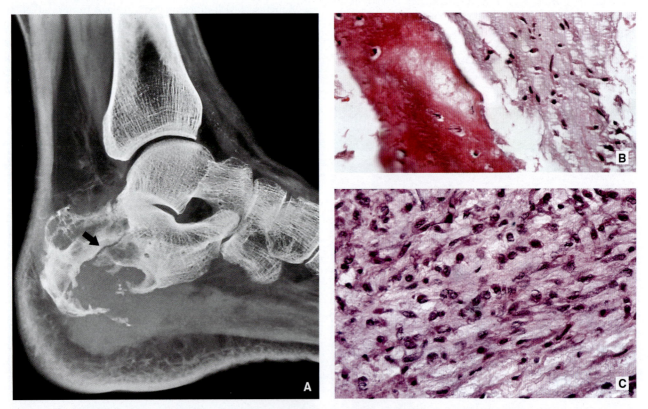

FIGURE 3.99 Histopathology of myxoid chondrosarcoma. (A) Lateral radiograph of the amputated specimen (same patient as shown in Fig. 3.98) shows a large osteolytic sharply marginated lesion in the posterior calcaneus, with a pathologic fracture (*arrow*). Soft-tissue extension of the tumor is clearly demonstrated. **(B)** Photomicrograph shows a myxoid pattern of cells, uniform in size, separated by abundant and pale basophilic matrix (*right*). The tumor invades the bone trabecula (*left*) (H&E, original magnification ×25). **(C)** At higher magnification, the tumor cells are rounded and elongated, fairly uniform in size, with prominent hyperchromatic nuclei. Note cartilaginous and myxoid features of the tumor (H&E, original magnification ×640).

Sites of Involvement:
- Most common location in the pelvis, femur, and humerus.

Clinical Features:
- Patients usually present with rapid onset of swelling and local tenderness superimposed on a long history of less severe discomfort.
- Paresthesia and pathologic fractures.
- Metastases to distant organs.

Imaging:
- Radiography shows biphasic pattern: long-standing benign-looking cartilage tumor and superimposed more aggressive appearing lesion exhibiting moth-eaten or permeative type of bone destruction (Figs. 3.100 and 3.101).
- CT and MRI similarly reveal two distinctive areas with different intrinsic characteristics, reflecting the coexistence of low-grade and high-grade cartilaginous tumors (Fig. 3.102).

Pathology:
Gross (Macroscopy):
- Both components, cartilaginous and noncartilaginous, are grossly evident in varying proportions (Figs. 3.103 to 3.106).
- Blue-gray lobulated low-grade cartilaginous component is located centrally with surrounding fleshy higher-grade component; note invasion of adjacent soft tissues.

Histopathology:
- Cartilaginous component is usually a low-grade chondrosarcoma (Figs. 3.107 and 3.108A).
- Characteristic abrupt demarcation between the two components (Fig. 3.108B) (in contrast to chondroblastic osteosarcoma where there is no abrupt demarcation between two components—osseous and cartilaginous, see Figs. 2.34 and 2.35).

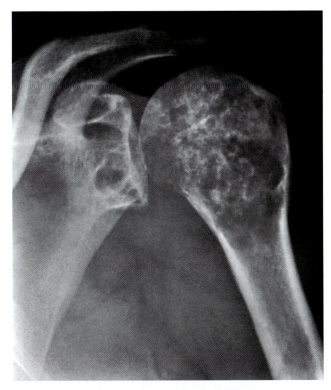

FIGURE 3.100 Radiography of dedifferentiated chondrosarcoma. Anteroposterior radiograph of the left shoulder of a 50-year-old man shows a lytic lesion in the humeral neck extending to the humeral head, containing typical chondroid calcifications. The distal part of the lesion exhibits more destructive pattern and deep endosteal scalloping.

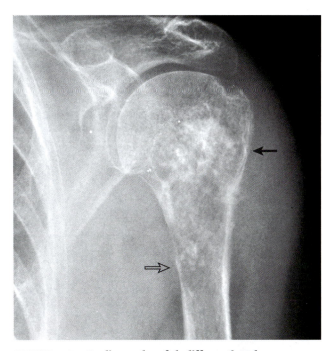

FIGURE 3.101 Radiography of dedifferentiated chondrosarcoma. A 70-year-old woman presented with a destructive lesion in the proximal left humerus associated with chondroid calcifications. The proximal part the lesion is consistent with a slow-growing tumor (*arrow*), whereas the distal part exhibits a more aggressive character including cortical destruction and a soft-tissue mass (*open arrow*). The excision biopsy revealed combination of grade 1 chondrosarcoma, MFH, and malignant giant cell tumor.

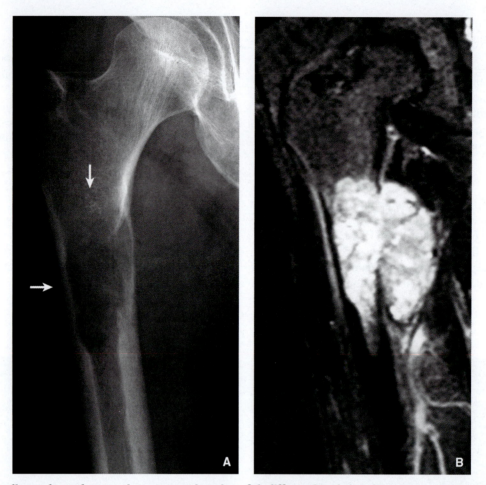

FIGURE 3.102 Radiography and magnetic resonance imaging of dedifferentiated chondrosarcoma. (A) Anteroposterior radiograph of the proximal right femur of a 60-year-old man shows a predominantly osteolytic destructive lesion in the subtrochanteric region (*arrows*). **(B)** Coronal STIR MR image shows the high signal intensity tumor breaking through the medial cortex to form a large soft-tissue mass.

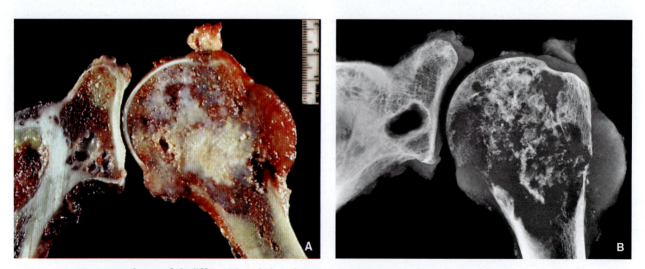

FIGURE 3.103 Gross specimen of dedifferentiated chondrosarcoma. (A) Resected surgical specimen of the left shoulder (patient had three-quarter amputation) shows lobules of cartilage invading humeral head and neck. Coarse calcifications are present proximally. Note more aggressive destruction at the distal part of the tumor, better demonstrated on the specimen radiograph **(B)** Radiograph of the resected specimen, in addition to the tumor in the proximal humerus, shows a benign lesion in the glenoid, proved to represent an intraosseous ganglion (same patient as shown in Fig. 3.100).

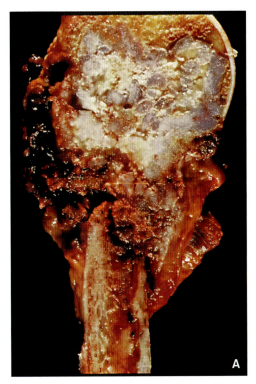
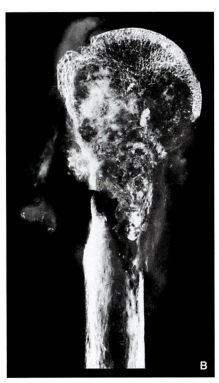

FIGURE 3.104 Gross specimen of dedifferentiated chondrosarcoma. (A) Resected surgical specimen of the proximal humerus and **(B)** specimen radiograph show biphasic appearance of cartilaginous tumor with a pathologic fracture through the more destructive portion of the lesion.

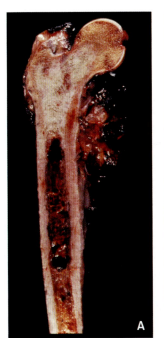
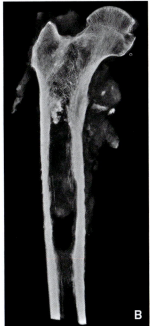

FIGURE 3.105 Gross specimen of dedifferentiated chondrosarcoma. (A) Resected surgical specimen of the right proximal femur and **(B)** specimen radiograph show biphasic appearance of cartilaginous tumor invading femoral neck and shaft. The distal part of the tumor is lytic, the cortex is markedly thickened, and there are endosteal erosions. Large soft-tissue mass is present medially. The calcified portion of the tumor in the femoral neck showed histopathologic features of enchondroma; the tissue from the femoral shaft showed mixture of grade 3 chondrosarcoma and MFH.

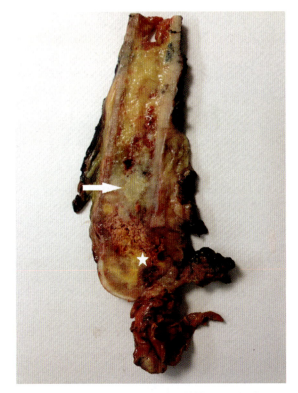

FIGURE 3.106 Gross specimen of dedifferentiated chondrosarcoma. In the tumor involving the distal femur, one can clearly distinguish two parts—gray-blue appearance of low-grade cartilaginous component (*arrow*) and yellow-tan to red-brown appearance of high-grade noncartilage sarcoma breaking through the cortex and extending into the soft tissues (*star*).

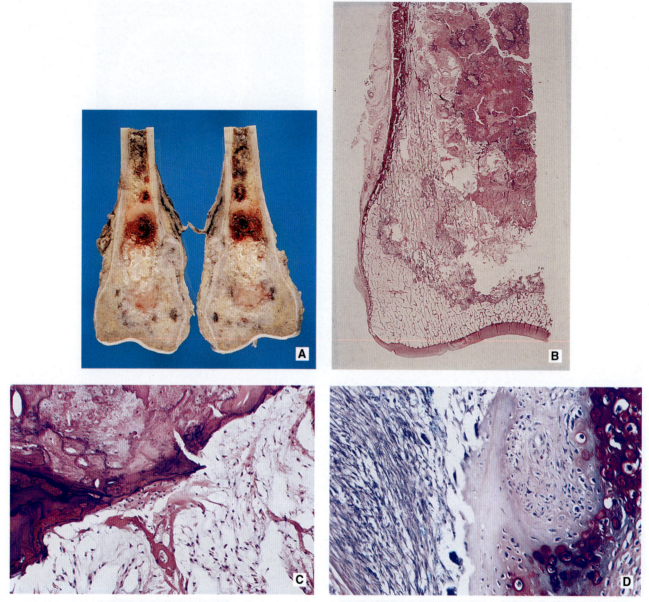

FIGURE 3.107 Gross specimen and histopathology of dedifferentiated chondrosarcoma. (A) Coronal section of the specimen of the distal femur shows calcified enchondroma (*round whitish areas in the center*), well-differentiated low-grade chondrosarcoma (*darker areas medially*), and dedifferentiated tumor (*rose areas distally*). Proximally note the hemorrhagic area (*red*). **(B)** Histologic overview of the medial half of the distal femur shows three different tumors: calcified enchondroma (*proximal middle*), well-differentiated chondrosarcoma (*section close to the medial cortex on the left*), and dedifferentiated tumor with osteoblastic differentiation (*distal middle*) (H&E, original magnification ×0.2). **(C)** Calcified enchondroma (*upper half*) is bordered by low-grade chondrosarcoma with myxoid component (H&E, original magnification ×25). **(D)** Two different tissues are clearly separated: on the right well-differentiated chondrosarcoma is abutting dedifferentiated part of the tumor formed of spindle cells and giant cells on the left.

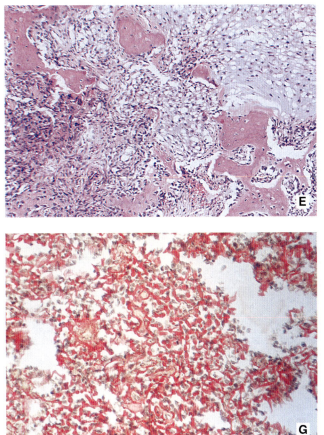
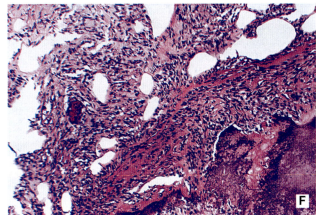
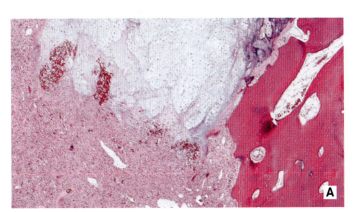

FIGURE 5.107 *(Continued).* **(E)** Another field of view shows well-differentiated chondrosarcoma (*upper right*) sharply demarcated from dedifferentiated tumor showing osteoblastic differentiation (*lower left*) (H&E, original magnification ×25). **(F)** Almost entirely cellular, dedifferentiated tumor tissue exhibits scanty tumor bone formation and remnants of cancellous bone (*lower right*) (H&E, original magnification ×25). **(G)** The dedifferentiated part of the tumor exhibits a delicate network of tumor osteoid (van Gieson, original magnification ×25).

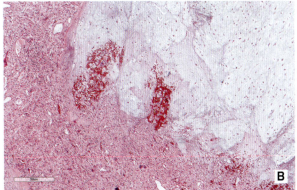

FIGURE 3.108 Histopathology of dedifferentiated chondrosarcoma. (A) There is an abrupt transition between low-grade cartilaginous tumor and high-grade spindle cell sarcoma (H&E, original magnification ×100). **(B)** On higher magnification, the character of two types of the cells is better appreciated (H&E, original magnification ×200).

- MFH is the most frequent component of the high-grade sarcoma; less common components are osteosarcoma, fibrosarcoma, rhabdomyosarcoma, and giant cell tumor (Figs. 3.109 and 3.110).

Genetics:
- Most common structural and numerical aberrations of chromosomes 1 and 9.
- Heterozygous mutations of the isocitrate dehydrogenase 1 and 2 genes were reported in both components in approximately 50% of these tumors.

Prognosis:
- Aggressive neoplasms; approximately 90% of patients develop distant metastases and died within 2 years.

Periosteal (Juxtacortical) Chondrosarcoma

Definition:
- A malignant cartilage tumor originating in periosteal location.

Epidemiology:
- Accounts for 4% of all malignant cartilage tumors.
- Adults in the third and fourth decade of life.
- Slight male predilection.

Sites of Involvement:
- Long bones, particularly the distal femur, and spine.

Clinical Findings:
- Asymptomatic or slightly painful slowly growing soft-tissue mass.

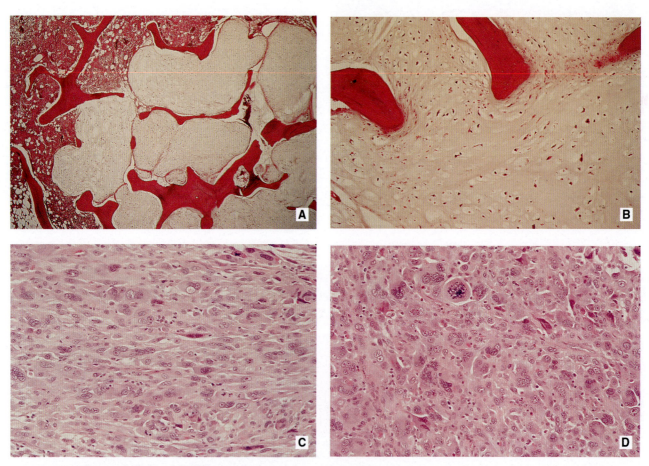

FIGURE 3.109 Histopathology of dedifferentiated chondrosarcoma. (A) Grade 1 chondrosarcoma invades marrow spaces of cancellous bone (*right 75%*). In addition, purely cellular dedifferentiated tumor tissue is present as well (*left 25%*) (van Gieson, original magnification ×12). **(B)** Higher magnification shows low-grade chondrosarcoma tissue flowing within the bone marrow spaces of cancellous bone (van Gieson, original magnification ×50). **(C)** In another field, spindle cell part of dedifferentiated tumor exhibits higher-grade malignant cells and nuclear pleomorphism (H&E, original magnification ×50). **(D)** Yet in another field, the dedifferentiated tissue represents a giant cell–rich variant of MFH (H&E, original magnification ×50) (same patient as in Fig. 3.104).

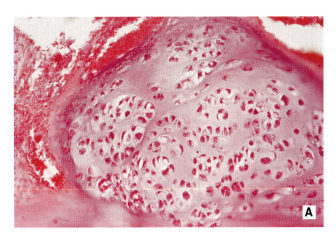
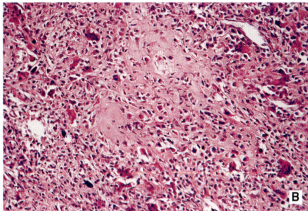
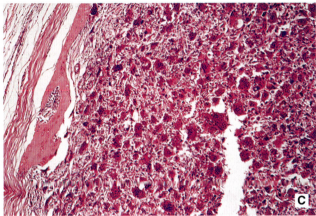

FIGURE 3.110 Histopathology of dedifferentiated chondrosarcoma. (A) In one part of the tumor, there is grade 2 chondrosarcoma with irregular distribution of chondrocytes (H&E, original magnification ×50). **(B)** The other part of the same tumor shows dedifferentiation with spindle cell tissue and tumor bone formation (*center*), typical for osteosarcoma. Some giant cells are also present (H&E, original magnification ×50). **(C)** Another field of view shows abnormal giant cells within the spindle cell tissue consistent with malignant giant cell tumor (H&E, original magnification ×350).

Imaging Findings:
- Same general features as central chondrosarcoma but outside the bone (Figs. 3.111 to 3.113).
- Occasionally, the adjacent bone may exhibit periosteal reaction or saucerization.

Pathology:
Gross (Macroscopy):
- Large (usually more than 5 cm) cartilaginous lobulated mass attached to the cortex; glistening appearance with gritty white areas of endochondral calcifications or ossifications (Fig. 3.114).

Histopathology:
- Similar to conventional chondrosarcoma (Figs. 3.115 to 3.117).
- Most lesions represent well-differentiated grade 1 or 2 cartilage malignancy.

Differential Diagnosis:
- ***Periosteal osteosarcoma***
  Similar appearance, but instead of chondroid calcifications within the tumor, tumor bone in form of fluffy ossifications.
  Histopathology shows tumor cells forming tumor osteoid or tumor bone.

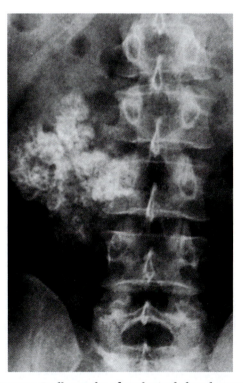

FIGURE 3.111 Radiography of periosteal chondrosarcoma. Anteroposterior radiograph of the lumbar spine shows a large calcified mass attached to the lateral aspect of the third lumbar vertebra.

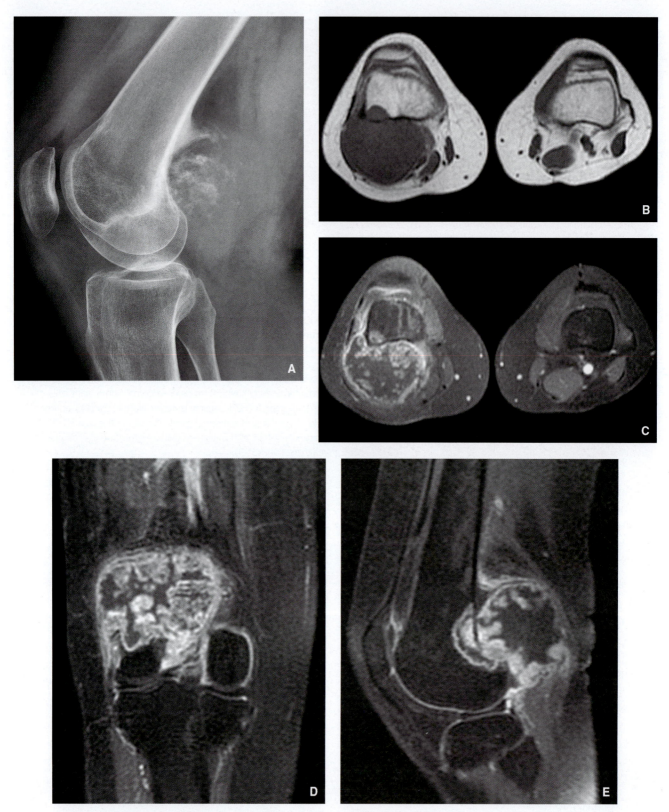

FIGURE 3.112 Radiography and magnetic resonance imaging of periosteal chondrosarcoma. (A) Lateral radiograph of the right knee of a 39-year-old man shows a large mass containing chondroid calcifications, abutting the posterior cortex of the distal femur. **(B)** Axial T1–weighted MR image and **(C)** axial T1–weighted fat-suppressed MRI obtained after intravenous administration of gadolinium show that the mass, exhibiting peripheral enhancement, is invading the lateral femoral condyle, better demonstrated on postcontrast coronal **(D)** and sagittal **(E)** fat-suppressed MR images.

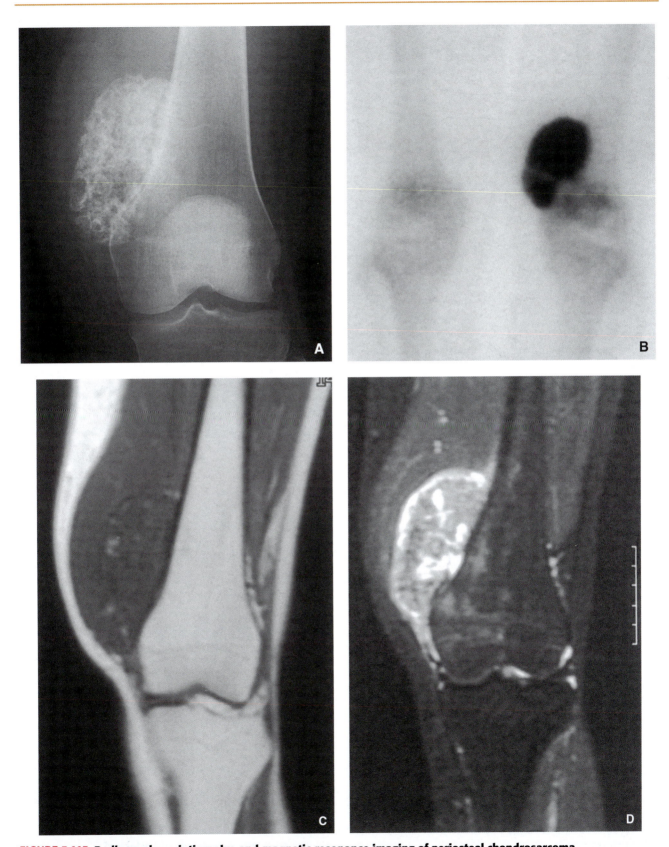

FIGURE 3.113 Radiography, scintigraphy, and magnetic resonance imaging of periosteal chondrosarcoma.
(A) Anteroposterior radiograph of the left knee of a 30-year-old woman shows a parosteal calcified mass at the medial cortex of the distal femur. **(B)** Radionuclide bone scan obtained after intravenous administration of 15mCi (555 MBq) of technetium-99m–labeled methylene diphosphonate shows markedly increased uptake of radiotracer within the mass. **(C)** Coronal T1–weighted MR image shows the mass to be isointense with the surrounding muscles displaying intermediate signal intensity. **(D)** On coronal T2–weighted fat-suppressed image, the mass becomes bright, but the central calcifications exhibit low signal intensity.

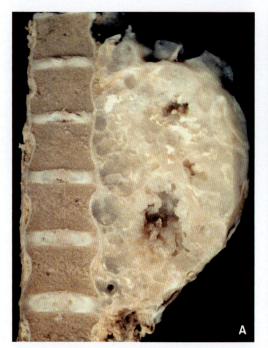
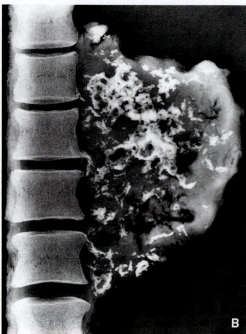

FIGURE 3.114 Gross specimen of periosteal chondrosarcoma. (A) Coronal section of a specimen of thoracolumbar spine junction shows a large mass adjacent to the five vertebral bodies. Note glistening cartilaginous matrix with focal calcifications. **(B)** Radiograph of the specimen better demonstrates chondroid calcifications. (From Bullough PG, Boachi-Adjei O. *Atlas of Spinal Diseases*. New York: Lippincott-Gower; 1988: 198, Fig. 14.29).

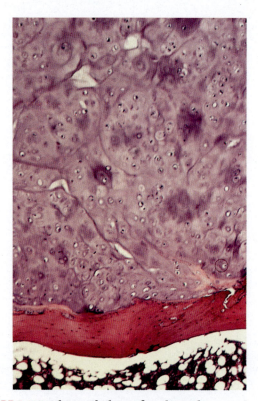

FIGURE 3.115 Histopathology of periosteal chondrosarcoma. Photomicrograph shows somewhat crowded but not atypical chondrocytes. The adjacent bone trabecula (*bottom*) shows scalloping but lack of invasion. These are the features of a low-grade tumor. (From Bullough PG, Boachi-Adjei O. *Atlas of Spinal Diseases*. New York: Lippincott-Gower; 1988:199, Fig. 14.30 A).

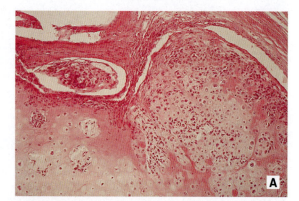
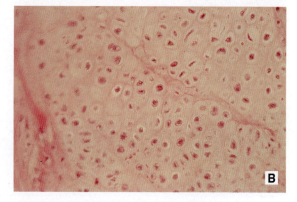

FIGURE 3.116 Histopathology of periosteal chondrosarcoma. (A) Lobulated chondroblastic tumor is clearly separated from the adjacent connective tissue (*top*) (H&E, original magnification ×12). **(B)** At higher magnification, there is obvious pleomorphism of the cells and hyperchromatism of the nuclei, consistent with malignancy (H&E, original magnification ×50).

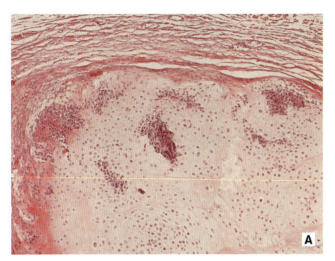
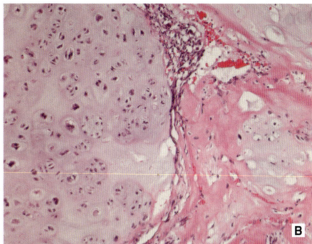
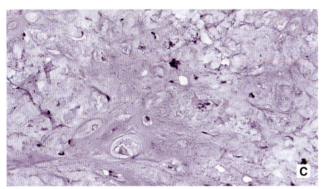

FIGURE 3.117 Histopathology of periosteal chondrosarcoma. (A) Hyaline cartilage with irregular cell arrangement and peripheral condensation of tumor cells is consistent with malignancy (H&E, original magnification ×50). **(B)** At higher magnification, in another area, high cellularity and conspicuous pleomorphism of the cells and nuclei are consistent with grade 2 chondrosarcoma (H&E, original magnification ×100). **(C)** On high magnification, note hypercellularity, atypical cells, and prominent myxoid component, consistent with grade 2 chondrosarcoma.

- *Periosteal chondroma*
  Smaller lesion (less than 5 cm in diameter).
  Histopathology shows lobules of mature hyaline cartilage and benign small and normochromic chondrocytes in lacunae.
- *Myositis ossificans*
  Imaging and histopathologic zonal phenomenon is diagnostic.

Soft-Tissue (Extraskeletal) Chondrosarcomas

Extraskeletal Myxoid Chondrosarcoma

Definition:
- Malignant soft-tissue tumor with characteristic multinodular architecture, myxoid matrix, and malignant chondroblast-like cells arranged in cords, clusters, and delicate networks.

Epidemiology:
- Rare tumor, accounting for less than 3% of soft-tissue sarcomas.
- Median age in the sixth decade.
- Male:female ratio 2:1.
- Rare cases in the pediatric population were described.

Sites of Involvement:
- Deep soft tissues of the proximal extremities and limb girdles.
- Most common location is the thigh, followed by trunk, paraspinal region, foot, popliteal fossa, buttocks, and neck.

Clinical Findings:
- Enlarging soft-tissue mass.
- In some cases, pain and tenderness.
- Large tumors may ulcerate the skin.

Imaging:
- Radiography shows soft-tissue mass with central chondroid calcifications, similar to conventional chondrosarcoma, in focal or uniform distribution (Fig. 3.118). Occasionally soft-tissue mass without visible calcifications (Fig. 3.119).
- Scintigraphy shows increased uptake of radiopharmaceutical tracer.
- Magnetic resonance imaging shows the mass to be isointense with the muscles on T1-weighted sequences and of high signal intensity on T2 weighting and water-sensitive sequences. After intravenous administration of gadolinium, there is heterogenous enhancement.

Pathology:
Gross (Macroscopy):
- Large, well-demarcated tumor with pseudocapsule.
- Median size about 7 cm; however, sizes may be variable (large size 20 to 25 cm have been reported).
- Cut section shows glistening multinodular architecture with gelatinous nodules separated by fibrous septa.
- Cystic changes, areas of hemorrhage, and necrosis can be seen.
- More cellular tumors have fleshy appearance.

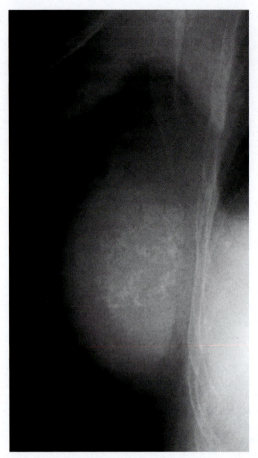

FIGURE 3.118 Radiography of soft-tissue chondrosarcoma. Conventional radiograph shows a large mineralized mass adjacent to the right lower ribs. Note the reverse zonal phenomenon that excludes the diagnosis of similarly appearing myositis ossificans, whereas extraskeletal osteosarcoma can be excluded because the matrix of the tumor exhibits typical chondroid calcifications in form of the dots, arcs, and rings.

Histopathology:

- Multinodular architecture with well-circumscribed pale-blue myxoid or chondromyxoid stroma, rich in sulfated proteoglycans separated by fibrous septa.
- Lobules show higher cellularity at the periphery.
- Hyaline cartilage is rarely present.
- Myxoid stroma is hypovascular.
- Undifferentiated mesenchymal tumor cells have uniform round to oval nuclei and fair amount of eosinophilic granular or vacuolated cytoplasm.
- Tumor cells form cords or clusters.
- Some tumor cells may show spindle or epithelioid features.
- Low mitotic figures (less than 2 per 10 HPF) in most of the cases (Fig. 3.120).
- Common areas of hemorrhage.

Immunophenotype:

- Positive for S-100 protein.
- Vimentin positive.
- Sometimes focally positive for cytokeratin and EMA.

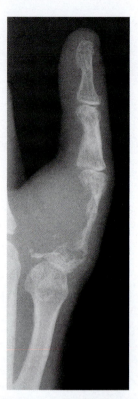

FIGURE 3.119 Radiography of soft-tissue chondrosarcoma. Oblique radiograph of the fifth finger of the left hand of a 47-year-old woman shows a soft-tissue mass invading and destroying the proximal phalanx. There are no visible calcifications present.

Genetics:

- Translocations t(9;22)(q22;q12).
- Translocations t(9;17)(q22;q11) less common.
- Translocations t(9;15)(q22;q21) described in a single case.
- Fusing the gene *NR4A3* to gene *TAF15* (*TAF 2N*, *TAFII68*, or *RBP56*) and gene *TCF12(HTF4)*.

Prognosis:

- Long survival, despite high local recurrence and metastases (to the lungs).

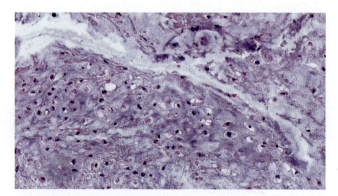

FIGURE 3.120 Histopathology of soft-tissue chondrosarcoma. Photomicrograph shows chondromyxoid stroma with variation of malignant cells exhibiting atypical mitotic figures (H&E, original magnification ×200).

- Tumor size greater than 10 cm is viewed as a negative factor.
- More cellular tumors with increased mitotic figures show more aggressive behavior.

Secondary Chondrosarcomas

Malignant Transformation of Osteochondroma

Epidemiology:
- The risk of malignant transformation is estimated as 1% in solitary lesions and 5% in multiple lesions.

Clinical Findings:
- Pain in the absence of fracture, bursitis, or pressure on nearby nerves.
- Sudden growth spurt of the lesion, particularly after skeletal maturity.

Imaging Features:
- Development of bulky cartilaginous cap (greater than 2 cm).
- Dispersed calcifications within the cartilaginous cap (Figs. 3.121 and 3.122).
- Development of soft-tissue mass.

Histopathologic Findings:
- Arises in the cap of osteochondroma (Fig. 3.123).
- Usually low-grade malignancy.
- Greater cellularity of the cartilage tissue.

- Uneven distribution of cells without cord- or column-like arrangement.
- Pleomorphism and cellular and nuclear atypia.
- Destruction of bone trabeculae of the stalk with invasion of the marrow spaces.

Malignant Transformation of Enchondroma

Epidemiology:
- Patients are usually younger than are those developing primary chondrosarcomas.

Clinical Findings:
- Development of pain in previously asymptomatic lesion in the absence of fracture, particularly in the patients with Ollier disease and Maffucci syndrome, rarely with solitary enchondroma.

Imaging Features:
- Thickening of the cortex at the site of the lesion.
- Deep endosteal scalloping.
- Destruction of the cortex and formation of soft-tissue mass (Fig. 3.124).

Histopathologic Findings:
- Similar to primary chondrosarcomas.
- Pleomorphic cells with hyperchromatism of the nuclei; entrapment and invasion of bone trabeculae and infiltration of marrow spaces (Fig. 3.125).

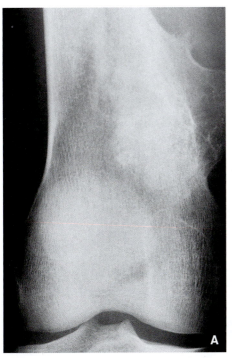
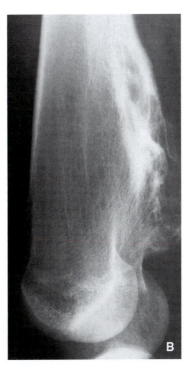
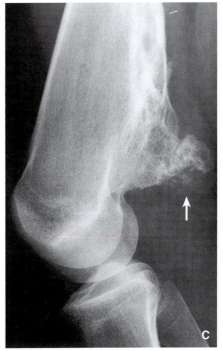

FIGURE 3.121 Radiography of secondary chondrosarcoma (malignant transformation of osteochondroma). A 28-year-old man had been diagnosed with having osteochondroma since age 14. Recently, he developed pain in the popliteal fossa and noticed a growing hard mass. **(A)** Anteroposterior and **(B)** lateral radiographs obtained in the past show a sessile osteochondroma arising from the posteromedial cortex of the distal femur. **(C)** Current lateral radiograph of the distal femur shows that the osteochondroma has enlarged. Also seen are dispersed calcifications in the cartilaginous cap (*arrow*), typical of malignant transformation to chondrosarcoma, that was proved on histopathologic examination.

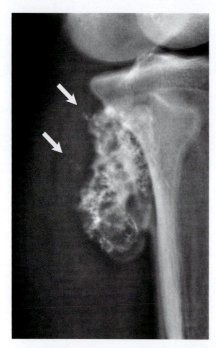

FIGURE 3.122 Radiography of secondary chondrosarcoma (malignant transformation of osteochondroma). Large osteochondroma is seen arising from the proximal fibula of a 32-year-old woman. Note dispersed calcifications within the thick cartilaginous cap (*arrows*).

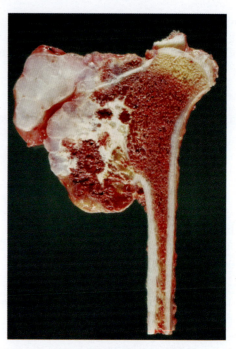

FIGURE 3.123 Gross specimen of secondary chondrosarcoma (malignant transformation of osteochondroma). Resected specimen shows a large osteochondroma arising from the fibula exhibiting a very thick cartilaginous cap (same patient as shown in Fig. 3.122). Note also flaring and destruction of the cortex. Histopathologic examination confirmed malignant transformation to chondrosarcoma.

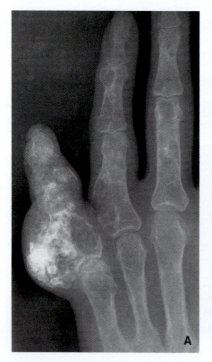
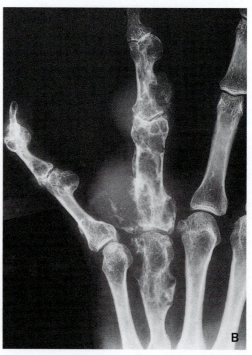

FIGURE 3.124 Radiography of secondary chondrosarcoma (malignant transformation of enchondroma). (A) A 38-year-old woman with known history of long-standing Ollier disease since childhood presented with pain and slowly enlarging mass at the dorsomedial aspect of the small finger of the right hand. The radiograph shows typical changes of this disorder with multiple enchondromas affecting phalanges and metacarpals. Note the destruction of the cortex of the proximal phalanx of the small finger and a soft-tissue mass containing chondroid calcifications, indicating malignant transformation to chondrosarcoma. **(B)** A 30-year-old man with Ollier disease presented with pain and enlarging mass at the base of the ring finger of the right hand. The radiograph shows characteristic changes of this disorder with multiple enchondromas affecting phalanges and metacarpals. Also noted is destruction of the cortex of the proximal and middle phalanges of the ring finger associated with soft-tissue masses, typical features of malignant transformation.

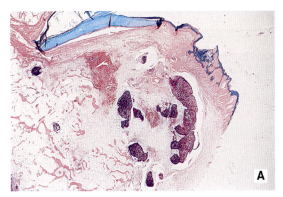
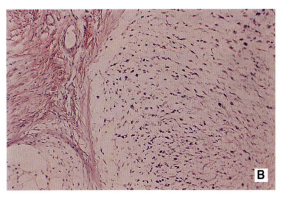

FIGURE 3.125 Histopathology of secondary chondrosarcoma (malignant transformation of enchondroma). (A) Longitudinal section of the distal phalanx of the left thumb with intact nail (*clear blue lamella*) of a patient with Ollier disease shows cancellous bone with large islands of malignant cartilage (*purple color*) proliferating into the surrounding soft tissues (*center*) (Giemsa, original magnification ×5). **(B)** At higher magnification, the malignant cartilage is composed of spindle cells in dense arrangement, with clearly polymorphic, hyperchromatic nuclei and myxoid matrix bordering the fibrous connective tissue (*upper left*) (Giemsa, original magnification ×20).

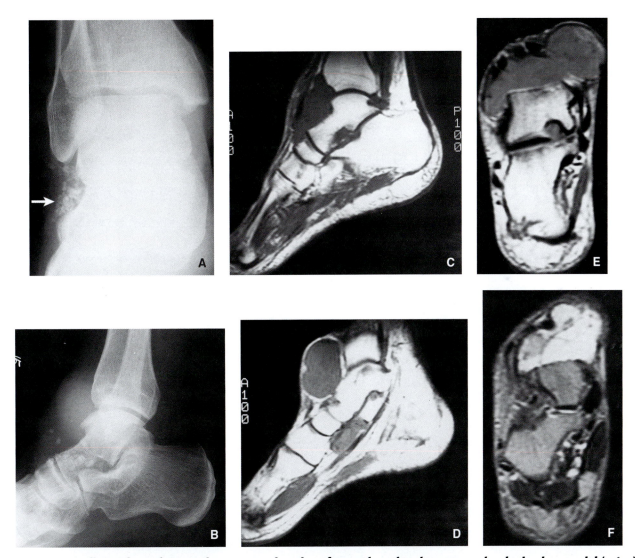

FIGURE 3.126 Radiography and magnetic resonance imaging of secondary chondrosarcoma developing in synovial (osteo) chondromatosis. (A) Anteroposterior and **(B)** lateral radiographs of the right ankle of a 64-year-old man with a long history of primary synovial (osteo)chondromatosis show a large soft-tissue mass on the dorsal aspect of the ankle joint, eroding the talus. Multiple calcifications, uniform in shape and size, are noted laterally (*arrow*). **(C)** Sagittal T1-weighted MR image shows the mass displaying intermediate signal intensity, isointense with the muscles. **(D)** Parasagittal T1-weighted MR image demonstrate the mass to be well encapsulated. **(E)** Coronal proton density–weighted MR image shows that the mass is continuous with the ankle joint. **(F)** Coronal T2-weighted MRI demonstrates the mass to be of high signal intensity. Punctate areas of low signal within the mass represent osteochondral bodies.

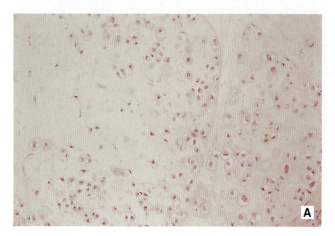
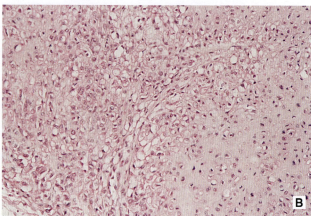
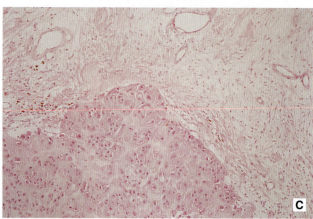

FIGURE 3.127 Histopathology of secondary chondrosarcoma developing in synovial (osteo)chondromatosis. (A) The chondrocytes with clearly pleomorphic and sometimes large nuclei (*lower right corner*) are unevenly distributed. This appearance of nuclear size and structure, however, does not indicate malignancy and may be the feature of uncomplicated synovial (osteo)chondromatosis (H&E, original magnification ×50). **(B)** Smaller parts of benign synovial lesion (*lower right*) border the cell-rich tissue of grade 2-3 secondary chondrosarcoma (H&E, original magnification ×50). **(C)** At the proliferation line of the tumor against the fibrous connective tissue, there is more cartilaginous matrix formation by the tumor cells (H&E, original magnification ×25).

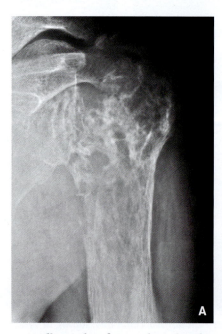
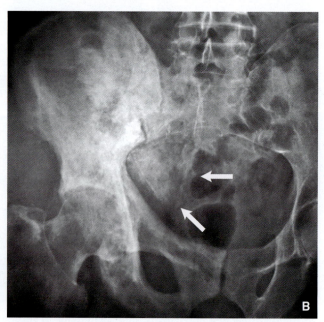

FIGURE 3.128 Radiography of secondary chondrosarcoma (malignant transformation of pagetic bone). (A) Anteroposterior radiograph of the left proximal humerus of a 78-year-old man with polyostotic Paget disease shows typical features of this disorder, consisting of cortical thickening and coarse trabeculation of medullary portion of the bone. Note chondroid calcifications and destruction of the medial cortex with tumor invading the soft tissues. **(B)** The radiograph of the pelvis in another patient, an 80-year-old woman with polyostotic Paget disease, shows involvement of the right ilium, ischium, and pubic bones. The tumor that developed in the ilium broke through the cortex and invaded the soft tissues. Note chondroid calcifications in the soft-tissue mass (*arrows*).

Chondrosarcoma Arising in Primary (Osteo)Chondromatosis

- Extremely rare (fewer than 50 documented cases).
- Difficult to distinguish from primary synovial chondrosarcoma.
- Clinical and imaging findings of development of a soft-tissue mass and destructive changes in the joint at the site of long-standing primary synovial (osteo)chondromatosis (Fig. 3.126).
- Histopathologic features of central grade 2–3 chondrosarcomas (Fig. 3.127).

Chondrosarcoma Arising in Pagetic Bone

- Extremely rare (most common malignancy is osteosarcoma, MFH, and fibrosarcoma).
- Imaging findings consist of cortical destruction of pagetic bone and formation of soft-tissue mass with chondroid type of calcifications (Fig. 3.128).
- Histopathologic findings consist of a typical mosaic pattern of Paget disease and malignant features of cartilage differentiation.

REFERENCES

Aisen AM, Martel W, Braunstein EM, McMillin KI, Phillips WA, Kling TF. MRI and CT evaluation of primary bone and soft-tissue tumors. *AJR Am J Roentgenol.* 1986;146:749–756.

Amary MF, Bacsi K, Maggiani F, et al. IDH1 and IDH2 mutations are frequent events in central chondrosarcoma and central and periosteal chondromas but not in other mesenchymal tumors. *J Pathol.* 2011;224:334–343.

Amary MF, Damato S, Halai D, et al. Ollier disease and Maffucci syndrome are caused by somatic mosaic mutations of IDH1 and IDH2. *Nat Genet.* 2011;43:1262–1265.

Angervall L, Enerback L, Knutson H. Chondrosarcoma of soft tissue origin. *Cancer.* 1973;32:507–513.

Aoki JA, Sone S, Fujioka F, et al. MR of enchondroma and chondrosarcoma: rings and arcs of Gd-DTPA enhancement. *J Comput Assist Tomogr.* 1991;15:1011–1016.

Armah HB, McGough RL, Goodman MA, et al. Chondromyxoid fibroma of rib with a novel chromosomal translocation: a report of four additional cases at unusual sites. *Diagn Pathol.* 2007;2:44–47.

Attwooll C, Tariq M, Harris M, Coyne D, Telford N, Varley JM. Identification of a novel fusion gene involving hTAFII68 and CHN a t(9;17) (q22;q11.2) translocation in an extraskeletal myxoid chondrosarcoma. *Oncogene.* 1999;18:7599–7601.

Azouz EM, Greenspan A, Marton D. CT evaluation of primary epiphyseal bone abscesses. *Skeletal Radiol.* 1993;22:17–23.

Bagley L, Kneeland JB, Dalinka MK, Bullough P, Brooks J. Unusual behavior of clear cell chondrosarcoma. *Skeletal Radiol.* 1993;22:279–282.

Bandiera S, Bacchini P, Bertoni F. Bizarre parosteal osteochondromatous proliferation of bone. *Skeletal Radiol.* 1998;27:154–156.

Bansal M, Goldman AB, DiCarlo EF, McCormack R. Soft tissue chondromas: diagnosis and differential diagnosis. *Skeletal Radiol.* 1993;22:309–315.

Bartsch O, Wuyts W, Van Hul W, et al. Delineation of a contiguous gene syndrome with multiple exostoses, enlarged parietal foramina, craniofacial dysostosis, and mental retardation, caused by deletion in the short arm of chromosome 11. *Am J Hum Genet.* 1996;58:734–742.

Beggs IG, Stoker DJ. Chondromyxoid fibroma of bone. *Clin Radiol.* 1982;33:671–679.

Berquist TH. Magnetic resonance imaging of primary skeletal neoplasms. *Radiol Clin North Am.* 1993;31:411–424.

Bertoni F, Boriani S, Laus M, Campanacci M. Periosteal chondrosarcoma and periosteal osteosarcoma. Two distinct entities. *J Bone Joint Surg Br.* 1982;64B:370–376.

Bertoni F, Picci P, Bacchini P, et al. Mesenchymal chondrosarcoma of bone and soft tissues. *Cancer.* 1983;52:533–541.

Bertoni F, Present D, Bacchini P, et al. Dedifferentiated peripheral chondrosarcomas. A report of seven cases. *Cancer.* 1989;63:2054–2059.

Bertoni F, Unni KK, Beabout JW, Sim FH. Chondrosarcomas of the synovium. *Cancer.* 1991;67:155–162.

Bierry G, Kerr DA, Nielsen GP, et al. Enchondromas in children: imaging appearance with pathological correlation. *Skeletal Radiol.* 2012;41:1223–1229.

Bird JE, Wang W-L, Deavers MT, Madewell J, Lewis VO. Enchondroma with secondary aneurysmal bone cyst. *Skeletal Radiol.* 2012;41:1475–1478.

Bjerkehagen B, Dietrich C, Reed W, et al. Extraskeletal myxoid chondrosarcoma: multimodal diagnosis and identification of a new cytogenetic subgroup characterized by t(9;17) (q22;q11). *Virchows Arch.* 1999;435:524–530.

Björnsson J, Unni KK, Dahlin DC, Beabout JW, Sim FH. Clear-cell chondrosarcoma of bone: observation in 47 cases. *Am J Surg Pathol.* 1984;8:223–230.

Blacksin MF, Ghelman B, Freiberger RH, Salvata E. Synovial chondromatosis of the hip: evaluation with air computed arthrotomography. *Clin Imaging.* 1990;14:315–318.

Bloem JL, Mulder JD. Chondroblastoma: a clinical and radiological study of 104 cases. *Skeletal Radiol.* 1985;14:1–9.

Borges AM, Huvos AG, Smith J. Bursa formation and synovial chondrometaplasia associated with osteochondromas. *Am J Clin Pathol.* 1981;75:648–653.

Boriani S, Bacchini P, Bertoni F, Campanacci M. Periosteal chondroma. A review of twenty cases. *J Bone Joint Surg Am.* 1983;65A:205–212.

Borys D, Cantor R. Mesenchymal chondrosarcoma of the chest wall. *Pathol Case Rev.* 2012;17:10–13.

Braunstein E, Martel W, Weatherbee L. Periosteal bone apposition in chondroblastoma. *Skeletal Radiol.* 1979;4:34–36.

Brien EW, Mirra JM, Herr R. Benign and malignant cartilage tumors of bone and joints: their anatomic and theoretical basis with an emphasis on radiology, pathology, and clinical biology. I. The intramedullary cartilage tumors. *Skeletal Radiol.* 1997;26:325–353.

Brien EW, Mirra JM, Luck JV Jr. Benign and malignant cartilage tumors of bone and joint: their anatomic and theoretical basis with an emphasis on radiology, pathology, and clinical biology. II. Juxtacortical cartilage tumors. *Skeletal Radiol.* 1999;28:1–20.

Brower AC, Moser RP, Gilkey FW, et al. Chondroblastoma. In: Moser RP, ed. *Cartilaginous Tumors of the Skeleton. AFIP Atlas of Radiologic-Pathologic Correlation, Fascicle II.* Philadelphia, PA: Hanley & Belfus; 1990:74–113.

Brower AC, Moser RP, Kransdorf MJ. The frequency and diagnostic significance of periostitis in chondroblastoma. *AJR Am J Roentgenol.* 1990;154:309–314.

Bruder E, Zanetti M, Boos N, von Hochstetter AR. Chondromyxoid fibroma of two thoracic vertebrae. *Skeletal Radiol.* 1999;28:286–289.

Buddingh EP, Naumann S, Nelson M, et al. Cytogenetic findings in benign cartilaginous neoplasms. *Cancer Genet Cytogenet.* 2003;141:164–168.

Bui KL, Ilaslan H, Bauer TW, Lietman SA, Joyce MJ, Sundaram M. Cortical scalloping and cortical penetration by small eccentric chondroid lesions in the long tubular bones: not a sign of malignancy? *Skeletal Radiol.* 2009;38:791–796.

Bullough PG. *Atlas of Orthopedic Pathology.* 2nd ed. New York: Gower; 1992:14.9.

Burnstein MI, Fisher DR, Yandow DR, Hafez GR, De Smet AA. Case report 502. Intra-articular synovial chondromatosis of shoulder with extra-articular extension. *Skeletal Radiol.* 1988;17:458–461.

Cannon CP, Nelson SD, Seeger L, Eckardt JJ. Clear cell chondrosarcoma mimicking chondroblastoma in a skeletally immature patient. *Skeletal Radiol.* 2002;31: 369–372.

Capanna R, Bertoni F, Bettelli G, et al. Dedifferentiated chondrosarcoma. *J Bone Joint Surg Am.* 1988;70A:60–69.

Cawte TG, Steiner GC, Beltran J, Dorfman HD. Chondrosarcoma of the short tubular bones of the hands and feet. *Skeletal Radiol.* 1998;27:625–632.

Chung EB, Enzinger FM. Chondromas of soft parts. *Cancer.* 1978;41: 1414–1424.

Codman EA. Epiphyseal chondromatous giant cell tumors of the upper end of the humerus. *Surg Gynecol Obstet.* 1931;52:543–548.

Cohen EK, Kressel HY, Frank TS, et al. Hyaline cartilage-origin bone and soft-tissue neoplasms: MR appearance and histologic correlation. *Radiology.* 1988;167: 477–481.

Collins PS, Han W, Williams LR, Rich N, Lee JF, Villavicencio JL. Maffucci's syndrome (hemangiomatosis osteolytica): a report of four cases. *J Vasc Surg.* 1992;16: 364–371.

Collins MS, Koyama T, Swee RG, Inwards CY. Clear cell chondrosarcoma: radiographic, computed tomographic, and magnetic resonance findings in 34 patients with pathologic correlation. *Skeletal Radiol.* 2003;32:687–694.

Crim JR, Seeger LL. Diagnosis of low-grade chondrosarcoma. *Radiology.* 1993;189:503–504.

Crotty JM, Monu JUV, Pope TL Jr. Synovial osteochondromatosis. *Radiol Clin North Am.* 1996;34:327–342.

Dahlin DC. Chondromyxoid fibroma of bone, with emphasis on its morphological relationship to benign chondroblastoma. *Cancer.* 1956;9:195–203.

Dahlin DC. Grading of bone tumors. In: Unni KK, ed. *Bone Tumors.* New York: Churchill Livingstone; 1988:35–45.

Dahlin DC, Beabout JW. Dedifferentiation of low-grade chondrosarcomas. *Cancer.* 1971;28:461–466.

Dahlin DC, Ivins JC. Benign chondroblastoma: a study of 125 cases. *Cancer.* 1972; 30:401–413.

Dahlin DC, Unni KK. *Bone Tumors: General Aspects and Data on 8,542 Cases.* 4th ed. Springfield, IL: Charles C. Thomas; 1986:18, 33–51, 227–259.

Davids JR, Glancy GL, Eilert RE. Fracture through the stalk of pedunculated osteochondromas. A report of three cases. *Clin Orthop* 1991;271:258–264.

De Beuckeleer LHL, De Schepper AMA, Ramon F. Magnetic resonance imaging of cartilaginous tumors: retrospective study of 79 patients. *Eur J Radiol.* 1995;21: 34–40.

De Beuckeleer LHL, De Schepper AMA, Ramon F. Magnetic resonance imaging of cartilaginous tumors: is it useful or necessary? *Skeletal Radiol.* 1996;25:137–141.

Demertzis JL, Kyriakos M, Conolly S, McDonald DJ. Surface-based chondroblastoma of the tibia: a unique presentation. *Skeletal Radiol.* 2015;44:1045–1050.

deSantos LA, Spjut HJ. Periosteal chondroma: a radiographic spectrum. *Skeletal Radiol.* 1981;6:15–20.

Devidayal A, Marvaha RK. Langer-Giedion syndrome. *Indian Pediatr.* 2006;43:174–175.

Dhondt E, Oudenhoven L, Khan S, et al. Nora's lesion, a distinct radiological entity? *Skeletal Radiol.* 2006;35:497–502.

Douis H, Saifuddin A. The imaging of cartilaginous bone tumours. I Benign lesions. *Skeletal Radiol.* 2012;41:1195–1212.

Douis H, Davies AM, James SL, Kindblom LG, Grimer RJ, Johnson KJ. Can MR imaging challenge the commonly accepted theory of the pathogenesis of solitary enchondroma of long bone? *Skeletal Radiol.* 2012;41:1537–1542.

Douis H, Jeys L, Grimer R, et al. Is there a role for diffusion-weighted MRI (DWI) in the diagnosis of central cartilage tumors? *Skeletal Radiol.* 2015;44:963–969.

El-Khoury GY, Bassett GS. Symptomatic bursa formation with osteochondromas. *AJR Am J Roentgenol.* 1979;133:895–898.

Enzinger FM, Shiraki M. Extraskeletal myxoid chondrosarcoma—an analysis of 34 cases. *Hum Pathol.* 1972;3:421–435.

Enzinger FM, Weiss SW. Cartilaginous tumors and tumorlike lesions of soft tissue. In: Enzinger FM, Weiss SW, eds. *Soft Tissue Tumors.* St. Louis, MO: Mosby-Year Book; 1988:861–881.

Epstein DA, Levin EJ. Bone scintigraphy in hereditary multiple exostoses. *AJR Am J Roentgenol.* 1978;130:331–333.

Erickson JK, Rosenthal DI, Zaleske DJ, Gebhardt MC, Cates JM. Primary treatment of chondroblastoma with percutaneous radiofrequency heat ablation: report of three cases. *Radiology.* 2001;221: 463–468.

Eustace S, Baker N, Lan H, Wadhwani A, Dorfman D. MR imaging of dedifferentiated chondrosarcoma. *Clin Imaging.* 1997;21:170–174.

Fairbank TJ. Dysplasia epiphysealis hemimelica (tarso-epiphyseal aclasis). *J Bone Joint Surg Br.* 1956;38B:237–257.

Fechner RE, Mills SE. *Tumors of the Bones and Joint.* Washington, DC: Armed Forces Institute of Pathology; 1993.

Feldman F. Cartilaginous tumors and cartilage-forming tumor-like conditions of the bones and soft tissues. In: Ranniger K, ed. *Bone Tumors.* Berlin, Germany: Springer-Verlag; 1977:177–220.

Feldman F, Hecht HL, Johnston AD. Chondromyxoid fibroma of bone. *Radiology.* 1970;94:249–260.

Flach HZ, Ginai AZ, Oosterhuis JW. Best cases from the AFIP. Maffucci syndrome: radiologic and pathologic findings. *Radiographics.* 2001;21:1311–1316.

Flemming DJ, Murphey MD. Enchondroma and chondrosarcoma. *Semin Musculoskelet Radiol.* 2000;4:59–71.

Fletcher CDM, Unni KK, Mertens E, eds. *World Health Organisation Classification of Tumours of Soft Tissue and Bone.* Lyon, France: ARC Press; 2013:234–246:264–274.

Frassica FJ, Unni KK, Beabout JW, Sim FH. Dedifferentiated chondrosarcoma. A report of the clinicopathological features and treatment of seventy-eight cases. *J Bone Joint Surg Am.* 1986;68A:1197–1205.

Garcia RA, Inward CY, Unni KK. Benign bone tumors—recent developments. *Semin Diagn Pathol.* 2011;28:73–85.

Garrison RC, Unni KK, McLeod RA, Pritchard DJ, Dahlin DC. Chondrosarcoma arising in osteochondroma. *Cancer.* 1981;49:1890–1897.

Geirnaerdt MJA, Bloem JL, Eulderink F, Hogendoorn PCW, Taminiau AH. Cartilaginous tumors: correlation of gadolinium-enhanced MR imaging and histopathologic findings. *Radiology.* 1993;186:813–817.

Geirnaerdt MJA, Hogendoorn PCW, Bloem JJ, Taminiau AHM, van der Woude H-J. Cartilaginous tumors: fast contrast-enhanced MR imaging. *Radiology.* 2000;214:539–546.

O'Connor PJ, Gibbon WW, Hardy G, Butt WP. Chondromyxoid fibroma of the foot. *Skeletal Radiol.* 1996;25:143–148.

Gitelis S, Block JA, Inerot SE. Clonal analysis of human chondrosarcoma. The 35th Annual Meeting, Orthopedic Research Society. *Orthop Trans.* 1989;13:443.

Giudici MA, Moser RP Jr, Kransdorf MJ. Cartilaginous bone tumors. *Radiol Clin North Am.* 1993;31:237–259.

Gohel VK, Dalinka MK, Edeiken J. Ischemic necrosis of the femoral head simulating chondroblastoma. *Radiology.* 1973;107:545–546.

Goldman RL, Lichtenstein L. Synovial chondrosarcoma. *Cancer.* 1964;17:1233–1240.

González-Lois C, Garcia-de-la-Torre JP, SantosBriz-Terrón A, Vila J, Manrique-Chico J, Martinez-Tello FJ. Intracapsular and para-articular chondroma adjacent to large joints: report of three cases and review of the literature. *Skeletal Radiol.* 2001;30:672–676.

Goodman SB, Bell RS, Fornasier VS, De Demeter D, Bateman JE. Ollier's disease with multiple sarcomatous transformation. *Hum Pathol.* 1984;15:91–93.

Green P, Wittaker RP. Benign chondroblastoma. Case report with pulmonary metastasis. *J Bone Joint Surg Am.* 1975;57A:418–420.

Greenfield GB, Arrington JA. *Imaging of Bone Tumors. A Multi-Modality Approach.* Philadelphia, PA: JB Lippincott; 1955:48–91.

Greenspan A. Tumors of cartilage origin. *Orthop Clin North Am.* 1989;20:347–366.

Greenspan A, Klein MJ. Radiology and pathology of bone tumors. In: Lewis MM, ed. *Musculoskeletal Oncology. A Multidisciplinary Approach.* Philadelphia, PA: WB Saunders; 1992:13–72.

Greenspan A, Unni KK, Matthews J II. Periosteal chondroma masquerading as osteochondroma. *Can Assoc Radiol J.* 1993;44:205–210.

Greenspan A, Jundt G, Remagen W. *Differential Diagnosis in Orthopaedic Oncology.* 2nd ed. Philadelphia, PA: Lippincott Williams & Wilkins; 2007:84–148; 212–249.

Griffiths HJ, Thompson RC Jr, Galloway HR, Everson LI, Suh J-S. Bursitis in association with solitary osteochondromas presenting as mass lesions. *Skeletal Radiol.* 1991;20:513–516.

Gunawan B, Weber M, Bergmann F, Wildberger J, Niethard FU, Füzesi L. Clonal chromosome abnormalities in enchondromas and chondrosarcomas. *Cancer Genet Cytogenet.* 2000;120:127–130.

Hameetman L, Szuhai K, Yavas A, et al. The role of EXT1 in nonhereditary osteochondroma: identification of homozygous deletions. *J Natl Cancer Inst.* 2007;99:396–406.

Hatano H, Ogose A, Hotta T, Otsuka H, Takahashi HE. Periosteal chondrosarcoma invading the medullary cavity. *Skeletal Radiol.* 1997;26:375–378.

Hau MA, Fox EJ, Rosenberg AE, Mankin HJ. Chondromyxoid fibroma of the metacarpal. *Skeletal Radiol.* 2001;30:719–721.

Hayes CW, Conway WF, Sundaram M. Misleading aggressive MR imaging: appearance of some benign musculoskeletal lesions. *Radiographics.* 1992;12:1119–1134.

Helliwell TR, O'Connor MA, Ritchie DA, Feldberg L, Stilwell JH, Jane MJ. Bizarre parosteal osteochondromatous proliferation with cortical invasion. *Skeletal Radiol.* 2001;30:282–285.

Helms C. Pseudocyst of the humerus. *AJR Am J Roentgenol.* 1979;131: 287–292.

Henderson ED, Dahlin DC. Chondrosarcoma of bone: a study of 280 cases. *J Bone Joint Surg Am.* 1963;45A:1450–1458.

Hensinger RN, Cowell HR, Ramsey PL, Leopold RG. Familial dysplasia epiphysealis hemimelica associated with chondromas and osteochondromas. Report of a kindred with variable presentations. *J Bone Joint Surg Am.* 1974;56A:1513–1516.

Hermann G, Abdelwahab IF, Klein MJ, et al. Synovial chondromatosis. *Skeletal Radiol.* 1995;24:298–300.

Hermann G, Klein MJ, Abdelwahab IF, Kenan S. Synovial chondrosarcoma arising in synovial chondromatosis of the right hip. *Skeletal Radiol.* 1997;26:366–369.

Hisaoka M, Hashimoto H. Soft tissue tumors: extraskeletal myxoid chondrosarcoma. *Atlas Genet Cytogenet Oncol Haematol.* 2004;8:334–335.

Hudson TM. Medullary (central) chondrosarcoma. In: Hudson TM, ed. *Radiologic Pathologic Correlation of Musculoskeletal Lesions.* Baltimore, MD: Williams & Wilkins; 1987:153–175.

Hudson TM, Chew FS, Manaster BJ. Scintigraphy of benign exostoses and exostotic chondrosarcoma. *AJR Am J Roentgenol.* 1983;140:581–586.

Hudson TM, Spriengfield DS, Spanier SS, Enneking WF, Hamlin DJ. Benign exostoses and exostotic chondrosarcomas: evaluation of cartilage thickness by CT. *Radiology.* 1984;152:595–599.

Huvos AG. Chondroblastoma and clear cell chondrosarcoma. In: Huvos AG, ed. *Bone Tumors. Diagnosis, Treatment and Prognosis.* 2nd ed. Philadelphia, PA: WB Saunders; 1991:295–318.

Huvos AG, Higinbotham NL, Marcove RC, O'Leary P. Aggressive chondroblastoma: review of the literature on aggressive behavior and metastases with a report of one new case. *Clin Orthop.* 1977;126:266–272.

Ilaslan H, Sundaram M, Unni KK. Vertebral chondroblastoma. *Skeletal Radiol.* 2003;32:66–71.

Ishida T, Dorfman HD, Habermann ET. Dedifferentiated chondrosarcoma of humerus with giant cell tumor-like features. *Skeletal Radiol.* 1995;24:76–80.

Ishida T, Yamamoto M, Goto T, Kawano H, Yamamoto A, Machinami R. Clear cell chondrosarcoma of the pelvis in a skeletally immature patient. *Skeletal Radiol.* 1999;28:290–293.

Jaffe HL. Juxtacortical chondroma. *Bull Hosp Joint Dis.* 1956;17:20–29.

Jaffe HL. *Tumors and Tumorous Conditions of the Bones and Joints.* Philadelphia, PA: Lea & Febiger; 1968.

Jaffe HL, Lichtenstein L. Benign chondroblastoma of bone: reinterpretation of so-called calcifying or chondromatous giant cell tumor. *Am J Pathol.* 1942;18:969–991.

Jaffe HL, Lichtenstein L. Chondromyxoid fibroma of bone: a distinctive benign tumor likely to be mistaken especially for chondrosarcoma. *Arch Pathol.* 1948;45:541–551.

Janzen L, Logan PM, O'Connell JX, Connel DG, Munk PL. Intramedullary chondroid tumors of bone: correlation of abnormal peritumoral marrow and soft-tissue MRI signal with tumor type. *Skeletal Radiol.* 1997;26:100–106.

Johnson S, Tetu B, Ayala AG, Chawla SP. Chondrosarcoma with additional mesenchymal component (dedifferentiated chondrosarcoma). A clinical study of 26 cases. *Cancer.* 1986;58:278–286.

Kahn S, Taljanovic MS, Speer DP, Graham AR, Dennis PD. Kissing periosteal chondroma and osteochondroma. *Skeletal Radiol.* 2002;31:235–239.

Kaim AH, Hügli R, Bonél HM, Jundt G. Chondroblastoma and clear cell chondrosarcoma: radiological and MRI characteristics with histopathological correlation. *Skeletal Radiol.* 2002;31:88–95.

Kaufman JH, Cedermark BJ, Parthasarathy KL, Didolkar MS, Bakshi SP. The value of ^{67}Ga scintigraphy in soft-tissue sarcoma and chondrosarcoma. *Radiology.* 1977;123:131–134.

Keating RB, Wright PW, Staple TW. Enchondroma protuberans of the rib. *Skeletal Radiol.* 1985;13:55–58.

Kenan S, Ginat DT, Steiner GC. Dedifferentiated high-grade osteosarcoma originating from low-grade central osteosarcoma of the fibula. *Skeletal Radiol.* 2007;36:347–351.

Kettelkamp DB, Campbell CJ, Bonfiglio M. Dysplasia epiphysealis hemimelica. A report of fifteen cases and a review of the literature. *J Bone Joint Surg Am.* 1966;48A:746–766.

King JW, Spjut HJ, Fechner RE, Vanderpool DW. Synovial chondrosarcoma of the knee joint. *J Bone Joint Surg Am.* 1967;49A:1389–1396.

Klein MJ. Chondrosarcoma. *Semin Orthop.* 1991;6:167–176.

Kransdorf MJ, Meis JM. Extraskeletal osseous and cartilaginous tumors of the extremities. *Radiographics.* 1993;13:853–884.

Kricun ME. *Imaging of Bone Tumors.* Philadelphia, PA: WB Saunders; 1993.

Kricun ME, Kricun R, Haskin ME. Chondroblastoma of the calcaneus: radiographic features with emphasis on location. *AJR Am J Roentgenol.* 1977;128:613–616.

Kroon HM, Bloem JL, Holscher HC, van der Woude HJ, Reijnierse M, Taminiau AHM. MR imaging of edema accompanying benign and malignant bone tumors. *Skeletal Radiol.* 1994;23:261–269.

Kurt AM, Unni KK, Sim FH, McLeod RA. Chondroblastoma of bone. *Hum Pathol.* 1989;20:965–976.

Lang IM, Azouz EM. MRI appearances of dysplasia epiphysealis hemimelica of the knee. *Skeletal Radiol.* 1997;26:226–229.

Lee KC, Davies AM, Cassar-Pullicino VN. Imaging the complications of osteochondroma. *Clin Radiol.* 2002;57:18–28.

Leffler SG, Chew FS. CT-guided percutaneous biopsy of sclerotic bone lesions: diagnostic yield and accuracy. *AJR Am J Roentgenol.* 1999;172:1389–1392.

Lichtenstein L, Hall JE. Periosteal chondroma: a distinctive benign cartilage tumor. *J Bone Joint Surg Am.* 1952;34A:691–697.

Lichtenstein L, Jaffe HL. Chondrosarcoma of the bone. *Am J Pathol.* 1943;19:553–589.

Liu J, Hudkins PG, Swee RG, Unni KK. Bone sarcomas associated with Ollier's disease. *Cancer.* 1987;59:1376–1385.

Ly JQ, Beall DP. A rare case of infantile Ollier's disease demonstrating bilaterally symmetric extremity involvement. *Skeletal Radiol.* 2003;32:227–230.

Ly JQ, LaGatta LM, Beall DP. Calcaneal chondroblastoma with secondary aneurysmal bone cyst. *AJR Am J Roentgenol.* 2004;182:130.

Maffucci A. Di un caso di encondroma el antioma multiplo. Contribuzone alla genesi embrionale dei tumori. *Movimento Med Chir Napoli.* 1881;3:399–412.

Maheshwari AV, Jelinek JS, Song AJ, et al. Metaphyseal and diaphyseal chondroblastomas. *Skeletal Radiol.* 2011; 40:1563–1573.

McCarthy EF, Dorfman HD. Chondrosarcoma of bone with dedifferentiation: a study of eighteen cases. *Hum Pathol.* 1982;13:36–40.

Mellon CD, Carter JE, Owen DB. Ollier's disease and Maffucci's syndrome: distinct entities or a continuum? *J Neurol.* 1988;235:376–378.

Meneses MF, Unni KK, Swee RG. Bizarre parosteal osteochondromatous proliferation of bone (Nora's lesion). *Am J Surg Pathol.* 1993;17:691–697.

Mercuri M, Picci P, Campanacci M, Rulli E. Dedifferentiated chondrosarcoma. *Skeletal Radiol.* 1995;24:409–416.

Michelsen H, Abramovici L, Steiner G, Posner M. Bizarre parosteal osteochondromatous proliferation (Nora's lesion) in the hand. *J Hand Surg Am.* 2004;29A:520–525.

Mirra JM, Ulich TR, Eckardt JJ, Bhuta S. "Aggressive" chondroblastoma. Light and ultramicroscopic findings after *en bloc* resection. *Clin Orthop.* 1983;178:276–284.

Mirra JM, Gold R, Downs J, Eckardt JJ. A new histologic approach to the differentiation of enchondroma and chondrosarcoma of the bones: a clinicopathologic analysis of 51 cases. *Clin Orthop.* 1987;2: 89–107.

Mirra JM, Picci P, Gold RH. *Bone tumors: Clinical, Radiologic and Pathologic Correlations.* Philadelphia, PA: Lea & Febiger; 1989.

Monda L, Wick MR. S-100 protein immunostaining in the differential diagnosis of chondroblastoma. *Hum Pathol.* 1985;16:287–293.

Moser RP. Cartilaginous tumors of the skeleton. In: *AFIP Atlas of Radiologic-Pathologic Correlation*. Vol. 2. Philadelphia, PA: Hanley & Belfus; 1990:190–197.

Moser RP, Brockmole DM, Vinh TN, Kransdorf MJ, Aoki J. Chondroblastoma of the patella. *Skeletal Radiol.* 1988;17:413–419.

Moser RP, Gilkey FW, Madewell JE. Enchondroma. In: Moser RP, ed. *Cartilaginous Tumors of the Skeleton. AFIP Atlas of Radiologic-Pathologic Correlation, Fascicle II*. Philadelphia, PA: Hanley & Belfus; 1990:8–34.

Mulder JD, Schütte HE, Kroon HM, Taconis WK. *Radiologic Atlas of Bone Tumors*. Amsterdam, the Netherlands: Elsevier; 1993:51–76.

Murphey MD, Flemming DJ, Boyea SR, Bojescul JA, Sweet DE, Temple HT. From the archives of the AFIP. Enchondroma versus chondrosarcoma in the appendicular skeleton: differentiation features. *Radiographics.* 1998;18:1213–1237.

Murphey MD, Choi JJ, Kransdorf MJ, Flemming DJ, Gannon FH. Imaging of osteochondroma: variants and complications with radiologic-pathologic correlation. *Radiographics.* 2000;20:1407–1434.

Murphey MD, Walker EA, Wilson AJ, Kransdorf MJ, Temple HT, Gannon FH. From the archives of the AFIP. Imaging of primary chondrosarcoma: radiologic-pathologic correlation. *Radiographics.* 2003;23:1245–1278.

Murphey MD, Vidal JA, Fanburg-Smith JC, Gajewski DA. Imaging of synovial chondromatosis with radiologic-pathologic correlation. *Radiographics.* 2007;27:1465–1488.

Nakashima Y, Unni KK, Shives TC, Swee RG, Dahlin DC. Mesenchymal chondrosarcoma of bone and soft tissue. A review of 111 cases. *Cancer.* 1986;57:2444–2453.

Nora FE, Dahlin DC, Beabout JW. Bizarre parosteal osteochondromatous proliferation of the hands and feet. *Am J Surg Pathol.* 1983;7:245–250.

Norman A, Sissons HA. Radiographic hallmarks of peripheral chondrosarcoma. *Radiology.* 1984;151:589–596.

Norman A, Steiner GC. Bone erosion in synovial chondromatosis. *Radiology.* 1986;161:749–752.

Ollier L. De la dyschondroplasie. *Bull Soc Lyon Med.* 1899;93:23–24.

Ontell F, Greenspan A. Chondrosarcoma complicating synovial chondromatosis: findings with magnetic resonance imaging. *Can Assoc Radiol J.* 1994;45:318–323.

Orndal C, Mandahl N, Rydholm A. Chromosome aberrations and cytogenetic intratumor heterogeneity in chondrosarcomas. *J Cancer Res Clin Oncol.* 1993;120:51–56.

Ozkoc G, Gonlusen G, Ozalay M, Kayaselcuk F, Pourbagher A, Tandogan RN. Giant chondroblastoma of the scapula with pulmonary metastases. *Skeletal Radiol.* 2006;35:42–48.

Park Y-K, Yang MH, Ryu KN, Chung DW. Dedifferentiated chondrosarcoma arising in an osteochondroma. *Skeletal Radiol.* 1995;24:617–619.

Pösl M, Werner M, Amling M, Ritzel H, Delling G. Malignant transformation of chondroblastoma. *Histopathology.* 1996;29:477–480.

Pritchard DJ, Lunke RJ, Taylor WF, Dahlin DC, Medley BE. Chondrosarcoma: clinicopathologic and statistical analysis. *Cancer.* 1980;45:149–157.

Ragsdale BD, Sweet DE, Vinh TN. Radiology as gross pathology in evaluating chondroid tumors. *Hum Pathol.* 1989;20:930–951.

Rahimi A, Beabout JW, Ivins JC, Dahlin DC. Chondromyxoid fibroma: clinicopathologic study of 75 cases. *Cancer.* 1972;30:726–736.

Resnick D, Cone RO III. The nature of humeral pseudocyst. *Radiology.* 1984;150: 27–28.

Resnik CS, Levine AM, Aisner SC, Young JW, Dorfman HD. Case report 522. Concurrent adjacent osteochondroma and enchondroma. *Skeletal Radiol.* 1989;18:66–69.

Safar A, Nelson M, Neff JR, et al. Recurrent anomalies of 6q25 in chondromyxoid fibroma. *Hum Pathol.* 2000;31:306–311.

Salvador AH, Beabout JW, Dahlin DC. Mesenchymal chondrosarcoma—observations on 30 new cases. *Cancer.* 1971;28:605–615.

Sanerkin NG. Definitions of osteosarcoma, chondrosarcoma and fibrosarcoma of bone. *Cancer.* 1980;46:178–185.

Sanerkin NG, Gallagher P. A review of the behaviour of chondrosarcoma of bone. *J Bone Joint Surg Br.* 1979;61B:395–400.

Saunders C, Szabo RM, Mora S. Chondrosarcoma of the hand arising in a young patient with multiple hereditary exostoses. *J Hand Surg Br.* 1997;22B:237–242.

Schajowicz F. Cartilage-forming tumors. In: Schajowicz F, ed. *Tumors and Tumorlike Conditions of Bone*. New York: Springer-Verlag; 1994:141–256.

Schajowicz F, Gallardo H. Chondromyxoid fibroma (fibromyxoid chondroma) of bone. *J Bone Joint Surg Br.* 1971;53B:198–216.

Schajowicz F, McGuire M. Diagnostic difficulties in skeletal pathology. *Clin Orthop.* 1989;240:281–308.

Schajowicz F, Sissons HA, Sobin LH. The World Health Organization's histologic classification of bone tumors. A commentary on the second edition. *Cancer.* 1995;75:1208–1214.

Sensarma A, Madewell JE, Meis J, et al. Regression of an enchondroma: a case report and proposed etiology. *Skeletal Radiol.* 2015;44:739–742.

Sirsat MV, Doctor VM. Benign chondroblastoma of bone. Report of a case of malignant transformation. *J Bone Joint Surg Br.* 1970; 52B:741–745.

Sjogren H, Orndal C, Tingby O, Meis-Kindblom JM, Kindblom LG, Stenman G. Cytogenetic and spectral karyotype analyses of benign and malignant cartilage tumours. *Int J Oncol.* 2004;24:1385–1391.

Spjut HJ, Dorfman HD, Fechner RE, Ackerman LV. Tumors of bone and cartilage. In: *Atlas of Tumor Pathology, Second Series, Fascicle 5*. Washington, DC: Armed Forces Institute of Pathology; 1971.

Stout AP, Verner EW. Chondrosarcoma of the extraskeletal soft tissues. *Cancer.* 1953;6:581–590.

Sun TC, Swee RG, Shives TC, Unni KK. Chondrosarcoma in Maffucci's syndrome. *J Bone Joint Surg Am.* 1985;67A:1214–1219.

Swarts SJ, Neff JR, Nelson M, Johansson S, Bridge JA. Chromosomal abnormalities in low grade chondrosarcoma and a review of the literature. *Cancer Genet Cytogenet.* 1997;98:126–130.

Tateishi U, Hasegawa T, Nojima T, Takegami T, Arai Y. MR features of extraskeletal myxoid chondrosarcoma. *Skeletal Radiol.* 2006;35:27–33.

Tetu B, Ordonez NG, Ayala AG, Mackay B. Chondrosarcoma with additional mesenchymal component (dedifferentiated chondrosarcoma). *Cancer.* 1986;58:287–298.

Unger EC, Kessler HB, Kowalyshyn MJ, Lackman RD, Morea GT. MR imaging of Maffucci syndrome. *AJR Am J Roentgenol.* 1988;150:351–353.

Unni KK. *Dahlin's Bone Tumors: General Aspects and Data on 11,087 Cases.* 5th ed. Philadelphia, PA: Lippincott-Raven; 1996:25-45;185–196.

Unni KK, Dahlin DC, Beabout JW, Sim FH. Chondrosarcoma: clear-cell variant: a report of 16 cases. *J Bone Joint Surg Am.* 1976;58A:676–683.

Uri DS, Dalinka MK, Kneeland JB. Muscle impingement: MR imaging of a painful complication of osteochondromas. *Skeletal Radiol.* 1996;25:689–692.

Vanel D, De Paolis M, Monti C, Mercuri M, Picci P. Radiological features of 24 periosteal chondrosarcomas. *Skeletal Radiol.* 2001;30:208–212.

Varma DGK, Kumar R, Carrasco CH, Guo S-Q, Richli WR. MR imaging of periosteal chondroma. *J Comput Assist Tomogr.* 1991;15:1008–1010.

Viala P, Vanel D, Larbi A, Cytevel C, Laredo J-D. Bilateral ischiofemoral impingement in a patient with hereditary multiple exostoses. *Skeletal Radiol.* 2012;41:1637–1640.

Wang L, Motoi T, Khanin R, et al. Identification of a novel, recurrent HEY1-NCOA2 fusion in mesenchymal chondrosarcoma based on genome-wide screen of exon level expression data. *Genes Chromosomes Cancer.* 2012;51:127–139.

Weatherall PT, Maale GE, Mendelsohn DB, Sherry CS, Erdman WE, Pascoe HR. Chondroblastoma: classic and confusing appearance at MR imaging. *Radiology.* 1994;190:467–474.

West OC, Reinus WR, Wilson AJ. Quantitative analysis of the plain radiographic appearance of central chondrosarcoma of bone. *Invest Radiol.* 1995;30:440–447.

White PG, Saunders L, Orr W, Friedman L. Chondromyxoid fibroma. *Skeletal Radiol.* 1996;25:79–81.

Wilson AJ, Kyriakos M, Ackerman LV. Chondromyxoid fibroma: radiographic appearance in 38 cases and in a review of the literature. *Radiology.* 1991;179:513–518. [Erratum, *Radiology* 1991;180:586.]

Wittkop B, Davies AM, Mangham DC. Primary synovial chondromatosis and synovial chondrosarcoma: a pictorial review. *Eur Radiol.* 2002;12:2112–2119.

Wootton-Georges SL. MR imaging of primary bone tumors and tumor-like conditions in children. *Magn Reson Imaging Clin N Am.* 2009;17:469–487.

Wuyts W, Van Hul W. Molecular basis of multiple exostoses: mutations in the EXT1 and EXT2 genes. *Hum Mutat.* 2000;15:220–227.

Yamaguchi T, Dorfman HD. Radiologic and histologic patterns of calcification in chondromyxoid fibroma. *Skeletal Radiol.* 1998;27:559–564.

Yamamura S, Sato K, Sugiura H, Iwata H. Inflammatory reaction in chondroblastoma. *Skeletal Radiol.* 1996;25:371–376.

CHAPTER 4

Fibrogenic, Fibro-osseous, and Fibrohistiocytic Lesions

These lesions represent a clinical spectrum ranging from very innocent lesions requiring no treatment at all to very aggressive and malignant neoplasms. All of these conditions have a common denominator, which is the fibroblast cell. In general, the *fibrous lesions* are composed of spindle cells (myofibroblasts and fibroclasts), which produce a collagenous matrix and so-called ground substance consisting of glucosaminoglycans, whereas the *fibrohistiocytic lesions* may or may not produce a collagenous matrix. Although some fibrous lesions, such as nonossifying fibroma or periosteal desmoid, are not regarded as tumors and are not categorized as miscellaneous lesions by World Health Organization (WHO), they are included here for the purpose of differential diagnosis (Table 4.1). Occasionally, nonossifying fibromas may involve several bones, in which case the condition is called disseminated nonossifying fibromatosis. Some of the patients with this presentation may exhibit on the skin café-au-lait spots with smooth border and develop neurofibromas affecting various nerves. This association is known as Jaffe-Campanacci syndrome. Benign fibrous histiocytoma is a lesion histopathologically very similar to nonossifying fibroma, but affecting older patients, seen in atypical locations, and frequently symptomatic. Fibrous dysplasia is classified by some authorities as a developmental abnormality, but now is considered to represent a genetically based sporadic disorder characterized by the replacement of normal lamellar cancellous bone by an abnormal fibrous tissue. Its polyostotic form may be associated with endocrine disturbances (leading to premature sexual development in girls) and skin pigmentation (café-au-lait spots with rough border), known as McCune-Albright syndrome, or with benign soft-tissue myxomas, known as Mazabraud syndrome. Furthermore, massive formation of cartilage may be observed in some lesions, accompanied by secondary calcifications, a condition known as fibrocartilaginous dysplasia. Desmoplastic fibroma represents locally aggressive lesion, classified by some investigators into the so-called intermediate category between benign and malignant tumors. Malignant fibrous tumors consisting of fibrosarcoma and malignant fibrous histiocytoma exhibit similar clinical, imaging, and histopathologic features. However, fibrosarcoma exhibits a characteristic herringbone tweed pattern and malignant fibrous histiocytoma the storiform pattern of cells arrangement. Fibrosarcomas range from the well-differentiated neoplasms, close in appearance to desmoplastic fibroma, to highly malignant tumors, close in appearance to fibroblastic osteosarcoma. Moreover, both fibrosarcomas and malignant fibrous histiocytomas may arise in the preexisting benign conditions such as a medullary bone infarct, Paget disease, or chronic draining sinus of osteomyelitis, as well as in the bones that had been previously irradiated. Angiomatoid fibrous histiocytoma, recently classified by WHO as a tumor of uncertain differentiation, is a rare lesion of low-grade malignancy, affecting predominantly children and young adults, involving mainly the soft tissues but occasionally seen in the bones.

A. Benign Fibrous Lesions
Fibrous Cortical Defect/Nonossifying Fibroma
Benign Fibrous Histiocytoma
Periosteal Desmoid (Cortical Desmoid)
Fibrous Dysplasia
   Monostotic
   Polyostotic
Fibrocartilaginous Dysplasia
Osteofibrous Dysplasia (Kempson-Campanacci Lesion)
Desmoplastic Fibroma (Desmoid Tumor of Bone)

B. Malignant Fibrohistiocytic Tumors
Fibrosarcoma
Malignant Fibrous Histiocytoma (Pleomorphic Undifferentiated Sarcoma)
Angiomatoid Fibrous Histiocytoma of Bone

Table 4.1 Differential Features of Various Fibrous Lesions with Similar Radiographic Appearances

Sex	Age	Location	Radiographic Appearance	Histopathology
Fibrous Dysplasia				
M/F	Any age (monostotic) First to third decades (polyostotic)	Femoral neck (frequent) Long bones Pelvis Ends of bones usually spared Polyostotic: unilateral in skeleton (frequent)	Radiolucent, ground glass, or smoky lesion Thinning of the cortex with endosteal scalloping "Shepherd's crook" deformity Accelerated growth	Woven (nonlamellar) type of bone in loose to dense fibrous stroma; bone trabeculae lacking osteoblastic activity ("naked trabeculae")
Nonossifying Fibroma				
M/F	First to third decades	Long bones (frequently posterior femur)	Radiolucent, eccentric lesion Scalloped, sclerotic border	Whorled pattern of fibrous tissue containing giant cells, hemosiderin, and lipid-filled histiocytes
Osteofibrous Dysplasia (Kempson-Campanacci Lesion)				
M/F	First to second decades	Tibia (frequently anterior aspect) Fibula Intracortical (frequent)	Osteolytic, eccentric lesion Scalloped, sclerotic border Anterior bowing of long bone	Woven and mature (lamellar) type of bone surrounded by cellular fibrous spindle cell growth in whorled or matted pattern; bone trabeculae rimmed by differentiated osteoblasts ("dressed trabeculae")
Ossifying Fibroma of Jaw				
F	Third to fourth decades	Mandible (90%) Maxilla	Expansive radiolucent lesion Sclerotic, well-defined borders	Uniformly cellular fibrous spindle cell growth with varying amounts of woven bone formation and small, round cementum-like bodies
Ossifying Fibroma (Sissons Lesion)				
M/F	Second decade	Tibia Humerus	Radiolucent lesion Sclerotic border Similar to osteofibrous dysplasia	Fibrous tissue containing rounded and spindle-shaped cells with scant intercellular collagen and small, partially calcified spherules resembling cementum-like bodies of ossifying fibroma of the jaw
Liposclerosing Myxofibrous Tumor				
M/F	Second to seventh decades	Intertrochanteric region of the femur	Radiolucent or partially sclerotic lesion with well-defined sclerotic border, occasional central matrix mineralization	Fibrous or myxofibrous areas with metaplastic curvilinear or circular woven bone ossicles and/or dystrophic mineralization in necrotic fat

From Greenspan A, Jundt G, Remagen W. *Differential Diagnosis in Orthopaedic Oncology*. 2nd ed., 295, Table 4-2.

A. BENIGN FIBROUS LESIONS

Fibrous Cortical Defect/Nonossifying Fibroma

Definition:

- Benign lesion of bone composed of spindle-shaped fibroblasts, arranged in a storiform pattern, with a variable admixture of multinucleated osteoclast-like giant cells, and occasionally lipid-bearing xanthomatous cells, chronic inflammatory cells, and hemosiderin-laden histiocytes.
- The name fibrous cortical defect is used when the lesion is confined to the cortex; if the lesion becomes large enough to extend into adjacent medullary cavity, then the term nonossifying fibroma (NOF) is used.

Epidemiology:
- Age ranged from 6 to 74 years old; 30% to 40% in children.
- Children of an average age of 4 years (54% of boys and 22% of girls) had a lesion involving the cortex, and majority of lesions regressed spontaneously over a period of approximately 2.5 years.

Site of Involvement:
- Approximately 40% lesions occur in the long bones, with the distal femur and distal and proximal tibia most commonly affected.
- As many as 25% of cases involve the pelvic bones, particularly the ilium.

Clinical Findings:
- Majority of patients are asymptomatic, and the lesion is accidentally discovered on imaging studies performed for other reasons.
- Larger lesion may cause pain that is probably secondary to microfractures or obvious pathologic fracture.
- Most pathologic fractures develop through the lesions that involve more than 50% of the transverse diameter of the bone.
- The vast majority of lesions are monostotic; approximately 8% of cases are polyostotic.
- Polyostotic lesions may be associated with Jaffe-Campanacci syndrome, a condition comprising nonossifying fibromatosis, neurofibromas, and café-au-lait spots.

Imaging:
- Radiography demonstrates eccentric, radiolucent lesion with sclerotic border centered within the metaphyseal or diaphyseal cortex (fibrous cortical defect) (Fig. 4.1), or extending into the adjacent medullary cavity (NOF) (Figs. 4.2 to 4.4); it may exhibits prominent trabeculations (see Fig. 4.2B).
- Scintigraphy shows minimal to mildly increased activity.
- Computed tomography demonstrates to better advantage the cortical thinning and medullary involvement (Fig. 4.5) and may delineate early pathologic fracture more precisely.
- Magnetic resonance imaging shows intermediate-to-low signal intensity on T1-weighted and intermediate-to-high signal intensity on T2-weighted and other water-sensitive sequences. After intravenous administration of gadolinium, the lesion exhibits a hyperintense border and signal enhancement (Fig. 4.6).

Pathology:
Gross (Macroscopy):
- Central or more often eccentric, well-circumscribed lesion with sclerotic and sometimes scalloped borders.
- The lesions are reddish-brown and frequently exhibit areas that are soft and yellow (Fig. 4.7A).
- The overlying cortex is thinned out and may be eroded (Fig. 4.7B).

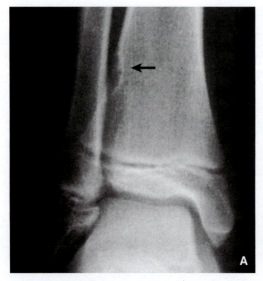 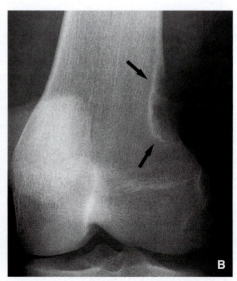

FIGURE 4.1 Radiography of fibrous cortical defect. (A) Small radiolucent lesion exhibiting a thin sclerotic border *(arrow)* is present in the lateral cortex of the distal tibia of a 13-year-old boy. **(B)** In another patient, a 21-year-old woman, note a radiolucent lesion with sclerotic border affecting the medial cortex of the distal femur *(arrows)*.

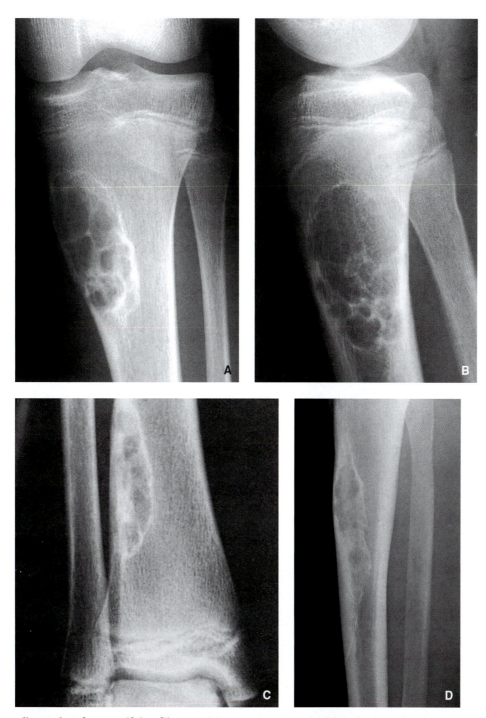

FIGURE 4.2 Radiography of nonossifying fibroma. (A) Anteroposterior and **(B)** lateral radiographs of a 12-year-old girl, show a large elliptical lobulated lesion eccentrically located in the proximal tibia exhibiting well-defined sclerotic border and prominent trabeculations. **(C)** Eccentrically located lesion in the distal tibia of an asymptomatic 15-year-old boy exhibits a slightly scalloped sclerotic border. **(D)** In another patient, an 8-year-old boy, lateral radiograph of the leg shows a long radiolucent lesion with sclerotic border affecting the anterior cortex of the proximal tibia and extending into the medullary cavity of bone, similar in appearance to osteofibrous dysplasia (see Figs. 4.39 and 4.40).

Histopathology:
- Stroma of spindle-shaped fibroblasts, arranged, at least focally, in a whorled, storiform pattern, with scattered variable number of small, multinucleated, osteoclast-type giant cells (Figs. 4.8 to 4.10).
- Foam (xanthoma) cells, with small, dark nuclei, are frequently but not always found, interspersed among the stromal cells individually or in small clusters (see Fig. 4.8C).
- Siderin-containing macrophages may be present (see Fig. 4.10A).
- Scattered inflammatory cells, mainly lymphocytes, are present (see Fig. 4.9B).
- Small stromal hemorrhages and hemosiderin may be present.

Prognosis:
- Excellent.
- Many lesions undergo spontaneous healing.
- Asymptomatic lesions usually do not need surgical intervention.
- Painful larger lesions or those that exhibit an impending or established pathologic fracture are adequately treated by curettage and bone grafting.

Differential Diagnosis:
- ***Monostotic fibrous dysplasia***
  Lesion centrally located in a long bone.
  Ground-glass or smoky appearance.
  Rind sign usually present.

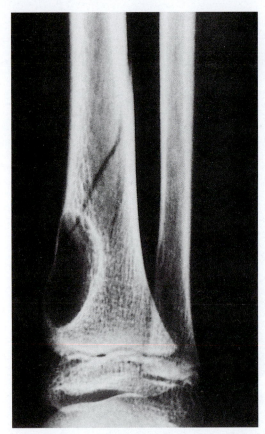

FIGURE 4.3 Radiography of nonossifying fibroma. A large radiolucent lesion in the distal tibia of a 10-year-old boy is complicated by a pathologic fracture.

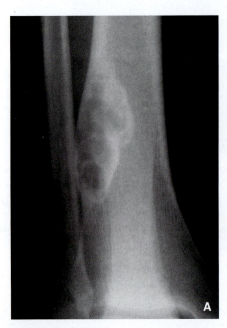
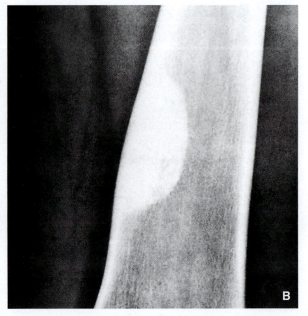

FIGURE 4.4 Radiography of nonossifying fibroma. (A) In a healing stage, the lesion may exhibit progressive sclerosis at periphery. **(B)** Completely healed lesion may persists as a sclerotic patch.

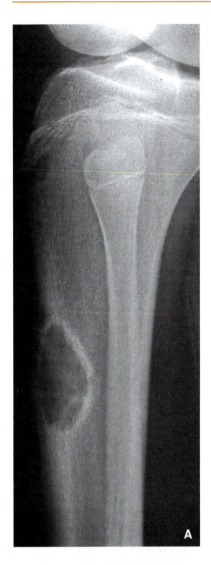
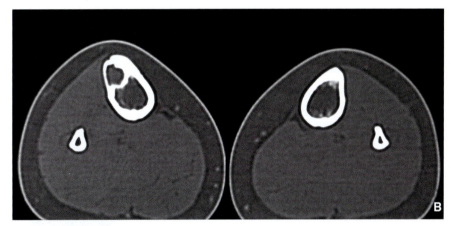
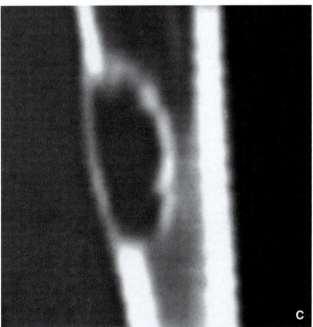

FIGURE 4.5 Radiography and computed tomography of nonossifying fibroma. **(A)** Oblique radiograph of the right tibia of a 14-year-old girl shows an elliptical radiolucent lesion with sclerotic border. **(B)** Axial CT section well demonstrates the extension of the lesion into the medullary portion of bone. **(C)** Coronal reformatted CT image shows the full extent of the lesion. Note the thinning of the anterior tibial cortex.

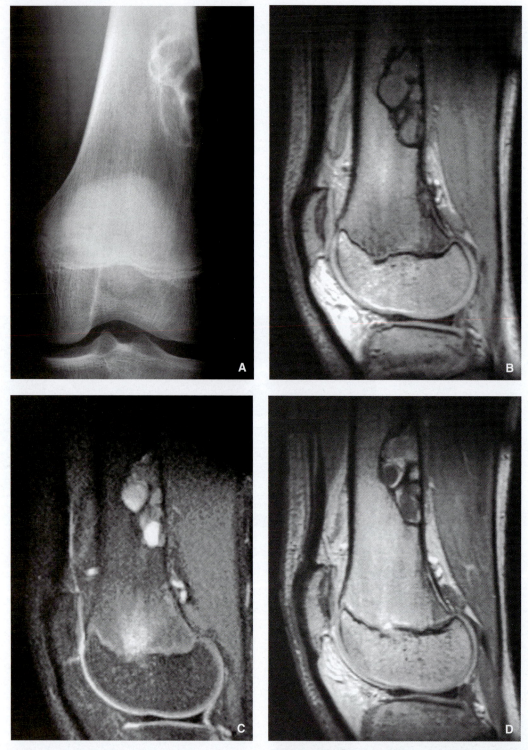

FIGURE 4.6 Radiography and magnetic resonance imaging of nonossifying fibroma. (A) Anteroposterior radiograph of the right knee shows an eccentric radiolucent lesion with sclerotic border abutting the posteromedial femoral cortex. **(B)** Sagittal T1-weighted MR image shows the lesion to be predominantly of intermediate signal intensity with low-signal border. **(C)** Sagittal T2-weighted MRI shows heterogeneous but predominantly high signal intensity of the lesion. **(D)** Sagittal T1-weighted fat-suppressed MRI obtained after intravenous administration of gadolinium shows slight heterogeneous enhancement of the lesion.

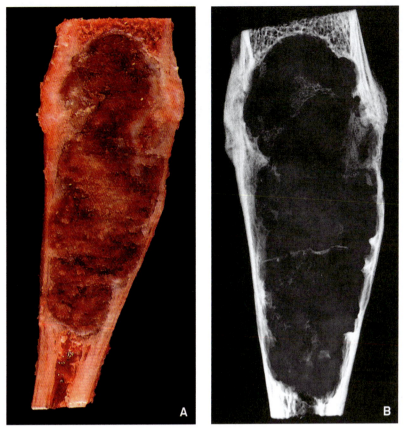

FIGURE 4.7 Gross specimen of nonossifying fibroma. (A) Section through the specimen of resected proximal fibula shows red-brownish in color lesion with lobulated margins. **(B)** Radiograph of the specimen demonstrates endosteal scalloping and thinning of the cortex. (From Bullough P. *Atlas of Orthopedic Pathology*. 2nd ed. New York: Gower Medical Publication; 1992, Figs. 15.40 and 15.41, p. 15.15).

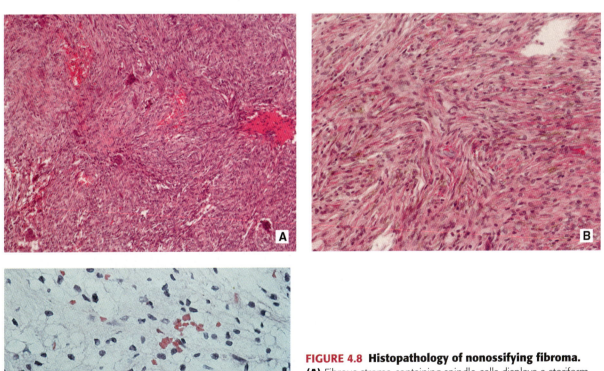

FIGURE 4.8 Histopathology of nonossifying fibroma. (A) Fibrous stroma containing spindle cells displays a storiform arrangement. Several osteoclast-like giant cells are also present (H&E, original magnification ×100). **(B)** On higher magnification, the storiform arrangement of slender cells is better appreciated (H&E, original magnification ×200). **(C)** In another field of view, several foam cells are conspicuous (H&E, original magnification ×400).

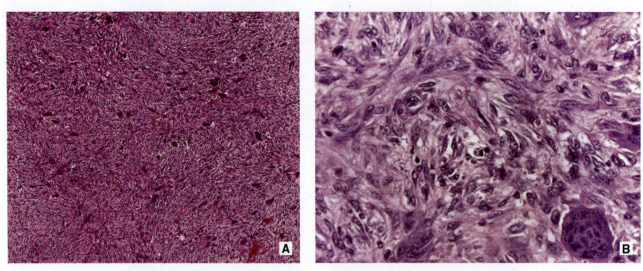

FIGURE 4.9 Histopathology of nonossifying fibroma. (A) Stroma of spindle-shaped fibroblasts is arranged, at least focally, in a whorled, storiform pattern. Note scattered variable number of multinucleated giant cells (H&E, original magnification ×50). **(B)** High-power magnification better depicts the spindle-shaped fibroblasts, scattered lymphocytes, and osteoclast-type giant cells (H&E, original magnification ×200).

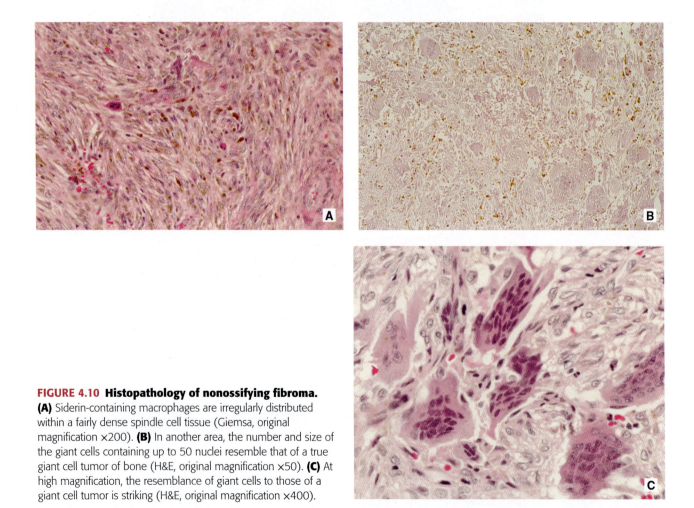

FIGURE 4.10 Histopathology of nonossifying fibroma. (A) Siderin-containing macrophages are irregularly distributed within a fairly dense spindle cell tissue (Giemsa, original magnification ×200). **(B)** In another area, the number and size of the giant cells containing up to 50 nuclei resemble that of a true giant cell tumor of bone (H&E, original magnification ×50). **(C)** At high magnification, the resemblance of giant cells to those of a giant cell tumor is striking (H&E, original magnification ×400).

Histopathology shows immature woven bone trabeculae within loose to dense fibrous stroma and conspicuous lack of osteoblastic activity ("naked trabeculae").
- *Osteofibrous dysplasia*
Majority of the patients are children.
Tibia is the primary site of involvement.
Affects the anterior cortex of bone.
Anterior bowing commonly present.
Histopathology shows woven and mature (lamellar) bone trabeculae being rimmed by the osteoblasts ("dressed trabeculae").
- *Giant cell tumor*
Occurs in skeletally matured patients.
Tumor invariably extends into the articular end of the bone.
Lack of sclerotic border.
Histopathology shows dual population of fibrocytic or monocytic mononuclear stromal cells and even distribution of giant cells throughout the lesion.
- *Langerhans cell histiocytosis*
Usually the lesion lacks the sclerotic border.
"Hole-within-hole" appearance may be observed.
Scalloping of endocortex may be present.
Fusiform thickening of the cortex and periosteal (usually lamellated) reaction is a common finding.
Histopathology shows agglomerates of small or large round cells without obvious cytoplasmic extensions. The nuclei are ovoid or kidney bean shaped and may exhibit longitudinal grooves. Langerhans cells are positive for CD1a. Electron microscopy is diagnostic because of the presence of racquet-shaped cytoplasmic organelles known as Birbeck granules.
- *Desmoplastic fibroma*
Expansive radiolucent lesion with nonsclerotic but usually sharply defined borders. Internal trabeculations are common. Honeycomb pattern of bone destruction may be present. Occasionally, soft-tissue extension may be encountered.
Histopathology shows very regular benign-looking spindle-shaped fibroblasts with elongated or ovoid nuclei interspersed in a densely collagenized matrix, which constitutes the greater portion of the tumor.
- *Chondromyxoid fibroma*
Proximal tibia is the preferential location.
Often erodes or balloons out of the cortex.
Periosteal reaction in form of well-defined buttress invariably present.
Histopathology shows lobulated areas of spindle-shaped or stellate cells distributed within abundant myxoid or chondroid intercellular matrix.

Benign Fibrous Histiocytoma

Definition:
- A benign neoplasm, which may develop within the bone, subcutaneous tissue, deep soft tissue, or in the parenchymal organs, composed of mixture of fibroblastic and histiocytic cells arranged in sheets of short fascicles and accompanied by inflammatory cells, foam cells, and siderophages.
- When located in the skin is also called dermatofibroma.

Epidemiology:
- May occur in any age, but adults over 25 years are most commonly affected.

Sites of Involvement:
- In the skeletal system—articular end of long bone, flat bones (pelvis, ribs).
- In the soft tissues—the lower limb and the head and neck region are the most common sites; most cases involve skin and subcutaneous tissue, but a few cases were described in muscle, mesentery, trachea, and kidney.

Clinical Findings:
- In the bones, presents as a painful mass.
- In the skin and soft tissues, most cases present as solitary, painless, and slowly enlarging mass.
- May occur after minor trauma or insect bites.

Imaging:
- Radiography shows well-defined radiolucent lesion with sclerotic borders, similar in appearance to NOF, occasionally exhibiting some degree of expansion (Fig. 4.11).
- Scintigraphy shows moderately increased uptake of radiopharmaceutical tracer (Fig. 4.12).
- Magnetic resonance imaging features are identical to those of NOF and show the lesion to be of intermediate signal intensity and isointense with the muscles on T1-weighted images and of high signal intensity on water-sensitive sequences.

Pathology:
Gross (Macroscopy):
- Osseous lesions similar to NOFs.
- Cutaneous lesions are elevated or pedunculated, measuring from a few millimeters to few centimeters.

Histopathology:
- Osseous lesions similar to NOFs but storiform pattern more prominent (Figs. 4.13 and 4.14).
- Cutaneous lesions consist of nodular spindle cell proliferation involving the dermis and occasionally subcutis.
- Borders of the tumor are sharply demarcated and typically interdigitate with dermal collagen ("collagen trapping").
- Tumor cells are cytologically bland and spindle shaped with elongated or plump vesicular nuclei and eosinophilic, ill-defined cytoplasm.
- There is no nuclear pleomorphism or hyperchromasia; mitoses may be seen.
- Stroma may show myxoid changes or hyalinization, and some xanthoma-like cells.

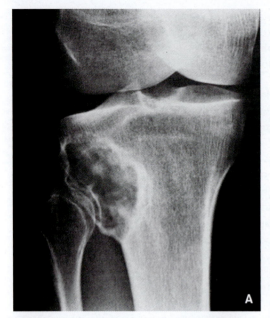
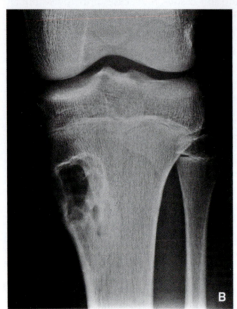
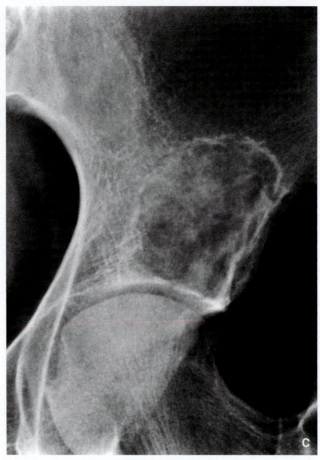

FIGURE 4.11 Radiography of benign fibrous histiocytoma. (A) A 37-year-old man presented with occasional pain in the right knee. An oblique radiograph of the knee shows a lobulated radiolucent lesion with well-defined sclerotic border, located eccentrically in the proximal tibia. **(B)** A 16-year-old boy presented with a painful tibial lesion, which on radiographic examination looked like a NOF. On the excision biopsy, the lesion was more consistent with benign fibrous histiocytoma (see Fig. 4.13). **(C)** A 42-year-old woman presented with left hip pain. The radiograph shows a well-defined lesion with sclerotic border located in the supra-acetabular portion of the ilium, similar in appearance to NOF. The excision biopsy was more consistent with benign fibrous histiocytoma.

- Deep fibrous histiocytomas usually are similar to cutaneous form but show more prominent storiform pattern and fewer secondary elements like xanthoma cells.

Immunohistochemistry:
- Positive for factor XIIIa, desmin, and CD34.

Prognosis:
- May recur locally if not incompletely excised.

Differential Diagnosis:
- ***Nonossifying fibroma***
  Younger age.
  Most of the time asymptomatic.
  Radiographically very similar to benign fibrous histiocytoma (BFH).
  Histopathology almost identical to BFH.
- ***Giant cell tumor***
  Invariably extends into the articular end of bone.
  Lack of sclerotic border.
  Histopathology including the dual population of fibrocytic or monocytic mononuclear stromal cells and uniformly distributed giant cells is diagnostic.
- ***Osteoblastoma***
  Younger age.
  Periosteal reaction very common.
  Central opacities.
  Histopathology showing trabeculae of woven bone surrounded by osteoblasts is diagnostic.
- ***Chondromyxoid fibroma***
  Younger age.
  Periosteal reaction very common.

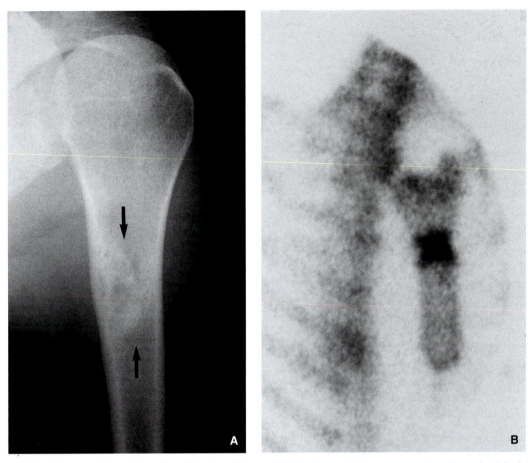

FIGURE 4.12 Radiography and scintigraphy of benign fibrous histiocytoma. (A) Anteroposterior radiograph of the left proximal humerus of a 26-year-old woman, who presented with chronic pain in this region, shows well-defined, partially sclerotic lesion (*arrows*). **(B)** Radionuclide bone scan demonstrates homogenously increased uptake of the radiopharmaceutical agent.

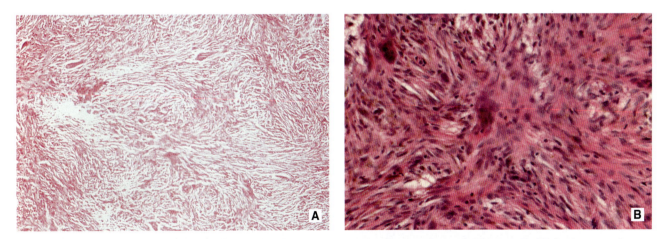

FIGURE 4.13 Histopathology of benign fibrous histiocytoma (same patient as shown in Fig. 4.11B). (A) Benign-appearing fibrous tissue displays prominent storiform pattern (H&E, original magnification ×100). **(B)** In another section, giant cells and some inflammatory cells are also present. The spindle cells do not exhibit atypical features (H&E, original magnification ×200).

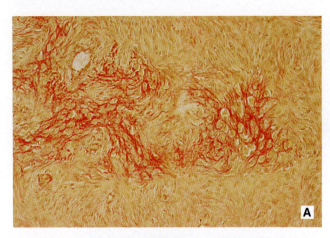
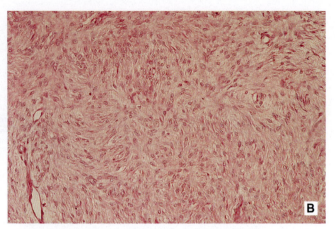

FIGURE 4.14 **Histopathology of benign fibrous histiocytoma. (A)** Spotty increase of collagen fiber formation *(center, red)* resembles primitive osteoid (van Gieson, original magnification ×20). **(B)** On higher magnification, densely arranged spindle cells exhibit a cartwheel-like arrangement *(center)* (H&E, original magnification ×50).

Ballooning out of the cortex.
Histopathology showing large lobulated areas of spindle-shaped or stellate cells distributed within abundant myxoid or chondroid intercellular matrix is diagnostic.

Periosteal Desmoid (Cortical Desmoid)

Definition:
- Tumor-like fibrous proliferation of the periosteum, with striking predilection for the posteromedial cortex of the distal femur.

Epidemiology:
- Age between 12 and 20 years.
- Predominantly the boys are affected.

Sites of Involvement:
- Posteromedial cortex of the medial femoral condyle at linea aspera.

Clinical Findings:
- Asymptomatic lesion discovered by serendipity, usually through the imaging studies done for trauma.

Imaging:
- Radiography and computed tomography shows cortical irregularity or saucer-like radiolucent defect with sclerosis at its base (Figs. 4.15 and 4.16). May mimic aggressive or malignant tumor–like osteosarcoma or Ewing sarcoma.
- Magnetic resonance imaging shows the lesion to be hypointense on T1-weighted images and hyperintense on T2-weighted and other water-sensitive sequences.

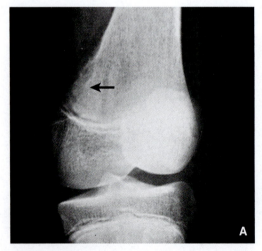
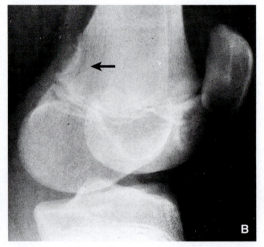

FIGURE 4.15 **Radiography of periosteal desmoid. (A)** Oblique radiograph of the left knee of a 12-year-old boy shows the classic appearance of this lesion. Note elliptical radiolucency within the cortex of the medial aspect of the distal femoral metaphysis at the linea aspera producing cortical irregularity *(arrow)*. **(B)** In another patient, an 11-year-old boy, a saucer-like defect is present in the medial cortex of the distal femoral metaphysis *(arrow)*.

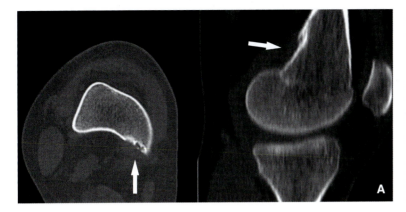
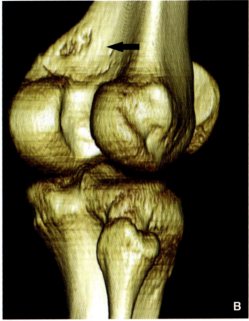

FIGURE 4.16 Computed tomography of periosteal desmoid. (A) Axial and sagittal reformatted CT images and **(B)** 3D reconstructed CT image with surface-rendering algorithm of the knee of a 17-year-old boy show well-marginated cortical defect in the posteromedial aspect of the distal femur *(arrows)*.

Histopathology:

- Fibroblastic spindle cells that produce a large amount of collagen. Large areas of hyalinization and fibrocartilage and small fragments of bone may be scattered within fibrous tissue (Fig. 4.17).

Prognosis:

- Excellent. Spontaneous regression in majority of cases.

Differential Diagnosis:

- *Osteosarcoma*
  Imaging studies show aggressive periosteal reaction; tumor bone in form of fluffy densities within the bone lesion and in the soft-tissue mass.
  Histopathology shows malignant cells forming tumor osteoid or tumor bone.
- *Ewing sarcoma*
  Imaging studies show permeative or moth-eaten bone destruction; onionskin-like periosteal reaction; usually large soft-tissue mass.
  Histopathology shows small uniform-sized round cells with indistinct borders, clear-to-light eosinophilic cytoplasm, and round and hyperchromic nuclei.
- *Periosteal chondroma*
  Usually exhibits chondroid calcifications and buttress of periosteal reaction.
  Histopathology shows chondrocytes located in the lacunae.

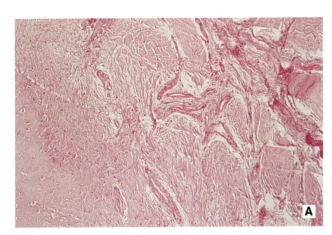
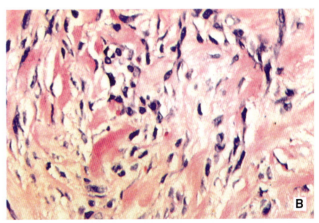

FIGURE 4.17 Histopathology of periosteal desmoid. (A) The cortical bone is made up of coarse plates of cell-rich woven bone merging with benign-appearing fibrous tissue (H&E, original magnification ×12). **(B)** Poorly organized but benign-appearing fibroblasts produce abundant collagen (H&E, original magnification ×25). (From Bullough P. *Atlas of Orthopedic Pathology*. 2nd ed. New York: Gower Medical Publication; 1992,15.20, Fig. 15.54).

- *Fibrous cortical defect*
  Imaging studies show sharply demarcated cortical lesion without periosteal reaction.
  Histopathology shows spindle-shaped fibroblasts arranged in a storiform pattern, with a variable admixture of multinucleated osteoclast-like giant cells and occasionally lipid-bearing xanthomatous cells.

Fibrous Dysplasia

Definition:
- Benign medullary fibro-osseous lesion, which may involve one (monostotic form) or more (polyostotic form) bones, characterized by the replacement of normal lamellar and cancellous bone by abnormal fibrous tissue containing trabeculae of immature woven bone.

Epidemiology:
- Children and adults.
- No gender predilection.
- Monostotic form most common (70% to 80%).

Sites of Involvement:
- Gnathic (jaw) bones most common.
- Long bones are more often affected in women.
- Ribs and skull are favored sites for men.
- In monostotic form, about 35% involve the skull, 33% the tibia and femur, and 20% the ribs.
- In polyostotic form, the femur, pelvic bones, and tibia are most commonly affected.

Clinical Findings:
- Polyostotic form can be confined to one extremity or one side of the body or be diffuse.
- Polyostotic form often manifest earlier in life than the monostotic form.
- The condition is often asymptomatic, but pain and pathologic fractures may be part of the clinical spectrum.
- Oncogenic osteomalacia may be associated.
- Polyostotic form may manifest as McCune-Albright syndrome, the condition marked by skin pigmentation (café-au-lait spots) and variety of endocrine abnormalities.
- If polyostotic form is associated with formation of soft-tissue myxomas, the condition is known as Mazabraud syndrome.
- If there is cartilage deposition within the lesion, the condition is known as fibrocartilaginous dysplasia (see below).

Imaging:
- The various amount of bone in the fibrous tissue that replaces the cancellous bone imparts a radiographic picture that ranges from radiolucency to radiodensity of the lesion (Fig. 4.18).
- More common radiographic presentation is a radiolucent lesion exhibiting a ground-glass, milky, or smoky appearance (see Fig. 4.18A).
- In the appendicular skeleton, the margins are usually well defined and surrounded by a rim of sclerotic bone (rind sign) (Fig. 4.19), but some lesions, including those in the craniofacial bones, may have indistinct borders.
- Cortex is usually thinned out (see Fig. 4.18A).
- "Shepherd's crook" deformity of the femur is a characteristic feature (Fig. 4.20).
- Skull lesions affect primarily the base, causing thickening and sclerosis of the sphenoid wings, sella, and the vertical portion of the frontal bones; less common the vault of the skull is affected (Fig. 4.21).
- Scintigraphy shows moderate to markedly increased activity of radiopharmaceutical agent (Figs. 4.22 and 4.23).
- CT accurately delineates the extent of bone involvement, with Hounsfield units in the range of between 70 and 400 HU (Figs. 4.24 to 4.28, see also Fig. 4.21).
- MRI shows the lesion to be of intermediate to low signal intensity on T1-weighed sequences and of high signal on T2-weighting and other water-sensitive sequences (Figs. 4.29 to 4.31). There is enhancement of the lesion after intravenous administration of gadolinium.
- In Mazabraud syndrome, MRI shows soft-tissue masses of intermediate signal intensity on T1-weighted images and homogenously bright on T2 weighting, representing myxomas (Fig. 4.32).

Pathology:
Gross (Macroscopy):
- Well-circumscribed white-tan lesion of gritty and leather-like consistency (Fig. 4.33).

Histopathology:
- Cellular fibrous tissue is surrounding the irregular, curvilinear bone trabeculae (Fig. 4.34).
- The bone trabeculae are discontinuous and are composed of woven bone that is formed directly from the spindle cells with no osteoblastic rimming ("naked trabeculae") (Figs. 4.35 and 4.36).
- In craniofacial tumors, the abnormal bone tends to fuse with the surrounding host cancellous bone.
- The spindle cells may be arranged in a storiform pattern and may be associated with collection of foamy macrophages mimicking xanthoma or fibroxanthoma.
- Collagen fibers (Sharpey-like fibers) are frequently seen extending from the fibrous tissue into the immature woven bone trabeculae (see Fig. 4.35B).
- Cementicle-like pattern, reminiscent of cementifying fibroma of the jaw, is occasionally present (Fig. 4.37).
- Cystic changes mimicking aneurysmal bone cyst are occasionally encountered.
- Occasionally encountered are foam cells, multinucleated giant cells, and myxoid changes.

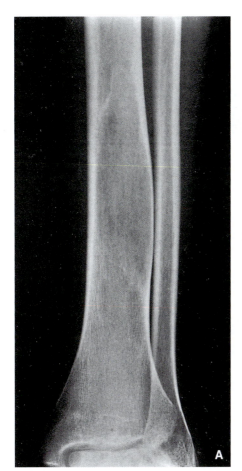
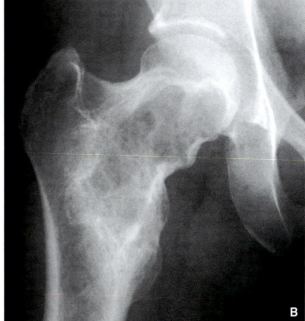
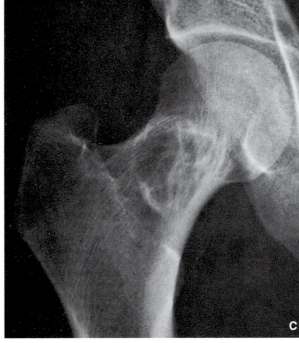

FIGURE 4.18 Radiography of monostotic fibrous dysplasia. (A) Anteroposterior radiograph of the distal leg of a 17-year-old girl shows a solitary focus of fibrous dysplasia in the diaphysis of tibia. Note the "ground-glass" appearance of the lesion and thinning of the lateral cortex. **(B)** Anteroposterior radiograph of the right hip of a 22-year-old woman shows a radiolucent lesion with sclerotic border extending from the femoral neck into the intertrochanteric region. **(C)** Anteroposterior radiograph of the right hip of a 25-year-old man shows more sclerotic appearance of the lesion affecting the femoral neck.

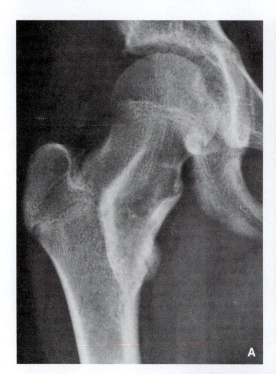
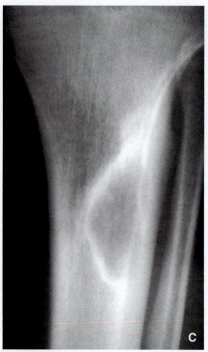
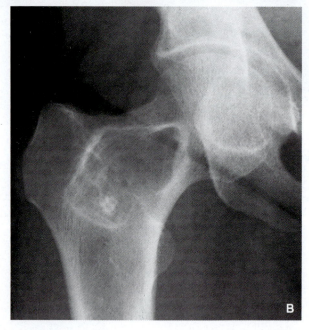

FIGURE 4.19 Radiography of monostotic fibrous dysplasia. **(A)** Anteroposterior radiograph of the right hip shows a radiolucent lesion with sclerotic border (rind sign) located in the femoral neck. **(B)** In another patient, a similar rind sign marks a focus of fibrous dysplasia. **(C)** Yet in another patient, a focus of fibrous dysplasia in the left proximal tibia exhibits characteristic rind sign.

Chapter 4 • Fibrogenic, Fibro-osseous, and Fibrohistiocytic Lesions

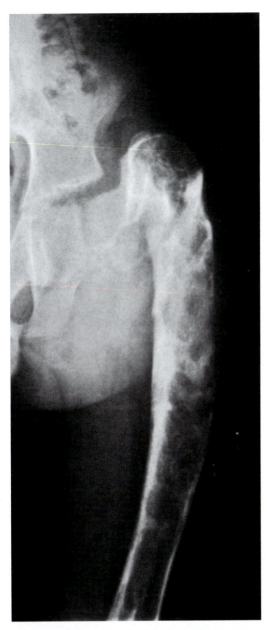

FIGURE 4.20 Radiography of polyostotic fibrous dysplasia. A "shepherd's crook" deformity, seen here in the proximal femur in a 12-year-old boy, is often the result of multiple pathologic fractures.

Genetics:
- Mutation in the *GNAS1* gene (20q13) that encodes the alpha-subunit of the stimulatory G protein–alpha (GS-alpha).
- Mutation of the G proteins (guanine nucleotide–binding protein).
- Trisomy 12 and structural aberrations of 12p13 were described.

Prognosis:
- Good.
- Therapy ranges from observation to surgical intervention.

Differential Diagnosis:
Monostotic Form
- ***Osteofibrous dysplasia***
  Tibia most often affected, particularly anterior cortex; anterior bending is common.
  Histopathology showing "dressed trabeculae" (woven bone trabeculae surrounded by outer zone of lamellar transformation with prominent osteoblastic activity) is diagnostic.
- ***Nonossifying fibroma***
  Radiography shows eccentric location in bone and sclerotic, often lobulated border.
  Histopathology showing bland monomorphous spindle cells admixed with histiocytic and giant cells, and storiform arrangement is usually diagnostic.
- ***Liposclerosing myxofibrous tumor of bone***
  Radiographically the lesion may look identical to focus of fibrous dysplasia (FD).
  Characteristic location in the femoral neck and intertrochanteric region.
  Histopathology showing a complex mixture of elements, including lipoma, fibroxanthoma, myxoma, myxofibroma, cartilage, and fat necrosis, is diagnostic.
- ***Pachydysostosis***
  Rare condition that invariably affects the fibula in children of ages 4 weeks to 4 years. Radiolucent lesion is associated with thinning of the cortex, as well as widening of the bone and bowing deformity.

Polyostotic Form
- ***Ollier disease***
  May show similar to polyostotic FD, a unilateral involvement of the skeleton.
  Imaging studies show marked deformities of the bones associated with growth stunting; intracortical chondromas frequently present; common involvement of the hands.
  Histopathology showing lobules of hyaline cartilage of variable cellularity and uniformly translucent intercellular matrix, coupled with chondrocytes located in the lacunae, and lack of woven bone trabeculae is diagnostic.

Fibrocartilaginous Dysplasia

Definition:
- Disorder consisting of massive chondroid differentiation in FD.

Epidemiology:
- Occurs in patients ranged from 4 to 26 years, with average age of 17.5 years.
- Equal male-to-female ratio.

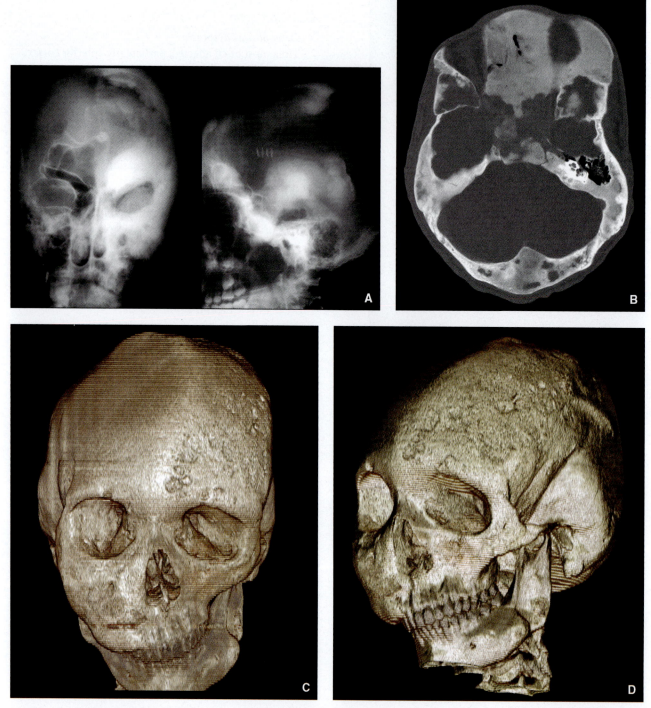

FIGURE 4.21 Radiography and computed tomography of polyostotic fibrous dysplasia. (A) Anteroposterior and lateral radiographs of the skull, **(B)** axial CT, and 3D CT reconstructed in shaded surface display images viewed from the front **(C)** and side **(D)** of a 25-year-old man show extensive involvement of the facial bones and vault of the skull (calvaria), termed *leontiasis ossea*.

Chapter 4 • Fibrogenic, Fibro-osseous, and Fibrohistiocytic Lesions   **199**

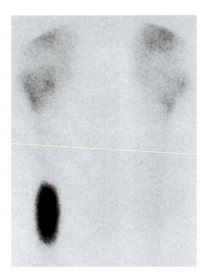

FIGURE 4.22 Scintigraphy of monostotic fibrous dysplasia. Radionuclide bone scan performed in a 24-year-old woman with solitary lesion in the right tibia shows markedly increased focal uptake of the radiopharmaceutical tracer.

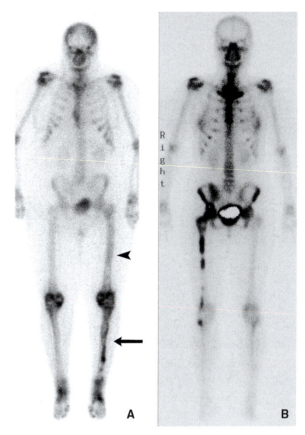

FIGURE 4.23 Scintigraphy of polyostotic fibrous dysplasia. **(A)** Total body radionuclide bone scan performed in a 50-year-old woman shows markedly increased uptake of the radiotracer in the left tibia and fibula (*arrow*) and only slight activity of the lesion in the left femur (*arrowhead*). **(B)** Total body radionuclide bone scan performed in another patient with polyostotic disease shows several areas of significantly increased uptake of the radiopharmaceutical agent.

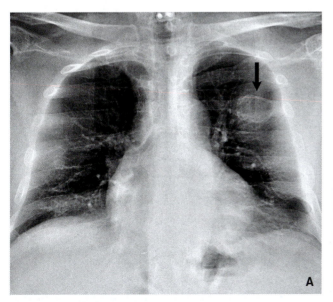
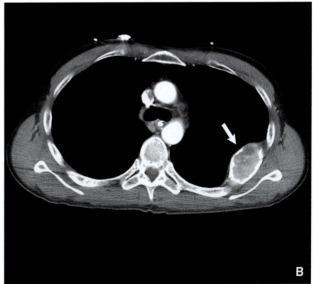

FIGURE 4.24 Radiography and computed tomography of monostotic fibrous dysplasia. **(A)** Anteroposterior radiograph and **(B)** axial CT of the chest of a 56-year-old man show an expansive lesion affecting the fifth left posterior rib (*arrows*).

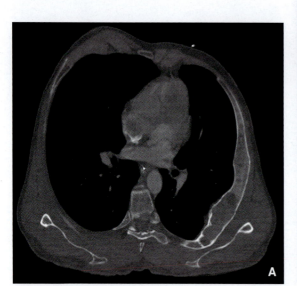
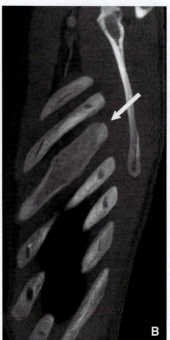
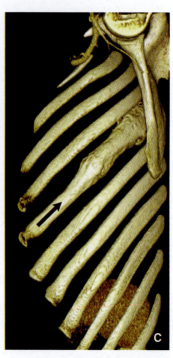

FIGURE 4.25 Computed tomography of monostotic fibrous dysplasia. (A) Axial, **(B)** sagittal reformatted, and **(C)** 3D reconstructed CT images show a lesion affecting posterior portion of the fourth left rib of a 42-year-old man (*arrows*). Observe characteristic expansion of the bone and thinning of the cortex.

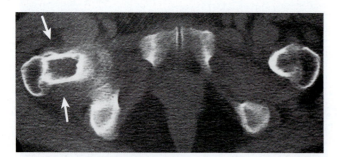

FIGURE 4.26 Computed tomography of monostotic fibrous dysplasia. Axial computed tomography section through the proximal femora shows a low-attenuated lesion in the neck of the right femur with a thick sclerotic rim (*arrows*).

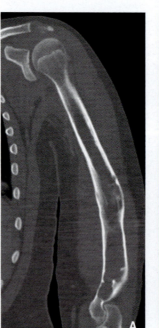
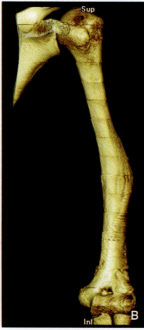

FIGURE 4.27 Computed tomography of monostotic fibrous dysplasia. (A) Coronal reformatted CT image and **(B)** three-dimensional reconstructed in shaded surface display CT image show solitary lesion affecting the mid-to-distal diaphysis of the left humerus of a 13-year-old boy.

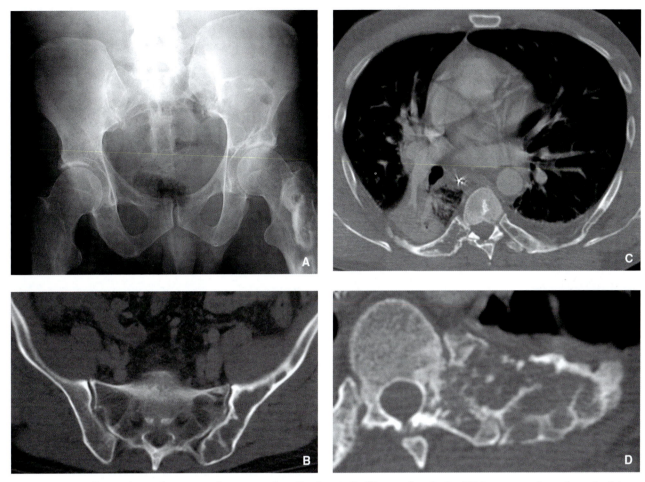

FIGURE 4.28 Radiography and computed tomography of polyostotic fibrous dysplasia. (A) Anteroposterior radiograph of the pelvis shows multiple lesions in the left ilium and proximal left femur. The involvement of the sacrum is not well demonstrated. **(B)** Axial CT section of the pelvis precisely shows the extent of involvement of the left ilium and sacrum. **(C)** Axial CT section of the chest shows foci of fibrous dysplasia in the posterior ribs. **(D)** Magnified coned-down CT image of one of the affected ribs shows details of this condition: observe the multiloculated appearance, expansion of the bone, pseudosepta, thinning of the cortex, and a pathologic fracture.

Sites of Involvement:
- Most common location in the femur, humerus, and tibia.

Clinical findings:
- Identical to those of polyostotic FD.

Imaging:
- Radiography shows typical features of FD including ground-glass appearance and thinning of the cortex, associated with intralesional chondroid in type (stippled, comma-shaped, and ring-like) calcifications (Fig. 4.38).

Pathology:
Gross (Macroscopy):
- Similar to FD with foci of bluish-gray cartilage.

Histopathology:
- Typical findings of FD with hyaline cartilage islands in juxtaposition to fibro-osseous elements; moderate atypia of chondrocytes may be present.

Differential Diagnosis:
- **Ollier disease**
  Imaging studies show marked deformities of the bones associated with growth stunting; presence of intracortical chondromas; common involvement of the hands.
  Histopathology showing lobules of hyaline cartilage of variable cellularity and uniformly translucent intercellular matrix, together with chondrocytes located in the lacunae, and lack of curvilinear woven bone trabeculae, is diagnostic.

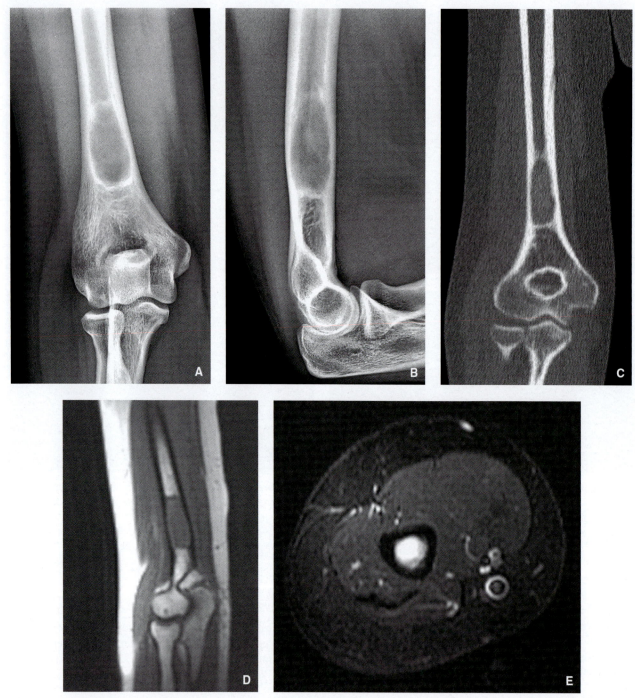

FIGURE 4.29 Radiography, computed tomography, and magnetic resonance imaging of monostotic fibrous dysplasia.
(A) Anteroposterior and **(B)** lateral radiographs of the right elbow show a radiolucent lesion with sclerotic border in the distal humeral shaft of a 26-year-old woman. **(C)** Coronal reformatted CT image shows low-attenuated intramedullary lesion. Note thinning of the cortex.
(D) Sagittal T1-weighted MR image shows the lesion to be of intermediate signal intensity, isointense with the surrounded skeletal muscles.
(E) Axial inversion recovery (IR) MR image shows the lesion exhibiting high signal intensity.

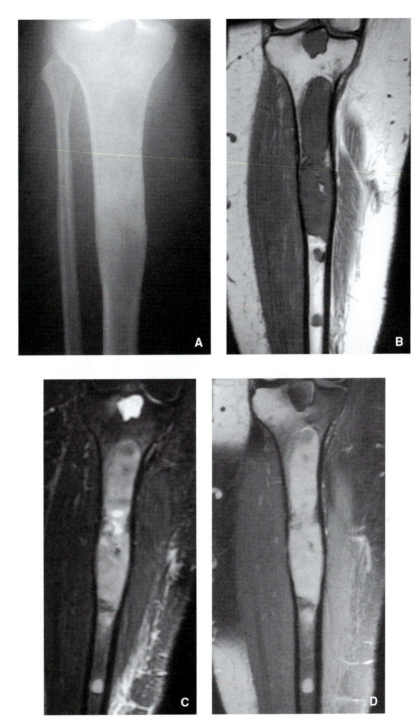

FIGURE 4.30 Radiography and magnetic resonance imaging of polyostotic fibrous dysplasia. (A) Anteroposterior radiograph of the proximal right leg of a 23-year-old woman shows a long lesion in the tibia exhibiting "ground-glass" appearance. The bone is mildly expanded, and the cortex is thin. **(B)** Coronal T1-weighted MR image shows the lesion to be multifocal exhibiting intermediate signal intensity isointense with the skeletal muscles. **(C)** Coronal T2-weighted MRI shows heterogeneous signal of the lesion ranging from intermediate-to-high intensity. **(D)** Coronal T1-weighted fat-suppressed MRI obtained after intravenous administration of gadolinium shows enhancement of the lesion.

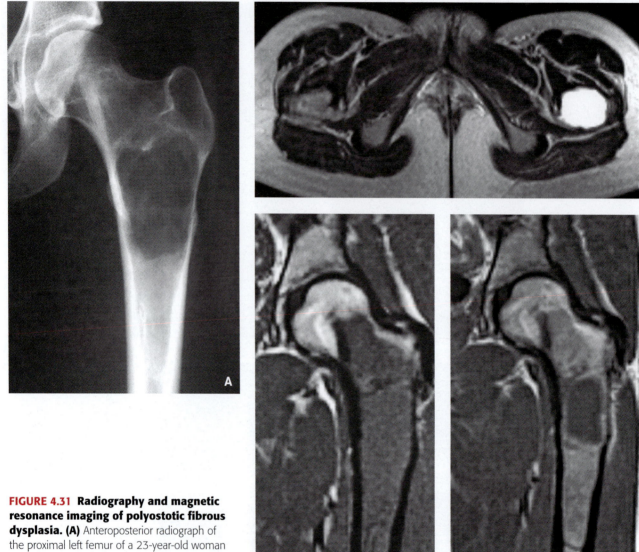

FIGURE 4.31 Radiography and magnetic resonance imaging of polyostotic fibrous dysplasia. (A) Anteroposterior radiograph of the proximal left femur of a 23-year-old woman shows a radiolucent lesion in the subtrochanteric region of the bone. **(B)** Coronal T1-weighted MR image demonstrates the full extent of the lesion, which is of intermediate-to-low signal intensity. Note that the lesion is much larger than shown by radiography. **(C)** Axial T2-weighted MRI shows high signal intensity of the lesion. **(D)** Coronal T1-weighted MR image obtained after intravenous administration of gadolinium shows mild central enhancement.

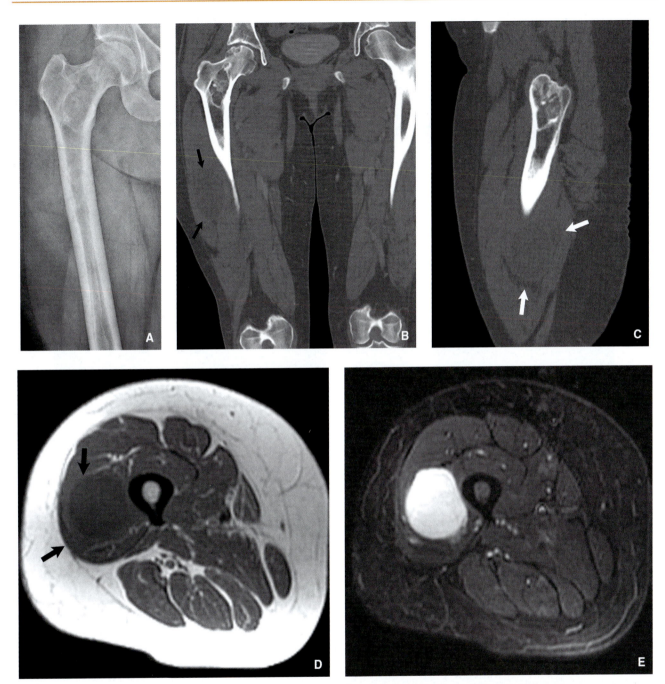

FIGURE 4.32 Radiography, computed tomography, and magnetic resonance imaging of Mazabraud syndrome.
(A) Anteroposterior radiograph of the right femur of a 49-year-old woman shows several radiolucent lesions in the proximal part of the bone.
(B) Coronal and **(C)** sagittal reformatted CT images, in addition to osseous lesions, demonstrate a well-defined soft-tissue mass (*arrows*).
(D) Axial T1-weighted MR image shows a soft-tissue mass to be of intermediate signal intensity (*arrows*), isointense with the skeletal muscles. **(E)** Axial inversion recovery (IR) image shows the mass becoming bright.

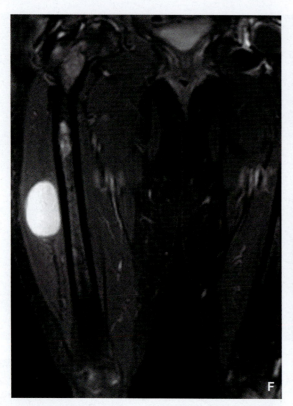 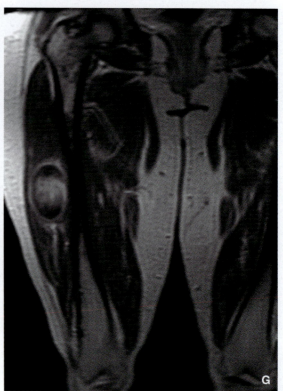

FIGURE 4.32 *(Continued).* **(F)** Coronal T2-weighted fat-suppressed MR image shows the soft-tissue mass to be homogenously of high signal intensity. **(G)** Coronal T1-weighted fat-suppressed MR image obtained after intravenous injection of gadolinium shows mild enhancement of the mass, proven on excision biopsy to represent a benign myxoma.

- *Fibrocartilaginous mesenchymoma*
  Occurs in young patients (mean age 13 years). Radiography shows a radiolucent lesion with scalloped borders, extending to or abutting the growth plate; after skeletal maturity, the lesion may extend into the articular end of the bone. Chondroid calcifications may be present.
  Histopathology shows two components of the lesion—cartilage structured similarly to the growth plate, and spindle cell tissue exhibiting subtle to moderate pleomorphism and some collagen formation. Characteristic feature, however, is the presence of numerous curved cartilage particles surrounded by spindle cell stroma, giving the tumor on H&E staining a "shrimp cocktail" appearance.
- *Chondrosarcoma*
  Imaging studies show thickening of the cortex, deep endosteal scalloping, periosteal reaction, and occasionally soft-tissue mass.
  Histopathology showing pleomorphism, hyperchromatism, nuclear atypia, and production of malignant cartilage by the tumor cells, accompanied by infiltration of haversian systems, and entrapment of bone trabeculae is diagnostic.

Osteofibrous Dysplasia (Kempson-Campanacci Lesion)

Definition:
- Self-limited benign fibro-osseous lesion of the bone.

Epidemiology:
- Rare lesion that accounts for less than 1% of all bone tumors.
- Majority of cases have been described during infancy and early childhood.

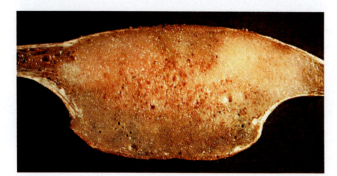

FIGURE 4.33 Gross specimen of fibrous dysplasia. Resected segment of the rib shows yellow-reddish expansive lesion. Observe thinning of the cortex. (From Bullough P. *Atlas of Orthopedic Pathology*. 2nd ed. New York: Gower Medical Publication; 1922:14.2, Fig. 14.2)

Chapter 4 • Fibrogenic, Fibro-osseous, and Fibrohistiocytic Lesions **207**

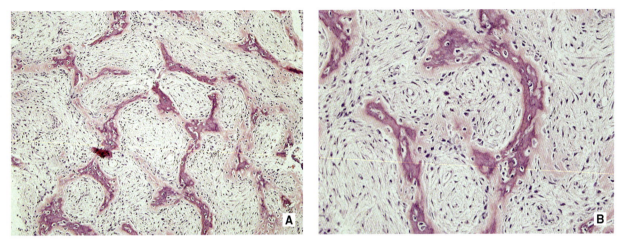

FIGURE 4.34 Histopathology of fibrous dysplasia. (A) Characteristic curvilinear-shaped bone trabeculae are scattered within the spindle cell stroma (H&E, original magnification ×100). **(B)** Typical C-shaped woven bone trabeculae contain several osteocytes. Observe lack of osteoblastic rimming (H&E, original magnification ×200).

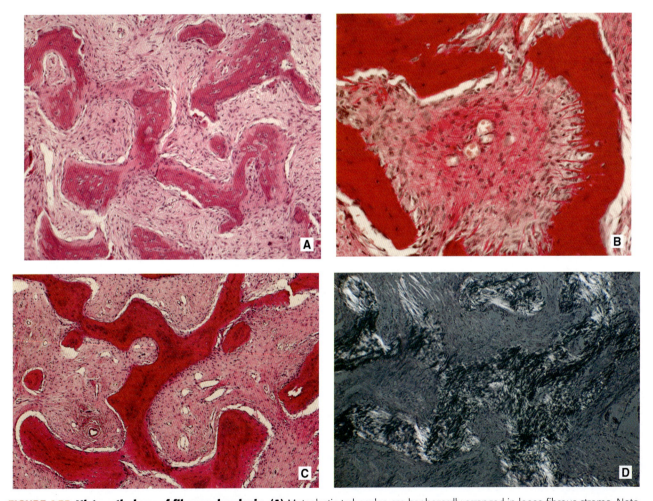

FIGURE 4.35 Histopathology of fibrous dysplasia. (A) Metaplastic trabeculae are haphazardly arranged in loose fibrous stroma. Note lack of osteoblastic activity (H&E, original magnification ×200). **(B)** Collagen fibers, reminiscent of Sharpey fibers, extend from the fibrous stroma into the bone trabeculae. Again, observe the absence of osteoblastic rimming (van Gieson, original magnification ×400). **(C)** In a background of collagenized fibrous tissue, irregularly shaped woven bone trabeculae lacking osteoblastic rimming have been formed (H&E, original magnification ×50). **(D)** Viewed under polarized light, the woven structure of immature bone and the collagen fibers are conspicuous (H&E, polarized light, original magnification ×50).

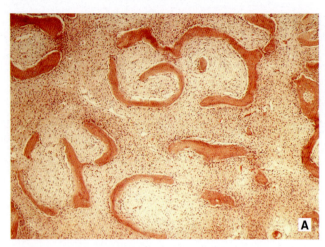 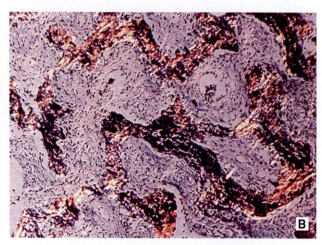

FIGURE 4.36 Histopathology of fibrous dysplasia. (A) Immature woven bone trabeculae resembling Chinese characters are irregularly scattered within the fibrous stroma. Note conspicuous absence of osteoblastic activity (H&E, original magnification ×100). **(B)** Under polarized light, these characteristic features of fibrous dysplasia are better appreciated (H&E, polarized light, original magnification ×200). (Courtesy of Peter Bullough, M.D., New York.)

- Commonly seen in boys during the first two decades of life with precipitous drop-off thereafter.

Sites of Involvement:
- Proximal or middle-third of the tibia (mainly anterior cortex of the diaphysis) is the most common site (90%).
- Much less common sites are the fibula, ulna, and radius.

Clinical Findings:
- Most common presenting symptoms are swelling or painless deforming (bowing) of the involved segment of the limb.

Imaging:
- Radiography demonstrates well-delineated, frequently scalloped, occasionally saw-toothed, or bubbly multiloculated mixed radiolucent and sclerotic intracortical lesion, extending into the medullary cavity (Figs. 4.39 to 4.41).
- Magnetic resonance imaging shows on T1 weighting a heterogeneous but predominantly low signal intensity lesion, whereas on T2-weighted and other water-sensitive sequences, the lesion becomes of intermediate-to-low signal intensity (Fig. 4.42). After intravenous administration of gadolinium, there is always noted significant enhancement (Fig. 4.43).

Pathology:
Gross (Macroscopy):
- Varies in size from less than 1 to greater than 10 cm.
- Typically solid, gritty, yellow, or white lesion, confined to the expanded and attenuated cortex.

Histopathology:
- Irregular, curvilinear trabeculae of woven bone that at the periphery display more mature lamellar bone (so-called zonal architecture), rimmed by prominent osteoblasts, and merging with preexisting cancellous bone (Figs. 4.44 to 4.46).
- Scattered osteoclasts may be seen (see Fig. 4.44B).
- Intervening stroma is composed of benign-appearing spindle-shaped cells embedded in a collagenous matrix.
- Mitoses are extremely rare.
- Occasionally seen are xanthomatous changes, hyalinization, hemorrhage, and cyst formation.

Immunohistochemistry:
- Positive for vimentin, occasionally positive for S-100 protein and Leu7.
- Isolate single stromal cells may express positivity for keratin; however, clusters of epithelial cells, as seen in well-differentiated adamantinoma, are absent.

FIGURE 4.37 Histopathology of fibrous dysplasia. Variant of classic histopathologic appearance with small, discrete, almost osteocyte-free foci of calcified matrix that resemble the cementicles usually seen in cementifying fibroma of the jaw. The scanty spindle cell stroma shows the typical passing of the collagen fibers into the bone trabeculae (H&E, original magnification ×25).

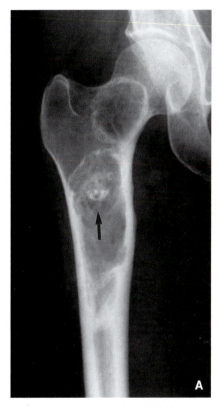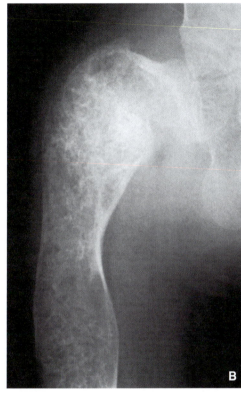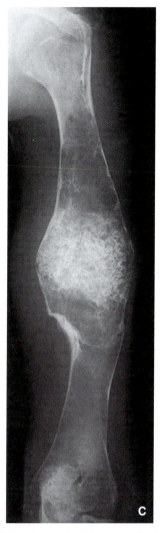

FIGURE 4.38 Radiography of fibrocartilaginous dysplasia. (A) Two separate foci of fibrous dysplasia affecting the right femur display a rind sign (*proximal lesion*) and chondroid calcifications (*distal lesion*) (*arrow*). **(B)** In another patient, a 10-year-old boy, more extensive cartilaginous differentiation is present in the lesion affecting the entire right femur. **(C)** Anteroposterior radiograph of the left humerus of a 19-year-old man shows extensive involvement of almost entire bone with cartilage formation in the midportion of the diaphysis.

Genetics:
- Trisomies 7, 8, 12, and 22 have been demonstrated.

Prognosis:
- Natural history of osteofibrous dysplasia is that of gradual growth during the first decade of life with stabilization or resolution at about 15 years of age.
- Progression of osteofibrous dysplasia-like adamantinoma to classic adamantinoma has been shown in few patients.

Differential Diagnosis:
- *Monostotic fibrous dysplasia*
  Radiography commonly shows centrally located lesion exhibiting ground-glass or smoky appearance, associated with thinning of the cortex. Characteristic rind sign is usually present.
  Histopathology shows characteristic absence of osteoblasts on the surface of the woven bone trabeculae ("naked trabeculae").
- *Nonossifying fibroma*
  Radiography similar to osteofibrous dysplasia; however, histopathology showing bland monomorphous spindle cells admixed with histiocytic cells arranged in a swirling storiform pattern and possessing clear or foamy cytoplasm, and the presence of multinucleated giant cells, is diagnostic.
- *Adamantinoma*
  Radiography shows elongated osteolytic cortical defect separated by areas of sclerosis, exhibiting a soap-bubble appearance, and occasionally saw-toothed area of cortical destruction.
  Histopathology shows biphasic appearance consisting of an epithelial component intimately admixed in various proportions with a fibrous component. Immunohistochemistry showing the cells of adamantinoma strongly marked by antibodies to cytokeratins is diagnostic for this tumor.

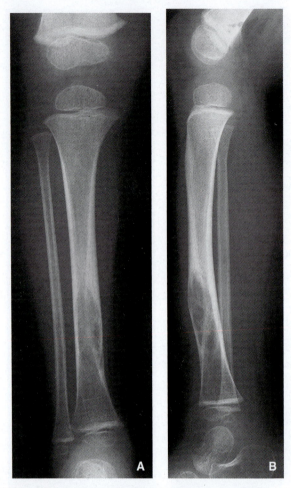

FIGURE 4.39 Radiography of osteofibrous dysplasia. **(A)** Anteroposterior and **(B)** lateral radiographs of the right leg of a 2-year-old boy demonstrate a cortical lesion with medullary extension in the distal tibia.

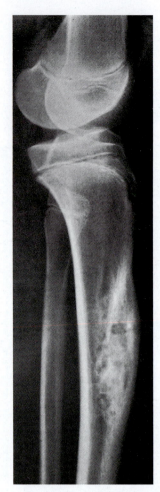

FIGURE 4.40 Radiography of osteofibrous dysplasia. Lateral radiograph of the leg of a 14-year-old boy shows mostly sclerotic lesion affecting the anterior tibia.

- Pathologic fracture or deformity of the affected bone can occasionally be a presenting symptom.

Imaging:
- Usually well-defined, radiolucent lesion that may expand the host bone (Figs. 4.47 to 4.49).
- Intralesional trabeculation is common (see Fig. 4.47B,C).
- Larger lesion often destroys the cortex with extension into soft tissue (see Fig. 4.48).
- Features of more aggressive growth pattern with irregular, ill-defined margins, and pathologic fracture may be present (see Fig. 4.48).
- Honeycombed or moth-eaten patterns have been described.
- Erosive, destructive pattern may mimic more aggressive and even malignant lesions (see Figs. 4.48 and 4.49).
- Magnetic resonance imaging shows low signal intensity on T1-weighted sequences and heterogeneous but predominantly intermediate-to-low signal on T2 weighting with tumor enhancement on the contrast studies (see Fig. 4.49).

Desmoplastic Fibroma (Desmoid Tumor of Bone)

Definition:
- Rare, locally aggressive, solitary tumor, microscopically composed of well-differentiated myofibroblasts with abundant collagen production by the tumor cells.

Epidemiology:
- Rare, 0.1% of all primary bone tumors, and 0.3% of all benign bone tumors.
- It tends to occur in adolescent and young adults (younger than 40 years) with near equal gender distribution.

Sites of Involvement:
- May involve any bone but is most common in the mandible.

Clinical findings:
- Pain and swelling of the affected area are the most common symptoms.

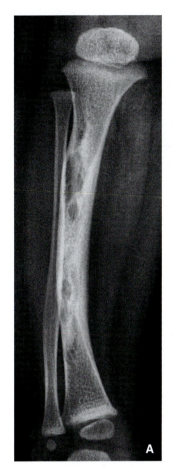
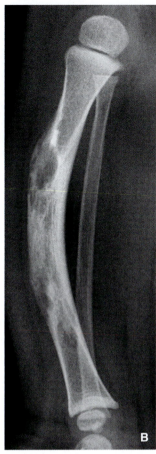

FIGURE 4.41 Radiography of osteofibrous dysplasia.
(A) Anteroposterior and **(B)** lateral radiographs of a 10-month-old girl show mixed lytic and sclerotic lesion affecting the midportion of the tibial diaphysis. Note characteristic anterior bowing of the tibia.

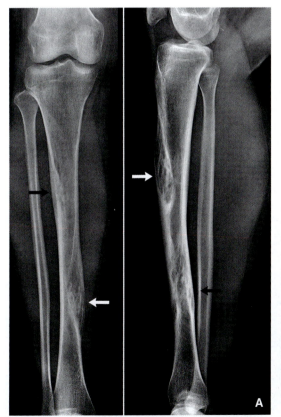
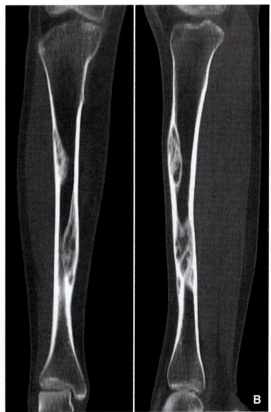

FIGURE 4.42 Radiography, computed tomography, and magnetic resonance imaging of osteofibrous dysplasia.
(A) Anteroposterior and lateral radiographs of the right leg of a 14-year-old girl show fusiform in shape, trabeculated, predominantly cortical lesions affecting diaphysis of the tibia (*arrows*). **(B)** Coronal and sagittal reformatted CT images demonstrate sharply demarcated mixed high- and low-attenuated lesions without evidence of periosteal reaction or soft-tissue mass.

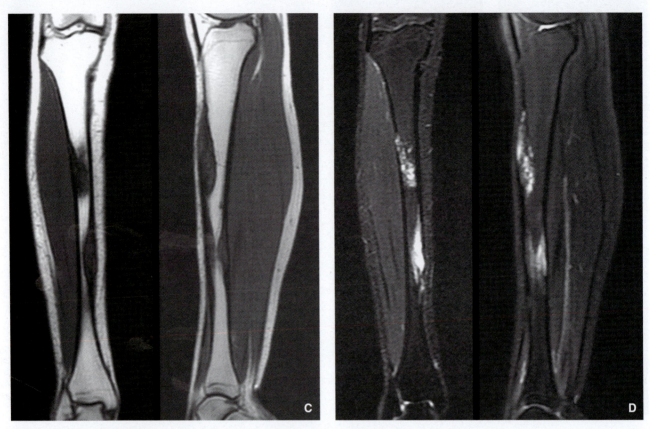

FIGURE 4.42 *(Continued).* **(C)** Coronal and sagittal T1-weighted MR images show the lesions to be of intermediate signal intensity. **(D)** Coronal and sagittal STIR MR images show the lesions exhibiting high signal intensity.

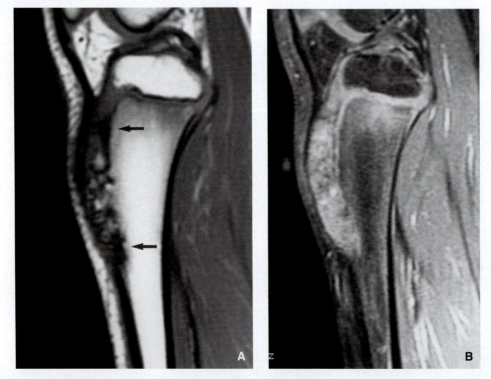

FIGURE 4.43 Magnetic resonance imaging of osteofibrous dysplasia. (A) Sagittal T1-weighted MR image shows oblong lesion involving anterior cortex of the tibia, exhibiting heterogeneous signal intensity (*arrows*). **(B)** Sagittal T1-weighted fat-suppressed MRI obtained after intravenous administration of gadolinium shows significant enhancement of the lesion.

Chapter 4 • Fibrogenic, Fibro-osseous, and Fibrohistiocytic Lesions   213

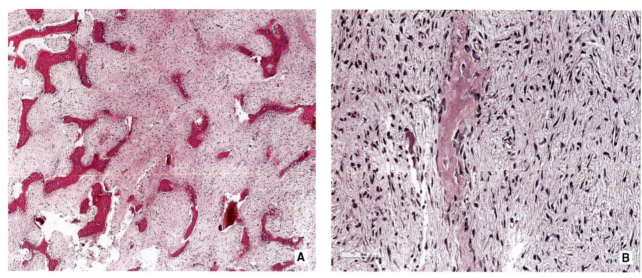

FIGURE 4.44 Histopathology of osteofibrous dysplasia. (A) Irregular in shape curvilinear trabeculae, displaying centrally woven bone and at periphery more mature lamellar architecture, merge with preexisting cancellous bone (H&E, original magnification ×50). **(B)** Under higher magnification, observe scattered osteoclasts and prominent rimming of bone trabecula by the osteoblasts (H&E, original magnification ×100).

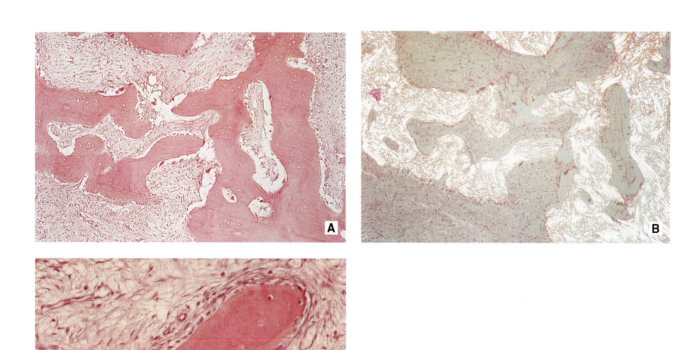

FIGURE 4.45 Histopathology of osteofibrous dysplasia. (A) Plump, irregular woven bone trabeculae, displaying at the periphery lamellar bone, are scattered in a moderately dense spindle cell stroma. Note prominent osteoblastic activity (H&E, original magnification ×25). **(B)** Viewed under polarized light, lamellar bone *(light green)* and woven bone *(darker areas)* are clearly discernable (H&E, polarize light, original magnification ×25). **(C)** High-magnification photomicrograph shows clearly the osteoblastic rimming of bone trabecula (H&E, original magnification ×200).

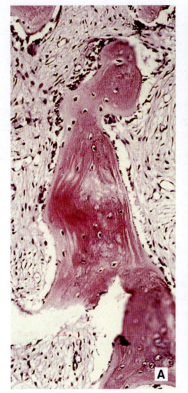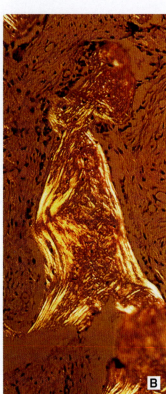

FIGURE 4.46 Histopathology of osteofibrous dysplasia. (A) Woven bone trabecula shows on the periphery a zone of lamellar transformation (zonal architecture) rimmed by the osteoblasts (H&E, original magnification ×400). **(B)** Under polarized light, this characteristic feature of osteofibrous dysplasia is more conspicuous (H&E, polarized light, original magnification ×400). (Courtesy of Peter Bullough, M.D., New York).

Pathology:

Gross (Macroscopy):

- Solid in consistency tumor expanding the bone, with yellowish-tan-to-creamy color (Fig. 4.50).

Histopathology:

- Composed of spindle cells (fibroblasts/myofibroblasts) within an abundant, dense matrix of collagen (Fig. 4.51).
- Degree of cellularity is variable, but cellular atypia and pleomorphism are minimal or absent.
- Mitoses are rare.
- Mast cells may be present.
- Borders of the tumor, especially in soft tissue, are irregular with finger-like projections infiltrating adipose tissue and skeletal muscle.
- Lesion is moderately vascular with small- to medium-sized capillaries and well-developed arterioles regularly dispersed throughout.

Immunohistochemistry:

- Nuclear beta-catenin is occasionally present but generally less than 10% of cells.
- Negativity for MDM2 and CDK4.

Genetics:

- Trisomies 8 and 20 have been detected by FISH analyses.
- Rearrangement involving chromosomes 11 and 19 at G-banding analysis.
- Deletion in 11q13.
- In contrast to desmoid-type fibromatosis of soft tissue, there are no mutations in exon 3 of CTNNB1 encoding beta-catenin.

Prognosis:

- Locally aggressive behavior without capacity to metastasize.
- Recurrence following curettage and resection are 72% and 17%, respectively.
- Local recurrence has been reported as late as 8 years following primary surgery.

Differential Diagnosis:

- **Aneurysmal bone cyst**
  Imaging studies show eccentric expansive lesion with solid buttress of periosteal reaction. Fluid–fluid levels are characteristic.

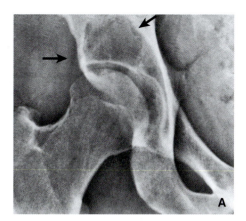
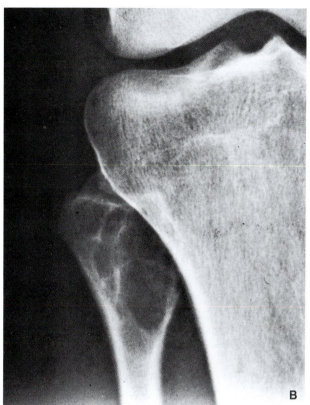
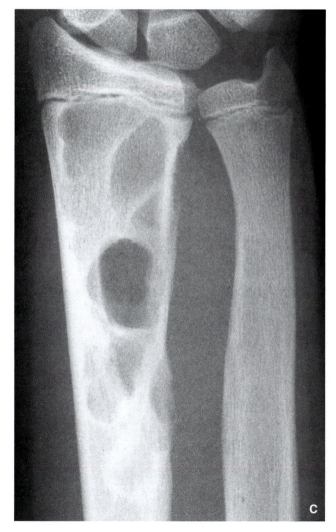

FIGURE 4.47 Radiography of desmoplastic fibroma.
(A) Radiolucent lesion with nonsclerotic but sharply defined borders is seen in the supra-acetabular region of the right ilium *(arrows)*. **(B)** Radiolucent trabeculated lesion occupies the proximal end of the right fibula of a 17-year-old girl. **(C)** Radiolucent trabeculated lesion is present in the metadiaphyseal region of the distal radius of a 15-year-old boy.

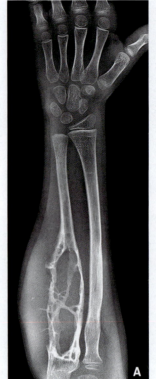
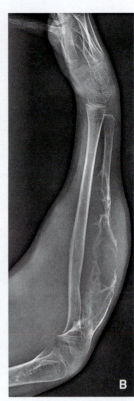

FIGURE 4.48 Radiography of desmoplastic fibroma.
(A) Anteroposterior and **(B)** lateral radiographs of the left forearm of an 8-year-old boy show aggressive osteolytic, expansive, trabeculated lesion in the proximal ulna. Note a pathologic fracture of the posterior cortex and soft-tissue extension of the tumor.

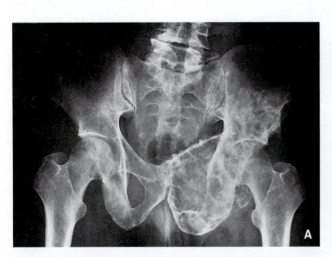
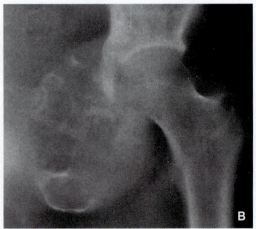

FIGURE 4.49 Radiography, computed tomography, and magnetic resonance imaging of desmoplastic fibroma.
(A) Anteroposterior radiograph of the pelvis of a 67-year-old man shows an expansive lytic lesion that involves the left ischium and pubis and extends into the supra-acetabular region of the ilium. **(B)** Conventional tomography shows the lytic nature of the tumor and its expansive character.

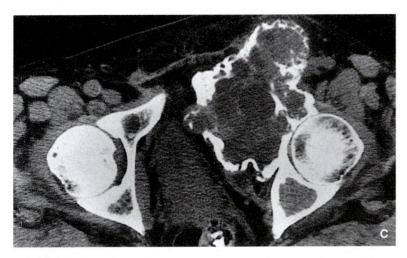

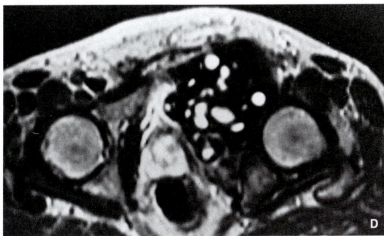

FIGURE 4.49 *(Continued).* **(C)** Computed tomography section through the hip joints shows a lobulated appearance of the tumor exhibiting thick sclerotic border. **(D)** Axial T2-weighted MR image demonstrates heterogeneity of the signal from the tumor. The bulk of the tumor displays low-to-intermediate signal intensity with several foci of high signal.

Histopathology shows multiple blood-filled spaces alternating with more solid areas composed of fibrous, richly vascular connective tissue.

- *Simple bone cyst*
  Imaging studies show centrally located, well-circumscribed radiolucent lesion with sclerotic margin, without periosteal reaction. "Fallen fragment" or "trap door" sign is characteristic.
  Histopathology show wall of the lesion exhibiting fibrous tissue or flattened single-cell lining.

- *Chondromyxoid fibroma*
  Imaging studies show findings very similar to those of an aneurysmal bone cyst, but since the lesion is solid, there is lack of fluid–fluid levels.
  Histopathology showing large lobulated areas of spindle-shaped or stellate cells distributed within abundant myxoid or chondroid intercellular matrix is diagnostic.

- *Giant cell tumor*
  Imaging studies show eccentrically located radiolucent lesion with geographic type of bone destruction and without periosteal reaction, extending to the articular end of the bone.

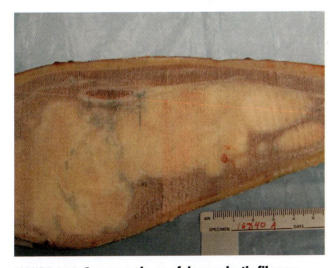

FIGURE 4.50 Gross specimen of desmoplastic fibroma. Resected specimen of the radius shows expansive lobulated yellowish-tan solid fibrous tumor.

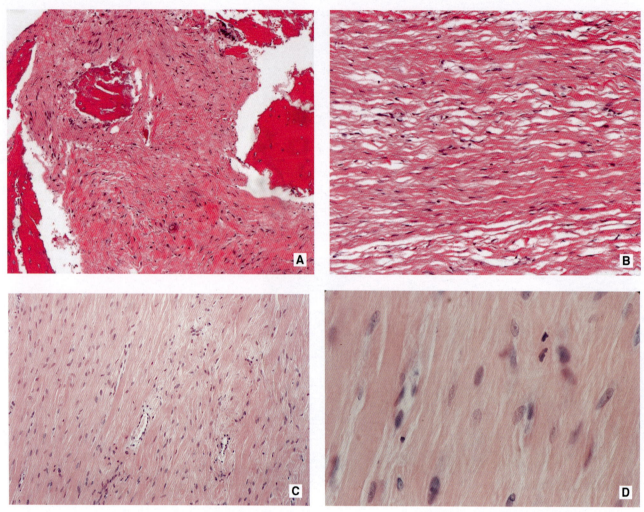

FIGURE 4.51 Histopathology of desmoplastic fibroma. (A) Densely collagenized stroma with spindle-shaped cell traps and destroys the preexisting bone trabeculae (H&E, original magnification ×50). **(B)** Higher-power magnification shows spindle cells (fibroblasts and myofibroblasts) within abundant collagenized matrix (H&E, original magnification ×100). **(C)** Photomicrograph of another patient shows densely collagenized stroma containing spindle-shaped fibroblasts with uniform in size appearing nuclei (H&E, original magnification ×40). **(D)** At higher magnification, the cells producing the abundant collagen show no evidence of atypia (H&E, original magnification ×150).

Histopathology showing a dual population of fibrocytic or monocytic mononuclear stromal cells, and of giant cells that are uniformly distributed throughout the tumor, is diagnostic.

- *Monostotic fibrous dysplasia*

  Imaging studies show centrally located radiolucent lesion exhibiting ground-glass or smoky appearance, without periosteal reaction; typical thinning of the cortex; characteristic rind sign.

  Histopathology showing immature woven bone trabeculae without osteoblastic rimming ("naked trabeculae") scattered within the fibrous stroma is diagnostic.

B. MALIGNANT FIBROHISTIOCYTIC TUMORS

Fibrosarcoma

Definition:
- Spindle cell malignant tumor exhibiting histologically a characteristic fascicular or "herringbone" pattern.

Epidemiology:
- Constitute about 5% of all primary malignant bone neoplasms.
- Usually occurs in the third to sixth decades of life.
- Equal gender distribution.

Sites of Involvement:
- Femur, humerus, tibia, and pelvic bones.

Clinical Findings:
- Pain and localized swelling, ranging in duration from a few weeks to several months.
- In about 25% of cases, the pathologic fracture is the first symptom of the tumor.

Imaging:
- Radiography shows a lytic lesion with wide zone of transition exhibiting moth-eaten or permeative type of bone destruction; there is usually no periosteal reaction; soft-tissue mass is often present (Fig. 4.52); preservation of small sequestrum-like bone fragments of cortical and spongy bone within destructive lesion.
- MRI shows no characteristic features to distinguish this tumor from the other lytic osseous neoplasms.

Pathology:
Gross (Macroscopy):
- Solid tumor with trabeculated tan-to-white cut surface.
- Poorly differentiated tumors exhibit more fleshy consistency with foci of hemorrhage and necrosis, commonly breaking the cortex and extending into the soft tissues (Fig. 4.53).

Histopathology:
- Uniformly distributed spindle-shaped cells arranged in a fascicular or "herringbone" pattern and variable amount of collagen production (Fig. 4.54).
- The cells have hyperchromatic nuclei with an increased ratio of nucleus to cytoplasm.
- Mitotic activity including bizarre mitoses may be present.
- Myxoid changes may be seen.
- Higher-grade lesions tend to be more cellular showing pleomorphism, less collagen production, and areas of necrosis.

Genetics:
- Gain of chromosomes 1q, 4q, 5p, 8q, 12p, 15q, 16q, 17q, 20q, 22q, and Xp.
- Gain of the *platelet-derived growth factor beta* (*PDGF-B*) gene, located at 22q12.3-q13.1.
- Losses at chromosomes 6q, 8p, 9p, 10, 13q, and 20p.
- Homozygous deletion of *CDKN2A*.
- Recurrent coamplification of KIT, PDGFRA, and KDR.

Prognosis:
- Common metastases to the lungs and other bones.
- Survival rates 5 to 10 years are 34% and 28%, respectively, depending upon age, grade of malignancy, location, and stage of the tumor.

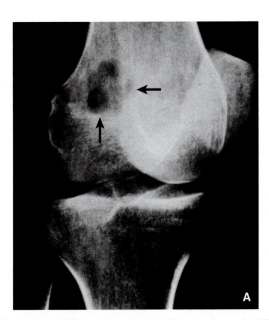
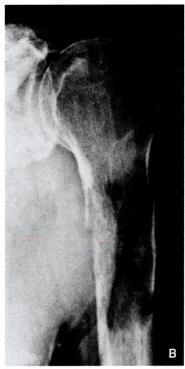

FIGURE 4.52 Radiography of fibrosarcoma. (A) Oblique radiograph of the right knee of a 28-year-old woman shows a purely destructive osteolytic lesion in the intercondylar fossa of the distal femur (*arrows*). Note the absence of reactive sclerosis and lack of periosteal reaction. **(B)** Anteroposterior radiograph of the left proximal humerus of a 62-year-old man shows an osteolytic lesion in the shaft of the bone associated with a pathologic fracture. Again observe lack of reactive sclerosis and lack of periosteal reaction, the characteristic features of this tumor.

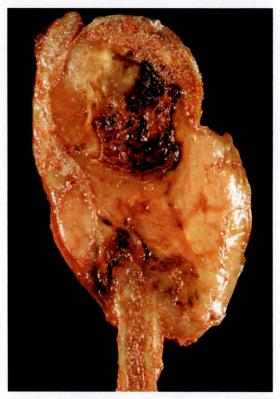

FIGURE 4.53 Gross specimen of fibrosarcoma. Resected specimen of the humerus shows a solid tumor at the proximal end of bone, breaking the cortex and extending into the soft tissues. Observe focal areas of hemorrhage (*dark red*). (From Bullough P. *Atlas of Orthopedic Pathology*. 2nd ed. New York: Gower Medical Publication;1992:17.3, Fig. 17.5)

Differential Diagnosis:

- **Giant cell tumor**

  Imaging studies show geographic rather than moth-eaten or permeative type of bone destruction; the lesion invariably extends into the articular end of the bone.

  Histopathology showing a dual population of fibrocytic or monocytic mononuclear stromal cells coupled with numerous giant cells uniformly distributed throughout the tumor is diagnostic.

- **Plasmacytoma**

  Imaging studies may show similar appearance to fibrosarcoma, but the tumor occurs in much older population.

  Histopathology showing extended sheets of atypical plasmacytoid cells replacing the normal fatty and hematopoietic bone marrow is diagnostic.

- **Telangiectatic osteosarcoma**

  Imaging studies show purely lytic lesion with aggressive periosteal reaction. MRI shows characteristic fluid–fluid levels.

  Histopathology showing blood-filled cystic spaces divided by solid septa containing malignant cells forming tumor osteoid or tumor bone is diagnostic.

- **Fibroblastic osteosarcoma**

  Imaging studies show similar appearance to the conventional osteosarcoma but less radiopacities within the lesion; aggressive periosteal reaction (sunburst and Codman triangle); soft-tissue mass.

  Histopathology showing predominantly spindle-shaped fibroblasts arranged in sheets, with deeply stained nuclei, and presence of tumor osteoid or tumor bone is diagnostic.

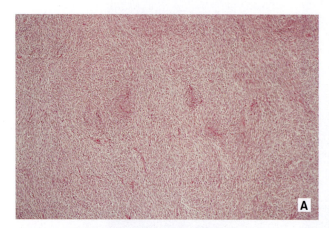
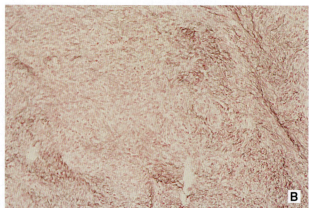

FIGURE 4.54 Histopathology of fibrosarcoma. (A) Interwoven bundles of spindle cells with a moderate degree of pleomorphism are consistent with grade 2 malignancy (H&E, original magnification ×25). **(B)** Using reticulin fiber stain, the uneven distribution of the fibers is conspicuous (Novotny reticulin stain, original magnification ×50).

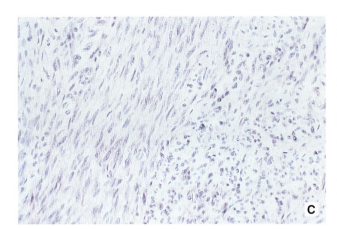 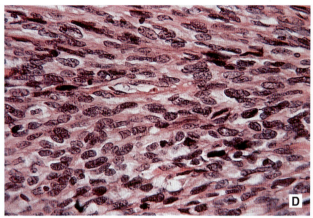

FIGURE 4.54 *(Continued).* **(C)** The cells and fiber bundles are cut longitudinally (*center*) and across the axis (*left and right*), producing characteristic for this tumor herringbone pattern (Giemsa, original magnification ×50). **(D)** At high magnification, the herringbone pattern is more obvious (H&E, original magnification ×400).

- *Osteolytic metastasis*

  Imaging studies may show identical features to that of fibrosarcoma; however, histopathology showing morphologic features of carcinomas (lytic metastases usually denote spread of primary carcinomas of the lung, kidney, breast, or thyroid) is diagnostic.

Malignant Fibrous Histiocytoma (Pleomorphic Undifferentiated Sarcoma)

Definition:
- A malignant neoplasm, more common in soft tissues than in bones, composed of spindle and pleomorphic cells exhibiting a storiform pattern of arrangement.

Epidemiology:
- More common in men than in women.
- Age of patients between the second to eighth decades.
- Higher incidence in adults over 40 years of age.
- May arise as a secondary bone tumor as a complication of Paget disease, bone infarct, or after irradiation of osseous or extraosseous lesions.

Sites of Involvement:
- Predilection for the long bones of the lower extremities, particularly the femur (30% to 45%), followed by the tibia and humerus.
- Most commonly presents as a solitary lesion; rare multifocal presentation.

Clinical findings:
- Local pain and swelling.
- Pathologic fracture may be the initial presenting symptom.

Imaging:
- Radiography, very similar to that of fibrosarcoma, shows a purely lytic lesion with very little or no reactive sclerosis, and usually no periosteal reaction (Fig. 4.55).
- MRI findings, also identical to those of fibrosarcoma, include intermediate or low signal intensity on T1-weighted sequences, heterogeneous but predominantly high signal on T2 weighting, and tumor enhancement after administration of gadolinium (Fig. 4.56).

Pathology:
Gross (Macroscopy):
- Varies from tan to grayish-white in color, from soft to solid, firm mass.

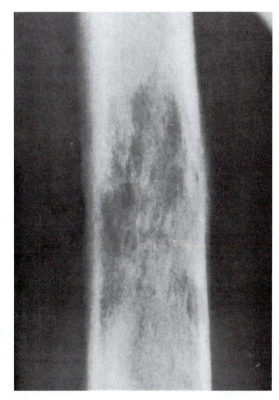

FIGURE 4.55 Radiography of malignant fibrous histiocytoma. A purely lytic destructive lesion with wide zone of transition and lack of reactive sclerosis is present in the femoral shaft.

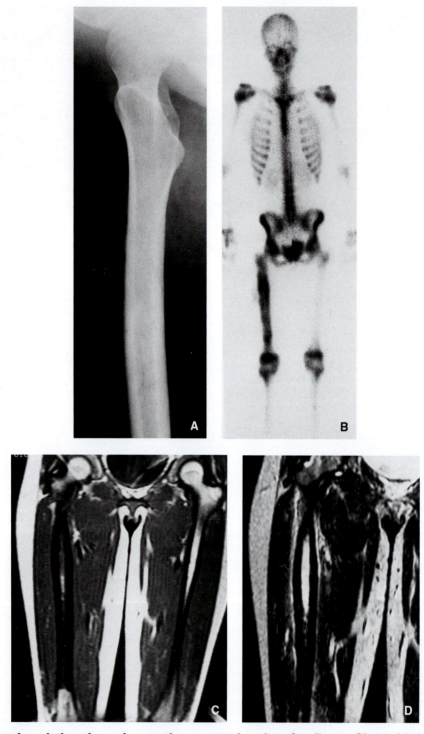

FIGURE 4.56 Radiography, scintigraphy, and magnetic resonance imaging of malignant fibrous histiocytoma. (A) Oblique radiograph of the right femur of a 16-year-old girl demonstrates fusiform thickening of the cortex and permeative type of bone destruction. **(B)** Radionuclide bone scan shows increased uptake of the radiopharmaceutical tracer in the right femur. **(C)** Coronal T1-weighted MR image shows the extent of the tumor involving about 75% of the length of the femur. **(D)** Coronal T2-weighted MRI shows that the tumor exhibits high signal intensity.

- Areas of yellowish discoloration representing necrosis and hemorrhage are frequently seen.
- Margins of the tumor are irregular, and often cortical destruction and soft-tissue infiltration are present (Fig. 4.57).

Histopathology:

- Mixed population in various proportion of spindle and histiocytoid cells arranged in storiform pattern, exhibiting marked cytologic and nuclear pleomorphism and atypia as well as mitotic activity (Fig. 4.58).
- Multinucleated osteoclast-like giant cells (often atypical), foamy macrophages, and chronic inflammatory cells, predominantly lymphocytes, may be present (Fig. 4.59).
- Areas of thick coarse collagen occasionally may be present, the feature that may be misinterpreted as neoplastic osteoid.
- Foci of reactive osteoid or primitive bone formation at the periphery (juxtaperiosteal).

Genetics:

- Loss of heterozygosity at chromosome region 9p21-22.
- Mutation in *p53* gene was reported in secondary malignant fibrous histiocytoma (MFH) associated with bone infarction.

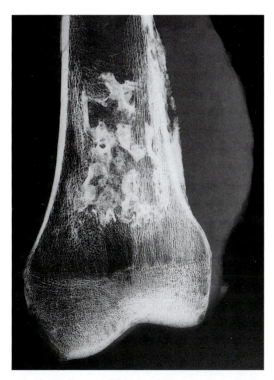

FIGURE 4.57 Malignant fibrous histiocytoma complicating the medullary bone infarct. Radiograph of the resected specimen of the distal femur of a 39-year-old woman with known multiple idiopathic bone infarctions shows serpentine coarse calcifications in the medullary portion of bone. In addition, observe bone destruction, aggressive periosteal reaction, and soft-tissue mass histopathologically proven to represent secondary MFH.

Prognostic Factors:
- Tendency to metastasize, particularly to the lungs (45% to 50%).
- Favorable prognostic factors are younger age at manifestation (under 40 years), lower histologic grade, and adequate surgical resection margins.

Differential Diagnosis:
- *Telangiectatic osteosarcoma*

  See differential diagnosis of Fibrosarcoma.
- *Plasmacytoma*

  See differential diagnosis of Fibrosarcoma.
- *Osteolytic metastasis*

  See differential diagnosis of Fibrosarcoma.
- *Giant cell tumor*

  See differential diagnosis of Fibrosarcoma.

Angiomatoid Fibrous Histiocytoma of Bone

Definition:
- Predominantly a soft tissue, rarely metastasizing tumor, which occasionally may affect the bones, consisting of lobulated sheets of spindle cells having fibrohistiocytic features, pseudoangiomatoid cystic spaces filled with blood, and prominent lymphoplasmacytic rim. Currently is classified by WHO as a tumor of uncertain differentiation. Originally described as angiomatoid "malignant" fibrous histiocytoma, the lesion was renamed due to its very rare malignant behavior.

Epidemiology:
- Typically affects children and young adults, with a mean age of 20 years.
- Equal gender distribution.

Sites of Involvement:
- Extremities, following by the structures of the trunk, head, and neck (deep dermis and subcutis).
- About 66% occurring in areas of normal lymphoid tissue.
- Uncommon in bones.

Clinical Findings:
- Anemia, weight loss, fever.
- Extremely rare pain and local tenderness.
- Slow growth rate and rare metastases.
- May be mistaken for hematoma or hemangioma.

Imaging:
- Lack of characteristic features.

Pathology:
Gross (Macroscopy):

- Circumscribed, firm in consistency, tan-gray mass resembling lymph nodes, ranged in size from 1 to 12 cm; may appear multinodular with blood-filled cystic spaces.

Histopathology:

- Spindled or epithelioid cells, generally uniform, with ovoid vesicular nuclei.

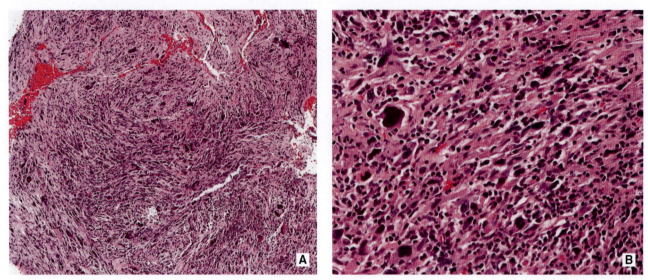

FIGURE 4.58 **Histopathology of malignant fibrous histiocytoma. (A)** Proliferation of mixed population of spindle and histiocytoid cells show marked pleomorphism (H&E, original magnification ×50). **(B)** Higher magnification demonstrates anaplastic cytomorphology of the tumor to better advantage (H&E, original magnification ×100).

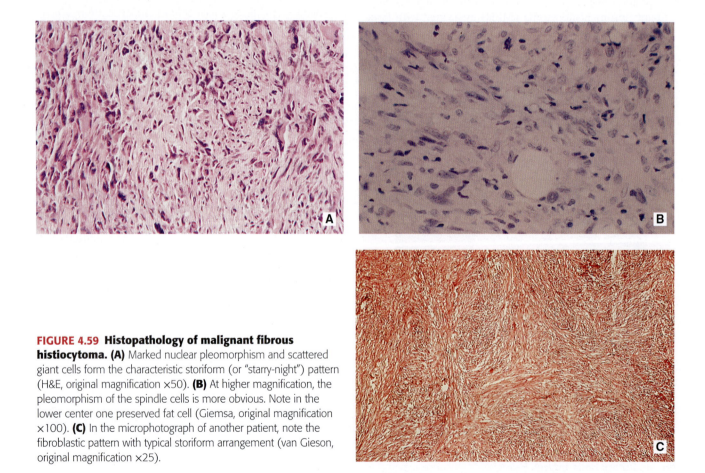

FIGURE 4.59 **Histopathology of malignant fibrous histiocytoma. (A)** Marked nuclear pleomorphism and scattered giant cells form the characteristic storiform (or "starry-night") pattern (H&E, original magnification ×50). **(B)** At higher magnification, the pleomorphism of the spindle cells is more obvious. Note in the lower center one preserved fat cell (Giemsa, original magnification ×100). **(C)** In the microphotograph of another patient, note the fibroblastic pattern with typical storiform arrangement (van Gieson, original magnification ×25).

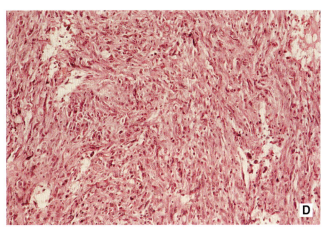
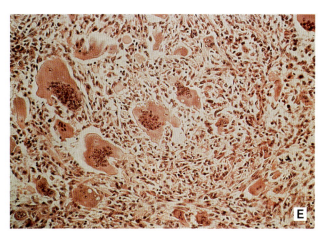

FIGURE 4.59 *(Continued).* **(D)** In another field of view, observe histiocytic pattern with giant cells (H&E, original magnification ×25). **(E)** At higher magnification, note several various in size multinucleated giant cells of osteoclast type (H&E, original magnification ×250).

- Thick fibrous pseudocapsule with pericapsular lymphocytic and plasma cells infiltrate, and pseudoangiomatous spaces filled with blood (Fig. 4.60A).
- Multinodular proliferation of eosinophilic, histiocytoid, and myoid cells (Fig. 4.60B).
- Cellular pleomorphism and increased mitotic activity may be seen.

Immunohistochemistry:
- Positivity for vimentin.
- Positivity for EMA, CD68, CD99, and desmin in 50% of cases.
- Positivity for KP-1 in 15% of cases.

- Negativity for S-100 protein, CD21, CD31, CD34, CD35, Factor VIII, keratins, and lysozyme.
- Negativity for HMB45, MyoD1, myoglobin, and myogenin (myf4).

Genetics:
- Translocations t(12;16) (q13;p11) and t(12;22) (q13;q12).
- *FUS-ATF1* fusion gene in t(12;16) (q13;p11).
- *EWSR1-ATF1* fusion gene in t(12;22) (q13;q12).

Prognosis:
- Indolent behavior, with 2% to 11% of local recurrence after excision and less than 1% metastases.

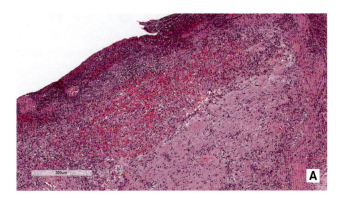
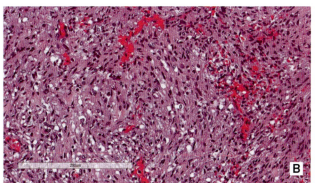

FIGURE 4.60 Histopathology of angiomatoid malignant fibrous histiocytoma. (A) Lymphoplasmacytic and fibrohistiocytic components of the tumor are surrounded by a thick fibrous pseudocapsule. Note several pseudoangiomatoid cystic spaces filled with blood (H&E, original magnification ×40). **(B)** At higher magnification, observe pseudoangiomatoid cystic spaces within the tumor consisting of eosinophilic, histiocytoid, and myoid cells (H&E, original magnification ×100).

REFERENCES

Albright F, Butler AM, Hampton AO, Smith P. Syndrome characterized by osteitis fibrosa disseminata, areas of pigmentation and endocrine dysfunction with precocious puberty in females. *N Engl J Med*. 1937;216:727–731.

Alguacil-Garcia A, Alonso A, Pettigrew NM. Osteofibrous dysplasia (ossifying fibroma) of the tibia and fibula and adamantinoma. *Am J Clin Pathol*. 1984;82: 470–474.

Bahk W-J, Kang Y-K, Lee A-H, Mirra JM. Desmoid tumor of bone with enchondromatous nodules, mistaken for chondrosarcoma. *Skeletal Radiol*. 2003;32:223–226.

Bancroft LW, Kransdorf MJ, Menke DM, O'Connor MI, Foster WC. Intramuscular myxoma: characteristic MR imaging features. *AJR Am J Roentgenol*. 2002;178:1255–1259.

Barnes GR Jr, Gwinn JL. Distal irregularities of the femur simulating malignancy. *AJR Am J Roentgenol*. 1974;122:180–185.

Bernal K, Nelson M, Neff JR, Nielsen SM, Bridge JA. Translocations (2;11) (q31;q12) is recurrent in collagenous fibroma (desmoplastic fibroblastoma). *Cancer Genet Cytogenet*. 2004;149:161–163.

Bertoni F, Calderoni P, Bacchini P, Campanacci M. Desmoplastic fibroma of bone: a report of six cases. *J Bone Joint Surg Br*. 1984;66B:265–268.

Bertoni F, Calderoni P, Bacchini P, Sudanese A. Benign fibrous histiocytoma of bone. *J Bone Joint Surg Am*. 1986;68A:1225–1230.

Bertoni F, Capanna R, Calderoni P, Bacchini P, Campanacci M. Primary central (medullary) fibrosarcoma of bone. *Semin Diagn Pathol*. 1984;1:185–198.

Bertoni F, Unni KK, McLeod RA, Sim FH. Xanthoma of bone. *Am J Pathol*. 1988;90: 377–384.

Bianco P, Rimminuci M, Majolagbe A, et al. Mutations of the *GNAS1* gene, stromal cell dysfunction, and osteomalacic changes in non-McCune-Albright fibrous dysplasia of bone. *J Bone Miner Res*. 2000;15:120–128.

Blau RA, Zwick DL, Westphal RA. Multiple nonossifying fibromas. *J Bone Joint Surg Am*. 1988;70A:299–304.

Boland PJ, Huvos AG. Malignant fibrous histiocytoma of bone. *Clin Orthop*. 1986;204:130–134.

Bridge JA, Dembinski A, Deboer J, et al. Clonal chromosomal abnormalities in osteofibrous dysplasia. Implications for histopathogenesis and its relationship with adamantinoma. *Cancer*. 1994;73:1746–1752.

Bridge JA, Swarts SJ, Buresh C, et al. Trisomies 8 and 20 characterize a subgroup of benign fibrous lesions arising in both soft tissue and bone. *Am J Pathol*. 1999;154:729–733.

Brower AC, Culver JE Jr, Keats TE. Histological nature of the cortical irregularity of the medial posterior distal femoral metaphysis in children. *Radiology*. 1971;99:389–392.

Bufkin WJ. The avulsive cortical irregularity. *AJR Am J Roentgenol*. 1971;112:487–492.

Bullough PG, Vigorita VJ. *Atlas of Orthopaedic Pathology with Clinical and Radiologic Correlations*. 2nd ed. New York: Gowen Medical Publishing; 1992.

Cabral CEL, Guedes P, Fonseca T, Rezende JF, Cruz Júnior LC, Smith J. Polyostotic fibrous dysplasia associated with intramuscular myxomas: Mazabraud's syndrome. *Skeletal Radiol*. 1998;27:278–282.

Caffey J. On fibrous defects in cortical walls of growing tubular bone: their radiologic appearance, structure prevalence, natural course and diagnostic significance. *Adv Pediatr*. 1955;7:13–51.

Camilleri AE. Craniofacial fibrous dysplasia. *J Laryngol Otol*. 1991;105:662–666.

Campanacci M. Osteofibrous dysplasia of the long bones. A new clinical entity. *Ital J Orthop Traumatol*. 1976;2:221–237.

Campanacci M, Laus M. Osteofibrous dysplasia of the tibia and fibula. *J Bone Joint Surg Am*. 1981;63A:367–375.

Campanacci M, Laus M, Boriani S. Multiple non-ossifying fibromata with extraskeletal anomalies: a new syndrome? *J Bone Joint Surg Br*. 1983;65-B:627–632.

Campbell CJ, Hawk T. A variant of fibrous dysplasia (osteofibrous dysplasia). *J Bone Joint Surg Am*. 1982;64A:231–236.

Capanna R, Bertoni F, Bacchini P, Bacci G, Guerra A, Campanacci M. Malignant fibrous histiocytoma of bone: the experience at the Rizzoli Institute. Report of 90 cases. *Cancer*. 1984;54:177–187.

Choi IH, Kim CJ, Cho T-J, et al. Focal fibrocartilaginous dysplasia of long bones: report of eight additional cases and literature review. *J Pediatr Orthop*. 2000;20:421–427.

Clarke BE, Xipell JM, Thomas DP. Benign fibrous histiocytoma of bone. *Am J Surg Pathol*. 1985;9:806–815.

Cohen DM, Dahlin DC, Pugh DG. Fibrous dysplasia associated with adamantinoma of the long bones. *Cancer*. 1962;15:515–521.

Costa MJ, Weiss SW. Angiomatoid malignant fibrous histiocytoma. A follow-up study of 108 cases with evaluation of possible histologic predictors of outcome. *Am J Surg Pathol*. 1990;14:1126–1132.

Crim JR, Gold RH, Mirra JM, Eckardt JJ, Bassett LW. Desmoplastic fibroma of bone: radiographic analysis. *Radiology*. 1989;172:827–832.

Cunningham BJ, Ackerman LV. Metaphyseal fibrous defects. *J Bone Joint Surg*. 1956;38:797–808.

Czerniak B, Rojas-Corona RR, Dorfman HD. Morphologic diversity of long bone adamantinoma. The concept of differentiated (regressing) adamantinoma and its relationship to osteofibrous dysplasia. *Cancer*. 1989;64:2319–2334.

Dahlin DC, Ivins JC. Fibrosarcoma of bone: a study of 114 cases. *Cancer*. 1969;23:35–41.

Dahlin DC, Unni KK. *Bone tumors: General Aspects and Data on 8,542 Cases*. 4th ed. Springfield, IL: Charles C. Thomas; 1986:141–148.

Dahlin DC, Unni KK, Matsuno T. Malignant (fibrous) histiocytoma of bone—fact or fancy? *Cancer*. 1977;39:1508–1516.

DeSmet A, Travers H, Neff JR. Chondrosarcoma occurring in a patient with polyostotic fibrous dysplasia. *Skeletal Radiol*. 1981;7:197–201.

DiCaprio MR, Enneking WF. Fibrous dysplasia. Pathophysiology, evaluation, and treatment. *J Bone Joint Surg*. 2005;87:1848–1864.

Dorfman HD, Ishida T, Tsuneyoshi M. Exophytic variant of fibrous dysplasia (fibrous dysplasia protuberans). *Hum Pathol*. 1994;25:1234–1237.

Dorfman HD, Norman A, Wolff H. Fibrosarcoma complicating bone infarction in a caisson worker: case report. *J Bone Joint Surg Am*. 1966;48A:528–532.

Dreizin D, Glenn C, Jose J. Mazabraud syndrome. *Am J Orthop*. 2012;41:332–335.

Endo M, Kawai A, Kobayashi E, et al. Solitary intramuscular myxoma with monostotic fibrous dysplasia as a rare variant of Mazabraud's syndrome. *Skeletal Radiol*. 2007;36:523–529.

Enzinger FM. Angiomatoid malignant fibrous histiocytoma: a distinct fibrohistiocytic tumor of children and young adults simulating a vascular neoplasm. *Cancer*. 1979;44:2147–2157.

Evans GA, Park WM. Familial multiple non-osteogenic fibromata. *J Bone Joint Surg Br*. 1978;60B:416–419.

Fanburg-Smith JC, Miettinen M. Angiomatoid "malignant" fibrous histiocytoma: clinicopathologic study of 158 cases and further exploration of the myoid phenotype. *Hum Pathol*. 1999;30:1336–1343.

Fechner RE, Mills SE. *Atlas of Tumor Pathology. Tumors of the Bones and Joints, 3rd Series, Fascicle 8*. Washington, DC: Armed Forces Institute of Pathology; 1993.

Feldman F, Lattes R. Primary malignant fibrous histiocytoma (fibrous xanthoma) of bone. *Skeletal Radiol*. 1977;1:145–160.

Flanagan AM, Delaney D, O'Donnell P. Benefits of molecular pathology in the diagnosis of musculoskeletal disease. Part II of a two-part review: bone tumors and metabolic disorders. *Skeletal Radiol*. 2010;39:213–224.

Fletcher CDM. Pleomorphic malignant fibrous histiocytoma: fact or fiction? A critical reappraisal based on 159 tumors diagnosed as pleomorphic sarcoma. *Am J Surg Pathol*. 1992;16:213–228.

Fletcher CDM, Unni KK, Mertens E, eds. *World Health Organization Classification of Tumours of Soft Tissue and Bone*. Lyon, France: IARC Press; 2013:352–365.

Friedland JA, Reinus WR, Fisher AJ, Wilson AJ. Quantitative analysis of the plain radiographic appearance of nonossifying fibroma. *Invest Radiol.* 1995;30:474–479.

Galli SJ, Weintraub HP, Proppe KH. Malignant fibrous histiocytoma and pleomorphic sarcoma in association with medullary bone infarcts. *Cancer.* 1978;41:607–619.

Gebhardt MC, Campbell CJ, Schiller AL, Mankin HJ. Desmoplastic fibroma of bone. A report of eight cases and review of the literature. *J Bone Joint Surg Am.* 1985;67A:732–747.

Greenfield GB, Arrington JA. *Imaging of Bone Tumors. A Multimodality Approach.* Philadelphia, PA: JB Lippincott; 1995.

Greenspan A, Klein MJ. Radiology and pathology of bone tumors. In: Lewis MM, ed. *Musculoskeletal Oncology. A Multidisciplinary Approach.* Philadelphia, PA: WB Saunders; 1992.

Greenspan A, Unni KK. Case report 787. Desmoplastic fibroma. *Skeletal Radiol.* 1993;22:296–299.

Greenspan A, Jundt G, Remagen W. *Differential Diagnosis in Orthopaedic Oncology.* 2nd ed. Philadelphia, PA: Lippincott Williams & Wilkins; 2007.

Gross ML, Soberman N, Dorfman HD, Seimon LP. Case report 556. Multiple nonossifying fibromas of long bones in a patient with neurofibromatosis. *Skeletal Radiol.* 1989;18:389–391.

Hamada T, Ito H, Araki Y, et al. Benign fibrous histiocytoma of the femur: review of three cases. *Skeletal Radiol.* 1996;25:25–29.

Hauben EI, Jundt G, Cleton-Jansen AM, et al. Desmoplastic fibroma of bone: an immunohistochemical study including beta-catenin expression and mutational analysis for beta-catenin. *Hum Pathol.* 2005;36:1025–1030.

Hazelbag HM, Wessels JW, Mollevangers P, et al. Cytogenetic analysis of adamantinoma of long bones: further indications for a common histogenesis with osteofibrous dysplasia. *Cancer Genet Cytogenet.* 1997;97:5–11.

Hermann G, Klein M, Abdelwahab IF, Kenan S. Fibrocartilaginous dysplasia. *Skeletal Radiol.* 1996;25:509–511.

Hoshi H, Futami S, Ohnishi T, et al. Gallium-67 uptake in fibrous dysplasia of the bone. *Ann Nucl Med.* 1990;4:35–38.

Hudson TM, Stiles RG, Monson DK. Fibrous lesions of bone. *Radiol Clin North Am.* 1993;31:279–297.

Huvos A. *Bone Tumors: Diagnosis, Treatment and Prognosis,* 2nd ed. Philadelphia, PA: WB Saunders; 1991:677–693.

Huvos AG, Higinbotham NL. Primary fibrosarcoma of bone: a clinicopathologic study of 130 patients. *Cancer.* 1975;35:837–847.

Huvos AG, Heilweil M, Bretsky SS. The pathology of malignant fibrous histiocytoma of bone. A study of 130 patients. *Am J Surg Pathol.* 1985;9:853–871.

Huvos AG, Higinbotham NL, Miller TR. Bone sarcomas arising in fibrous dysplasia. *J Bone Joint Surg Am.* 1972;64A:1047–1056.

Huvos AG, Higinbotham NL, Miller TR. Bone sarcomas arising in fibrous dysplasia. *J Bone Joint Surg Am.* 1972;54A:1047–1056.

Huvos AG, Woodard HQ, Heilweil M. Postradiation malignant fibrous histiocytoma of bone. A clinicopathologic study of 20 patients. *Am J Surg Pathol.* 1986;10:9–18.

Inamo Y, Hanawa Y, Kin H, Okuni M. Findings on magnetic resonance imaging of the spine and femur in a case of McCune-Albright syndrome. *Pediatr Radiol.* 1993;23:15–18.

Inwards CY, Unni KK, Beabout JW, Sim FH. Desmoplastic fibroma of bone. *Cancer.* 1991;68:1978–1983.

Ishida T, Dorfman HD. Massive chondroid differentiation in fibrous dysplasia of bone (fibrocartilaginous dysplasia). *Am J Surg Pathol.* 1993;17:924–930.

Iwasko N, Steinbach LS, Disler D, et al. Imaging findings in Mazabraud's syndrome: seven new cases. *Skeletal Radiol.* 2002;31:81–87.

Jaffe HL. Fibrous cortical defect and non-ossifying fibroma. In: *Tumors and Tumorous Conditions of the Bones and Joints.* Philadelphia, PA: Lea & Febiger; 1958:76–91.

Jaffe HL, Lichtenstein L. Non-osteogenic fibroma of bone. *Am J Pathol.* 1942;18: 205–221.

Jee W-H, Choe B-Y, Kang H-S, et al. Nonossifying fibroma: characteristics at MR imaging with pathologic correlation. *Radiology.* 1998;209:197–202.

Jee W-H, Choi K-H, Choe B-Y, et al. Fibrous dysplasia: MR imaging characteristics with radiopathologic correlations. *AJR Am J Roentgenol.* 1996;167: 1523–1527.

Johnson CB, Gilbert EE, Gottlieb LI. Malignant transformation of polyostotic fibrous dysplasia. *South Med J.* 1979;72:353–356.

Kahn LB. Adamantinoma, osteofibrous dysplasia and differentiated adamantinoma. *Skeletal Radiol.* 2003;32:245–258.

Kahn LB, Webber B, Mills E, Anstey L, Heselson NG. Malignant fibrous histiocytoma (malignant fibrous xanthoma: xanthosarcoma) of bone. *Cancer.* 1978;42:640–651.

Kaushik S, Smoker WRK, Frable WJ. Malignant transformation of fibrous dysplasia into chondroblastic osteosarcoma. *Skeletal Radiol.* 2002;31:103–106.

Kawaguchi K, Oda Y, Sakamoto A, et al. Molecular analysis of $p53$, MDM_2, and H-ras genes in osteosarcoma and malignant fibrous histiocytoma of bone in patients older than 40 years. *Mod Pathol.* 2002;15:878–888.

Keeney GL, Unni KK, Beabout JW, Pritchard DJ. Adamantinoma of long bones. *Cancer.* 1989;64:730–737.

Kempson RL. Ossifying fibroma of the long bones. A light and electron microscopic study. *Arch Pathol.* 1966;82:218–233.

Khanna M, Delaney D, Tirabosco R, Saifuddin A. Osteofibrous dysplasia, osteofibrous dysplasia-like adamantinoma, and adamantinoma: correlation of radiological imaging features with surgical histology and assessment of the use of radiology in contributing to needle biopsy diagnosis. *Skeletal Radiol.* 2008;37:1077–1084.

Koplas MC, Lefkowitz RA, Bauer TW, et al. Imaging findings, prevalence and outcome of de novo and secondary malignant fibrous histiocytoma of bone. *Skeletal Radiol.* 2010;39:791–798.

Kransdorf MJ, Murphey MD. Case 12: Mazabraud syndrome. *Radiology.* 1999;212: 129–132.

Kransdorf MJ, Murphey MD, Sweet DE. Liposclerosing myxofibrous tumor: a radiologic-pathologic-distinct fibro-osseous lesion of bone with a marked predilection for the intertrochanteric region of the femur. *Radiology.* 1999;212:693–698.

Kransdorf MJ, Utz JA, Gilkey FW, Berrey BH. MR appearance of fibroxanthoma. *J Comput Assist Tomogr.* 1988;12:612–615.

Kumar R, Madewell JE, Lindell MM, Swischuk LE. Fibrous lesions of bones. *Radiographics.* 1990;10:237–256.

Kumar R, Swischuk LE, Madewell JE. Benign cortical defect: site for an avulsion fracture. *Skeletal Radiol.* 1986;15:553–555.

Kyriakos M, McDonald DJ, Sundaram M. Fibrous dysplasia with cartilaginous differentiation ("fibrocartilaginous dysplasia"): a review, with an illustrative case followed for 18 years. *Skeletal Radiol.* 2004;33:51–62.

Levine SM, Lambiase RE, Petchprapa CN. Cortical lesions of the tibia: characteristic appearances at conventional radiography. *Radiographics.* 2003;23:157–177.

Lichtenstein L, Jaffe HL. Fibrous dysplasia of bone. *Arch Pathol.* 1942;33:777–816.

Lichtman EA, Klein MJ. Case report 302. Desmoplastic fibroma of the proximal end of the left femur. *Skeletal Radiol.* 1985;13:160–163.

Link TM, Haeussler MD, Poppek S, et al. Malignant fibrous histiocytoma of bone: conventional X-ray and MR imaging features. *Skeletal Radiol.* 1998;27:552–558.

Luna A, Martinez S, Bossen E. Magnetic resonance imaging of intramuscular myxoma with histological comparison and a review of the literature. *Skeletal Radiol.* 2005;34:19–28.

Mangham DC, Williams A, Lalam RK, Brundler MA, Leahy MG, Cool WP. Angiomatoid fibrous histiocytoma of bone: a calcifying sclerosing variant mimicking osteosarcoma. *Am J Surg Pathol.* 2010;34:279–285.

Markel SF. Ossifying fibroma of long bone. *Am J Clin Pathol.* 1978;69:91–97.

Matsuno T. Benign fibrous histiocytoma involving the ends of long bone. *Skeletal Radiol.* 1990;19:561–566.

Mazabraud A, Semat P, Roze R. A propos de l'association de fibro-myxomes des tissus mous à la dysplasie fibreuse des os. *Presse Med.* 1967;75:2223–2228.

Mertens F, Romeo S, Bovee JV, et al. Reclassification and subtyping of so-called malignant fibrous histiocytoma of bone: comparison with cytogenetic features. *Clin Sarcoma Res.* 2011;1:10–13.

Mesiter P, Konrad E, Hohne N. Incidence and histological structure of the storiform pattern in benign and malignant fibrous histiocytomas. *Virchows Arch A Pathol Anat Histol.* 1981;393:93–101.

Mirra JM. Fibrohistiocytic tumors of intramedullary origin. In: Mirra JM, Picci P, Gold RH, eds. *Bone tumors: Clinical, Pathologic, and Radiologic Correlations.* Philadelphia, PA: Lea & Febiger; 1989:691–799.

Mirra JM, Gold RH. Fibrous dysplasia. In: Mirra JM, Picci P, Gold RH, eds. *Bone Tumors.* Philadelphia, PA: Lea & Febiger; 1989:191–226.

Mirra JM, Bullough PG, Marcove RC, Jacobs B, Huvos AG. Malignant fibrous histiocytoma and osteosarcoma in association with bone infarcts. *J Bone Joint Surg Am.* 1974;56A:932–940.

Mirra JM, Gold RH, Marafiote R. Malignant (fibrous) histiocytoma arising in association with a bone infarct in sickle-cell disease: coincidence or cause-and-effect? *Cancer.* 1977;39:186–194.

Mirra JM, Gold RH, Rand F. Disseminated nonossifying fibromas in association with café-au-lait spots (Jaffe-Campanacci syndrome). *Clin Orthop.* 1982;168:192–205.

Moser RP Jr, Sweet DE, Haseman DB, Madewell JE. Multiple skeletal fibroxanthomas: radiologic-pathologic correlation of 72 cases. *Skeletal Radiol.* 1987;16:353–359.

Mulder JD, Schütte HE, Kroon HM, Taconis WK. *Radiologic Atlas of Bone Tumors.* Amsterdam, the Netherlands: Elsevier; 1993:607–625.

Murphey MD, Gross TM, Rosenthal HG. Musculoskeletal malignant fibrous histiocytoma: radiologic-pathologic correlation. *Radiographics.* 1994;14:807–826.

Park Y, Unni KK, McLeod RA, Pritchard DJ. Osteofibrous dysplasia: clinicopathologic study of 80 cases. *Hum Pathol.* 1993;24:1339–1347.

Pennes DR, Braunstein EM, Glazer GM. Computed tomography of cortical desmoid. *Skeletal Radiol.* 1984;12:40–42.

Prieto VG, Reed JA, Shea CR. Immunohistochemistry of dermatofibroma and benign fibrous histiocytomas. *J Cutan Pathol.* 1995;22:336–341.

Rabhan WN, Rosai J. Desmoplastic fibroma. Report of ten cases and review of the literature. *J Bone J Surg Am.* 1968;50A:487–502.

Ragsdale BD. Polymorphic fibro-osseous lesions of bone: an almost site-specific diagnostic problem of the proximal femur. *Hum Pathol.* 1993;24:505–512.

Resnick D, Greenway G. Distal femoral cortical defects, irregularities, and excavations: a critical review of the literature with the addition of histologic and paleopathologic data. *Radiology.* 1982;143:345–354.

Riley GM, Greenspan A, Poirier VC. Fibrous dysplasia of a parietal bone. *J Comput Assist Tomogr.* 1997;21:41–43.

Riminucci M, Collins MT, Fedarko NS, et al. FGF-23 in fibrous dysplasia of bone and its relationship to renal phosphate wasting. *J Clin Invest.* 2003;112:683–692.

Ritschl P, Hajek PC, Pechmann U. Fibrous metaphyseal defects. Magnetic resonance imaging appearances. *Skeletal Radiol.* 1989;18:253–259.

Ritschl P, Karnel F, Hajek PC. Fibrous metaphyseal defects—determination of their origin and natural history using a radiomorphological study. *Skeletal Radiol.* 1988;17:8–15.

Romeo S, Bovee JV, Kroon HM, et al. Malignant fibrous histiocytoma and fibrosarcoma of bone: a re-assessment in the light of currently employed morphological, immunohistochemical and molecular approaches. *Virchows Arch.* 2012;461:561–570.

Rosenberg AE. Malignant fibrous histiocytoma: past, present, and future. *Skeletal Radiol.* 2003;32:613–618.

Ruggieri P, Sim FH, Bond JA, Unni KK. Malignancies in fibrous dysplasia. *Cancer.* 1994;73:1411–1424.

Sakamoto A, Oda Y, Iwamoto Y, Tsuneyoshi M. A comparative study of fibrous dysplasia and osteofibrous dysplasia with regards to Gsalpha mutation at the Arg201 codon: polymerase chain reaction-restriction fragment length polymorphism analysis of paraffin-embedded tissues. *J Mol Diagn.* 2000;2:67–72.

Schajowicz F. Histological typing of bone tumors. *World Health Organization International Histological Classification of Tumors.* Berlin, Germany: Springer-Verlag; 1993.

Schajowicz F. *Tumors and Tumor Like Lesions of Bone. Pathology, Radiology, and Treatment.* 2nd ed. Berlin, Germany: Springer-Verlag; 1994.

Schajowicz F, Sissons HA, Sobin LH. The World Health Organization's histologic classification of bone tumors. A commentary on the second edition. *Cancer.* 1995;75:1208–1214.

Schwartz DT, Alpert M. The malignant transformation of fibrous dysplasia. *Am J Med Sci.* 1964;247:1–20.

Schwartz AM, Ramos RM. Neurofibromatosis and multiple nonossifying fibroma. *AJR Am J Roentgenol.* 1980;135:617–619.

Seiss SW, Enzinger FM. Malignant fibrous histiocytoma: an analysis of 200 cases. *Cancer.* 1978;41:2250–2260.

Selby S. Metaphyseal cortical defects in the tubular bones of growing children. *J Bone Joint Surg Am.* 1961;43A:395–400.

Shelton III CH, Nimityongskul P, Richardson PH, Brogdon BG. Progressive painful bowing of the right leg. *Acad Radiol.* 1995;2:351–353.

Singnurkar A, Phancao JP, Chatha DS, Stern J. The appearance of Mazabraud's syndrome on 18F-FDG PET/CT. *Skeletal Radiol.* 2007;36:1085–1089.

Sissons HA, Kancherla PL, Lehman WB. Ossifying fibroma of bone. Report of two cases. *Bull Hosp Jt Dis Orthop Inst.* 1983;43:1–14.

Smith J. Radiation-induced sarcoma of bone: clinical and radiographic findings in 43 patients irradiated for soft tissue neoplasms. *Clin Radiol.* 1982;33:205–221.

Smith ME, Costa MJ, Weiss SW. Evaluation of CD68 and other histiocytic antigens in angiomatoid malignant fibrous histiocytoma. *Am J Surg Pathol.* 1991;15:757–763.

Soule EH, Enriquez P. Atypical fibrous histiocytoma, malignant fibrous histiocytoma, malignant histiocytoma, and epithelioid sarcoma. A comparative study of 65 tumors. *Cancer.* 1972;30:128–143.

Spanier SS, Enneking WF, Enriquez P. Primary malignant fibrous histiocytoma of bone. *Cancer.* 1975;36:2084–2098.

Spjut HJ, Dorfman HD, Fechner RE, Ackerman LV. *Tumors of bone pathology. Atlas of tumor pathology, 2nd series, Fascicle 5.* Washington, DC: Armed Forces Institute of Pathology; 1971:249–292.

Springfield DS, Rosenberg AE, Mankin HJ, Mindell ER. Relationship between osteofibrous dysplasia and adamantinoma. *Clin Orthop.* 1994;309:234–244.

Steiner GC. Fibrous cortical defect and non-ossifying fibroma of bone: a study of the ultrastructure. *Arch Pathol.* 1974;97:205–210.

Sugiura I. Desmoplastic fibroma. Case report and review of the literature. *J Bone Joint Surg Am.* 1976;58A:126–130.

Sundaram M, McDonald DJ, Merenda G. Intramuscular myxoma: a rare but important association with fibrous dysplasia of bone. *AJR Am J Roentgenol.* 1989;153:107–108.

Sweet DE, Vinh TN, Devaney K. Cortical osteofibrous dysplasia of long bone and its relationship to adamantinoma. *Am J Surg Pathol.* 1992;16:282–290.

Taconis WK, Schütte HE, van der Heul RO. Desmoplastic fibroma of bone: a report of 18 cases. *Skeletal Radiol.* 1994;23:283–288.

Tarkkanen M, Larramendy ML, Bohling T, et al. Malignant fibrous histiocytoma of bone: analysis of genomic imbalances by comparative genomic hybridisation and C-MYC expression by immunohistochemistry. *Eur J Cancer.* 2006;42:1172–1180.

Totty WG, Murphy WA, Lee JKT. Soft tissue tumors: MR imaging. *Radiology.* 1986;160:135–141.

Toyosawa S, Yuki M, Kishino M, et al. Ossifying fibroma vs fibrous dysplasia of the jaw: molecular and immunological characterization. *Mod Pathol.* 2007;20:389–396.

Trombetta D, Macchia G, Mandahl N, et al. Molecular genetic characterization of the 11q13 breakpoint in a desmoplastic fibroma of bone. *Cancer Genet.* 2012;205:410–413.

Ueda Y, Blasius S, Edel G, Wuisman P, Bocker W, Roessner A. Osteofibrous dysplasia of long bones—a reactive process to adamantinomatous tissue. *J Cancer Res Clin Oncol*. 1992;118:152–156.

Unni KK. Fibrous and fibrohistiocytic lesions of bone. *Semin Orthop*. 1991;6:177–186.

Unni KK. Fibrous and fibrohistiocytic lesions of bone. *Semin Orthop*. 1991;6:177–186.

Unni KK. *Dahlin's Bone Tumors: General Aspects and Data on 11,087 Cases*. 5th ed. New York: Lippincott-Raven; 1996.

Unni KK, Dahlin DC, Beaubout JW, Ivins JC. Adamantinoma of long bones. *Cancer*. 1974;34:1796–1805.

Utz JA, Kransdorf MJ, Jelinek JS, Moser RP, Berrey BH. MR appearance of fibrous dysplasia. *J Comput Assist Tomogr*. 1989;13:845–851.

Vanhoenacker FM, Hauben E, De Beuckeleer LH, et al. Desmoplastic fibroma of bone: MRI features. *Skeletal Radiol*. 2000;29:171–175.

Volpicelli ER, Fletcher CDM. Desmin and CD34 positivity in cellular fibrous histiocytoma: an immunohistochemical analysis of 100 cases. *J Cutan Pathol*. 2012;39:747–752.

Weiss SW, Dorfman HD. Adamantinoma of long bones. *Hum Pathol*. 1977;8:141–153.

Weiss SW, Enzinger FM. Malignant fibrous histiocytoma: an analysis of 200 cases. *Cancer*. 1978;41:2250–2266.

Weiss SW, Bratthauer GL, Morris PA. Post-radiation malignant fibrous histiocytoma expressing cytokeratin: implications for the immunodiagnosis of sarcomas. *Am J Surg Pathol*. 1988;12:554–558.

Wold LE. Fibrohistiocytic tumors of bone. In: Unni KK, ed. *Bone Tumors*. New York: Churchill Livingstone; 1988:183–197.

Wood GS, Beckstead JH, Turner RR, Hendrickson MR, Kempson RL, Warnke RA. Malignant fibrous histiocytoma tumor cells resemble fibroblasts. *Am J Surg Pathol*. 1986;10:323–335.

Yabut SM, Kenan S, Sissons HA, Lewis MM. Malignant transformation of fibrous dysplasia. *Clin Orthop*. 1988;228:281–289.

Yamamoto Y, Takakuwa Y, Kuroda M, et al. A p53 gene mutation in malignant fibrous histiocytoma associated with bone infarction. *Tohoku J Exp Med*. 2011;225:215–220.

Yamazaki T, Maruoka S, Takahashi S, et al. MR findings of avulsive cortical irregularity of the distal femur. *Skeletal Radiol*. 1995;24:43–46.

Young JWR, Aisner SC, Levine AM, Resnik CS, Dorfman HD. Computed tomography of desmoid tumors of bone: desmoplastic fibroma. *Skeletal Radiol*. 1988;17:333–337.

Zoccali C, Teori G, Erba F. Mazabraud's syndrome: a new case and review of the literature. *Int Orthop*. 2009;33:605–610.

CHAPTER 5

Round Cell Lesions

Langerhans cell histiocytosis (LCH), previously called eosinophilic granuloma, and categorized together with Hand-Schuller-Christian disease and Letterer-Siwe disease as histiocytosis X, is a lesion now classified by World Health Organization (WHO) into a group of histiocytic and dendritic cell disorders. Recently, it has been verified that the primary proliferative element in this disease is a Langerhans cell, a mononuclear cell of the dendritic type, that is derived from precursors in the skin and bone marrow. The condition may manifest as a solitary lesion or as multifocal disorder. Rosai-Dorfman disease, a sinus histiocytosis with massive lymphadenopathy, may occasionally affect the bones. Erdheim-Chester disease is a rare disseminated histiocytic disorder of unknown cause affecting the musculoskeletal system and various visceral organs including the heart and lungs. Some investigators raised the hypothesis of possible association of this disorder with LCH.

Round small cell malignancies of bone form a heterogeneous group of neoplasms, distinguished from most other malignancies of bone by the fact that the tumors form a pure cellular growth without production of tumor matrix. The common denominator is an undifferentiated, small round basophilic (bluish), cytoplasm-scant, stroma-poor, highly cellular tumor. These malignancies include Ewing sarcoma/primitive neuroectodermal tumors (PNET) family, lymphoma (non-Hodgkin and Hodgkin), mesenchymal chondrosarcoma, small cell osteosarcoma, myeloma, metastatic neuroblastoma, and some other metastatic lesions (Table 5.1). Ewing sarcoma, along with Askin tumor and primitive neuroectodermal tumor is currently regarded by WHO as a single entity (Ewing sarcoma family tumors). These lesions are characterized by various degrees of neuroectodermal differentiation and by common histopathologic, immunohistochemical, and molecular properties (Table 5.2). The term malignant lymphoma refers to a group of neoplasms that are composed of lymphoid cells in various stages of maturation. According to WHO, malignant lymphomas of bone are subdivided into those that affect one skeletal site with or without regional lymph nodes involvement, those that affect multiple bones without lymph node or visceral involvement, those that present as a primary bone tumor but reveal nodal or visceral lesions at staging examination, and those with a known lymphoma and positive bone biopsy. The first two groups are considered to represent primary lymphomas of bone. Furthermore, lymphomas are subdivided into non-Hodgkin and Hodgkin lymphomas. Recently, WHO adopted the Revised European-American Classification of Lymphoid Neoplasms (REAL) that originally was proposed by the International Lymphoma Study Group. This classification defines distinct disease entities based on a combination of morphologic, immunophenotypic, genetic, and clinical features (Table 5.3). Myeloma, a tumor originating in the bone marrow, also referred to as multiple myeloma, plasma cell myeloma, or plasmacytoma, is the most common primary malignancy of bone. This tumor is often associated with the presence of abnormal proteins in the blood and urine and occasionally with the presence of amyloid in the tumor tissue and other organs.

A. Benign Round Cell Lesions
Langerhans Cell Histiocytosis (LCH, Eosinophilic Granuloma)
Rosai-Dorfman Disease
Erdheim-Chester Disease (Lipogranulomatosis)

B. Malignant Round Cell Tumors
Ewing Sarcoma/Primitive Neuroectodermal Tumor (PNET)
Malignant Lymphoma of Bone
Multiple Myeloma (Plasma Cell Myeloma, Plasmacytoma)

TABLE 5.1 Small Round Cell Tumors of Bone

Tumor	Histopathologic Features
Ewing sarcoma	Small, uniform-sized cells with almost clear cytoplasm, round, slightly hyperchromatic nuclei. Cell borders indistinct.
Large cell (atypical) Ewing sarcoma	Larger cells, with better delimited contours, more cytoplasm with eosinophilic "histiocytoid" appearance, nuclei may contain very prominent nucleoli; atypical variant merges into small cell Ewing sarcoma.
Primitive (peripheral) neuroectodermal tumor (PNET) of bone	Similar to Ewing sarcoma. Focal Homer-Wright rosettes, often in tumor association with a fibrillary intercellular background. Reticulin fibers surrounding large groups of cells in a basket-like distribution.
Askin tumor of bone (thoracopulmonary or thoracospinal variant of PNET)	Similar to Ewing sarcoma. Focal Homer-Wright rosettes. Compact sheets of cells with dark nuclei; nesting arrangement of cells with intervening fibrovascular stroma; serpiginous bands of cells with necrosis. May or may not display neural differentiation.
Malignant lymphoma	Aggregates of malignant lymphoid cells, typically mixture of small lymphocytic cells and large histiocytic cells. Cells are rounded, ovoid, and pleomorphic, displaying basophilic cytoplasm. Nuclei contain scanty chromatin, sometimes cleaved or horseshoe shaped with prominent nucleoli.
Myeloma	Sheets of atypical plasmacytoid cells frequently bi- and trinucleated. Round nuclei possess dense, coarse chromatin with cartwheel-like distribution. Prominent nuclei eccentrically located in a strongly basophilic cytoplasm.
Small cell osteosarcoma	Loose aggregations of small round cells with ovoid nuclei separated by collagenous bands of fine eosinophilic matrices. Occasional spindling of tumor cells. Focal production of osteoid or bone.
Mesenchymal chondrosarcoma	Small, round, uniform-sized cells with round or ovoid nuclei and scant cytoplasm, occasionally interspersed with spindle-shaped cells. Areas of well-differentiated cartilage containing foci of calcification.
Metastatic neuroblastoma	Very similar to PNET, including Homer-Wright rosettes; a fibrillary intercellular background; long, thin tapering cytoplasmatic extensions creating appearance of a "pear" or "carrot" cells; and higher degree of neural differentiation.
Metastatic primitive alveolar rhabdomyosarcoma	Similar to Ewing sarcoma. Alternating areas of cellularity and myxoid changes. Round or oval, occasionally spindled or tapered cells with scant eosinophilic cytoplasm.

From Greenspan A, Jundt G, Remagen W. *Differential Diagnosis in Orthopaedic Oncology*. 2nd ed. p. 324, Table 5-1. Modified from Triche T, Cavazzana A. Round cell tumors of bone. In: Unni KK, ed. *Bone Tumors*. New York: Churchill Livingstone, 1988;199–223; from Meis-Kindblom JM, Stenman G, Kindblom L-G. Differential diagnosis of small round cell tumors. *Semin Diagn Pathol.* 1996;13:213–214; and from Llombart-Bosch A, Contesso G, Peydro-Olaya A. Histology, immunohistochemistry, and electron microscopy of small round cell tumors of bone. *Semin Diagn Pathol.* 1996;13:153–170.

A. BENIGN ROUND CELL LESIONS

Langerhans Cell Histiocytosis (LCH, Eosinophilic Granuloma)

Definition:
- Monostotic or polyostotic histiocytic and dendritic monoclonal cell disorder characterized by neoplastic proliferation of Langerhans cells that normally populate the skin, mucosal surfaces, lymph nodes, and other tissues

Epidemiology:
- Relatively rare disorder, accounting for less than 1% of all osseous lesions.
- Age distribution ranging from the first month of life to eighth decade, with 80% to 85% of cases seen in patients under the age of 30, and 60% under the age of 10.
- Males are affected twice as often as females.

Sites of Involvement:
- Any bone may be affected, although there is predilection to involve the bones of the skull, particularly the calvaria.
- Other commonly involved sites include the femur, the bones of the pelvis, ribs, vertebrae, and the mandible.

Clinical Findings:
- Pain and swelling of the affected area occur most commonly.
- In cases of temporal bone involvement, the presenting features can overlap with those of otitis media and mastoiditis.
- Mandibular involvement may result in loosening and loss of teeth.
- Involvement of vertebral body may result in compression fracture and possible neurologic impairment.
- Fever, elevated sedimentation rate, and leukocytosis may be present.

TABLE 5.2 Small Round Cell Tumors of Bone and Typical Immunohistochemistry Results

Tumor	bcl-2	CK	Vim	Des	NF	CD99	CD57	NSE	CD45	Light Chains κ or λ	Syn	CD138
Ewing sarcoma	−	+/a	+	−	−/a	+	(+)	−	−	−	−	−
PNET/Askin tumor	−	−	+	−	(+)	+	(+)	+	−	−	+	−
Malignant lymphoma	+	−	+	−	−	(+)	(+)	−	+	+/−	−	(+)
Myeloma	+	−	−/+	−	−	(+)	−	−	−/+	+	−	+
Small cell osteosarcoma	−	−	+	−	−	−	−	−	−	−	−	−
Mesenchymal chondrosarcoma	−	−	+	−	−	+	−	−	−	−	−	−
Metastatic neuroblastoma	−	−	−	−	+	−	(+)	+	−	−	+	−
Rhabdomyosarcoma	−	−	(+)	+	−	−	−	(+)	−	−	−	−
Synovial sarcoma	+	+	+	−	−	+	−	−	−	−	−	(+)
Desmoplastic small round cell tumor	−	+	+	+	−	(+)	+	+	−	−	+	−

From Greenspan A, Jundt G, Remagen W. *Differential Diagnosis in Orthopaedic Oncology*. 2nd ed. p. 333, Table 5-2.

TABLE 5.3 Revised European-American Lymphoma Classification

B-Cell Lymphomas	T-Cell and Natural Killer Cell Neoplasms	Hodgkin Disease
Precursor B-cell neoplasm • Precursor B-lymphoblastic leukemia or lymphoma Mature B-cell neoplasm • B-cell chronic lymphocytic leukemia, prolymphocytic leukemia, small lymphocytic leukemia • Lymphoplasmacytoid lymphoma • Mantle cell lymphoma • Follicle center lymphoma • Marginal zone B-cell lymphoma • Hairy cell lymphoma • Diffuse large cell B-cell lymphoma • Burkitt lymphoma • High-grade B-cell lymphoma	Precursor T-cell neoplasm • Precursor T-lymphoblastic lymphoma or leukemia Peripheral T-cell and natural killer cell neoplasm • T-cell chronic lymphocytic leukemia • Large granular lymphocyte leukemia • Mycosis fungoides, Sézary syndrome • Peripheral T-cell lymphoma • Angioimmunoblastic T-cell lymphoma • Angiocentric lymphoma • Adult T-cell lymphoma • Anaplastic large cell lymphoma	Nodular lymphocyte predominance (paragranuloma) Nodular sclerosis Mixed cellularity Lymphocyte depletion Lymphocyte-rich classic Hodgkin disease

From Greenspan A, Jundt G, Remagen W. *Differential Diagnosis in Orthopaedic Oncology*. 2nd ed. p. 335, Table 5-3. Modified from Krishnan A, Shirkhoda A, Tehranzadeh J, et al. Primary bone lymphoma: radiographic—MR imaging correlation. *Radiographics*. 2003;23:1371–1387, with permission.

- Single or multiple lesions restricted to the skeleton have been termed eosinophilic granuloma.
- Multifocal bone disease associated with exophthalmos and diabetes insipidus is known as Hand-Schuller-Christian disease.
- Letterer-Siwe disease (nonlipid reticulosis) is a condition that usually affects very young children (<2 years old) and consists of disseminated bone lesions, anemia, lymphadenopathy, and splenomegaly.

Imaging:
- Radiography shows well-defined, lytic lesions; however, in a minority of cases, the lesions may exhibit wide zone of transition and permeative type of bone destruction (Figs. 5.1 to 5.3). More sclerotic appearance is seen in later stages of the disease (Fig. 5.4). Some lesions may show slanting or beveling of the edges. Scalloping of the endocortex is a common finding (see Fig. 5.1B).
- Cortical involvement may elicit an aggressive lamellated (onion-skin) type of periosteal reaction (Fig. 5.5A, see also Fig. 5.1A).
- Scintigraphy generally shows increased uptake of the radiopharmaceutical tracer (see Fig. 5.6B), but about 35% of lesions show normal radionuclide bone scan.
- Magnetic resonance imaging shows the lesion to be of intermediate signal intensity on T1-weighted images and of high signal on T2 weighting. After intravenous administration of gadolinium, there is significant enhancement of the lesions (Figs. 5.5 to 5.8).

Pathology:

Gross (Macroscopy):
- Involved tissue is soft and red in color.

Histopathology:
- Proliferating Langerhans cells are arranged in aggregates, sheets, or individually within a loose fibrous stroma, exhibiting indistinct cytoplasmic borders and eosinophilic to clear cytoplasm (Fig. 5.9).
- The nuclei are translucent, ovoid, coffee bean or kidney shaped with typical longitudinal grooves (Fig. 5.9C).

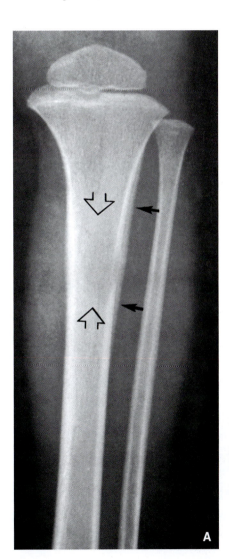
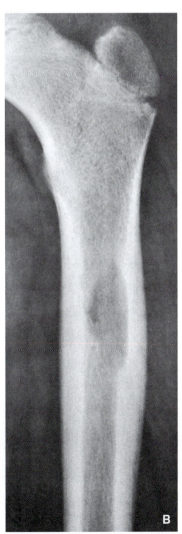

FIGURE 5.1 Radiography of Langerhans cell histiocytosis. (A) Anteroposterior radiograph of the lower leg of a 4-year-old boy shows a lesion in the diaphysis of the left tibia (*open arrows*). Observe a permeative type of bone destruction and a lamellated (onionskin) type of periosteal reaction (*arrows*), very similar to that seen in Ewing sarcoma. **(B)** Anteroposterior radiograph of the proximal right femur of a 3-year-old boy shows an osteolytic lesion causing endosteal scalloping. Note fusiform thickening of the cortex and solid uninterrupted periosteal reaction.

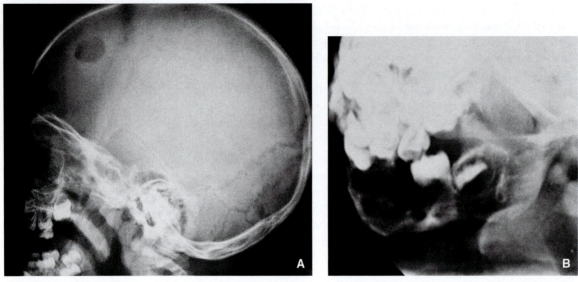

FIGURE 5.2 Radiography of Langerhans cell histiocytosis. (A) Lateral radiograph of the skull of a 2.5-year-old boy with disseminated disease shows an osteolytic lesion in the frontal bone with a sharply outlined borders, exhibiting a "punched-out" appearance. Uneven involvement of the inner and outer tables results in beveled presentation. **(B)** A 3-year-old girl with extensive skeletal involvement had a large destructive lesion in the mandible. Note the characteristic appearance of a floating tooth, which resulted from destruction of supportive alveolar bone.

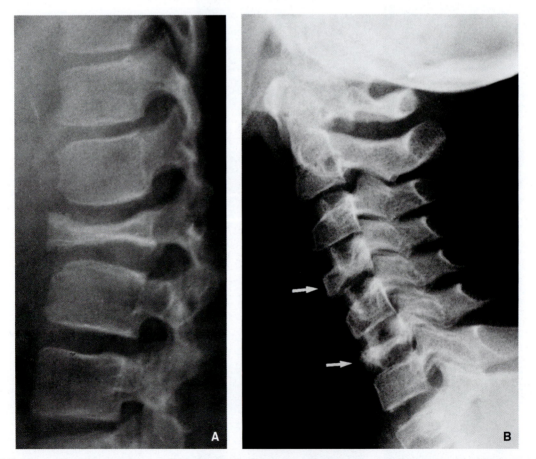

FIGURE 5.3 Radiography of Langerhans cell histiocytosis. (A) Vertebra plana represents collapse of vertebral body secondary to destruction of bone by granulomatous lesion. Note the preservation of intervertebral disk space. **(B)** In another patient, lateral radiograph of the cervical spine shows compression fractures of the vertebral bodies C4 and C6 (*arrows*).

- Chromatin is either diffusely dispersed or condensed along the nuclear membranes.
- Langerhans cells are frequently admixed with inflammatory cells including large numbers of eosinophils, lymphocytes, neutrophils, and plasma cells (Figs. 5.10 and 5.11).
- Necrosis may be found in a minority of cases, and if it is prominent, is usually the complication of a pathologic fracture.
- Mitotic figures may be seen; however, atypical forms are absent.
- In older or polyostotic lesions, lipid-bearing foam cells can be observed (see Fig. 5.9D).
- Special stains may reveal abundant droplets of sudanophilic fat peripherally or in the middle of the giant cell cytoplasm, so-called Touton cells.

Immunohistochemistry:
- Langerhans cells are positive for CD1a, S-100 protein (see Figs. 5.10C and 5.11C,D), and Langerin/CD207, but negative for CD68 and CD45.

Electron Microscopy:
- Intracytoplasmic "tennis racquet"–shaped inclusion bodies (organelles), known as Birbeck granules, are diagnostic for this disorder (Fig. 5.12).

Prognosis:
- Treatment and prognosis of LCH depends on the site and size of the lesion, the age of the patient, and the presence or absence of multifocal disease.

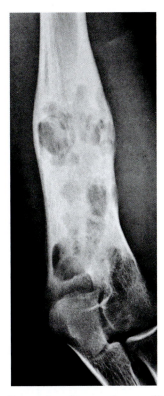

FIGURE 5.4 Radiography of Langerhans cell histiocytosis. The healing stage of the lesion, as seen here in the distal humerus of a 16-year-old girl, exhibits predominantly sclerotic changes with interspersed radiolucent foci, thickening of the cortex, and well-organized periosteal reaction. In this stage, the lesion mimics chronic osteomyelitis.

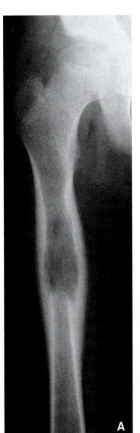
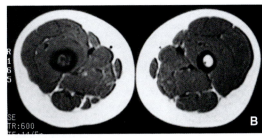
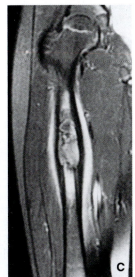

FIGURE 5.5 Radiography and magnetic resonance imaging of Langerhans cell histiocytosis. (A) Anteroposterior radiograph of the right femur of a 13-year-old boy demonstrates a radiolucent lesion in the proximal femoral diaphysis with a lamellated periosteal reaction. **(B)** Axial T1-weighted MRI shows the lesion to be of low signal intensity. Observe marked thickening of the cortex. **(C)** Coronal T1-weighted MR image obtained after intravenous administration of gadolinium shows marked enhancement of the lesion and soft tissues adjacent to the thickened cortex.

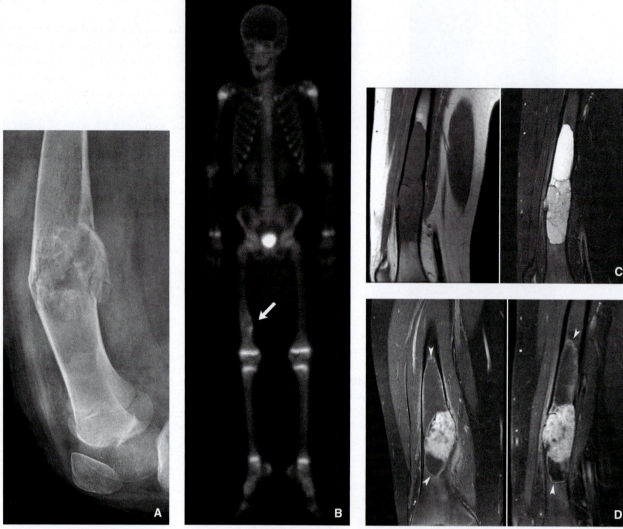

FIGURE 5.6 Radiography, scintigraphy, and magnetic resonance imaging of Langerhans cell histiocytosis. (A) Lateral radiograph of the right knee of a 9-year-old boy shows an osteolytic lesion in the diaphysis of the distal femur with a pathologic fracture. **(B)** Whole-body radionuclide bone scan obtained after intravenous injection of 15 mCi of ^{99m}Tc-labeled methylene diphosphonate shows mildly increased uptake of the radiopharmaceutical agent at the site of the lesion (*arrow*). There are no additional lesions present. **(C)** Sagittal T1-weighted and sagittal STIR MR images demonstrate sharply demarcated lesion exhibiting low signal intensity on T1 weighting and high signal intensity on STIR sequence. **(D)** Coronal and sagittal T1-weighted fat-suppressed MR images obtained after intravenous administration of gadolinium show significant enhancement of the lesion. The solid, enhancing lesion is surrounded proximally and distally by intramedullary cyst formation with a thin enhancing peripheral rim (*arrowheads*), a rare feature of this disorder.

- Monostotic disease is usually managed by curettage; however, tumors located in areas difficult to excise may be treated with low dose of radiation.
- Single- or multi-agent therapy may be administered in the setting of disseminated disease.
- Complete resolution may follow treatment or occasionally may occur spontaneously.

Differential Diagnosis:
Monostotic Form

- **Ewing sarcoma**
  In early stages the imaging features may be indistinguishable from those of LCH; however, clinical so-called tempo-phenomenon (rapid progression and disappearance of the lesion of LCH vs. slower progression of the tumor in Ewing sarcoma) is a very useful sign. Soft-tissue mass is usually much more prominent.
  Histopathology shows small, uniform-sized cells with indistinct borders and clear-to-slightly eosinophilic cytoplasm and hyperchromatic nuclei. Lack of Langerhans cells.
- **Osteomyelitis**
  Imaging features are similar to those of LCH, but clinical and laboratory findings are helpful.
  Histopathology showing typical inflammatory changes, and lack of Langerhans cells is diagnostic.

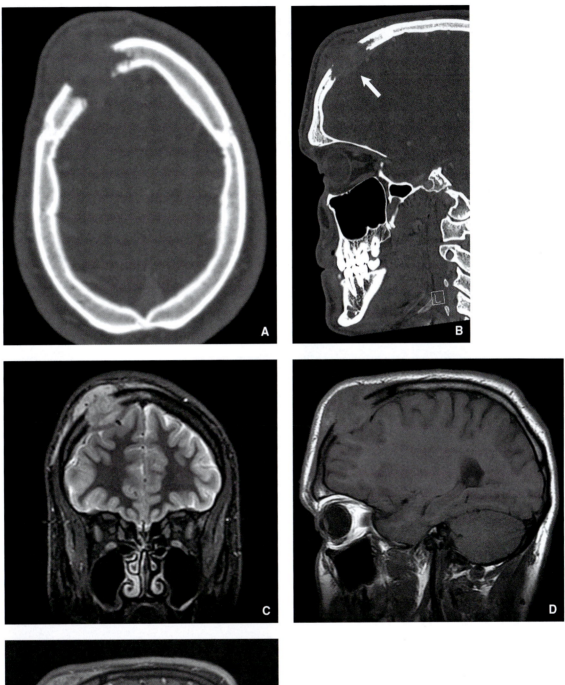
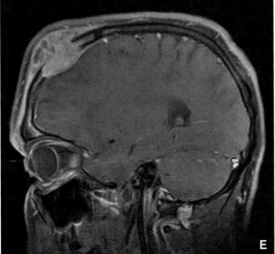

FIGURE 5.7 Computed tomography and magnetic resonance imaging of Langerhans cell histiocytosis. Axial **(A)** and sagittal **(B)** reformatted CT images of the skull of a 19-year-old man show a destructive lesion in the right frontal bone associated with a soft-tissue mass (*arrow*). **(C)** Coronal T2-weighted fat-suppressed MR image shows a soft-tissue mass to better advantage, displaying high signal intensity. The mass is compressing the right frontal lobe. **(D)** Sagittal T1-weighted and **(E)** sagittal T1-weighted fat-suppressed MRI obtained after intravenous administration of gadolinium show slight enhancement of both the intraosseous lesion and the soft-tissue mass.

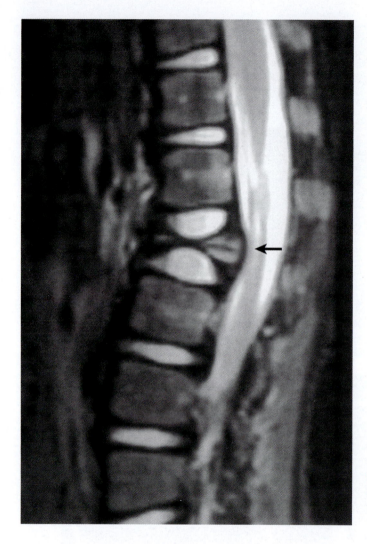

FIGURE 5.8 Magnetic resonance imaging of Langerhans cell histiocytosis. A sagittal T2-weighted MR image shows compression of the ventral aspect of the thecal sac by fractured vertebral body (*arrow*).

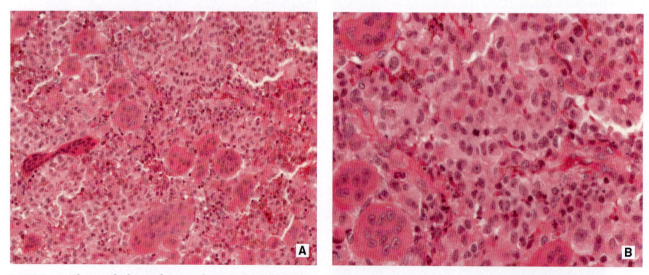

FIGURE 5.9 Histopathology of Langerhans cell histiocytosis. (A) Densely arranged large Langerhans cells and giant cells are infiltrated by numerous eosinophilic granulocytes (H&E, original magnification ×100). **(B)** At higher magnification large pale histiocyte-like Langerhans cells and numerous giant cells containing up to 10 nuclei (*left*) are clearly discernible. In addition, sparse lymphocytes and eosinophils are present (H&E, original magnification ×400).

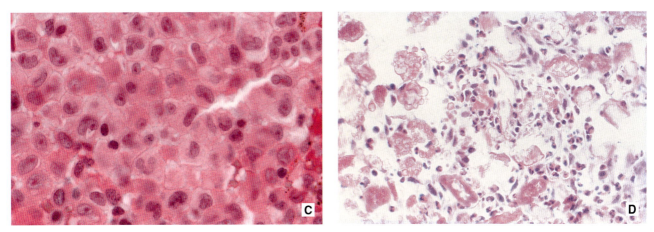

FIGURE 5.9 *(Continued).* **(C)** At high power, the indentations of oval nuclei of Langerhans cell are clearly visible (H&E, original magnification ×630). **(D)** In another field of view, mulberry-like foam cells (*left and upper right*), eosinophilic granulocytes, and hyaline bodies prevail (H&E, original magnification ×50).

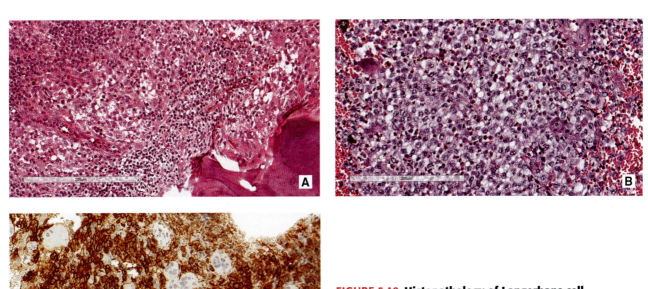

FIGURE 5.10 Histopathology of Langerhans cell histiocytosis. (A) Aggregates of ovoid to round histiocyte-like Langerhans cells are present. Note also prominent eosinophilia and foci of hemorrhage (H&E, original magnification ×100). **(B)** Higher magnification shows Langerhans cells in a mixed inflammatory background of lymphocytes, plasma cells, and eosinophils (H&E, original magnification ×200). **(C)** Immunohistochemistry shows membrane-based positivity of Langerhans cells for CD1a (original magnification ×200).

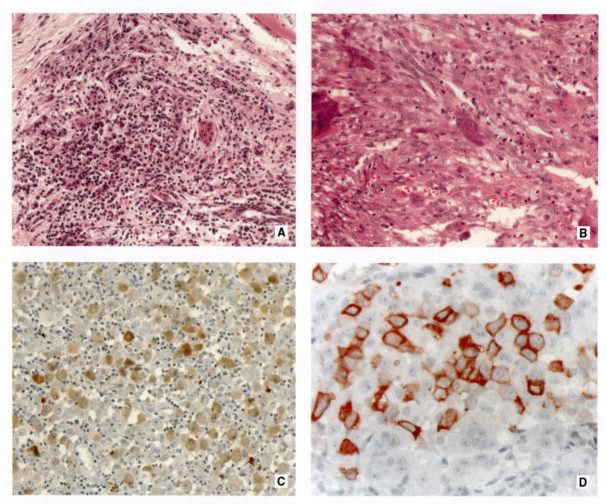

FIGURE 5.11 Histopathology of Langerhans cell histiocytosis. (A) In a later stage of development, nonspecific inflammatory cells, particularly lymphocytes, predominate. Some giant cells may also be present (H&E, original magnification ×100). **(B)** In another field, Langerhans cells show a more spindle-shaped appearance. Scattered eosinophils and giant cells are also present (H&E, original magnification ×200). **(C)** Both cytoplasm and nuclei of the tumor cells are positive for S-100 protein (biotin–streptavidin peroxidase, original magnification ×200). **(D)** On higher magnification observe cytoplasmic and membranous positivity of Langerhans cells for CD1a (ABC peroxidase, original magnification ×400).

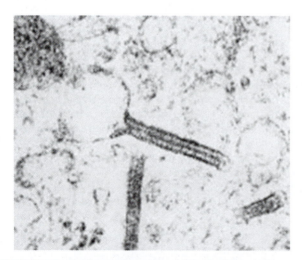

FIGURE 5.12 Electron microscopy of Langerhans cell histiocytosis. Intracytoplasmic tennis racquet–shaped inclusions known as Birbeck granules are pathognomonic for this disorder (EM, original magnification ×64,000).

Polyostotic Form

- ***Brown tumors of hyperparathyroidism***

    Although the imaging features may resemble those of LCH, the patients are usually much older. Other characteristic features of hyperparathyroidism are present, such as subperiosteal and chondral resorption, osteopenia, rugger–jersey spine, and soft-tissue calcifications.

    Histopathology of brown tumors, which are composed of reactive stromal cells in which multinucleated giant cells are arranged in clusters, and the presence of large aggregates of hemosiderin pigment, is characteristic. Additional findings of intracortical tunneling and resorption of cancellous and compact bone, large number of osteoclasts resorbing bone trabeculae, and paratrabecular marrow fibrosis are diagnostic.

Rosai-Dorfman Disease

Definition:
- Also known as sinus histiocytosis with massive lymphadenopathy, this rare, proliferative, histiocytic disease of unknown etiology is characterized by the enlargement of lymph node sinuses caused by an aggregation of histiocytic cells that exhibit marked lymphophagocytosis (numerous phagocytized lymphocytes are present in the cytoplasm).

Epidemiology:
- Majority of patients are teenagers and young adults.
- Mean age of presentation is 20 years.
- No gender preference.
- Solitary lesion in bones was described in young children.

Sites of Involvement:
- Tibia, femur, clavicle, skull, maxilla, calcaneus, metacarpals, and sacrum.

Clinical Findings:
- Fever and massive cervical lymphadenopathy are the most common symptoms at presentation.
- Other symptoms include weight loss, malaise, and night sweats.
- Quite often the disease fully manifests after a short period of a nonspecific fever and pharyngitis.
- Primary or secondary involvement of extranodal sites, including the skeleton, is common.

Imaging:
- Skeletal involvement manifests by the presence of solitary or multifocal defects with poorly or well-demarcated (sclerotic) borders.
- The intramedullary lesions are associated with cortical erosion, complete cortical disruption, periosteal reaction, or a combination of these features.
- Radiographic manifestations and clinical symptoms may suggest an inflammatory disorder, such as osteomyelitis.
- Scintigraphy using gallium scanning shows increased uptake of the radiopharmaceutical agent.
- FDG-PET scanning shows increased metabolism.

Pathology:
Histopathology:
- In typical cases, the sinuses of lymph nodes are filled with large, pale histiocytic cells of varying size.
- These cells have prominent eosinophilic cytoplasm, indistinct borders, and round or oval nuclei with a very fine chromatin pattern and a single small nucleolus.
- Nuclear grooves are not present, and some of these cells may have several nucleoli.
- Occasionally, cells with multilobulated nuclei may be present.
- Mitotic figures are rare; atypical mitoses are not present.
- The most striking and diagnostically important feature of histiocytic cells is prominent emperipolesis or lymphophagocytosis (i.e., the presence of well-preserved lymphocytes within the histiocytic cell cytoplasm) (Fig. 5.13A).
- In addition to lymphocytes, a smaller number of phagocytized plasma cells, neutrophils, and red cells are also present.
- Extranodal disease, including skeletal system, has all these features except that histiocytic cells, instead of growing in sinuses, form irregular geographic areas separated by other inflammatory cells.

Immunohistochemistry:
- Histiocytic cells are positive for S-100 protein (Fig. 5.13B) but negative for CD1a.

Prognosis:
- This disease is considered a histologically benign, proliferative, histiocytic disorder with a variable, but occasionally fatal, outcome.

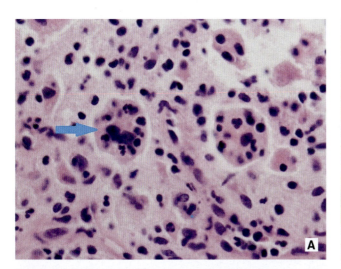
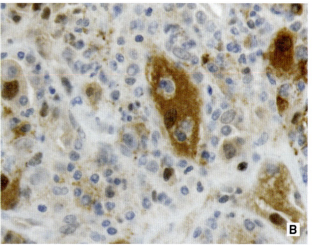

FIGURE 5.13 Histopathology of Rosai-Dorfman disease. (A) Large histiocytic cell with well-preserved lymphocytes within its cytoplasm (*blue arrow*), also known as emperipolesis or lymphophagocytosis, is a pathognomonic feature of this disorder (H&E, original magnification ×400). **(B)** Immunohistochemistry demonstrates strong positivity of large histiocytes to S-100 protein (original magnification ×400).

- The majority of patients have indolent regressive or clinically stable disease after several years.
- Fatal outcome of the disease is associated with the severe involvement of extranodal sites (lungs and kidney).

Differential Diagnosis:
- **Osteomyelitis**
  Although imaging findings may occasionally mimic those of Rosai-Dorfman disease, the histopathologic findings of classic inflammatory and infectious features as described in the prior text are diagnostic.

Erdheim-Chester Disease (Lipogranulomatosis)

Definition:
- Rare disseminated histiocytic disorder of unknown cause characterized by infiltration of musculoskeletal system and various organs including the heart, lungs, and skin by lipid-laden histiocytes leading to fibrosis and osteosclerosis.

Epidemiology:
- Slight male predominance.
- Age range between 7 and 84 years with mean age of 53.

Sites of Involvement:
- Mostly affects the major long bones with sparing of the articular ends.
- Rarely the flat bones can be involved.
- Extraskeletal involvement may occur, for example, kidney, heart, lungs, and skin.

Clinical Features:
- Mild bone pain sometimes associated with soft-tissue swelling.
- Extraskeletal manifestations may include general weakness, fever, weight loss, abdominal pain, shortness of breath, neurologic dysfunction, exophthalmos, diabetes insipidus, kidney failure, hepatosplenomegaly, and eyelid xanthomas.

Imaging:
- Radiography shows medullary sclerosis and cortical thickening of the long bones with sparing of the articular ends (Fig. 5.14).
- Scintigraphy shows increased uptake of the radiopharmaceutical tracer.
- Magnetic resonance imaging shows the lesion to be of low signal intensity on T1-weighted sequences with heterogeneous signal on T2 weighting and marked enhancement on contrast studies.

Pathology:
Gross (Macroscopy):
- Lesions appear yellow in color and variably firm.

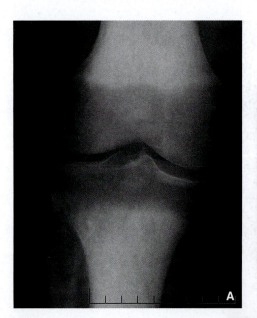
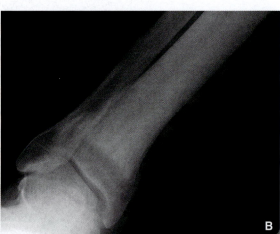
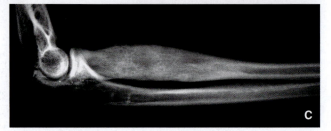

FIGURE 5.14 Radiography of Erdheim-Chester disease. **(A)** Anteroposterior radiograph of the right knee shows characteristic sclerosis of the long bones sparing the epiphysis of the distal femur and proximal tibia. **(B)** Similar features are noted in the distal tibia of the same patient. **(C)** In another patient, the lateral radiograph of the forearm shows sclerotic changes of the shaft of the radius. Again observe sparing of the articular end of bone.

Histopathology:

- Diffuse infiltration of bone marrow by foamy histiocytes, lymphocytes, plasma cells, and Touton giant cells, associated with dense fibrosis (Fig. 5.15A,C).
- Reactive sclerosis of cortical and cancellous bone with irregular cement lines resembling features of Paget disease (Fig. 5.15B).

Electron Microscopy:

- Histiocytes with indented nuclei with abundant intracytoplasmic lipid vacuoles and sparse mitochondria, lysosomes, and endoplasmic reticulum.
- Negative for Birbeck granules.

Immunohistochemistry:

- Foamy macrophages and giant cells positive for lysozyme, Mac387, CD68 (Kp-1) (Fig. 5.15D), CD4, alpha-1-antichymotrypsin, alpha-1-antitrypsin, and S-100 protein (variable).
- Negative for CD1a.

Genetics:

- *BRAF* V600E mutations seen in 50% of cases.
- Chromosome translocation t(12;15;20;)(q11;q24;p13.3).

Differential Diagnosis:

- *Lymphoma*

  Imaging studies show sclerotic changes more often in the vertebrae and the ribs, rarely in the long bones; thickening of the cortex; periosteal reaction is seen in more than 50% of cases.

  Histopathology showing aggregates of pleomorphic malignant lymphoid cells with large cleaved or horseshoe-shaped nuclei possessing prominent nucleoli is diagnostic.

- *Sclerotic metastasis*

  Imaging studies may closely mimic the appearance of Erdheim-Chester disease, although metastatic disease is more patchy in distribution; unusual sites for that disorder such as skull, vertebrae, ribs, and pelvic bones will also be affected.

  Histopathology, occasionally showing the origin of metastatic lesion (prostate, seminoma, osteosarcoma, neurogenic tumor), and immunohistochemistry (particularly application of cytokeratins) are diagnostic.

- *Paget disease*

  Imaging studies show invariably involvement of the articular end of the long bones. Cortical thickening and coarse trabecular pattern of cancellous bone are characteristic.

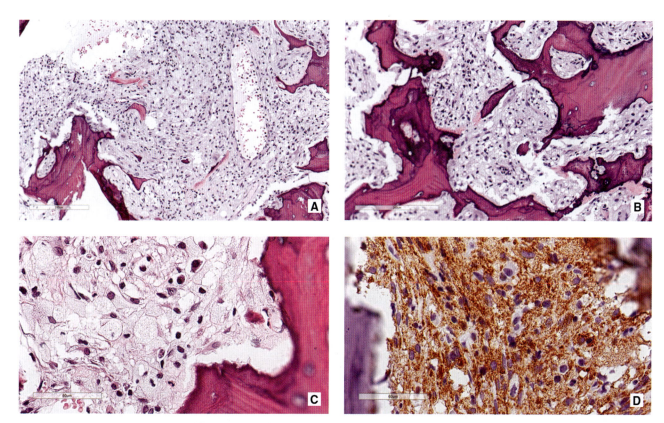

FIGURE 5.15 **Histopathology of Erdheim-Chester disease. (A)** Observe accumulation of foamy histiocytes in bone (H&E, original magnification ×100). **(B)** Diffuse infiltration of foamy histiocytes between bone trabeculae that show sclerotic changes, and in some areas resemble mosaic pattern of Paget disease (H&E, original magnification ×200). **(C)** Under high-power magnification the details of the foamy macrophages are better appreciated (H&E, original magnification ×400). **(D)** Immunohistochemistry shows positivity of foamy macrophages for CD68 (original magnification ×400).

Histopathology showing mosaic pattern of cement lines is diagnostic.

- **Camurati-Engelmann disease (Progressive diaphyseal dysplasia)**

  Imaging features of bilateral symmetrical fusiform diaphyseal sclerosis with thickening of the cortex, narrowing of the medullary canal, and sparing of the metaphyses and epiphyses are characteristic.

  Histopathology shows active new bone formation on the endosteal surface of the cortex and some periosteal new bone formation. Thick-walled vessels and admixed lymphocytes and plasma cells may be seen in the stroma.

- **Ribbing disease (Hereditary multiple diaphyseal sclerosis)**

  Imaging and histopathologic findings very similar to those of Camurati-Engelmann disease.

B. MALIGNANT ROUND CELL TUMORS

Ewing Sarcoma/Primitive Neuroectodermal Tumor (PNET)

Definition:
- Small round cell sarcomas (belong to the group of pediatric small blue cell tumors) that show varying degrees of neuroectodermal differentiation.
- Term Ewing sarcoma is used for those tumors that lack neuroectodermal differentiation.
- Term PNET is used for tumors with neuroectodermal differentiation.

Epidemiology:
- Ewing sarcoma accounts for 11% to 12% of all primary malignant bone tumors.
- It is the second most common sarcoma of bone in children.
- Male-to-female ratio of 3:2.
- Nearly 80% of patients are younger than 20 years, and the peak incidence is during the second decade of life (median age 13 years).

Sites of Involvement:
- Diaphysis or metaphyseal–diaphyseal portion of long bones.
- The pelvic bones and ribs are also common locations.

Clinical Features:
- Painful mass in the involved area is the most common clinical symptom.
- Fever, weight loss, anemia, leukocytosis, and increased sedimentation rate are often present.

Imaging:
- Radiography shows a lytic lesion exhibiting moth-eaten or permeative type of bone destruction, associated with aggressive, frequently lamellated (onionskin) type of

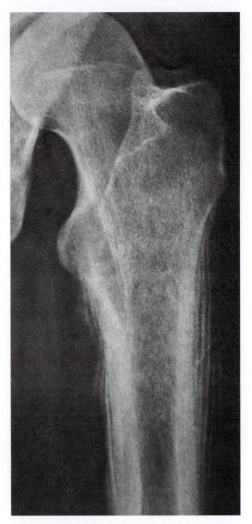

FIGURE 5.16 Radiography of Ewing sarcoma. Anteroposterior radiograph of the right proximal femur of a 20-year-old woman shows permeative lesion associated with characteristic for this tumor onionskin periosteal reaction.

periosteal reaction (Fig. 5.16); saucerization of the cortex is a characteristic feature (Fig. 5.17); soft-tissue mass, commonly disproportionally larger than the bone lesion (Fig. 5.18); small number of cases may show mineralization within the tumor (Fig. 5.19).
- Scintigraphy shows significant uptake of radiopharmaceutical agent.
- Computed tomography shows to better advantage the soft-tissue mass (Fig. 5.20).
- Magnetic resonance imaging shows low-to-intermediate signal intensity on T1-weighted sequences, and heterogeneous but predominantly high signal on T2-weighting and other water-sensitive sequences. After administration of gadolinium there is invariably significant enhancement of the osseous component and soft-tissue mass (Figs. 5.21 and 5.22).
- FDG-PET images show hypermetabolic foci of activity within the tumor (Figs. 5.23 to 5.25).

Pathology:

Gross (Macroscopy):
- Tan-gray and often necrotic and hemorrhagic mass.

Histopathology:
- Most tumors are composed of uniform small round cells with scanty clear or eosinophilic cytoplasm and indistinct cytoplasmic membranes; the prominent septa composed of fibrous connective tissue divide the tumor tissue into the lobules (Fig. 5.26).
- The nuclei are round and slightly hyperchromatic, containing fine chromatin (Figs. 5.27 and 5.28A).
- Some tumor cells are larger, have prominent nucleoli, and irregular contours.
- The cytoplasm of the tumors commonly contains PAS-positive glycogen (diastase sensitive) (Figs. 5.28B).
- Tumor cells do not form reticulin fibers (Fig. 5.28C).
- In some cases, Homer-Wright rosettes are present.
- Necrosis is common with residual viable cells frequently perivascular in distribution.
- Reactive bone formation may be present, particularly at the periphery of the tumor.

Immunohistochemistry:
- Positive: Fli-1, CD99 (Fig. 5.29), vimentin, and neuron-specific enolase (NSE) (Fig. 5.30).
- Negative: S-100 protein, CD45, muscular, and vascular markers.

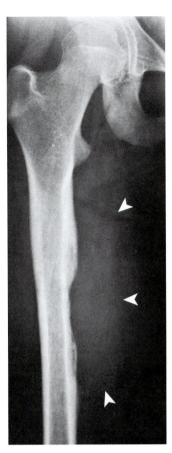

FIGURE 5.17 Radiography of Ewing sarcoma. Anteroposterior radiograph of the right femur of a 12-year-old girl shows saucerization of the medial cortex of the diaphysis, a feature characteristic for this malignancy. Note a large soft-tissue mass (*arrowheads*).

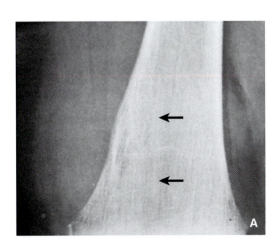
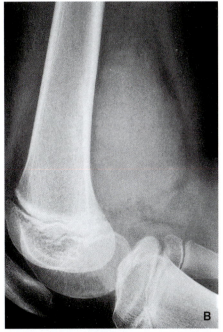

FIGURE 5.18 Radiography of Ewing sarcoma. (A) Bone destruction (*arrows*) is almost imperceptible on this magnification study of the distal femoral diaphysis of a 10-year-old girl. **(B)** Lateral radiograph of the distal femur, however, shows a large soft-tissue mass adjacent to the posterior cortex.

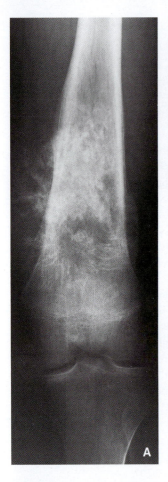
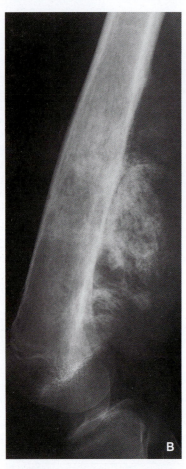

FIGURE 5.19 Radiography of Ewing sarcoma.
Anteroposterior **(A)** and lateral **(B)** radiographs of the left femur of a 17-year-old boy show a destructive lesion in the distal diaphysis exhibiting significant sclerosis. This presentation of Ewing sarcoma mimics features of osteosarcoma.

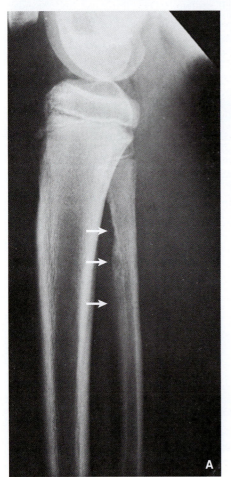
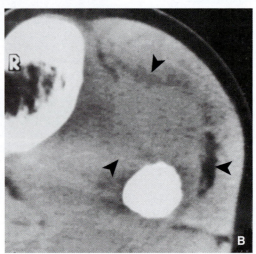

FIGURE 5.20 Radiography and computed tomography of Ewing sarcoma.
(A) Lateral radiograph of the proximal leg of a 12-year-old boy shows the typical appearance of this tumor affecting the diaphysis of the fibula. The poorly marginated lesion exhibits a permeative type of bone destruction associated with an aggressive periosteal reaction (*arrows*). Soft-tissue mass is not well appreciated on this study.
(B) Axial CT section through the tumor demonstrates a large soft-tissue mass (*arrowheads*). Observe complete obliteration of the marrow cavity by tumor.

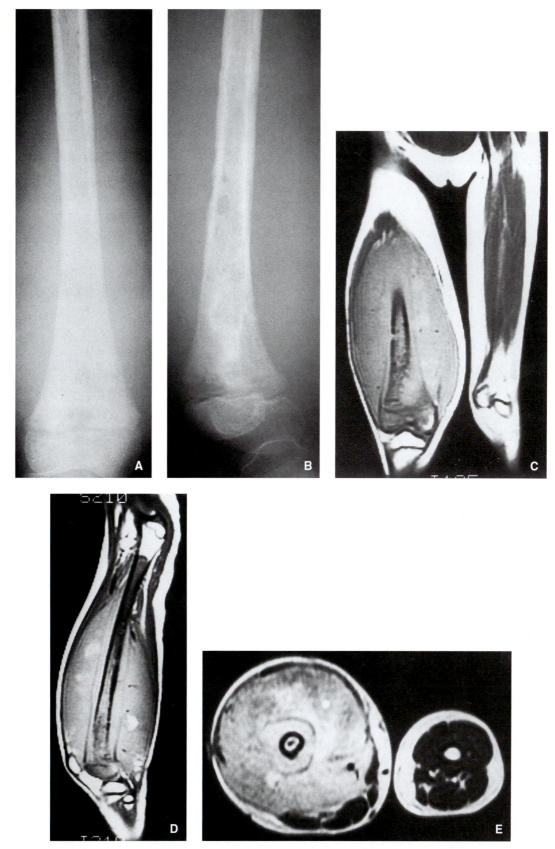

FIGURE 5.21 Radiography and magnetic resonance imaging of Ewing sarcoma. Anteroposterior **(A)** and lateral **(B)** radiographs of the right distal femur of a 7-year-old girl show a lesion in the metaphysis and diaphysis exhibiting a permeative type of bone destruction, associated with a large soft-tissue mass. Coronal **(C)** and sagittal **(D)** T1-weighted MR images demonstrate the intraosseous and extraosseous extent of the tumor. **(E)** Axial T2-weighted MRI shows heterogeneous but mostly high signal intensity of the soft-tissue mass.

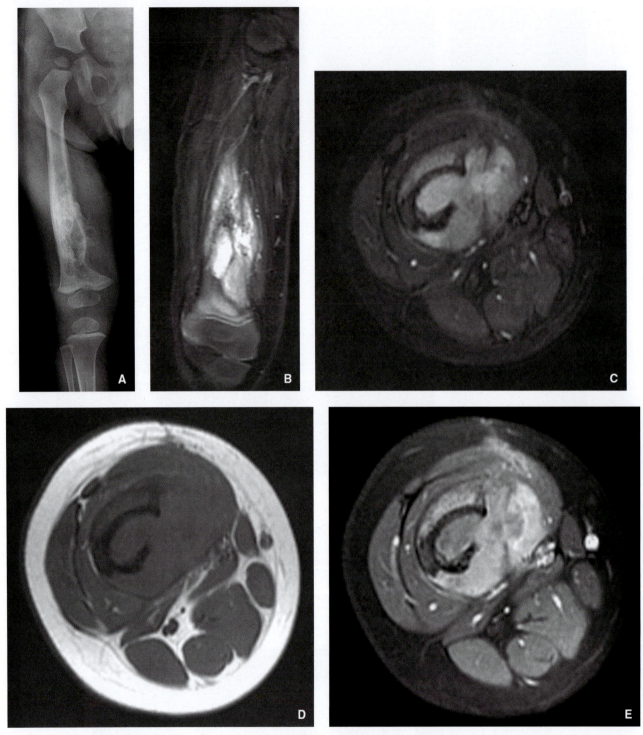

FIGURE 5.22 Radiography and magnetic resonance imaging of Ewing sarcoma. (A) Anteroposterior radiograph of the right femur of a 2-year-old boy shows a destructive lesion of the distal diaphysis with periosteal reaction and a soft-tissue mass. **(B)** Coronal and **(C)** axial STIR MR images show the tumor to exhibit heterogenous, but predominantly high signal intensity. **(D)** Axial T1-weighted and **(E)** T1-weighted fat-suppressed MR image obtained after intravenous administration of gadolinium show significant enhancement of both intramedullary tumor and soft-tissue mass.

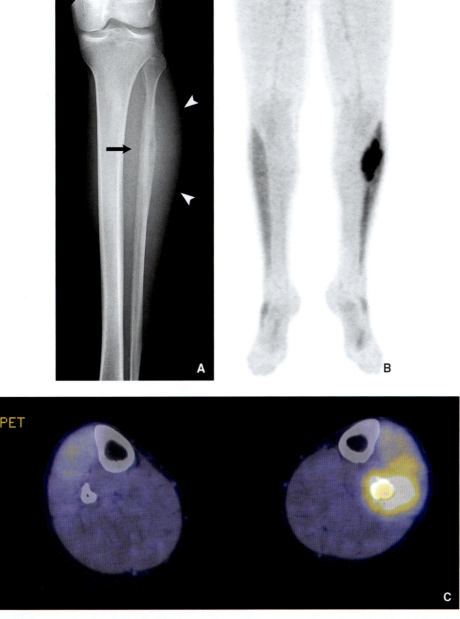

FIGURE 5.23 Radiography, PET, and PET-CT of Ewing sarcoma. (A) Anteroposterior radiograph of the left leg of a 23-year-old man shows a slightly expansive lesion in the proximal fibula (*arrow*) associated with a soft-tissue mass (*arrowheads*). **(B)** 18FDG PET scan of the lower extremities and **(C)** fused PET-CT image show a hypermetabolic focus corresponding to the site of the tumor.

Genetics:
- Recurrent chromosomal translocations involving chromosomes 11 and 22:
  [t(11,22) (q24;q12)]—85% (expression of chimeric *EWS/FLI-1* protein).
  [t(21;22) (q22;q12)]—10% to 15%.
  [t(7;22), t(17;22), t(2;22)]—1%.

Prognosis:
- Has improved with adjuvant therapy.
- Important prognostic features include the stage, anatomic location, and the size of the tumor.
- Patients with tumors that are already metastatic at the time of the diagnosis, particularly if they are large and arising in the pelvic bones, tend to do poorly.

Differential Diagnosis:
- ***Osteosarcoma***
  Although this tumor may appear similar to Ewing sarcoma, imaging studies shows more often metaphyseal rather than diaphyseal location; Codman triangle and sunburst type of periosteal reaction is more common than is onionskin; sclerotic changes (tumor bone) predominate in conventional tumors.

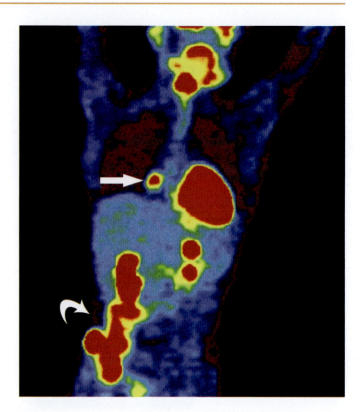

FIGURE 5.24 PET of Ewing sarcoma. Whole-body 18FDG PET scan of a 9-year-old girl shows hypermetabolic tumor in the right ilium (*curved arrow*) and a metastatic nodule in right lung (*arrow*). (Courtesy of Frieda Feldman M.D. and Ronald van Heertum, M.D., New York.)

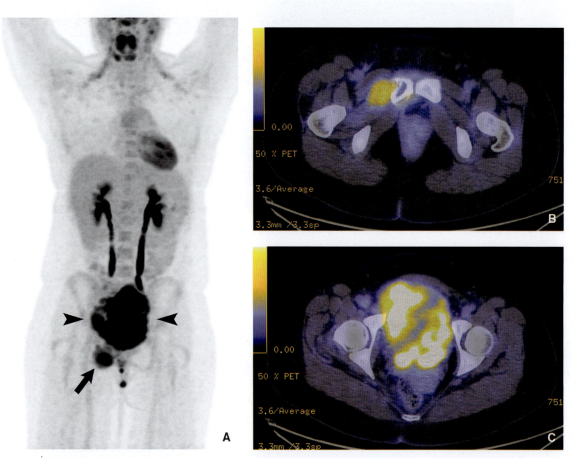

FIGURE 5.25 PET, PET-CT, and MRI of Ewing sarcoma. (A) Total body 18FDG PET scan of a 19-year-old woman shows small extrapelvic (*arrow*) and large intrapelvic (*arrowheads*) hypermetabolic foci. **(B)** Fused PET-CT image shows destructive lesion in the right pubic bone and extrapelvic mass. **(C)** Fused PET-CT image obtained more proximally demonstrates a large intrapelvic mass.

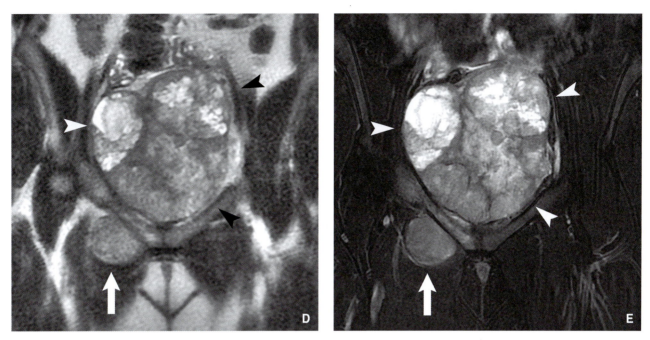

FIGURE 5.25 *(Continued).* Coronal T1-weighted **(D)** and T2-weighted **(E)** MR images demonstrate the tumor within the right pubic bone, and the full extent of the extrapelvic (*arrow*) and intrapelvic (*arrowheads*) soft tissue involvement.

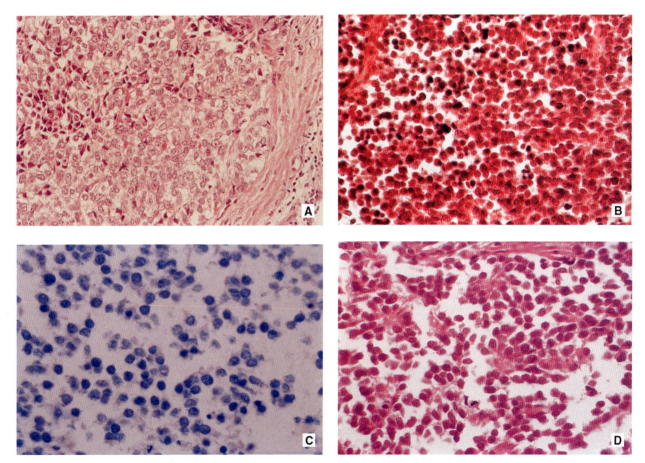

FIGURE 5.26 Histopathology of Ewing sarcoma. (A) Densly packed small cells with round nuclei and indistinct cell borders are characteristic for this tumor. A prominent septum composed of a fibrous connective tissue is also visible (*right*) (H&E, original magnification ×50). **(B)** At higher magnification the uniform aspect of the round nuclei without clear cytoplasmic outline is striking (H&E, original magnification ×100). **(C)** With Giemsa staining, the cytoplasm is more distinct. The nuclei are homogenously darkly stained (Giemsa, original magnification ×100). **(D)** With alcohol fixation, the details of the cells are better preserved (H&E, original magnification ×100).

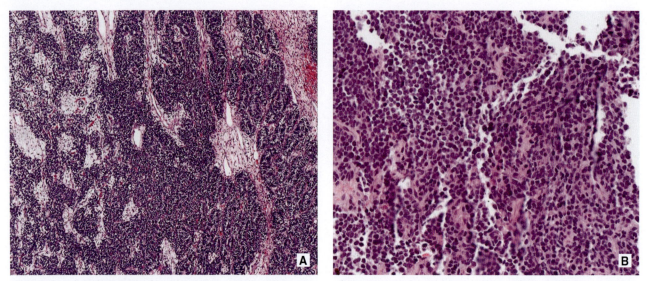

FIGURE 5.27 Histopathology of Ewing sarcoma. (A) Prominent septa composed of fibrous connective tissue divide the tumor consisting of the small round cells with darkly stained nuclei into the lobules (H&E, original magnification ×100). **(B)** Uniform aspect of small round cells containing round nuclei, scanty clear or eosinophilic cytoplasm, and indistinct cytoplasmic outlines are typical for this tumor (H&E, original magnification ×200).

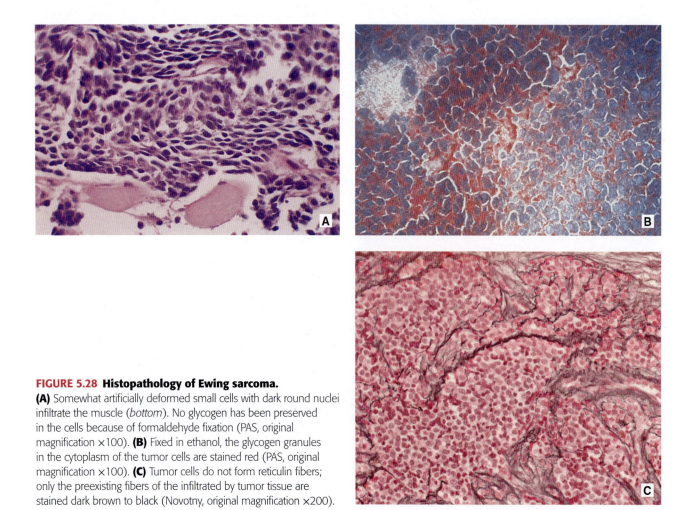

FIGURE 5.28 Histopathology of Ewing sarcoma.
(A) Somewhat artificially deformed small cells with dark round nuclei infiltrate the muscle (*bottom*). No glycogen has been preserved in the cells because of formaldehyde fixation (PAS, original magnification ×100). **(B)** Fixed in ethanol, the glycogen granules in the cytoplasm of the tumor cells are stained red (PAS, original magnification ×100). **(C)** Tumor cells do not form reticulin fibers; only the preexisting fibers of the infiltrated by tumor tissue are stained dark brown to black (Novotny, original magnification ×200).

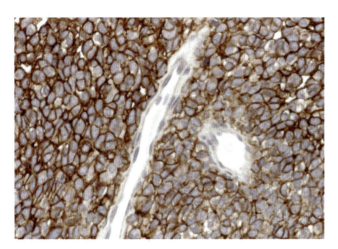

FIGURE 5.29 Histopathology of Ewing sarcoma. Immunohistochemistry shows positive reaction of the tumor cells with CD99, however, the endothelial cells (*center*) do not react (biotin–streptavidin peroxidase, original magnification ×400).

Histopathology showing malignant cells forming tumor osteoid or tumor bone is diagnostic.

- ***Osteomyelitis***

Imaging features of the soft-tissue mass, which is diffuse with ill-defined borders as opposed to one in Ewing sarcoma, which is more circumscribed, are characteristic.

Histopathology showing typical inflammatory and infectious features as described in the previous text is diagnostic.

- ***Langerhans cell histiocytosis***

Imaging features of the solitary lesion may be very similar to those of Ewing sarcoma; however, the soft-tissue mass is usually smaller; slanting or beveling of the edges of the lesion and "hole-in-hole" appearance are characteristic.

Histopathology showing typical Langerhans cells, and EM identification of Birbeck granules is diagnostic.

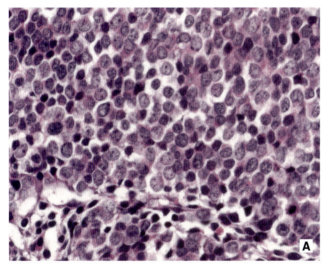

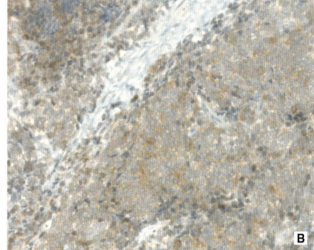

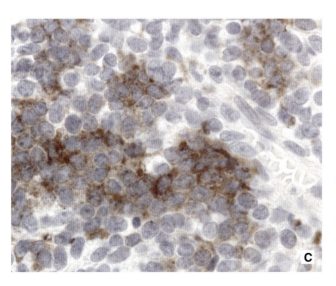

FIGURE 5.30 Histopathology of PNET. (A) The malignant cells and their nuclei are identical to those of Ewing sarcoma (H&E, original magnification ×400). **(B)** Almost all tumor cells are positive for neuron-specific enolase (NSE) (biotin–streptavidin peroxidase, original magnification ×200). **(C)** Some cells of the tumor also exhibit a positive reaction for synaptophysin (biotin–streptavidin peroxidase, original magnification ×400).

Malignant Lymphoma of Bone

Definition:
- Malignant lymphoma is a neoplasm composed of malignant lymphoid cells in various stages of maturation, affecting bones and extraosseous structures, including lymph nodes and visceral organs. It is subdivided into non-Hodgkin lymphoma and Hodgkin lymphoma.

Epidemiology:
- Primary lymphoma of bones is not common, accounting for approximately 7% of all bone malignancies and 5% of extranodal involvement.
- Lymphoma usually affects the patients between the second and seventh decades, with peak incidence between the ages 35 and 45 years.
- Occasionally, young children may be affected, causing difficulty in diagnostic differentiation from Ewing sarcoma.

Sites of Involvement:
- Affects portion of the bone with persistent bone marrow.
- The femur is the most commonly involved single site.
- The tibia, pelvic bones, and the spine are the other common sites of involvement.

Clinical Features:
- Majority of patients present with bone pain.
- Some patients may present with palpable mass.
- Patients with primary lymphoma of bone rarely present with systemic symptoms like fever or night sweats.
- Some patients may be asymptomatic; disproportion between overall good clinical condition and extensive local disease is a helpful feature in differential diagnosis.
- Lymphoma involving bone may be separated into four groups:
  1. A single skeletal site, with or without regional lymph node involvement.
  2. Multiple bones are involved, but there is no visceral or lymph node involvement.
  3. Patients present with a bone involvement, but workup shows affliction of lymph nodes and other visceral sites.
  4. Patients with known lymphoma and consecutive positive bone biopsy.
  5. Patients belonging to groups 1 and 2 are considered to have primary lymphoma of bone.

Imaging:
- Shaft of the long bones is primarily affected.
- Tumor tends to involve a large portion of bone; it is not unusual to see destruction of more than half of the bone.
- The type of bone destruction may be geographic, moth-eaten, or permeative (Fig. 5.31).
- The lesion is poorly demarcated with a wide zone of transition.
- There may be variable degree of sclerosis; rarely, the tumor is entirely sclerotic (Figs. 5.32 and 5.33) or entirely lytic (see Fig. 5.31A); most of the time, there is mixture of sclerotic and lytic areas (see Fig. 5.31C,D).
- Cortex is frequently destroyed, and there may be soft-tissue mass present.
- If the cortex is not involved, the marrow destruction may not be obvious on radiography.
- Radionuclide bone scan is almost always positive (see Fig. 5.36B).
- Computed tomography and magnetic resonance imaging are more sensitive than radiography to demonstrate the full intramedullary involvement and the presence of a soft-tissue mass (Figs. 5.34 to 5.37).
- FDG-PET and PET-CT demonstrate hypermetabolic activity (see Fig. 5.37D,E).

Pathology:
Gross:
- Large portion of bone is involved with cortical destruction.
- The lesion is soft fish-fleshy in appearance with occasional areas of necrosis.

Histopathology:
- Diffuse growth pattern of aggregates of malignant rounded or ovoid large lymphoid cells within the marrow spaces inducing resorption of bone trabeculae (Fig. 5.38).
- Mixture of the small lymphocytic cells and a larger histiocytic cells.
- Depending on the type of lymphoma, the infiltrate may be monomorphic or polymorphic.
- Nuclei are large, contain relatively scanty chromatin, sometimes indented (cleaved) or horseshoe shaped with prominent nucleoli (Figs. 5.39 and 5.40).
- Reticulin fibers are usually present forming a uniformly distributed net around the tumor cells (Fig. 5.41).
- Basophilic cytoplasm with well-defined outlines (see Fig. 5.40A,B).
- Fibroblastic component often prominent, sometimes associated with spindling of the lymphoid cells.
- Crush artifacts on bone biopsy specimens are characteristic.
- The histopathologic findings of Hodgkin lymphoma consist of mixed-cell pattern including lymphocytes, neutrophilic granulocytes, histiocytes, and plasma cells (Fig. 5.42).
- Characteristic features of Hodgkin lymphoma are Reed-Sternberg cells (Fig. 5.43).

Immunohistochemistry:
- Positivity for CD45 or CD20 and CD3 (B-cell and T-cell markers) (see Fig. 5.40C).
- Hodgkin and Reed-Sternberg cells are positive for CD15 and CD30 (see Fig. 5.43C).

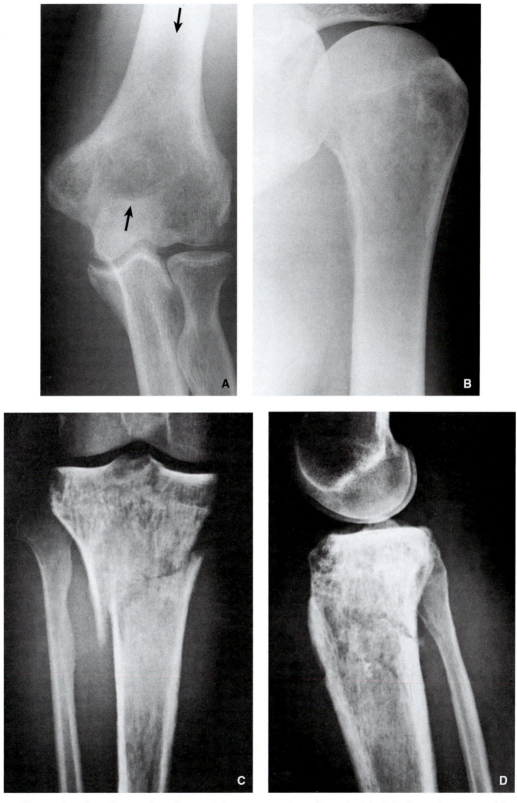

FIGURE 5.31 Radiography of malignant lymphoma. (A) Anteroposterior radiograph of the left elbow of a 42-year-old man shows a large lytic lesion in the distal humerus (*arrows*). **(B)** Anteroposterior radiograph of the left shoulder of a 30-year-old man shows a permeative pattern of bone destruction in the proximal humerus accompanied by a lamellated periosteal reaction. Antroposterior **(C)** and lateral **(D)** radiographs of the right knee of a 47-year-old woman show a mixed sclerotic and lytic lesion of the proximal tibia, associated with a pathologic fracture.

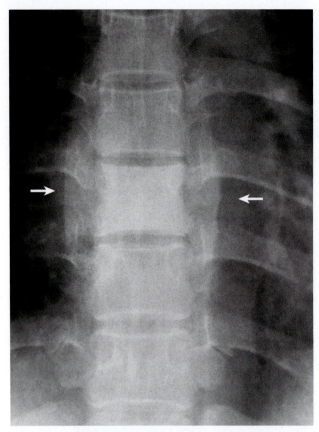

FIGURE 5.32 Radiography of malignant lymphoma. Anteroposterior radiograph of the lower thoracic spine of a 32-year-old man shows sclerotic T7 vertebra. Observe bulging of the paraspinal line (*arrows*).

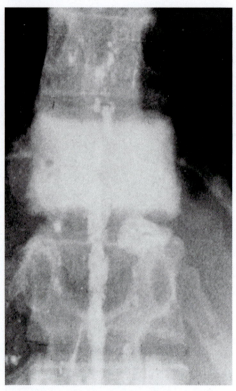

FIGURE 5.33 Radiography of Hodgkin lymphoma. Anteroposterior radiograph of the lower lumbar spine of a 35-year-old man shows sclerotic T10 vertebra ("ivory vertebra"). (From Bullough PG. *Atlas of Orthopedic Pathology*. 2nd ed. New York: Gower; 1992, p. 17.16, reprinted from Greenspan A, Jundt G, Remagen W. *Differential Diagnosis in Orthopaedic Oncology*. 2nd ed. p. 343, Fig. 5-38).

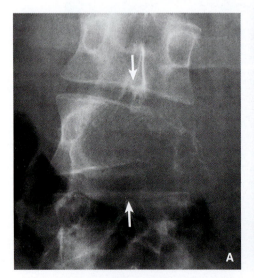
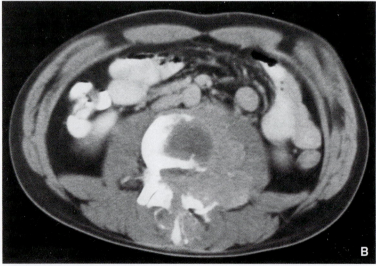

FIGURE 5.34 Radiography and computed tomography of malignant lymphoma. (A) Anteroposterior radiograph of the upper lumbar spine of a 45-year-old man shows a destructive lesion of the L3 vertebra (*arrows*). **(B)** Axial computed tomography section shows the full extent of the lesion in the bone and a large soft-tissue mass.

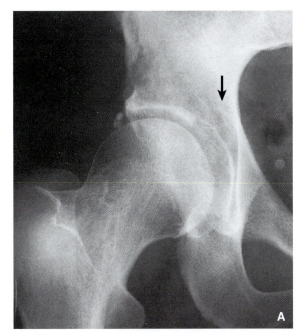
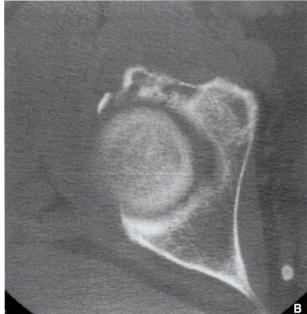
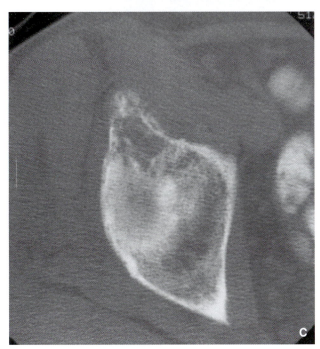

FIGURE 5.35 Radiography and computed tomography of malignant lymphoma. (A) Anteroposterior radiograph of the right hip of a 36-year-old man shows a very subtle osteolytic lesion of the acetabulum (*arrow*). **(B, C)** Two CT sections demonstrate more clearly the involvement of the anterior column and the roof of the acetabulum.

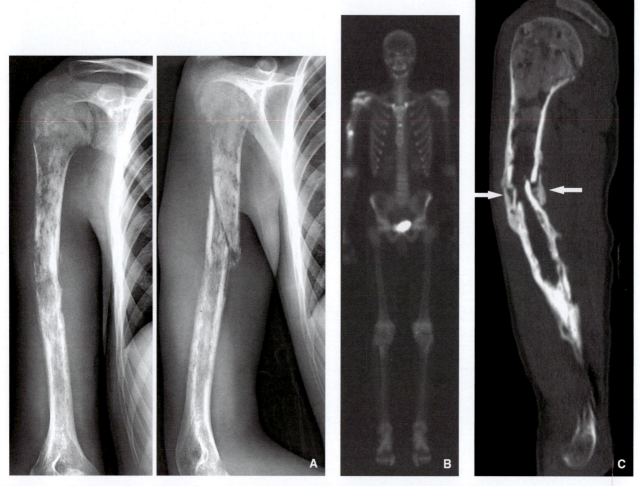

FIGURE 5.36 Radiography, scintigraphy, and computed tomography of malignant lymphoma. (A) Anteroposterior and oblique radiographs of the right humerus of a 20-year-old man show a long lesion exhibiting permeative and moth-eaten type of bone destruction. Periosteal reaction is secondary to a healing pathologic fracture. **(B)** Total body radionuclide bone scan shows increased uptake of radiopharmaceutical tracer at the site of the lesion, with most significant accumulation at the level of a pathologic fracture. **(C)** Sagittal reformatted CT image demonstrates endosteal scalloping and early callus formation at the site of a pathologic fracture (*arrows*).

Prognosis:

- Prognosis of lymphoma depends upon cell type and stage of disease.
- Patients older than 60 years have a worse overall survival and a worse progression-free period.
- Patients with immunoblastic subtype have a worse survival than those with the centroblastic mono/polymorphic subtype or the centroblastic multilobulated subtype.

Differential Diagnosis:

- **Osteosarcoma**

  Occurs in younger age group than lymphoma; the lesion is more commonly metaphyseal rather than diaphyseal; periosteal reaction in form of sunburst or Codman triangle; soft-tissue mass shows fluffy areas of tumor bone formation.

  Histopathology showing malignant cells forming tumor osteoid or tumor bone is diagnostic.

- **Ewing sarcoma**

  Occurs in younger age group than lymphoma; lamellated (onionskin) periosteal reaction more commonly present; often soft-tissue mass is disproportionally larger than the bone lesion.

  Histopathology showing uniform small round cells with scanty eosinophilic cytoplasm and indistinct cytoplasmatic membranes coupled with PAS-positive glycogen is diagnostic.

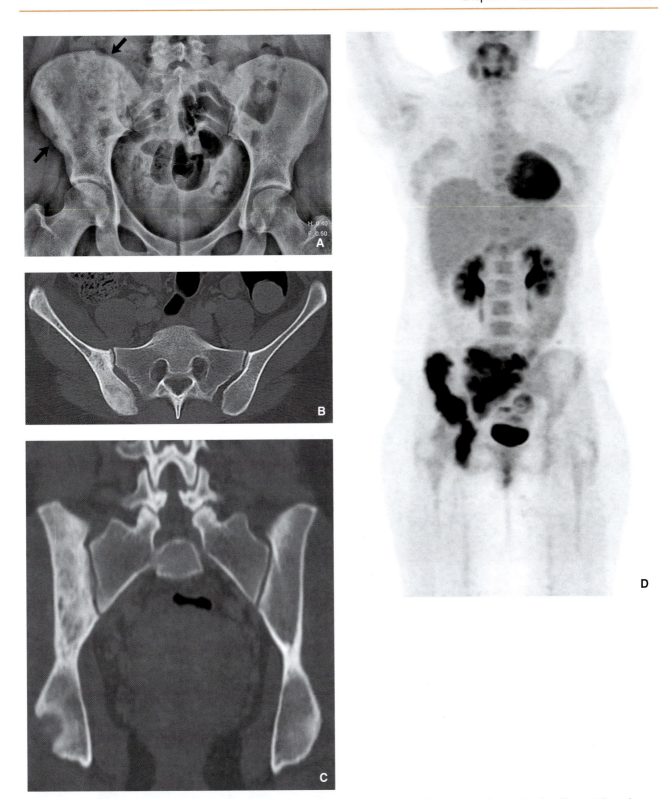

FIGURE 5.37 Radiography, computed tomography, magnetic resonance imaging, PET, and PET-CT of malignant lymphoma.
(A) Anteroposterior radiograph of the pelvis of a 19-year-old woman shows sclerosis of the right ilium (*arrows*). **(B)** Direct axial and **(C)** coronal reformatted CT images confirm diffuse involvement of the ilium. **(D)** Total body PET scan shows hypermetabolic tumor involving the right ilium, right ischium, and right-sided sacrum.

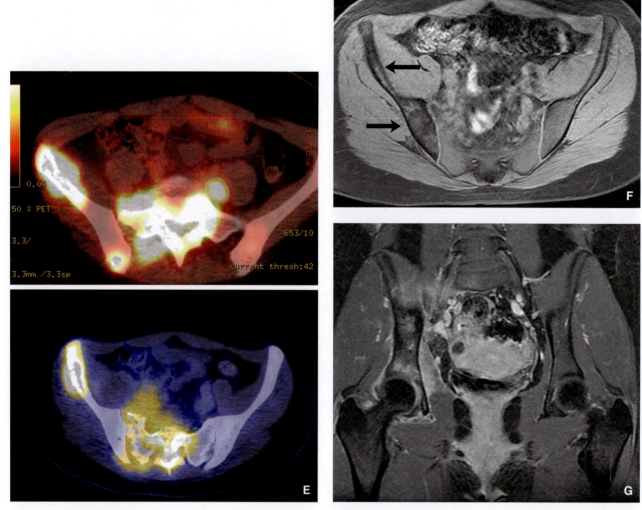

FIGURE 5.37 *(Continued).* **(E)** Two axial fused FDG PET-CT images confirm the location of the tumor in the ilium, ischium, and sacrum. **(F)** Axial T1-weighted MR image shows the tumor to be of intermediate-to-low signal intensity (*arrows*). **(G)** Coronal T1-weighted fat-suppressed MRI obtained after intravenous injection of gadolinium demonstrates heterogenous enhancement of the tumor.

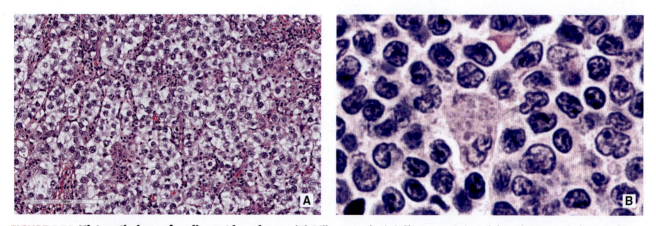

FIGURE 5.38 Histopathology of malignant lymphoma. (A) Diffuse neoplastic infiltrate consisting of densely arranged pleomorphic lymphoma cells (H&E, original magnification ×100). **(B)** Pleomorphic round cells with large nuclei and well-demarcated cytoplasmic outline are characteristic for large B-cell lymphoma. In the center observe the focal necrosis (H&E, original magnification ×600).

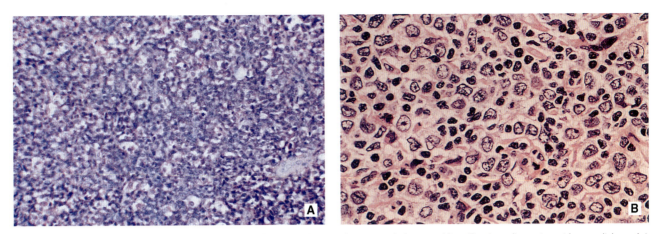

FIGURE 5.39 Histopathology of malignant lymphoma. (A) Densely arranged pleomorphic cells of medium size with roundish nuclei are present, some exhibiting a clear cytoplasm. The cells are larger and more pleomorphic than those of Ewing sarcoma (Giemsa, original magnification ×50). **(B)** At high magnification, the mixed cell population and the cleaved nuclei with prominent nucleoli are conspicuous (H&E, original magnification ×500). (From Bullough PG. *Atlas of Orthopedic Pathology*. 2nd ed. New York: Gower; 1992:17.15.)

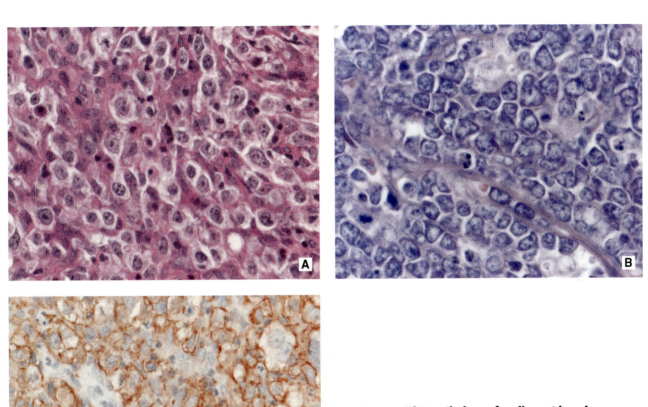

FIGURE 5.40 Histopathology of malignant lymphoma. (A) In diffuse large B-cell lymphoma, observe round cells with well-defined cytoplasmic outline and large nuclei with one to three nucleoli (H&E, original magnification ×400). **(B)** With Giemsa staining, the basophilic darkly staining cytoplasm of the tumor cells and nuclear details are better delineated. Cleaved nuclei, nuclear polymorphism, and prominent nucleoli distinguish this tumor from Ewing sarcoma (Giemsa, original magnification ×630). **(C)** The tumor cells react with the B-cell marker CD20 (biotin–streptavidin peroxidase, original magnification ×400).

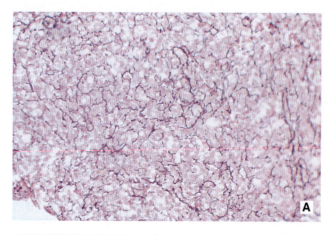
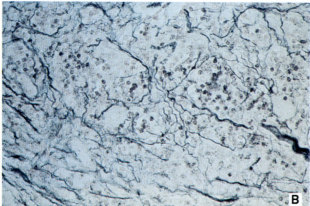

FIGURE 5.41 Histopathology of malignant lymphoma.
(A) With reticulin fiber staining, a fine black-appearing net surrounding the individual cells is clearly discernable (Novotny, original magnification ×50). **(B)** At higher magnification, abundant reticulin fibers form a dense network surrounding individual and small group of cells (Gomori silver stain, original magnification ×100).

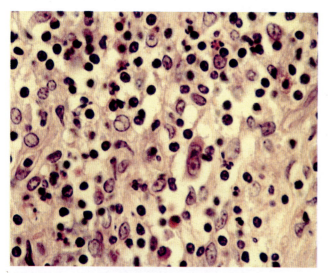

FIGURE 5.42 Histopathology of Hodgkin lymphoma.
Fibrous stroma with mixed cellular infiltrate of small round cells and large histiocytes is characteristic for this tumor (H&E, original magnification ×400). (From Bullough PG. *Atlas of Orthopedic Pathology*. 2nd ed. p. 17.16, Fig. 17.45).

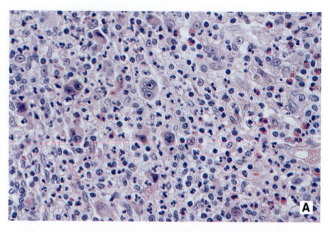
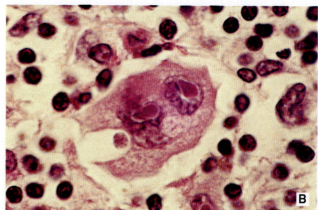
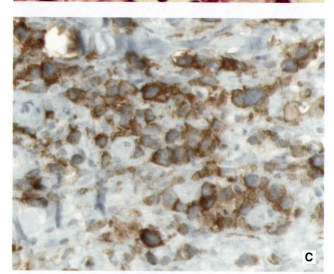

FIGURE 5.43 Histopathology of Hodgkin lymphoma.
(A) Pleomorphic round cells are seen together with scattered Reed-Sternberg cells (H&E, original magnification ×400). **(B)** High-power photomicrograph shows a binucleate Reed-Sternberg cell with prominent eosinophilic nucleoli (H&E, original magnification ×1,000). **(C)** Immunohistochemically, both Hodgkin and Reed-Sternberg cells are positive for CD30 (biotin–streptavidin peroxidase, original magnification ×400). (A and B: From Bullough PG. *Atlas of Orthopedic Pathology*. 2nd ed. New York: Gower; 1992:17.16.)

- *Paget disease*
  Occurs in much older age group than lymphoma; articular end of bones invariably affected; coarse trabecular pattern of cancellous bone is characteristic.
  Histopathology showing pathognomonic mosaic pattern of cement lines is diagnostic.
- *Metastasis*
  Imaging appearance of solitary metastatic lesion may be very similar to lymphoma; periosteal reaction and soft-tissue mass, however, are less common.
  Histopathology occasionally showing the origin of metastatic lesion, and immunohistochemistry studies (particularly application of cytokeratins) is diagnostic.

Multiple Myeloma (Plasma Cell Myeloma, Plasmacytoma)

Definition:
- Usually multicentric tumor that originates in the bone marrow, consisting of monoclonal neoplastic proliferation of plasma cells, and characterized by osteolytic lesions, bone pain, hypercalcemia, a monoclonal gammopathy, and deposition of abnormal immunoglobulin chains (amyloid) in different organs.

Epidemiology:
- Most common primary malignant tumor of the bone.
- Accounts for 27% of biopsied bone tumors.
- Most common in the sixth and seventh decades of life, with median age of 68 in males and 70 in females.
- Rare in patients younger than 40 years (<10%).

Sites of Involvement:
- Most commonly affects the skull, mandible, vertebrae, ribs, pelvic bones, femur, clavicle, and scapula.

Clinical Features:
- Bone pain, malaise, fatigue, weight loss, fever, hypercalcemia, and anemia.
- Anemia is a consequence of bone marrow destruction and renal damage with loss of erythropoietin.
- Renal failure is the result of tubular lesions (Bence Jones proteinuria with formation of tubular cast) due to monoclonal light chain proteinuria, hypercalcemia, and occasional amyloidosis.
- Patients may show recurrent bacterial infections due to decreased production of normal immunoglobulin, which is replaced with neoplastic clone.
- A pathologic fracture may be the first symptom.
- If lumbar or thoracic regions of the spine are affected, neurologic symptoms prevail.
- M-component of monoclonal immunoglobulin can be found in the serum or urine in 99% of the patients.
- Ratio of serum albumins to globulins is reversed because of the high concentration of monoclonal immunoglobulin produced by the myeloma cells (IgG, 65%; IgA, 20%; IgD, 2%; IgM and IgE, <1%).
- Biclonal gammopathies are found in 1% of cases and monoclonal light chain (Bence Jones protein) is found in the serum in 75% of the cases.
- Diagnostic criteria of symptomatic plasma cell myeloma:
  - M protein in serum or urine.
  - Bone marrow contains clonal plasma cells.
  - Related organ or tissue impairment.
- Diagnostic criteria of asymptomatis (smoldering) myeloma:
  - M-protein in serum at myeloma levels (>30 g/dL).
  - 10% or more clonal plasma cells in the bone marrow.
  - No related organ or tissue impairment (end-organ damage or bone lesions) or myeloma-related symptoms.

POEMS syndrome: polyneuropathy, organomegaly (liver, spleen), endocrine disturbances (amenorrhea, gynecomastia, impotence, diabetes mellitus, hypothyroidism), monoclonal gammopathy (lambda light chains), and skin changes (hyperpigmentation, hirsutism).

Imaging:
- Radiography shows variety of patterns, depending upon site of involvement and type of the lesion (Fig. 5.44); most characteristic are "punched-out" lesions (Fig. 5.45) and endosteal scalloping (Fig. 5.46); sclerotic lesions are present in <1% of patients.
- Scintigraphy shows either very minimal or lack of uptake of the radiopharmaceutical tracer.
- Computed tomography shows low-attenuated lesions and endosteal scalloping (Fig. 5.47).
- Magnetic resonance imaging shows lesions to be of intermediate signal intensity on T1 weighting and of homogenously high signal on T2-weighted and other water-sensitive sequences (Fig. 5.48).

Pathology:
Gross (Macroscopy):
- Grayish-pink soft friable mass.
- Bone may be diffusely involved or in form of discrete nodules.
- Common expansion of the affected bone with extraosseous extension.
- Some tumor masses may have a gray, waxy appearance due to extensive amyloid deposition.

Histopathology:
- Round or oval plasma cells show a spectrum of variable features of cellular maturity (Fig. 5.49).
- Well-differentiated tumors exhibit sheets of closely packed cells, which resemble normal plasma cells with eccentric nuclei, clustered chromatin with cartwheel pattern, and prominent nucleoli; the cytoplasm is basophilic, abundant, and dense and shows distinct outlines; there is little intercellular matrix (Fig. 5.50).
- Mitotic figures are rare.

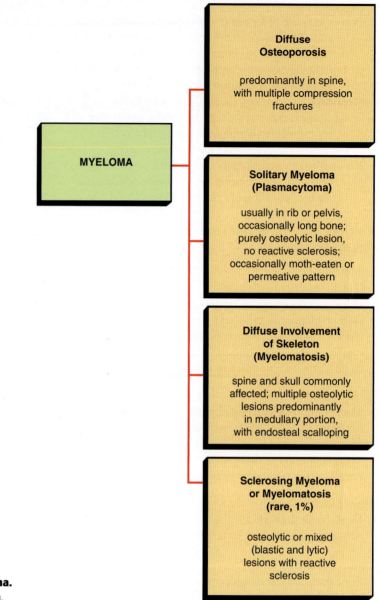

FIGURE 5.44 Radiography of multiple myeloma.
Variants of the radiographic presentation of myeloma.

- The tumor cells may accumulate immune globulins in cytoplasm and show morular appearance or "Mott cells"; extracellular globules of polymerized globules called Russell bodies may be seen.
- Less-differentiated tumors show cells with nuclei exhibiting less clumping chromatin, enlarged nucleoli, and indistinct cytoplasmic membrane.
- Poorly differentiated tumors show atypical cells, with occasional double nuclei, brisk mitotic activity, and atypical mitotic figures (Fig. 5.51).

Immunohistochemistry:
- Positive for CD138 (see Fig. 5.50D), CD38, and MUM1 (multiple myeloma oncogene 1).
- Characteristic feature is expression of monotypic cytoplasmic Ig and lack of surface Ig.
- Monotypic expression of kappa or lambda immunoglobulin by the tumor cells establishes the diagnosis of malignancy (see Fig. 5.50B).
- Frequently expresses the natural killer antigen CD56/58 and CD117, which are not expressed in normal reactive plasma cells.
- Majority of myelomas lack the pan-B antigens CD19 and CD20.
- May show positivity for EMA.
- Cyclin D1 protein may be expressed in 35% to 40% of cases and is associated with translocations t(11;14)(q13;32).

Genetics:
- Gains of chromosomes 1q, 3q, 9q, 11q, and 15q.
- Losses of chromosome 13 at 13q14 observed in 60% of cases.
- Deletion of gene *TP53* at 17q13 reported in 25% of cases. (related to poor outcome).

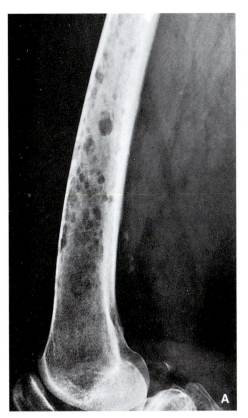
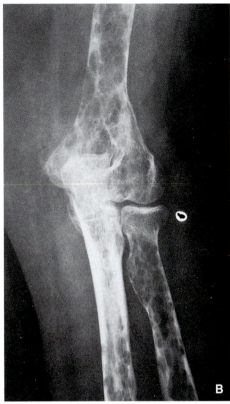

FIGURE 5.45 Radiography of multiple myeloma. (A) Lateral radiograph of the distal femur of a 65-year-old woman shows multiple "punched-out" lytic lesions. **(B)** Anteroposterior radiograph of the left elbow of the same patient demonstrates several lytic lesions in the distal humerus, proximal radius, and proximal ulna exhibiting endosteal cortical scalloping.

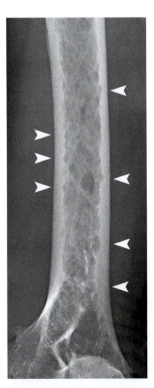

FIGURE 5.46 Radiography of multiple myeloma. Magnified radiograph of the distal humerus of a 72-year-old man shows characteristic for this malignancy endosteal scalloping (*arrowheads*).

- Translocations t(11;14)(q13;q32).
- Translocations targeting Ig heavy chain locus (IgH), which targets several different well-characterized partner genes mainly in chromosome bands 4p16.3 (FGFR3/MMSET), 6p21(CCND3), 11q13 (CCND1), 16q23 (MAF), and 20q11 (MAFB).

Prognostic Factors:
- Multiple myeloma is generally an incurable disease (median survival 3 years; 10% survival at 10 years).
- Renal insufficiency, higher stage and degree of marrow replacement by tumor cells, increased proliferative activity, and certain karyotypic abnormalities are associated with shorter survival time.
- Translocations t(4;14) and t(14;16) and deletion 17q13 (*TP53*) are associated with poorer prognosis.

Differential Diagnosis:
Plasmacytoma:

- **Osteolytic metastasis**
  Imaging appearance may be similar to solitary plasmacytoma; however, scintigraphy shows increased uptake of the radiopharmaceutical tracer.
  Histopathology, particularly immunohistochemistry studies are diagnostic.

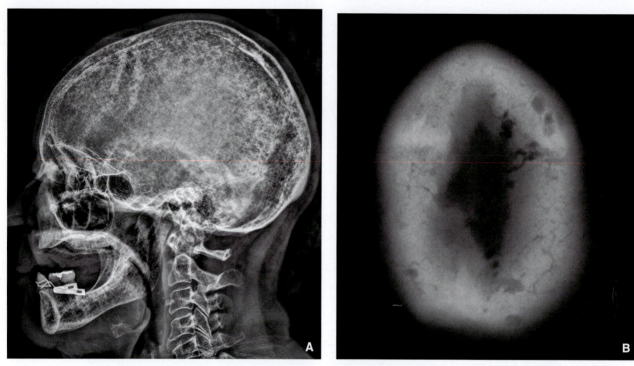

FIGURE 5.47 Radiography and computed tomography of multiple myeloma. (A) Lateral radiograph of the skull of a 76-year-old woman shows extensive involvement of the calvaria. Observe also "punched-out" lesions in the mandible, not an unusual site of involvement. **(B)** Computed tomography section of the skull shows "punched-out" low-attenuated lesions in the occiput.

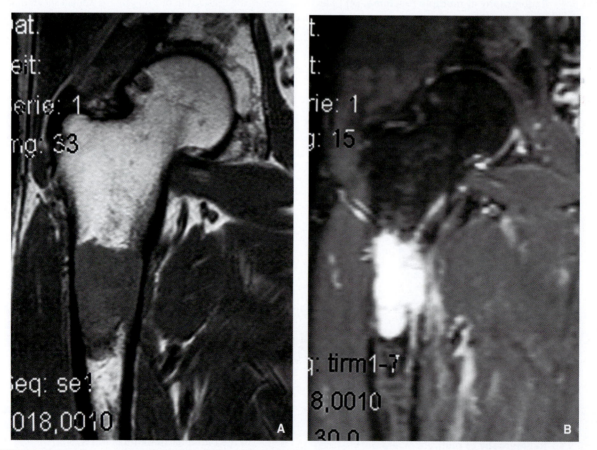

FIGURE 5.48 Magnetic resonance imaging of plasmacytoma. (A) Coronal T1-weighted MR image of the right hip of a 53-year-old man shows a lesion in the proximal femur exhibiting intermediate signal intensity isointense with the skeletal muscles. **(B)** Coronal T2-weighted MRI shows the tumor to be of homogeneous high signal intensity.

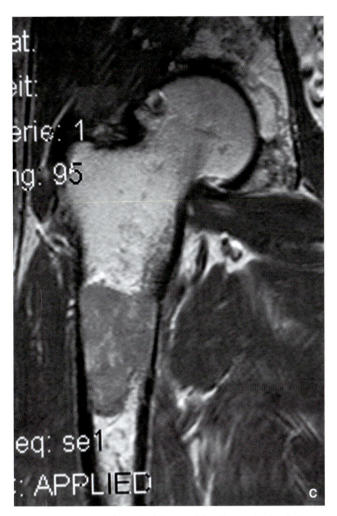

FIGURE 5.48 *(Continued).* **(C)** T1-weighted MRI obtained after intravenous administration of gadolinium shows slight enhancement of the tumor.

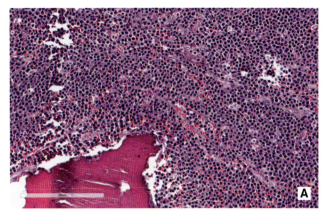

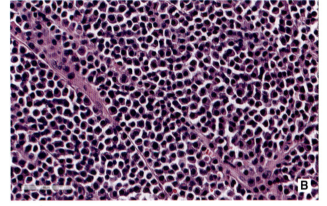

FIGURE 5.49 **Histopathology of multiple myeloma.**
(A) Well-differentiated mature-looking plasma cells are characteristic for low-grade malignancy (H&E, original magnification ×100).
(B) High magnification shows tumor cells with eccentric round nuclei, dense chromatin, and abundant cytoplasm (H&E, original magnification ×400).

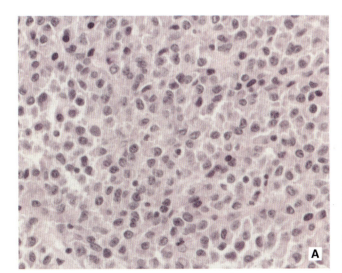

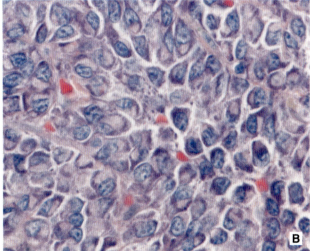

FIGURE 5.50 **Histopathology of multiple myeloma. (A)** In grade 2 malignancy the tumor cells exhibit plasma cell–like features with eccentric nuclei and enlarge eosinophilic cytoplasm with juxtanuclear halo. Few cells exhibit a "spoke-wheel" chromatine pattern. Most tumor cells contain clearer and larger, slightly pleomorphic nuclei with eosinophilic nucleoli (H&E, original magnification ×400). **(B)** In Giemsa-stained preparation basophilic cytoplasm and perinuclear halos are better demonstrated (Giemsa, original magnification ×630).

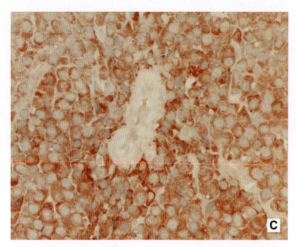 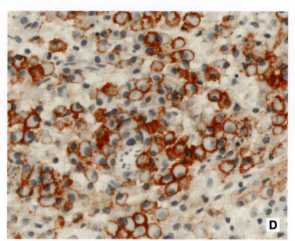

FIGURE 5.50 *(Continued).* **(C)** Immunohistochemistry shows tumor cells exhibiting a monoclonal expression of lambda light chains (biotin–streptavidin peroxidase, original magnification ×400). **(D)** The collagen type I–binding protein syndecan-1 (CD1 38) is typically present in myeloma cells (biotin–streptavidin peroxidase, original magnification ×400).

- *Fibrosarcoma*
  Imaging appearance may be similar to solitary plasmacytoma; however, scintigraphy shows increased uptake of the radiopharmaceutical tracer.
  Histopathology showing fascicles of spindle cells exhibiting characteristic "herringbone tweed" pattern is diagnostic.

Multiple Myeloma:

- *Osteolytic metastases*
  Morphology of lytic metastatic lesions may be identical to multiple myeloma on the imaging studies; however, skeletal scintigraphy showing significant uptake of radiopharmaceutical tracer is diagnostic differentiation feature.
  Histopathology may show identifying features of primary carcinoma.

- *Brown tumors of hyperparathyroidism*
  Multiple lytic bone lesions representing brown tumors may look on imaging studies similar to the lesions of multiple myeloma; however, MRI shows often low signal intensity of the brown tumors, reflecting magnetic susceptibility to hemosiderin.
  Histopathology showing clusters of multinucleated giant cells within fibroblastic, and reactive stroma in addition to clumps of hemosiderin pigment is diagnostic.

- *Gaucher disease*
  Imaging studies show reactive periostitis, Erlenmeyer flask deformity, intramedullary bone infarcts, and osteonecrotic changes.
  Histopathology showing infiltration of the bone marrow spaces by large macrophages (Gaucher cells) possessing round to ovoid nuclei and abundant striped cytoplasm that has a characteristic "crumpled tissue paper" appearance is diagnostic.

- *Diffuse osteoporosis*
  Imaging studies show lack of endosteal scalloping.
  Histopathology showing lack of malignant cells is diagnostic.

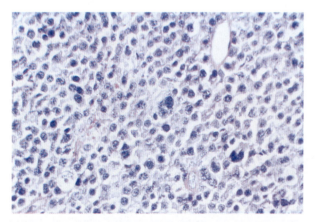

FIGURE 5.51 **Histopathology of multiple myeloma.** In grade 3 malignancy, between the normal-appearing plasma cells (fewer than the number illustrated in Figure 5.49A) are scattered pleomorphic cells with clearer nuclei. Numerous giant cells with two or more nuclei are also present (Giemsa, original magnification ×100).

REFERENCES

Adams HJA, Kwee TC, Vermoolen MA, et al. Whole-body MRI for the detection of bone marrow involvement in lymphoma: prospective study in 116 patients and comparison with FDG-PET. *Eur Radiol.* 2013;23:2271–2278.

Aggarwal S, Goulatia RK, Sood A, et al. POEMS syndrome: a rare variety of plasma cell dyscrasia. *AJR Am J Roentgenol.* 1990;155:339–341.

Algra PR, Bloem JL. Magnetic resonance imaging of metastatic disease and multiple myeloma. In: Bloem JL, Sartoris DJ, eds. *MRI and CT of the Musculoskeletal System.* Baltimore, MD: Williams & Wilkins; 1992:218.

Antonmattei S, Tetalman MR, Lloyd TV. The multiscan appearance of eosinophilic granuloma. *Clin Nucl Med.* 1979;4:53–55.

Arico M, Danesino C. Langerhans's cell histiocytosis: is there a role for genetics? *Haematologica.* 2001;86:1009–1014.

Baraga JJ, Amrani KK, Swee RG, Wold L, Unni KK. Radiographic features of Ewing's sarcoma of the bones of the hands and feet. *Skeletal Radiol.* 2001;30:121–126.

Bardwick PA, Zvaifler NJ, Gill GN, Newman D, Greenway GD, Resnick DL. Plasma-cell dyscrasia with polyneuropathy, organomegaly, endocrinopathy, M-protein and skin changes: the POEMS syndrome. Report on two cases and review of the literature. *Medicine (Baltimore).* 1980;59:311–322.

Bataille R, Chevalier J, Rossi M, Sany J. Bone scintigraphy in plasma-cell myeloma. A prospective study of 70 patients. *Radiology.* 1982;145:801–804.

Baur A, Stäbler A, Lamerz R, Bartl R, Reiser M. Light chain deposition disease in multiple myeloma: MR imaging features correlated with histopathologic findings. *Skeletal Radiol.* 1998;27:173–176.

Beackley MC, Lau BP, King ER. Bone involvement in Hodgkin's disease. *AJR Am J Roentgenol.* 1972;114:559–563.

Beltran J, Aparisi F, Marti Bonmati L, Rosenberg ZS, Present D, Steiner GC. Eosinophilic granuloma: MR manifestations. *Skeletal Radiol.* 1993;22:157–161.

Bertoni F, Bacchini P, Ferruzzi A. Small round-cell malignancies of bone: Ewing's sarcoma, malignant lymphoma, and myeloma. *Semin Orthop.* 1991;6:186–195.

Bessler W, Antonucci F, Stamm B, Stuckmann G, Vollrath T. Case report 646. POEMS syndrome. *Skeletal Radiol.* 1991;20:212–215.

Birbeck MS, Breathnach AS, Everall JD. An electron microscopic study of basal melanocytes and high-level clear cell (Langerhans cell) in vitiligo. *J Invest Dermatol.* 1961;37:51–64.

Bisciegla M, Cammisa M, Suster S, Colby TV. Erdheim-Chester disease: clinical and pathologic spectrum of four cases. *Adv Anat Pathol.* 2003;10:160–171.

Blomery P, Wong SO, Lade S, Prince HM. Erdheim-Chester disease harboring the BRAF V600E mutation. *J Clin Oncol.* 2012;30:e331–e332.

Bohne WHO, Goldman AB, Bullough P. Case report 96. Chester-Erdheim disease (lipogranulomatosis). *Skeletal Radiol.* 1979;4:164–167.

Boston HC Jr, Dahlin DC, Ivins JC, Cupps RE. Malignant lymphoma (so-called reticulum cell sarcoma) of bone. *Cancer.* 1974;34:1131–1137.

Brandon C, Martel W, Weatherbee L, Capek P. Case report 572. Osteosclerotic myeloma (POEMS syndrome). *Skeletal Radiol.* 1989;18:542–546.

Braunstein EM. Hodgkin's disease of bone: radiographic correlation with the histologic classification. *Radiology.* 1980;137:643–646.

Breyer III RJ, Mulligan ME, Smith SE, Line BR, Badros AZ. Comparison of imaging with FDG PET/CT with other imaging modalities in myeloma. *Skeletal Radiol.* 2006;35:632–640.

Brown TS, Paterson CR. Osteosclerosis in myeloma. *J Bone Joint Surg Br.* 1973;55-B:621–623.

Castellino RA. Hodgkin disease: practical concepts for the diagnostic radiologist. *Radiology.* 1986;159:305–310.

Cavazzana AO, Miser JS, Jefferson J, Triche TJ. Experimental evidence for a neural origin of Ewing's sarcoma of bone. *Am J Pathol.* 1987;127:507–518.

Chan K-W, Rosen G, Miller DR, Tan CT. Hodgkin's disease in adolescents presenting as a primary bone lesion. A report of four cases and review of the literature. *Am J Pediatr Hematol Oncol.* 1982;4:11–17.

Chickwava K, Jaffe R. Langerin (CD207) staining in normal pediatric tissues, reactive lymph nodes, and childhood histiocytic disorders. *Pediatr Dev Pathol.* 2004;7:607–614.

Chong ST, Beasley HS, Daffner RH. POEMS syndrome: radiographic appearance with MRI correlation. *Skeletal Radiol.* 2006; 35:690–695.

Coles WC, Schultz MD. Bone involvement in malignant lymphoma. *Radiology.* 1948;50:458–462.

Compere EL, Johnson WE, Coventry MB. Vertebra plana (Calve's disease) due to eosinophilic granuloma. *J Bone Joint Surg.* 1954;36:969–980.

Coombs RJ, Zeiss J, McKann K, Phillips E. Case report 360: multifocal Ewing tumor of the skeletal system. *Skeletal Radiol.* 1986;15:254–257.

da Costa CE, Annels NE, Faaij CM, Forsyth RG, Hogendoorn PC, Egeler RM. Presence of osteoclast-like multinucleated giant cells in the bone and nonostotic lesions of Langerhans cell histiocytosis. *J Exp Med.* 2005;201:687–693.

David R, Oria RA, Kumar R, et al. Radiologic features of eosinophilic granuloma of bone. *AJR Am J Roentgenol.* 1989;153:1021–1026.

de Graaf JH, Tamminga RY, Dam-Meiring A, Kamps WA, Timens W. The presence of cytokines in Langerhans' cell histiocytosis. *J Pathol.* 1996;180:400–406.

De Schepper AM, Ramon F, Van Marck E. MR imaging of eosiniphilic granuloma: report of 11 cases. *Skeletal Radiol.* 1993;22:163–166.

Dehner LP. Primitive neuroectodermal tumor and Ewing's sarcoma. *Am J Surg Pathol.* 1993;17:1–13.

Demicco EG, Rosenberg AE, Bjornsson J, Rybak LD, Unni KK, Nielsen GP. Primary Rosai-Dorfman disease of bone: a clinicopathologic study of 15 cases. *Am J Surg Pathol.* 2010;34:1324–1333.

Egeler RM, Annels NE, Hogendoorn PC. Langerhans cell histiocytosis: a pathologic combination of oncogenesis and immune dysregulation. *Pediatr Blood Cancer.* 2004;42:401–403.

Favara BE. Langerhans cell histiocytosis—pathobiology and pathogenesis. *Semin Oncol.* 1991;18:3–7.

Fisher AJ, Reinus WR, Friedland JA, Wilson AJ. Quantitative analysis of the plain radiographic appearance of eosinophilic granuloma. *Invest Radiol.* 1995;30:466–473.

Fishman EK, Kuhlman JE, Jones RJ. CT of lymphoma: spectrum of disease. *Radiographics.* 1991;11:647–669.

Fletcher CDM, Unni KK, Mertens E, eds. *World Health Organisation Classification of Tumours of Soft Tissue and Bone.* Lyon, France: IARC Press; 2013:281–296.

Fonseca R, Witzig TE, Gertz MA, et al. Multiple myeloma and the translocation t(11;14)(q13;32): a report on 13 cases. *Br J Haematol.* 1998;101:296–301.

Fonseca R, Blood EA, Oken MM, et al. Myeloma and t(11;14)(q13;32) evidence for biologically defined unique subset of patients. *Blood.* 2002;99:3735–3741.

Ford DR, Wilson D, Sothi S, Grimer R, Spooner D. Primary bone lymphoma—treatment and outcome. *Clin Oncol.* 2007;19:50–57.

Garber CZ. Reactive bone formation in Ewing's sarcoma. *Cancer.* 1951;4:839–845.

Gold RH, Mirra JM. Case report 101. Primary Hodgkin disease of humerus. *Skeletal Radiol.* 1979;4:233–235.

Greenspan A, Klein MJ. Radiology and pathology of bone tumors. In: Lewis MM, ed. *Musculoskeletal Oncology. A Multidisciplinary Approach.* Philadelphia: WB Saunders; 1992:13–72.

Grover SB, Dhar A. Imaging spectrum in sclerotic myelomas: an experience in three cases. *Eur Radiol.* 2000;10:1828–1831.

Hall FM, Gore SM. Osteosclerotic myeloma variant. *Skeletal Radiol.* 1988;17:101–105.

Haroche J, Charlotte F, Arnaud L, et al. High prevalence of BRAF V600E mutations in Erdheim-Chester disease but not in other non-Langerhans cell histiocytoses. *Blood.* 2012;120:2700–2703.

Heyning FH, Kroon HMJA, Hogendoorn PCW, Taminiau AH, van der Woude HJ. MR imaging characteristics in primary lymphoma of bone with emphasis on nonaggressive appearance. *Skeletal Radiol.* 2007;36:937–944.

Hillemanns M, McLeod RA, Unni KK. Malignant lymphoma. *Skeletal Radiol.* 1996;25:73–75.

Homann G, Weisel K, Mustafa DF, et al. Improvement of diagnostic confidence for detection of multiple myeloma involvement of the ribs by a new software generating rib unfolded images: Comparison with 5- and 1-mm axial images. *Skeletal Radiol.* 2015;44:971–979.

Hoover KB, Rosenthal DI, Mankin H. Langerhans cell histiocytosis. *Skeletal Radiol.* 2007;36:95–104.

Hoyer JD, Hanson CA, Fonseca R, Greipp PR, Dewald GW, Kurtin PJ. The (11;14)(q13;q32) translocation in multiple myeloma. A morphologic and immunohistochemical study. *Am J Clin Pathol.* 2000;113:831–837.

Ida K, Kobayashi S, Taki T, et al. EWS-FLI-1 and EWS-ERG chimeric mRNAs in Ewing's sarcoma and primitive neuroectodermal tumor. *Int J Cancer.* 1995;63:500–504.

Jaffe ES. Histiocytic and dendritic cell neoplasms: introduction. In: Jaffe ES, Harris NL, Stein H, Vardiman JW, eds. *World Health Organization Classification of Tumours. Pathology and Genetics of Tumours of Haematopoietic and Lymphoid Tissues.* Lyon, France: IARC Press; 2001:275–277.

Kaplan H. *Hodgkin Disease,* 2nd ed. Cambridge, UK: Harvard University Press; 1980:85–92.

Kilpatrick SE, Wenger DE, Gilchrist GS, Shives TC, Wollan PC, Unni KK. Langerhans cell histiocytosis (histiocytosis X) of bone: a clinicopathologic analysis of 263 pediatric patients and adult cases. *Cancer.* 1995;76:2471–2484.

Koura DT, Langston AA. Inherited predisposition to multiple myeloma. *Ther Adv Hematol.* 2013;4:291–297.

Kyle RA. Diagnostic criteria of multiple myeloma. *Hematol Oncol Clin N Am.* 1992;6:347–358.

Lichtenstein L. Histiocytosis X. I. Integration of eosinophilic granuloma of bone, Letterer-Siwe disese, and Schuller-Christian disease as related manifestations of single nosologic entity. *Arch Pathol.* 1953;56:84–102.

Lieberman PH, Jones CR, Steinman RM, et al. Langerhans cell (eosinophilic) granulomatosis. A clinicopathologic study encompassing 50 years. *Am J Surg Pathol.* 1996;20:519–552.

Lipshitz HI, Malthouse SR, Cunningham D, MacVicar AD, Husband JE. Multiple myeloma: appearance at MR imaging. *Radiology.* 1992;182:833–837.

Llombart-Bosch A, Contesso G, Henry-Amar M, et al. Histopathological predictive factors in Ewing's sarcoma of bone and clinicopathologic correlations. A retrospective study of 261 cases. *Virchows Arch A Pathol Pathol Anat.* 1986;409:627–640 (erratum published in *Virchows Arch A Pathol Pathol Anat* 1986;410:263).

Llombart-Bosch A, Lacombe MJ, Peydro-Olaya A, Perez-Bacete M, Contesso G. Malignant peripheral neuroectodermal tumors of bone other than Askin's neoplasm: characterization of 14 new cases with immunohistochemistry and electron microscopy. *Virchows Arch A Pathol Pathol Anat.* 1988;412:421–430.

Lukes RJ, Buttler JJ. Pathology and nomenclature of Hodgkin disease. *Cancer Res.* 1966;26:1063–2083.

Major N, Helms CA, Richardson WJ. The "mini brain" plasmacytoma in a vertebral body on MRI. *AJR Am J Roentgenol.* 2000;175:261–263.

May WA, Lessnick SL, Braun BS, et al. The Ewing's sarcoma *EWS/FLI-1* fusion gene encodes a more potent transcriptional activator and is a more powerful transforming gene than *FLI-1*. *Mol Cell Biol.* 1993;13:7393–7398.

Mazor RD, Manevich-Mazor M, Shoenfeld Y. Erdheim-Chester disease: a comprehensive review of the literature. *Orphanet J Rare Dis.* 2013;8:137–140.

Melamed JW, Martinez S, Hoffman CJ. Imaging of primary multifocal osseous lymphoma. *Skeletal Radiol.* 1997;26:35–41.

Meyer JE, Schulz MD. "Solitary" myeloma of bone: a review of 12 cases. *Cancer.* 1974;34:438–440.

Meyer JS, Harty MP, Mahboubi S, et al. Langerhans cell histiocytosis: presentation and evolution of radiologic findings with clinical correlation. *Radiographics.* 1995;15:1135–1146.

Moll RH, Lee I, Gould VE, Berndt R, Roessner A, Franke WW. Immunocytochemical analysis of Ewing's tumors. Patterns of expression of intermediate filaments and desmosomal proteins indicate cell type heterogeneity and pluripotential differentiation. *Am J Pathol.* 1987;127:288–304.

Mulligan ME, Badros AZ. PET/CT and MR imaging in myeloma. *Skeletal Radiol.* 2007;36:5–16.

Mulligan ME, Kransdorf MJ. Sequestra in primary lymphoma of bone: prevalence and radiologic features. *AJR Am J Roentgenol.* 1993;160:1245–1248.

Mulligan ME, McRae GA, Murphey MD. Imaging features of primary lymphoma of bone. *AJR Am J Roentgenol.* 1999;173:1691–1697.

Murakami I, Gogusev J, Fournet JC, Glorion C, Jaubert F. Detection of molecular cytogenetic aberrations in Langerhans cell histiocytosis of bone. *Hum Pathol.* 2002;33:555–560.

Ostrowski ML, Unni KK, Banks PM, et al. Malignant lymphoma of bone. *Cancer.* 1986;58:2646–2655.

Reinus WR, Kyriakos M, Gilula LA, Brower AC, Merkel K. Plasma cell tumors with calcified amyloid deposition mistaken for chondrosarcoma. *Radiology.* 1993;189:505–509.

Resnick D, Greenway GD, Bardwick PA, Zvaifler NJ, Gill GN, Newman DR. Plasma cell dyscrasia with polyneuropathy, organomegaly, endocrinopathy, M-protein, and skin changes: the POEMS syndrome. Distinctive radiographic abnormalities. *Radiology.* 1981;140:17–22.

Ruzek KA, Wenger DE. The multiple faces of lymphoma of the musculoskeletal system. *Skeletal Radiol.* 2004;33:1–8.

Schajowicz F. Ewing's sarcoma and reticulum cell sarcoma of bone: with special reference to the histochemical demonstration of glycogen as an aid to differential diagnosis. *J Bone Joint Surg Am.* 1959;41A:349–356.

Shirley SK, Gilula LA, Segal GP, Foulkes MA, Kissane JM, Askin FB. Roentgenographic-pathologic correlation of diffuse sclerosis in Ewing's sarcoma of bone. *Skeletal Radiol.* 1984;12:69–78.

Siegelman SS. Taking the X out of histiocytosis X. *Radiology.* 1997;204:322–324.

Stäbler A, Baur A, Bartl R, Munker R, Lamerz R, Reiser MF. Contrast enhancement and quantitative signal analysis in MR imaging of multiple myeloma: assessment of focal and diffuse growth patterns in marrow correlated with biopsies and survival rates. *AJR Am J Roentgenol.* 1996;167:1029–1036.

Steiner GC. Neuroectodermal tumor versus Ewing's sarcoma. Immunohistochemical and electron microscopic observations. *Curr Top Pathol.* 1989;80:1–29.

Steiner GC, Matano S, Present D. Ewing's sarcoma of humerus with epithelial differentiation. *Skeletal Radiol.* 1995;24:379–382.

Sun T, Akalin A, Rodacker M, Braun T. CD20 positive T cell lymphoma: is it a real entity? *J Clin Pathol.* 2004;57:442–444.

Symss NP, Cugati G, Vasudevan MC, Ramamurthi R, Pande A. Intracranial Rosai Dorfman disease: report of three cases and literature review. *Asian J Neurosurg.* 2010;5:19–30.

Treglia G, Salsano M, Stefanelli A, Mattoli MV, Giordano A, Bonomo L. Diagnostic accuracy of 18F-FDG-PET and PET/CT in patients with Ewing sarcoma family tumours: a systematic review and meta-analysis. *Skeletal Radiol.* 2012;41:249–256.

Triche T, Cavazzana A. Round cell tumors of bone. In: Unni KK, ed. *Bone Tumors.* New York: Churchill Livingstone; 1988:199–223.

Triche TJ, Askin FB, Kissane JM. Neuroblastoma, Ewing's sarcoma and the differential diagnosis of small, round blue cell tumors. In: Finegold M, ed. *Pathology of Neoplasia in Children and Adolescents.* Philadelphia, PA: WB Saunders; 1986:145–156.

Unni KK. *Dahlin's Bone Tumors: General Aspects and Data on 11,087 cases.* 5th ed. New York: Lippincott-Raven; 1996.

Uranishi M, Iida S, Sanda T, et al. Multiple myeloma oncogene 1 (MUM1)/interferon regulatory factor 4 (IRF4) upregulates monokine induced by interferon-gamma (MIG) gene expression in B-cell malignancy. *Leukemia.* 2005;19:1471–1478.

Vencio EF, Jenkins RB, Schiller JL. et al. Clonal cytogenetic abnormalities in Erdheim-Chester disease. *Am J Surg Pathol.* 2007;31:319–321.

Veyssier-Belot C, Cacoub P, Caparros-Lefebvre D, et al. Erdheim-Chester disease. Clinical and radiologic characteristics of 59 cases. *Medicine (Baltimore).* 1996;75:157–169.

Voss SD, Murphey MD, Hall FM. Solitary osteosclerotic plasmacytoma: association with demyelinating polyneuropathy and amyloid deposition. *Skeletal Radiol.* 2001;30:527–529.

Wang J, Chen C, Lau S, et al. CD3-positive large B-cell lymphoma. *Am J Surg Pathol.* 2009;33:505–512.

Williams CL. Detection of clonal histiocytes in Langerhans cell histiocytosis: biology and clinical significance. *Br J Cancer.* 1994;70(suppl 23):S29–S33.

Wright RA, Hermann RC, Parisi JE. Neurological manifestations of Erdheim-Chester disease. *J Neurol Neurosurg Psychiatry.* 1999;66:72–75.

Yu RC, Chu C, Buluwela L, Chu AC. Clonal proliferation of Langerhans cells in Langerhans cell histiocytosis. *Lancet.* 1994; 343:767–768.

Zelger B. Position paper. Langerhans histiocytosis: a reactive or neoplastic disorder? *Med Pediatr Oncol.* 2001;37:543–544.

CHAPTER 6

Vascular Lesions

Vascular lesions of bone constitute a spectrum of pathologic entities. These range from congenital vascular malformations, that is, errors of morphogenesis with nonproliferative capacity, which growth is parallel with growth of the patient (such as angiomatosis), to benign neoplasms that may be present at birth, and to highly malignant tumors that widely metastasize and have a low survival rate (such as angiosarcoma). In the past decade, immunohistochemistry studies have been conducted in attempts to discriminate between malformations and true tumors. The formers have been found to be negative for WT1 (a transcription factor initially isolated from a hereditary Wilms tumor encoded by the so-called Wilms tumor 1 [*WT1*] gene) and GLUT1 (an erythrocyte-type glucose transporter protein not present in normal vasculature and vascular malformations but found at sites of blood–tissue barriers and in vascular tumors). Furthermore, some investigators found somatic mutations in genes coding for the receptors *VEGFR2* and *VEGFR3* of the vascular endothelial growth factors, which play an important role in angiogenesis and vascular formation.

Benign vascular lesions are of either endothelial or pericytic origin. The first group includes hemangiomas, cystic angiomatosis, Gorham disease of bone, lymphangiomas, and lymphangiomatosis. The second group includes glomus tumor and its variants, glomangioma and glomangiomyoma. *Hemangiomas* are classified according to the type of vessels in the lesion as capillary, cavernous, venous, and mixed. Diffuse involvement of bones by hemangiomatous lesions is defined as *hemangiomatosis* or *angiomatosis*. When bone is extensively involved, particularly if there is formation of intramedullary cystic lesions, the term *cystic angiomatosis* is applied. *Gorham disease of bone*, also known as massive osteolysis, phantom bone disease, or disappearing bone disease, is characterized by progressive, localized bone resorption, probably caused by multiple or diffuse cavernous hemangiomas or lymphangiomas of bone or both. *Lymphangioma* is a rare disorder consisting of the lesion composed of sequestered, noncommunicating lymphoid tissue lined by lymphatic endothelium. *Glomus tumor* and its variants are rare lesions composed of rounded uniform cells often arranged in a brickwork-like pattern.

The locally aggressive and malignant tumors are quite uncommon and are mostly of endothelial origin, such as hemangioendothelioma and angiosarcoma. The existence of hemangiopericytoma as a distinct tumor is still a matter of debate. World Health Organization (WHO) classifies this lesion in the category of fibrous tumors changing its name to "myopericytoma."

A. Benign Vascular Lesions
Intraosseous Hemangioma
Epithelioid Hemangioma (Angiolymphoid Hyperplasia with Eosinophilia)
Cystic Angiomatosis
Gorham Disease (Disappearing Bone Disease, Massive Osteolysis)
Synovial Hemangioma
Lymphangioma, Lymphangiomatosis of Bone
Glomus Tumor

Variants of Glomus Tumor
  Glomangioma
  Glomangiomyoma
  Glomangiomatosis
  Symplastic Glomus Tumor
  Malignant Glomus Tumor

B. Malignant Vascular Tumors
Epithelioid Hemangioendothelioma
Angiosarcoma

A. BENIGN VASCULAR LESIONS

Intraosseous Hemangioma

Definition:
- Hemangioma is a benign lesion composed of newly formed blood vessels of capillary or cavernous type.

Epidemiology:
- Wide age distribution, ranging from the first to eighth decade of life, with nearly 70% of the cases diagnosed in patients between 30 and 60 years.
- They are rare in newborns and infants, and in reported cases, they have arisen in the skull bones.
- There is no sex predilection.
- The lesions are usually solitary, although multifocal involvement has been described (most commonly in the vertebral column).

Sites of Involvement:
- Craniofacial bones, predominantly calvaria (frontal and parietal regions)—50%, followed by the spine—20%.

Clinical Findings:
- Commonly asymptomatic.
- In the vertebrae may cause neurologic symptoms.

Imaging:
- On radiography, an osseous hemangioma in a long or short tubular bone is characterized by lace-like pattern, by coarse striations, or by focal lytic area (Fig. 6.1). In flat bones, they commonly expand the bone contour and produce rarefaction with radially oriented striations; overlying cortex is expanded and thinned, but complete cortical disruption and invasion into soft tissue are generally not present. In the vertebral body, hemangioma is characterized by either vertical striations (corduroy cloth pattern) or multiloculated lytic foci (honeycomb pattern) (Figs. 6.2 and 6.3). Characteristic sunburst appearance is seen in skull lesions with thickened trabeculae arranged in a spoke-wheel or web-like pattern. In concomitant involvement of the soft tissues, the hallmark is the phlebolith (see Fig. 6.8).
- Scintigraphy shows either photopenia or only moderate increase of uptake of radiopharmaceutical tracer.
- On computed tomography, "honeycomb" pattern may be observed in the long tubular and flat bones (Fig. 6.4), whereas vertebral hemangiomas characteristically exhibit pattern of a multiple dots ("polka-dot" appearance) (Fig. 6.5).
- Magnetic resonance imaging (MRI) generally reveals a high signal on T1-weighted and T2-weighted images (blood content of tumor vessels), with areas of trabecular

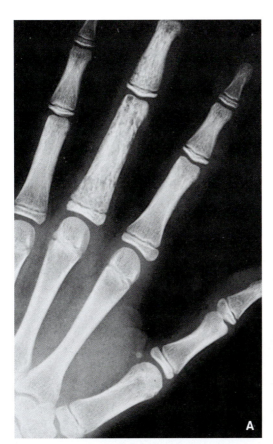 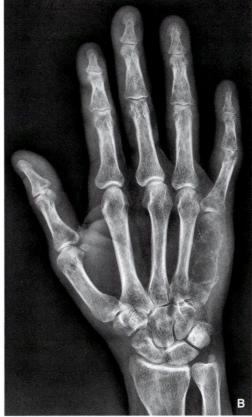

FIGURE 6.1 Radiography of intraosseous hemangioma. (A) Dorsovolar radiograph of the right hand of an 11-year-old girl shows a lace-like pattern of the lesion affecting the proximal and middle phalanx of the middle finger. **(B)** In another patient, a 50-year-old man, observe the lytic, expansive, bubble-like lesion affecting the fifth metacarpal bone of the left hand.

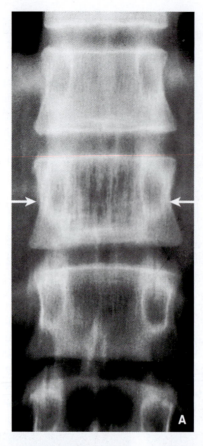
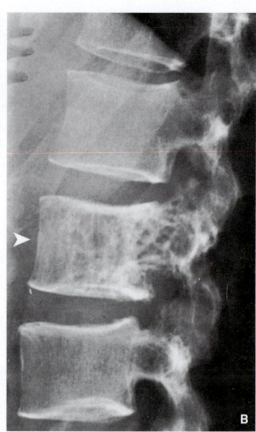

FIGURE 6.2 Radiography of intraosseous hemangioma. (A) Anteroposterior conventional tomogram demonstrates vertical striation of the lesion affecting L1 vertebra (*arrows*). **(B)** Lateral radiograph of the lumbar spine of another patient demonstrates a "honeycomb" pattern of the lesion affecting L2 vertebra (*arrowhead*).

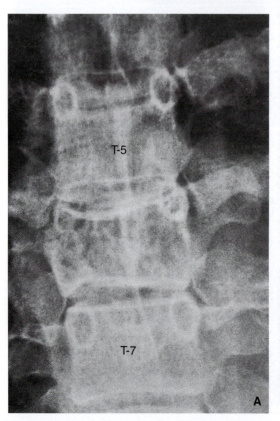
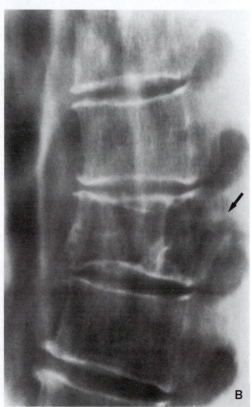

FIGURE 6.3 Radiography of intraosseous hemangioma. (A) Anteroposterior radiograph of the midthoracic spine of a 39-year-old woman shows a radiolucent lesion involving the body of T6 vertebra, extending into the pedicles. **(B)** Lateral radiograph demonstrates ballooning of the posterior cortex of the vertebra and extension of the lesion into the posterior elements (*arrow*).

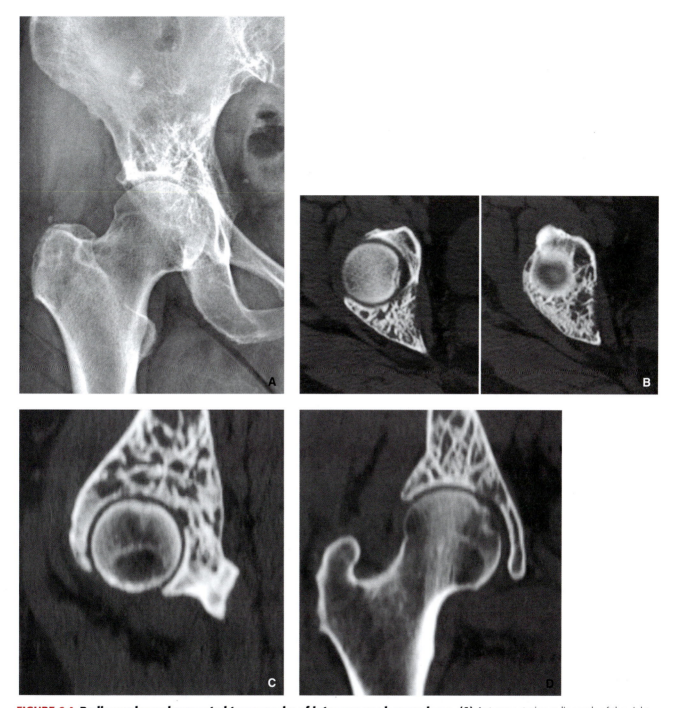

FIGURE 6.4 Radiography and computed tomography of intraosseous hemangioma. (A) Anteroposterior radiograph of the right hip of a 35-year-old woman shows mixed radiolucent and sclerotic lesion in the ilium extending into the acetabulum. **(B)** Two axial CT sections and **(C)** sagittal and **(D)** coronal reformatted CT images show a characteristic for hemangioma "honeycomb" pattern.

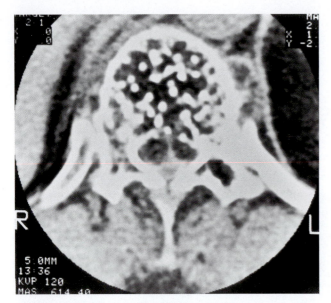

FIGURE 6.5 Computed tomography of intraosseous hemangioma. Axial CT section of a T10 vertebra shows coarse dots ("polka-dot" pattern) reflecting reinforced vertical trabeculae of the cancellous bone, characteristic for this lesion.

thickening imaged in low signal intensity regardless of the pulse sequence. After intravenous administration of gadolinium, there is always significant enhancement of the lesion (Figs. 6.6 to 6.10).

Pathology:

Gross:

- Brown-red or dark red, well demarcated, medullary lesion (Fig. 6.11).
- It may have a honeycomb appearance with sclerotic bone trabeculae interspersed among hemorrhagic cavities.

Histopathology:

- Hemangiomas are composed of conglomerate of thin-walled blood vessels (Fig. 6.12A,B).
- Vascular channels are lined by a single layer of flat endothelial cells (Fig. 6.12C).
- Vessels can have dilated open channels (cavernous hemangioma) or less commonly may be composed of capillary-sized vessels (capillary hemangioma).
- Majority of bone hemangiomas are of cavernous or mixed types (Fig. 6.13).

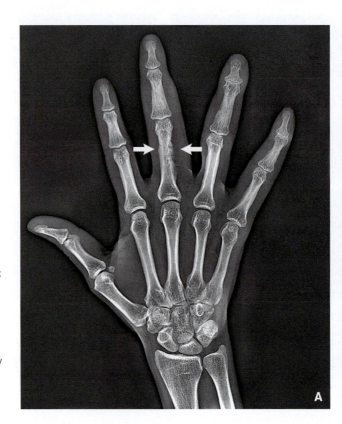
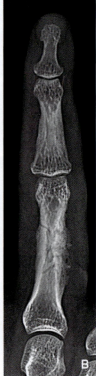

FIGURE 6.6 Radiography and magnetic resonance imaging of intraosseous and soft-tissue hemangioma.
(A) Dorsovolar radiograph of the left hand and **(B)** coned-down view of the middle finger of a 36-year-old woman show radiolucent channels traversing the medullary portion and the cortex of the proximal phalanx (*arrows*) associated with soft-tissue prominence.

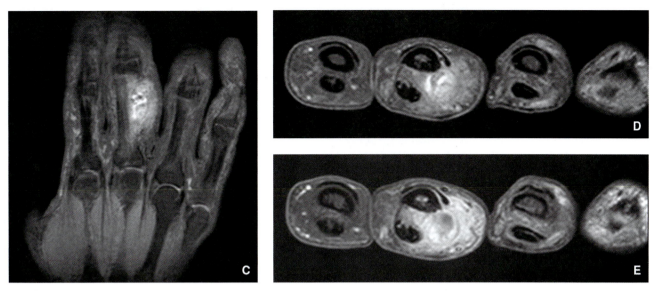

FIGURE 6.6 *(Continued).* **(C)** Coronal T2-weighted fat-suppressed MR image shows high signal intensity of the lesion affecting both the bone and the soft tissue. **(D)** Axial T1-weighted fat-suppressed and **(E)** axial T1-weighted fat-suppressed postcontrast MR images demonstrate significant enhancement of the lesion. (Courtesy of Robert Szabo, M.D., Sacramento, CA.)

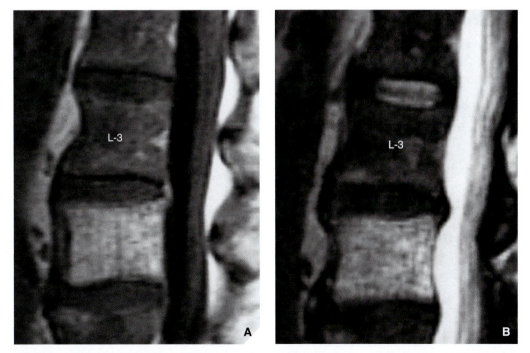

FIGURE 6.7 Magnetic resonance imaging of intraosseous hemangioma. (A) Sagittal T1-weighted and **(B)** T2-weighted MR images show high intensity signal of hemangioma of L4 vertebra.

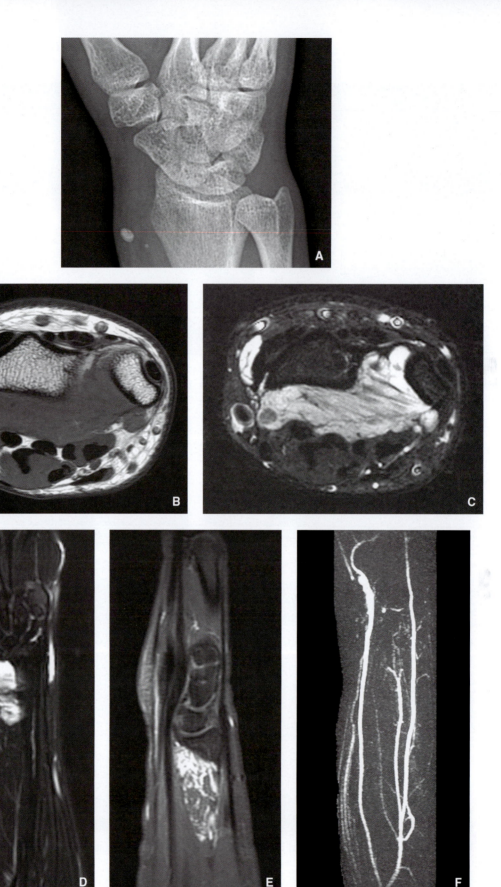

FIGURE 6.8 Radiography, magnetic resonance imaging, and magnetic resonance angiography of hemangiomatosis. (A) Oblique radiograph of the left wrist of a 21-year-old woman shows two phleboliths in the soft tissues adjacent to the distal radius. **(B)** Axial T1-weighted, **(C)** axial inversion recovery (IR), **(D)** coronal T2-weighted, and **(E)** sagittal T1-weighted fat-suppressed MR image obtained after intravenous administration of gadolinium show a tubular lobulated soft-tissue mass within the quadratus pronator muscle that extends into the radiocarpal and distal radioulnar joints, with intraosseous involvement of the distal ulna and volar aspect of the distal radius. **(F)** Coronal MR angiogram shows puddling of the contrast in the region of the distal radial artery at the site of hemangioma. (Courtesy of Robert Szabo, M.D., Sacramento, CA.)

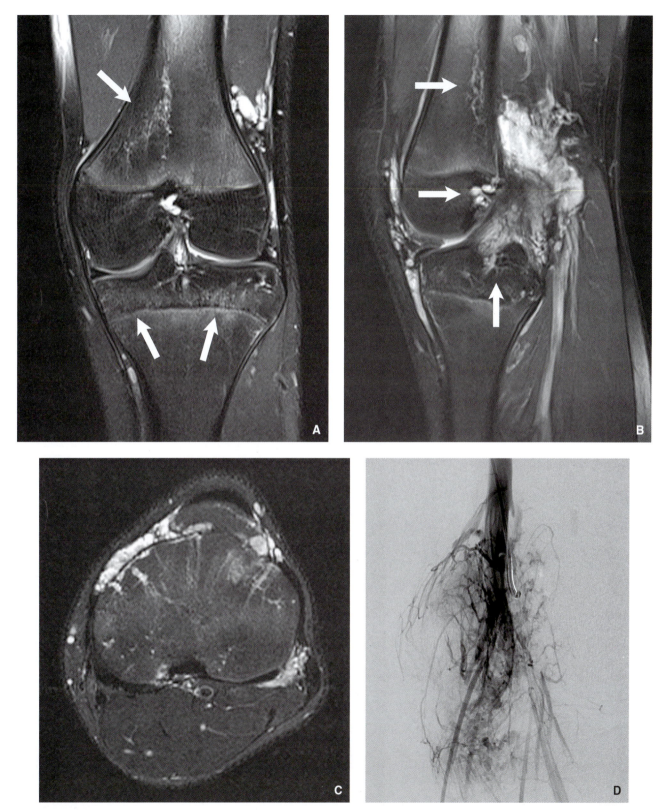

FIGURE 6.9 Magnetic resonance imaging and angiography of hemangiomatosis. (A) Coronal and **(B)** sagittal T2-weighted fat-suppressed MR images of the knee of a 14-year-old boy show high intensity lesions in the distal femur and proximal tibia (*arrows*), associated with soft-tissue involvement. **(C)** Axial T2-weighted MRI shows involvement of the knee joint. **(D)** Angiogram shows a hypervascular lesion affecting both osseous structures and soft tissues.

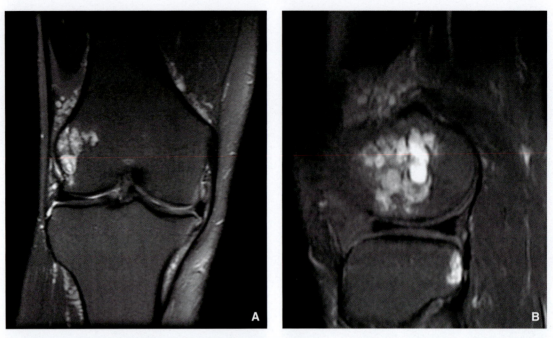

FIGURE 6.10 Magnetic resonance imaging of hemangiomatosis. (A) Coronal and **(B)** sagittal T2-weighted fat-suppressed MR images show multiple lesions affecting the osseous and soft-tissue structures of the knee of a 51-year-old man exhibiting high signal intensity.

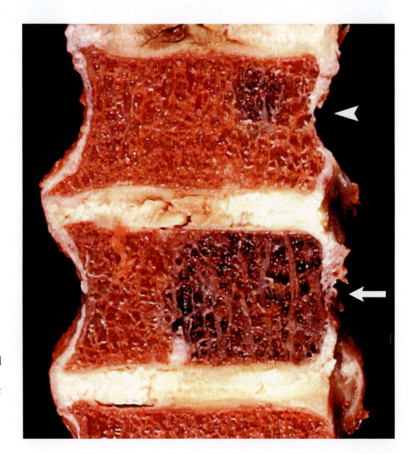

FIGURE 6.11 Gross specimen of hemangioma. Two red-brown hemangiomas of the vertebral bodies, one small (*arrowhead*) and one large (*arrow*) are well demarcated from the normal cancellous bone and exhibit coarse trabeculations. (From Bullough PG. *Atlas of Orthopedic Pathology with Clinical and Radiologic Correlations*. 2nd ed. New York: Gower Medical Publishing; 1992, p.16.11, Fig. 15.28.)

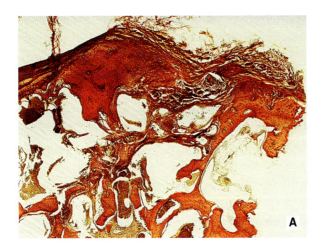
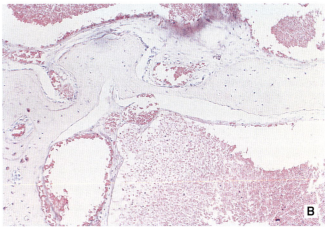
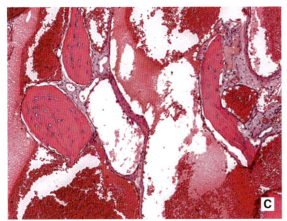

FIGURE 6.12 Histopathology of intraosseous hemangioma (cavernous type). (A) Cortical bone (*top*) and cancellous bone (*bottom*) stained red enclosing large, mostly empty vascular spaces (van Gieson, original magnification ×6). **(B)** At higher magnification, large vascular spaces filled with blood cells lie in the marrow spaces of cancellous bone. Surfaces of the trabeculae are lined with osteoblasts (H&E, original magnification ×25). **(C)** On high magnification, observe dilated open vascular spaces between bone trabeculae, some filled with blood, lined by a single layer of flat endothelial cells (H&E, original magnification ×200).

- Intercellular tissue is composed of loose connective tissue that may show myxoid change.
- Bone may be completely resorbed in affected area.
- Vascular channels of hemangioma are complete, are separate, and do not show anastomosing pattern.

Immunohistochemistry:
- Endothelial cells are positive for CD31, CD34, and factor VIII–related antigen.

Prognosis:
- Asymptomatic small hemangiomas require no treatment; some may undergo spontaneous regression.
- Symptomatic lesions or those that are large and may cause pathologic fracture or vertebral collapse require treatment; curettage and bone grafting usually is sufficient.

Differential Diagnosis:
- ***Aneurysmal bone cyst***
  Imaging shows the lesion ballooning out of the cortex, associated with periosteal reaction, usually in the form of well-defined buttress. Scintigraphy shows increased uptake in a ring-like pattern around the periphery of the lesion. MRI shows fluid–fluid levels. Histopathology showing blood-filled spaces alternating with solid areas composed of fibrous; richly vascular connective tissue containing clusters of giant cells is diagnostic.

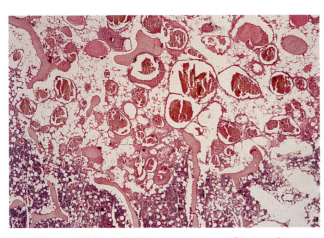

FIGURE 6.13 Histopathology intraosseous hemangioma (mixed type). Blood vessels of capillary character and partly of cavernous type lie between small bone trabeculae and border normal cancellous bone of the vertebra containing hematopoietic marrow (*below*) (H&E, original magnification ×25).

Epithelioid Hemangioma (Angiolymphoid Hyperplasia with Eosinophilia)

Definition:
- A benign but locally aggressive vascular neoplasm with endothelial phenotype and epithelioid morphology.

Epidemiology:
- Rare bone tumor (most common in skin and subcutis).
- Patient age range from 10 to 90 years with average age of 35 years.
- Male-to-female ratio of 1:1.4.

Sites of Involvement:
- Most common involvement of long tubular bones (40%), short tubular bones of lower extremities (18%), flat bones (18%), vertebrae (16%), and small bone of the hands (8%).
- Multifocal distribution can be seen.

Clinical Findings:
- Pain localized to involved anatomical site.

Imaging:
- Identical imaging features as of hemangioma (see above).

Pathology:
Gross (Macroscopy):
- Well-defined nodular, soft, solid, hemorrhagic mass.
- Most tumors less than 7 cm in size.
- May expand bone and extend into soft tissue.

Histopathology:
- Lobular architecture, infiltrates preexisting bone trabeculae.
- Periphery of the lobules may show small vessels lined by endothelial cells.
- Center of the lobules are more cellular and contain epithelioid cells with abundant eosinophilic cytoplasm.
- Epithelioid cells are large, plump, and have oval or kidney bean–shaped nuclei with uniformly distributed chromatin.
- Abundant eosinophilic cytoplasm with occasional one or two vacuoles.
- Cells with vacuoles may aggregate.
- Most tumors contain small well-formed vessels with open lumina surrounded by epithelioid cells sometimes arranged in tombstone-like pattern.
- Infrequent mitoses can be seen but without atypia.
- Loose connective stroma that may contain inflammatory component, mostly eosinophils.
- Intralesional hemorrhage may be seen.
- Osteoclast-type giant cells can be seen.

Immunohistochemistry:
- Positive for factor VIII, CD31, CD34, Fli-1, EGR, and ulex europaeus.
- May be positive for cytokeratin and epithelial membrane antigen (EMA).

Prognosis:
- Locally aggressive lesion, successfully treated with curettage or marginal bloc excision.
- Local recurrence rate of about 9%.

Differential Diagnosis:
- Same as for hemangioma (see above).

Cystic Angiomatosis

Definition:
- Rare condition, characterized by disseminated multifocal cystic in appearance hemangiomas affecting the skeleton, commonly associated with visceral involvement.

Epidemiology:
- Most cases are recognized in the first three decades of life.
- Male-to-female ratio of 2:1.

Sites of Involvement:
- Skull, spine, ribs, long bones (femur, tibia, fibula, humerus), and pelvic bones.
- Extraskeletal involvement includes soft tissues, lung, liver, and spleen.

Clinical Findings:
- Most of the time the patients are asymptomatic, the lesions detected incidentally by imaging studies obtained for other reasons (trauma).
- Patients may be symptomatic if there is concomitant visceral involvement.

Imaging:
- Radiography shows well-defined lytic lesions (Fig. 6.14), often with honeycomb or lattice work ("hole-within-hole") appearance (Fig. 6.15); the lesions may exhibit sclerotic border, and cortex may be thickened; periosteal reaction is rare.
- MRI shows the lesions to be of intermediate signal intensity on T1-weighted sequences, whereas T2 weighting shows mixture of high, low, and intermediate signal intensities.

Pathology:
Gross (Macroscopy):
- Resemble simple bone cyst with multiple communicating cavities lined by a dull, yellowish-gray membrane, separated by thickened bone trabeculae.

Histopathology:
- Indistinguishable from cavernous hemangiomas.
- Multiple dilated, thin-walled vascular channels lined by flat endothelial cells (Fig. 6.16).
- Occasionally osteoid and immature woven bone formation with osteoblasts rimming may be present.
- Admixture of dilated lymphatics can be seen.
- Sclerotic variant may show vessels with perivascular thick sclerotic bone.

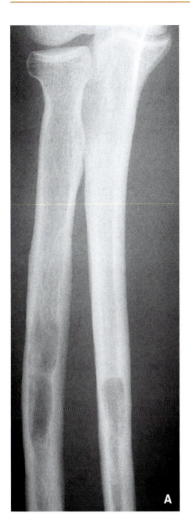
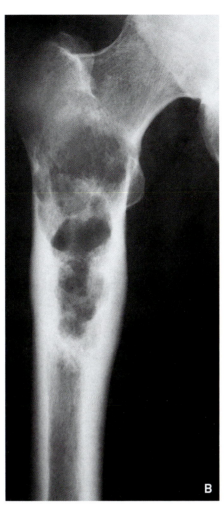

FIGURE 6.14 Radiography of cystic angiomatosis. **(A)** Several osteolytic lesions affect the shaft of the radius and ulna of a 25-year-old man. **(B)** In another patient, a 20-year-old man, several confluent lesions with peripheral sclerosis and cortical thickening are present within the right proximal femur.

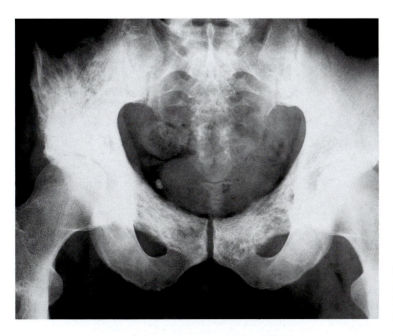

FIGURE 6.15 Radiography of cystic angiomatosis. Anteroposterior radiograph of the pelvis of a 28-year-old man shows several lesions in the right ilium and both pubic bones exhibiting a honeycomb pattern.

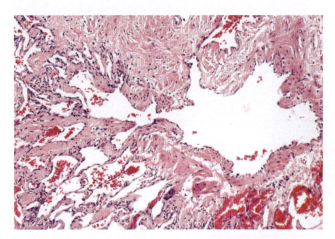

FIGURE 6.16 Histopathology of cystic angiomatosis. Observe large cystic spaces lined with single layer of flat endothelial cells, very similar to cavernous hemangioma (H&E, original magnification ×200).

Prognosis:
- Skeletal lesions are usually stable and may even regress with time.

Differential Diagnosis:
- **Pseudotumors of hemophilia**
   Radiography shows well-defined geographic in type destructive lytic lesions, sometimes septated or trabeculated, occasionally with sclerotic border and periosteal reaction; blow-out appearance may also be encountered; soft-tissue mass may be present with small bone fragments within it. Ultrasound shows a central anechoic area with increased echoes surrounding the lesion caused by fluid within the pseudotumor. MRI shows heterogeneous signal on T1-weighted sequences and high signal on T2 weighting with foci of low signal, with rim of low-to-intermediate signal on both sequences due to fibrous tissue containing hemosiderin.
   Histopathology shows blood clots within the cystic lesions, and fibrotic changes of the wall of the cysts; hemosiderin-laden macrophages may be seen.
- **Osteolytic metastases**
   Radiography shows predominantly lytic lesions without sclerotic border.
   Histopathology may show identifying features of primary carcinoma; however, immunohistochemistry studies may be needed to localize the primary site.
- **Brown tumors of hyperparathyroidism**
   Imaging features, particularly radiography, may closely resemble cystic angiomatosis; however, usually the other features of hyperparathyroidism are present, such as subperiosteal and chondral resorption, osteopenia, rugger jersey spine, and soft-tissue calcifications.
   Histopathology of brown tumors, that are composed of reactive stromal cells in which multinucleated giant cells are arranged in clusters, and the presence of large aggregate of hemosiderin pigment, is characteristic.

Gorham Disease (Disappearing Bone Disease, Massive Osteolysis)

Definition:
- Progressive, localized bone resorption, probably caused by multiple or diffuse cavernous hemangiomas or lymphangiomas, or both.

Epidemiology:
- Any age (from 1 month to 77 years), but more common in young adults.
- No gender preference.

Sites of Involvement:
- Shoulder girdle, skull, pelvic bones, ribs, spine, femur, radius, and metacarpals.

Clinical findings:
- Dull aching pain at the site of the lesion.
- Insidious onset of progressive weakness.
- Occasionally a pathologic fracture is the first clinical symptom.

Imaging:
- Radiographic presentation consists of lytic areas in the cancellous bone or concentric destruction of cortical bone, giving rise to a "sucked-candy" appearance (Fig. 6.17A); as the disease progresses, the bone becomes completely resorbed (Figs. 6.17B and 6.18A); lack of periosteal reaction; soft-tissue mass may be present.
- Scintigraphy initially positive, becomes negative with ongoing bone resorption.
- MRI shows intermediate signal intensity on T1-weighted sequences, high signal on T2 weighting, and significant enhancement after administration of gadolinium (Fig. 6.18B,C).

Histopathology:
- Increase in the number and size of the intraosseous capillaries, which form an anastomosing network of endothelium-lined channels (Fig. 6.19A).
- Increased osteoclastic activity (Fig. 6.19B,C).
- Replacement of bone by hypovascular fibrous connective tissue (Fig. 6.19D).

Prognosis:
- Clinical course generally protracted but rarely fatal.
- Progressive bone destruction.
- High morbidity and mortality when condition affects the base of the skull, ribs, sternum, vertebrae, or viscera.
- Recurrence following remission can occur.
- Self-limited in some cases.

Differential Diagnosis:
- **Osteolytic metastases**
   Imaging studies, particularly radiography, may show features resembling Gorham disease; however, scintigraphy will show increased uptake of the radiopharmaceutical agent.

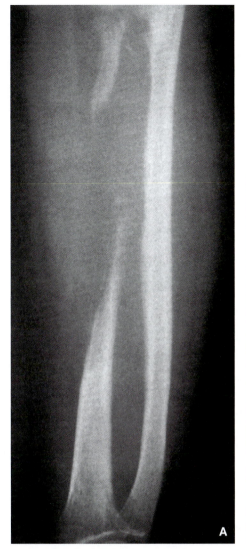 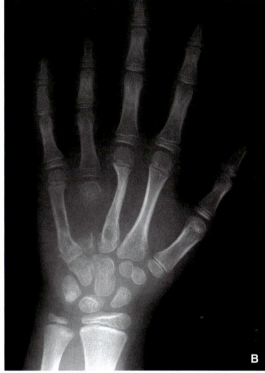

FIGURE 6.17 Radiography of the Gorham disease. (A) Anteroposterior radiograph of the right forearm of a 46-year-old woman shows osteolysis of the midportion of the shaft of the radius. Observe characteristic tapering of the proximal end of the radius that assumed "sucked-candy" appearance. **(B)** Dorsovolar radiograph of the left hand of a 9-year-old boy shows complete resorption of the diaphysis of the fourth metacarpal bone and pressure erosion of the ulnar aspect of the third metacarpal.

Histopathology may show identifying features of primary carcinoma; however, immunohistochemistry studies may be needed to localize primary site.
- *Angiosarcoma*
Radiography may show features similar to those of Gorham disease; however, histopathology showing typical malignant polygonal cells with large pleomorphic, and hyperchromatic nuclei is diagnostic.

Synovial Hemangioma

Synovial hemangioma, a rare benign lesion of the synovium, is discussed in the section devoted to the lesions of the joints (see the text that follows).

Lymphangioma, Lymphangiomatosis of Bone

Definition:
- Benign, usually diffuse or multiple cavernous/cystic vascular lesion composed of dilated lymphatic channels, most likely representing hamartomatous malformation.

Epidemiology:
- Mostly seen in infants and children (65%), and rarely manifest after the age of 20 years.
- No gender predilection.

Sites of Involvement:
- Diaphyses and metaphyses of long bones, most common in the tibia and humerus; skull, mandible, ilium, ribs, and vertebrae also occasionally affected.

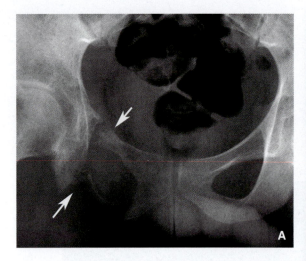
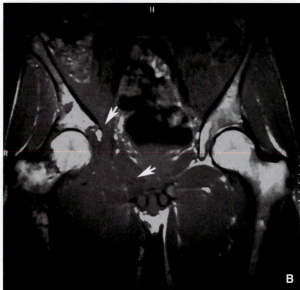
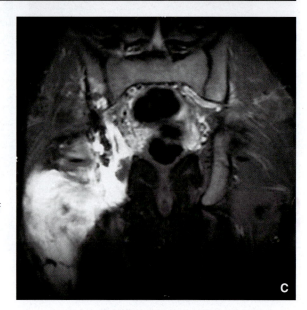

FIGURE 6.18 Radiography and magnetic resonance imaging of Gorham disease. (A) Anteroposterior radiograph of the lower pelvis shows bone resorption of the right superior and inferior pubic rami (*arrows*). **(B)** Coronal T1-weighted MRI shows bone destruction associated with soft-tissue mass (*arrowheads*). **(C)** Coronal T1-weighted fat-suppressed MR image obtained after intravenous administration of gadolinium shows extensive enhancement of the involved bone and soft-tissue mass.

- Multiple lymphangiomas of the ribs may be associated with chylothorax or chylopericardium.
- Lymphangiomatosis of the bone can be associated with soft-tissue (extraskeletal) lymphangiomas.

Clinical Findings:
- Lesions usually present as circumscribed painless swelling, which is soft and fluctuant in palpation.

Imaging:
- Radiography shows multiple, well-defined lytic lesions, commonly with sclerotic margin, without associated periosteal reaction, but occasionally with soft-tissue masses; in some cases, the margin may have a "soap-bubble" appearance, and in some cases, it may be quite poorly defined, with a moth-eaten pattern of bone destruction (Fig. 6.20).
- Lymphangiography is effective in demonstrating abnormal and dilated lymphatic channels filling the cystic bone lesions.
- MRI shows hyperintense foci on both T1- and T2-weighted sequences. There is no enhancement after intravenous gadolinium administration.

Pathology:
Gross (Macroscopy):
- Lymphangiomas vary from well-circumscribed lesions made up of one or more large interconnecting cysts to ill-defined, sponge-like compressible lesions composed of microscopic cysts.
- Dilated lymphatic spaces in bone.

Histopathology:
- Cavernous lymphangiomas are characterized by thin-walled, dilated lymphatic vessels of different size, which are lined by a flattened endothelium and frequently surrounded by lymphoid aggregates (Fig. 6.21).

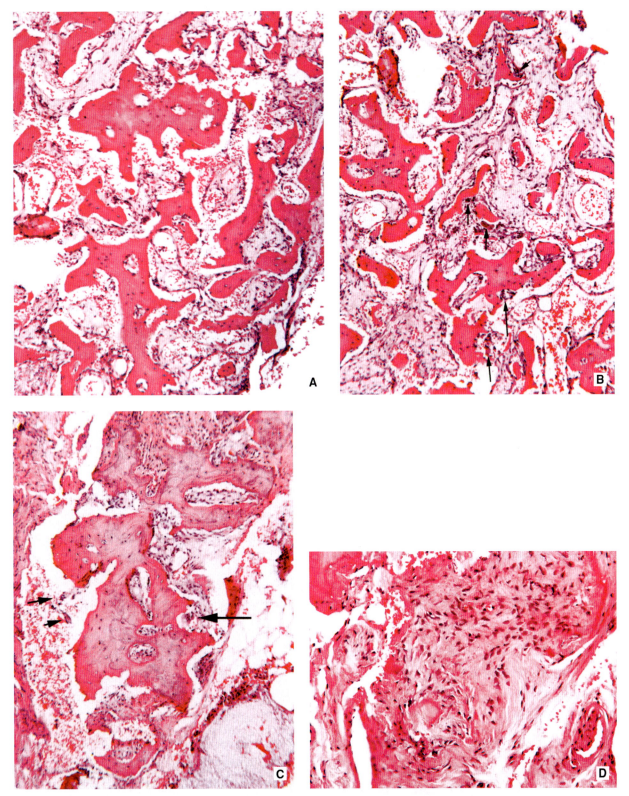

FIGURE 6.19 Histopathology of Gorham disease. (A) Irregular bone trabeculae exhibiting markedly increased vascularity are scattered within the fibrous stroma. **(B)** Trabeculae of cancellous bone immediately adjacent to the hypervascular areas show evidence of resorption by increased number of osteoclasts (*arrows*). **(C)** Trabeculae of compact bone also are being resorbed by the osteoclasts (*arrows*). **(D)** In the regions that are older or inactive, observe less vascular fibrous connective tissue. (Reprinted with permission from Klein MJ, Bonar SF, Freemont T, et al. *Atlas of Nontumor Pathology. Non-Neoplastic Diseases of Bones and Joints*. Washington, DC: AFIP; 2011, p. 869, Fig. 11-74A, and p. 870, Figs. 11-75 and 11-76.)

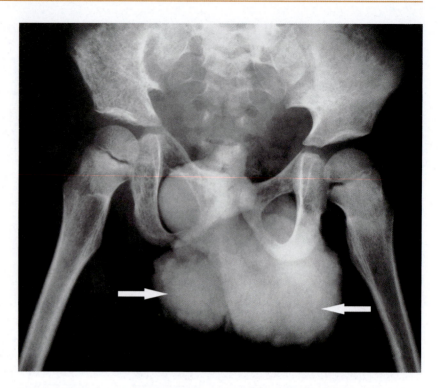

FIGURE 6.20 Radiography of skeletal lymphangiomatosis. A 2-year-old boy presented with multiple osseous lesions, particularly affecting the bones of the pelvis and proximal femora. Observe honeycomb and moth-eaten pattern of bone destruction. In addition to skeletal involvement, lymphangiomas were also present in the scrotum (*arrows*).

- The lumina may either be empty or contain eosinophilic material, chyle, proteinaceous fluid, lymphocytes, and sometimes erythrocytes.
- Larger vessels can be invested by a smooth muscle layer, and long-standing lesions may show fibrosis and inflammatory changes.
- Stromal mast cells are common, and hemosiderin deposition is frequently seen.

Immunohistochemistry:
- Positive for lymphatic lineage markers D2-40, VEGFR3.

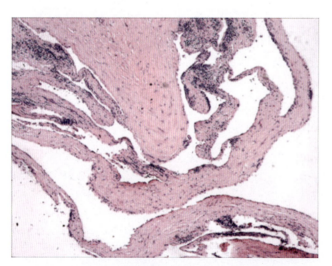

FIGURE 6.21 Histopathology of lymphangiomatosis. Note characteristic thin-walled dilated lymphatic vessels of varying size, lined by flattened endothelium (H&E, original magnification ×200).

Prognosis:
- Generally good prognosis.
- Lesions eventually stabilize and sclerose, but the profound bone deformity may persist.

Differential Diagnosis:
- **Metastatic neuroblastoma**
  Radiography shows ill-defined radiolucent lesions, commonly associated with periosteal reaction. MRI shows variable heterogeneous enhancement of the lesions on T1-weighted sequences after injection of gadolinium. Diagnostic imaging study is the positive MIBG (metaiodobenzylguanidine) scan.
  Histopathology showing small, round, blue tumor cells with round nuclei and scant cytoplasm, forming typical Homer-Wright rosettes is diagnostic. Foci of necrosis and calcifications may be present.
- **Langerhans cell histiocytosis**
  Imaging studies, particularly radiography, may show similar findings as in lymphangiomatosis, although periosteal reaction is usually present. MRI shows the lesions to be of intermediate-to-low signal intensity on T1-weighted sequences and enhancing after administration of gadolinium.
  Histopathology showing typical Langerhans cells, and EM identification of Birbeck granules is diagnostic.
- **Chronic recurrent multifocal osteomyelitis (CRMO)**
  Imaging studies show mixed radiolucent and radiodense lesions, occasionally bordered by rim of sclerosis, commonly within the clavicle, sternum, and metaphyses of the long bones.

Histopathology is nonspecific, including the presence of inflammatory changes associated with microsequestrations, active osteolytic resorption, and occasionally vasculitis.

- **Polyostotic fibrous dysplasia**

  Imaging studies show radiolucent lesions exhibiting smoky or ground-glass appearance; the cortex is typically thinned out.

  Histopathology showing metaplastic woven bone trabeculae without osteoblastic activity is diagnostic.

Glomus Tumor

Definition:
- Mesenchymal neoplasm composed of rounded uniform cells often arranged in a brickwork-like pattern that closely resemble the modified smooth muscle cells of the normal glomus body.

Epidemiology:
- Accounts for less than 2% of soft-tissue tumors, only occasionally arising primarily in bone (about 100 reported cases).
- Typically occurs in young adults, although may occur at any age.
- Ten percent of patients show multiple lesions.
- Malignant form (so-called symplastic glomus) is exceedingly rare.
- Subungual lesions are more common in female patients.

Sites of Involvement:
- Majority of lesions occur in the distal part of the extremities (the hand and the foot) particularly in the subungual region.
- Common site is the skin and superficial soft tissues.
- Rare cases were described in the stomach, lungs, mediastinum, and nerves.
- When primary in the bone, distal phalanges are preferential sites.
- Malignant forms mostly involve deep soft tissue.

Clinical Findings:
- Localized pain and exquisite point tenderness.
- Cutaneous forms are usually small (less than 1 cm), presenting as red-blue nodules that are often associated with a long history of pain, particularly with exposure to cold.
- Deep soft-tissue or visceral lesions may be asymptomatic or have symptoms related to involved organ.

Imaging:
- On radiography presents as a small, lytic bone defect with sharply marginated edges, usually located at the dorsal aspect of the phalanx.
- On CT, a nonspecific subungual mass is demonstrated with attenuation values similar to that of other soft-tissue lesions.
- On MRI, the lesion exhibits either isointense or hyperintense signal on T1-weighted sequences, whereas on T2 weighting, the lesion exhibits homogeneous high signal intensity. Strong enhancement is observed after intravenous injection of gadolinium.

Histopathology:
- The cells are small, uniform, and rounded, with centrally placed, round nuclei and amphophilic to lightly eosinophilic cytoplasm (Fig. 6.22).
- Each cell is surrounded by well-defined basal lamina.
- Some cases may exhibit oncocytic or epithelioid changes.
- Solid variant, which is most common, shows nests of glomus cells surrounding capillary-sized vessels, with stroma exhibiting hyalinization or myxoid changes.

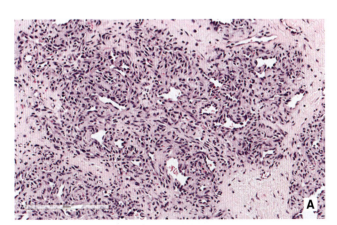 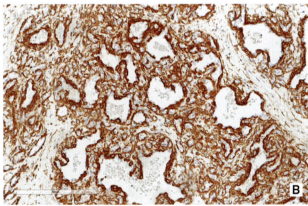

FIGURE 6.22 Histopathology of glomus tumor. (A) Characteristic small, uniform, rounded cells with well-defined cell membranes and centrally placed nuclei are surrounding the vascular capillaries (H&E, original magnification ×100). **(B)** The cells show immunopositivity for smooth muscle actin (SMA, original magnification ×200).

Variants of Glomus Tumor

Glomangioma
- A rare variant, constituting approximately 20% of all glomus tumors.
- Characterized by dilated veins surrounded by small clusters of glomus cells.

Glomangiomyoma
- Least common of all glomus tumor variants.
- Exhibits transition from typical glomus cells to elongated cells resembling mature smooth muscle.
- May show hemangiopericytoma-like vascular structures (glomangiopericytoma).

Glomangiomatosis
- Morphologically resemble diffuse angiomatosis but contain nests of glomus cells investing vessel walls.

Symplastic Glomus Tumor
- Shows prominent nuclear atypia in the absence of any other atypical features (e.g., large size, deep location, mitotic activity, necrosis).
- Marked nuclear atypia may be caused by degenerative changes.
- All reported cases behaved in benign fashion.

Malignant Glomus Tumor
- Extremely rare tumor.
- Marked nuclear atypia associated with any level of mitotic activity.
- Common atypical mitotic figures.
- Two types have been described:
  - In the first type, malignant component resembles leiomyosarcoma or fibrosarcoma.
  - In the second type, the malignant component consists of sheets of malignant-appearing round cells.
- Malignant glomus tumors are very aggressive with high probability to metastasize.

Immunohistochemistry:
- Expresses positivity for smooth muscle actin (SMA), pericellular collagen type IV, and H-caldesmon.
- Negative for desmin, CD34, cytokeratin, and S-100 protein.

Electron Microscopy:
- Glomus cells have short interdigitating cytoplasmic processes, bundles of thin actin-like filaments with dense bodies, and occasional attachments plaques to the cytoplasmic membrane, and prominent external lamina.

Genetics:
- *GLMN* (glomulin) gene mutation on chromosome 1p21-22.
- Biallelic inactivation of *NF1* gene due to loss of heterozygosity (LOH) underlies the pathogenesis of NF1-associated glomus tumors.
- Mitotic recombination of chromosome arm 17q has been identified.

Prognosis:
- Glomus tumor, glomuvenous malformation, and symplastic glomus tumor are benign lesions with excellent prognosis.
- Malignant glomus tumor is aggressive, with metastasis and death in up to 40% of patients.

B. MALIGNANT VASCULAR TUMORS

Epithelioid Hemangioendothelioma

Definition:
- Malignant vascular neoplasm of low-to-intermediate grade, with unpredictable clinical course, composed of endothelial phenotype with epithelioid features and a hyalinized, chondroid, or basophilic stroma.

Epidemiology:
- Rare tumor.
- May be solitary or multifocal and may involve many organs such as bone, lung, liver, and soft tissue.
- Wide age range from 10 to 75 years, with patients most commonly diagnosed during the second and third decades of life.
- Patients affected by multifocal disease are on average 10 years younger than those with solitary lesions.
- Equally affects male and female patients.

Sites of Involvement:
- May affect any bone, but most commonly those of lower extremities, followed by calvaria, pelvis, ribs, and spine.
- About 50% of cases show multicentric involvement of bones.

Clinical Findings:
- Most common symptoms are localized dull pain, tenderness, and swelling.

Imaging:
- Radiography shows osteolytic lesion with either narrow or wide zone of transition (Fig. 6.23A); variable degree of peripheral sclerosis may be present; occasionally, a soap-bubble appearance with expansion of bone is observed; soft-tissue extension may be present.
- MRI reveals a mixed signal on T1-weighted sequences, with moderately increased signal intensity on T2 weighting (Fig. 6.23B,C).

Pathology:
Gross (Macroscopy):
- Ovoid, rubbery, tan, and hemorrhagic masses.

Histopathology:
- Markedly pleomorphic epithelioid and spindle endothelial cells with abundant faintly eosinophilic or amphophilic cytoplasm and round or elongated hyperchromatic nuclei with prominent nucleoli (Fig. 6.24A,B).
- Intracytoplasmic vacuoles containing fragmented erythrocytes can be seen.

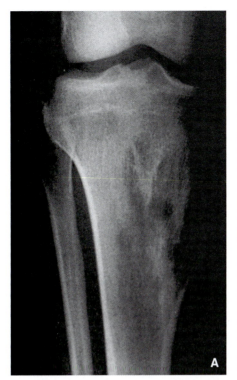
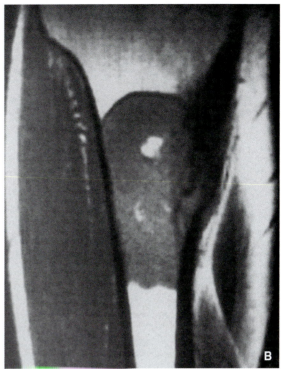
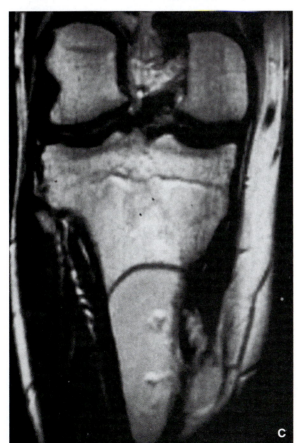

FIGURE 6.23 Radiography and magnetic resonance imaging of epithelioid hemangioendothelioma. **(A)** Anteroposterior radiograph of the proximal leg shows a radiolucent destructive lesion affecting medial aspect of the tibia. The cortex is destroyed. **(B)** Coronal T1-weighted MRI shows an intermediate signal intensity of the tumor replacing bone marrow. Small foci of high signal represent hemorrhagic areas. **(C)** Coronal T2-weighted MR image demonstrate heterogeneous but predominantly high signal intensity of the tumor that extends into the soft tissues.

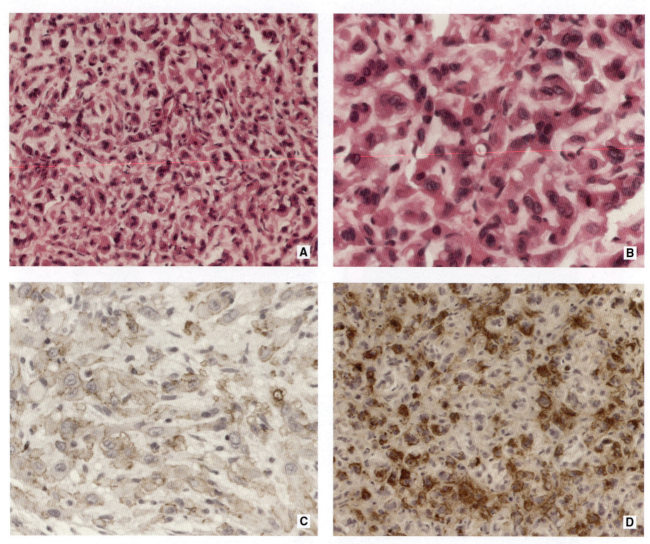

FIGURE 6.24 Histopathology of epithelioid hemangioendothelioma. (A) A pale-staining myxoid stroma is filled with single or cord-like proliferating plump epithelial cells that exhibit lack of obvious pleomorphism or significant mitotic activity (H&E, original magnification ×200). **(B)** Eosinophilic tumor cells contain intracytoplasmic vacuoles (H&E, original magnification ×400). **(C)** Immunohistochemistry shows intracytoplasmic vacuoles and membranous CD34 positivity (biotin–streptavidin peroxidase, original magnification ×400). **(D)** Also positive reaction is present to the endothelial marker FVIII-related antigen (biotin–streptavidin peroxidase, original magnification ×200).

- Tumor cells are arranged in cords and nests embedded in myxoid to hyalinized stroma, which may resemble chondroid matrix.
- Some cases may show nuclear pleomorphism and increased mitotic activity.
- Interanastomosing vascular channels often arranged in an antler-like pattern.
- Stroma varies from fibrous to myxoid.
- Small foci of hemorrhage or necrosis may be present.
- Vascular spaces may not be prominent.

Immunohistochemistry:
- Positive for CD31, CD34, Fli-1, factor VIII, D2-40, EGR, and may be positive for keratin and epithelial membrane antigen (EMA) (Fig. 6.24C,D).

Genetics:
- Translocation t(1;3)(p36;3:q25), the result in gene fusion of *WWTR1* in 3q25 and *CAMTA1* in 1p36.

Prognosis:
- Clinical course is variable.
- Involvement of more than one bone indicates worse prognosis.
- Histopathologic features are not of value in predicting the clinical course.

Differential Diagnosis:
- **Fibrosarcoma**
  Imaging features of fibrosarcoma may look similar to epithelioid hemangiosarcoma; however, histopathologic findings of sarcomatous spindle cells that form variable amount of collagen and particularly long fascicles of cells forming a "herringbone" pattern are diagnostic.
- **Metastasis**
  Imaging features of metastatic lesion may look similar to epithelioid hemangioendothelioma, and even

histopathology may show epithelioid morphology; however, immunohistochemical studies will be negative for CD34 and CD31.
- ***Plasmacytoma***
Imaging features of endosteal scalloping, and usually normal radionuclide bone scan, together with characteristic histopathologic findings showing extended sheets of population of atypical plasmacytoid cells, are diagnostic.

Angiosarcoma

Definition:
- High-grade vascular neoplasm composed of poorly formed blood vessels with endothelial differentiation.

Epidemiology:
- Represents less than 1% of malignant bone tumors.
- Age range between 20 and 80 years, with peak incidence during the third to fifth decade.
- Male-to-female ratio of 2:1.

Sites of Involvement:
- Wide skeletal distribution.
- Commonly (60%) involves long tubular bones (tibia, femur, humerus), pelvic bones, and axial skeleton, mainly the spine.
- Tendency to develop multifocal lesions in bone.

Clinical Features:
- Painful mass.
- Metastases to the lungs and other visceral organs occur in approximately 66% of cases.

Imaging:
- Imaging features similar to those of hemangioendothelioma, but more often, the tumor exhibits a wide zone of transition; cortical permeation and soft-tissue mass commonly present (Fig. 6.25).

Pathology:
Gross (Macroscopy):
- Firm, fleshy, and bloody mass; can erode the bone and extend to the soft tissues (Fig. 6.26).

Histopathology:
- Tissue ranging from well-differentiated lesions mimicking hemangiomas to poorly differentiated tumors difficult to diagnose as being of vascular nature.
- Tissue composed of tumor cells forming blood vessels that exhibit complicated infoldings and anastomoses (Fig. 6.27).
- Plump endothelial cells that line the blood vessels display features of frank malignancy showing nuclear hyperchromatism and atypical mitoses (Fig. 6.28A,B).
- Solid areas contain spindle and epithelioid cells encircled by reticulin fibers (Fig. 6.28C,D).

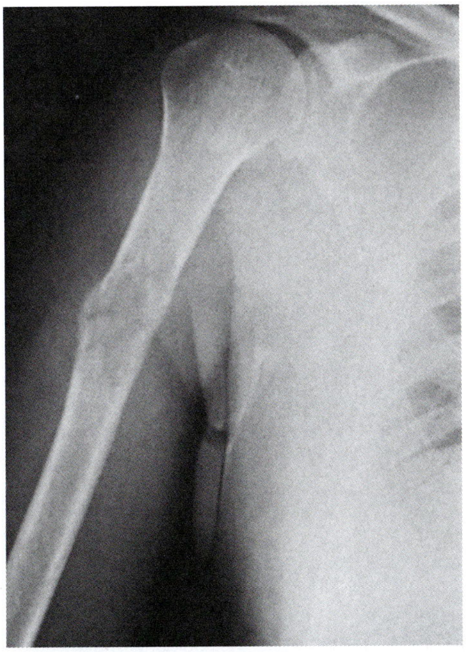

FIGURE 6.25 Radiography of angiosarcoma. An osteolytic lesion with wide zone of transition is present in the proximal right humerus of a 42-year-old man. Observe a pathologic fracture through the tumor and soft-tissue extension.

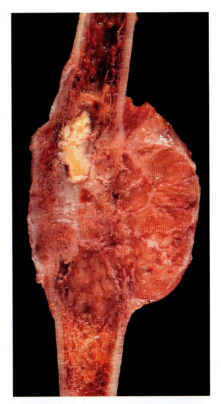

FIGURE 6.26 Gross specimen of angiosarcoma. Fleshy vascular tumor arising in the marrow cavity of the humerus invades the cortex and forms a large soft-tissue mass. (Courtesy of Peter Bullough, M.D., New York.)

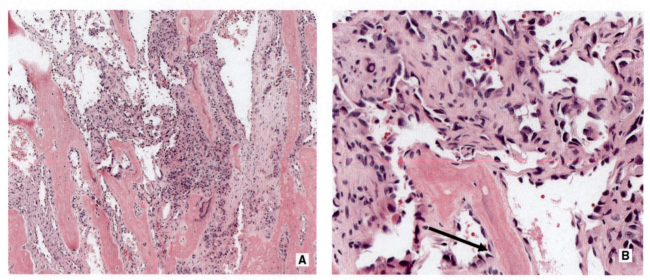

FIGURE 6.27 Histopathology of angiosarcoma. (A) Low-power view shows the pleomorphic tumor cells forming anastomosing vascular channels infiltrate between the bone trabeculae (H&E, original magnification ×100). **(B)** High-power view demonstrates that the tumor composed of plump hyperchromatic intraluminal cells invades the bone trabecula (*arrow*) (H&E, original magnification ×200).

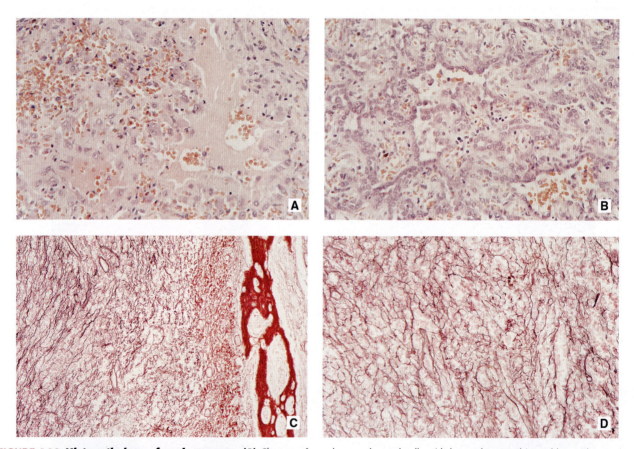

FIGURE 6.28 Histopathology of angiosarcoma. (A) Clusters of very large polygonal cells with large pleomorphic and hyperchromatic nuclei border blood-filled vascular spaces. Observe also the solid areas of the tumor (H&E, original magnification ×50). **(B)** In another field of view, the vascular spaces are larger and more prominent, pointing to the vascular nature of the tumor (H&E, original magnification ×50). **(C)** Reticulin fiber stain shows that the tumor cells lie corona-like within the rims of reticulin fibers (*black*). Note newly formed trabecular woven bone (*right*) (Novotny, original magnification ×25). **(D)** At higher magnification, the interconnecting network of vascular spaces each bound by the rim of reticulin fibers (*black*) is seen, surrounding a seam of large tumor cells (Novotny, original magnification ×50).

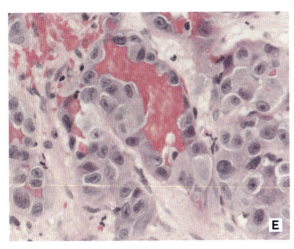 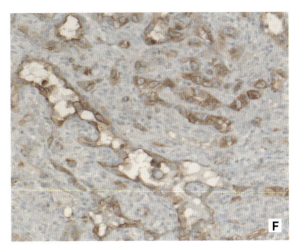

FIGURE 6.28 *(Continued)*. (E) Large epithelioid-appearing tumor cells line vascular spaces and protrude into the lumen (H&E, original magnification ×630). **(F)** Tumor cells lining vascular spaces and infiltrating the surrounding stroma are positive for CD31. Note luminar shedding of the tumor cells (biotin–streptavidin peroxidase, original magnification ×200).

- Reactive bone formation can be seen at the periphery of the tumor.
- Poorly differentiated tumors show more atypia, atypical mitotic figures, and necrosis.
- Some tumors may show epithelioid features mimicking carcinoma (Fig. 6.28E).
- Some tumors may show predominant spindle cell morphology mimicking primary bone sarcomas, such as undifferentiated pleomorphic sarcoma.
- Extravasated red blood cells may be seen, and scattered deposits of hemosiderin may also be present.
- Variable inflammatory infiltrates, predominantly composed of lymphocytes, may be seen.

Immunohistochemistry:
- Positive for vimentin, CD34, CD31 (Fig. 6.28F), factor VIII, and ulex europaeus.

Electron Microscopy:
- Endothelial cells contain Weibel-Palade bodies.

Genetics:
- Chromosomal translocations t(1;14)(p21;q24) were reported.
- Mutations of *PTPRB* and *PLCG1*.
- Genomic amplification of *MYC* was reported in radiation-induced angiosarcoma as well as in the primary angiosarcoma.

Prognosis:
- Poor prognosis.

Differential Diagnosis:
- Same as for epithelioid hemangioendothelioma.

REFERENCES

Abdelwahab IF. Sclerosing hemangiomatosis: a case report and review of the literature. *Br J Radiol.* 1991;64:894–897.

Abrahams TG, Bula W, Jones W. Epithelioid hemangioendothelioma of bone. *Skeletal Radiol.* 1992;21:509–513.

Assoun J, Richardi G, Railhac JJ, et al. CT and MRI of massive osteolysis of Gorham. *J Comput Assist Tomogr.* 1994;18:981–984.

Baker ND, Greenspan A, Neuwirth M. Symptomatic vertebral hemangiomas: a report of four cases. *Skeletal Radiol.* 1986;15:458–463.

Baudrez V, Galant C, Vande Berg BC. Benign vertebral hemangioma: MR-histological correlation. *Skeletal Radiol.* 2001;30:442–446.

Behjati S, Tarpey PS, Sheldon H, et al. Recurrent *PTPRB* and *PLCG1* mutations in angiosarcoma. *Nat Genet.* 2014;46:376–379.

Bergman AG, Rogers GW, Hellman B, Lones MA. Case report 841. Skeletal cystic angiomatosis. *Skeletal Radiol.* 1994;23:303–305.

Bergstrand A, Hook O, Lidvall H. Vertebral haemangiomas compressing the spinal cord. *Acta Neurol Scand.* 1963;39:59–66.

Bjorkengren AG, Resnick D, Haghighi P, Sartoris DJ. Intraosseous glomus tumor: report of a case and review of the literature. *AJR Am J Roentgenol.* 1986;147:739–741.

Boutin RD, Spaeth HJ, Mangalic A, Sell JJ. Epithelioid hemangioendothelioma of bone. *Skeletal Radiol.* 1996;25:391–395.

Boyle WJ. Cystic angiomatosis of bone. *J Bone Joint Surg [Br].* 1972;54B:626–636.

Brems H, Park C, Maertens O, et al. Glomus tumors in neurofibromatosis type 1: genetic, functional, and clinical evidence of a novel association. *Cancer Res.* 2009;69:7393–7401.

Brouillard P, Boon LM, Mulliken JB, et al. Mutations in a novel factor, glomulin, are responsible for glomuvenous malformations ("glomangiomas"). *Am J Hum Genet.* 2002;70:866–874.

Carstens HB, Ghadially FN, Henderson DW, Stirling JW. Case for the panel. Weibel-Palade body-like lamellar structure in angiosarcoma. *Ultrastruct Pathol.* 1995;19:137–143.

Choma ND, Biscotti CV, Bauer TW, Mehta AC, Licata AA. Gorham's syndrome: a case report and review of the literature. *Am J Med.* 1987;83:1151–1156.

Cohen MD, Rougraff B, Faught P. Cystic angiomatosis of bone: MR findings. *Pediatr Radiol.* 1994;24:256–257.

Coldwell DM, Baron RL, Charnsangavej C. Angiosarcoma: diagnosis and clinical course. *Acta Radiol.* 1989;30:627–631.

Cooper PH. Is histiocytoid hemangioma a specific pathologic entity? *Am J Surg Pathol.* 1988;12:815–817.

Daoud A, Olivieri B, Feinberg D, et al. Soft tissue hemangioma with osseous extension: a case report and review of the literature. *Skeletal Radiol.* 2015;44:597-603.

Davis AT, Gua AM, Phillips NJ, Greenberg DD. A novel treatment for bone lesions of multifocal epithelioid sarcoma-like hemangioendothelioma. *Skeletal Radiol.* 2015;44:1013-1019.

Dorfman HD, Czerniak B. *Bone Tumors.* 1st ed. St. Louis, MO: CV Mosby; 1998:746–747.

Dunlap JB, Magenis RE, Davis C, Himoe E, Mansoor A. Cytogenetic analysis of a primary bone angiosarcoma. *Cancer Genet Cytogenet.* 2009;194:1–3.

Enzinger FM, Weiss SW. Benign tumors and tumorlike lesions of blood vessels. In: Enzinger FM, Weiss SW, eds. *Soft Tissue Tumors.* 3rd ed. St. Louis, MO: CV Mosby; 1995.

Errani C, Zhang L, Panicek DM, Healey JH, Antonescu CR. Epithelioid hemangioma of bone and soft tissue: a reappraisal of a controversial entity. *Clin Orthop Relat Res.* 2011;470:1498–1506.

Errani C, Zhang L, Sung YS, et al. A novel WWTR1-CAMTA1 gene fusion is consistent abnormality in epithelioid hemangioendothelioma of different anatomic sites. *Genes Chromosomes Cancer.* 2011;50:644–653.

Errani C, Vanel D, Gambarotti M, Alberghini M, Picci P, Faldini C. Vascular bone tumors: a proposal of a classification based on clinicopathological, radiographic and genetic features. *Skeletal Radiol.* 2012;41:1495–1507.

Fayad L, Hazirolan T, Bluemke D, Mitchell S. Vascular malformations in the extremities: emphasis on MR imaging features that guide treatment options. *Skeletal Radiol.* 2006;35:127–137.

Fernandes BF, Al-Mujaini A, Petrogiannis-Haliotis T, Al-kandari A, Arthus B, Burnier MN. Epithelioid hemangioma (angiolymphoid hyperplasia with eosinophilia) of the orbit: a case report. *J Med Case Reports.* 2007;1:30–32.

Fletcher CDM, Unni KK, Mertens E, eds. *World Health Organization Classification of Tumours of Soft Tissue and Bone.* Lyon, France: IARC Press; 2013:281–296, 335–338.

Folpe AL. Glomus tumours. In: Fletcher CDM, Unni KK, Mertens F, eds. *World Health Organization Classification of Tumours. Pathology & Genetics. Tumours of Soft Tissue and Bone.* Lyon, France: IARC Press; 2002:136–137.

Folpe AL, Fanburg-Smith JC, Miettinen M, Weiss SW. Atypical and malignant glomus tumors: analysis of 52 cases, with a proposal for reclassification of glomus tumors. *Am J Surg Pathol.* 2001;25:1–12.

Friedman DP. Symptomatic vertebral hemangiomas: MR findings. *AJR Am J Roentgenol.* 1996;167:359–364.

Gaudino S, Martucci M, Colantonio R, et al. A systematic approach to vertebral hemangioma. *Skeletal Radiol.* 2015;44:25-36.

Gorham UV, Stout AP. Massive osteolysis (acute spontaneous absorption of bone, phantom bone, disappearing bone): its relation to haemangiomatosis. *J Bone Joint Surg Am.* 1955;37A:985–1004.

Gorham LW, Wright AW, Shultz HH, Mexon FC Jr. Disappearing bones: a rare form of massive osteolysis. *Am J Med.* 1954;17:674–682.

Greenspan A, Klein MJ, Bennett AJ, Lewis MM, Neuwirth M, Camins MB. Case report 242. Hemangioma of the T6 vertebra with a compression fracture, extradural block and spinal cord compression. *Skeletal Radiol.* 1978;10:183–188.

Griffith B, Yadam S, Mayer T, Mott M, van Holsbeeck M. Angiosarcoma of the humerus presenting with fluid-fluid levels on MRI: a unique imaging presentation. *Skeletal Radiol.* 2013;42:1611–1616.

Han BK, Ryu J-S, Moon DH, Shin MJ, Kim YT, Lee HK. Bone SPECT imaging of vertebral hemangioma. Correlations with MR imaging and symptoms. *Clin Nucl Med.* 1995;20:916–921.

Ignacio EA, Palmer KM, Mathur SC, Schwartz AM, Olan WJ. Residents' teaching files. Epithelioid hemangioendothelioma of the lower extremity. *Radiographics.* 1999;19:531–537.

Ishida T, Dorfman HD, Steiner GC, Norman A. Cystic angiomatosis of bone with sclerotic changes, mimicking osteoblastic metastases. *Skeletal Radiol.* 1994;23:247–252.

Italiano A, Thomas R, Breen M, et al. The miR--92 cluster and its target THBS1 are differentially expressed in angiosarcomas dependent on MYC amplification. *Genes Chromosomes Cancer.* 2012;51:569–578.

Jacobs JE, Kimmelstiel P. Cystic angiomatosis of the skeletal system. *J Bone Joint Surg Am.* 1953;35A:409–420.

Kleer CG, Unni KK, McLeod RA. Epithelioid hemangioendothelioma of bone. *Am J Surg Pathol.* 1996;20:1301–1311.

Kneeland JB, Middleton WD, Matloub HS, et. High resolution MR imaging of glomus tumor. *J Comput Assist Tomogr.* 1987;11:351–352.

Laredo JD, Reizine D, Bard M, Merland JJ. Vertebral hemangiomas: radiologic evaluation. *Radiology.* 1986;161:183–189.

Lateur L, Simoens CJ, Gryspeerdt S, Samson I, Mertens V, Van Damme B. Skeletal cystic angiomatosis. *Skeletal Radiol.* 1996;25:92–95.

Lomasney LM, Martinez S, Demos TC, Harrelson JM. Multifocal vascular lesions of bone: imaging characteristics. *Skeletal Radiol.* 1996;25:255–261.

Maki DD, Nesbit ME, Griffith HJ. Diffuse lymphangiomatosis of bone. *Australas Radiol.* 1999;43:535–538.

Manner J, Radlwimmer B, Hohenberger P, et al. MYC high level gene amplification is a distinctive feature of angiosarcomas after irradiation or chronic lymphedema. *Am J Pathol.* 2010;176:34–39.

Meyer JS, Hoffer FA, Barnes PD, Mulliken JB. Biological classification of soft-tissue vascular anomalies: MR correlation. *AJR Am J Roentgenol.* 1991;157:559–564.

Moukaddam H, Pollak J, Haims AH. MRI characteristics and classification of peripheral vascular malformations and tumors. *Skeletal Radiol.* 2009;38:535–547.

Mulliken JB, Glowacki J. Hemangiomas and vascular malformations in infants and children: a classification based on endothelial characteristics. *Plast Reconstr Surg.* 1982;69:412–420.

Mulliken JB, Zetter BR, Folkman J. In vitro characteristics of endothelium from hemangiomas and vascular malformations. *Surgery.* 1982;92:348–353.

Nielsen GP, Srivastava A, Kattapuram S, et al. Epithelioid hemangioma of bone revisited: a study of 50 cases. *Am J Surg Pathol.* 2009;33:270–277.

O'Connell JX, Kattapuram SV, Mankin HJ, Bhan AK, Rosenberg AE. Epithelioid hemangioma of bone. A tumor often mistaken for low-grade angiosarcoma or malignant hemangioendothelioma. *Am J Surg Pathol.* 1993;17:610–617.

O'Connell JX, Nielsen GP, Rosenberg AE. Epithelioid vascular tumors of bone: a review and proposal of a classification scheme. *Adv Anat Pathol.* 2001;8:74–82.

Ozel A, Uysal E, Dokucu AI, Erturk SM, Basak M, Cantisani V. US, CT and MRI findings in a case of diffuse lymphangiomatosis and cystic hygroma. *J Ultrasound.* 2008;11:22–25.

Patel DV. Gorham's disease or massive osteolysis. *Clin Med Res.* 2005;3:65–74.

Renjen P, Kovanlikaya A, Narula N, Brill PW. Importance of MRI in the diagnosis of vertebral involvement in generalized lymphangiomatosis. *Skeletal Radiol.* 2014;43:1633–1638.

Righi A, Gambarotti M, Picci P, et al. Primary pseudomyogenic hemangioendothelioma of bone: report of two cases. *Skeletal Radiol.* 2015;44:727-731.

Rigopoulou A, Saifuddin A. Intraosseous hemangioma of the appendicular skeleton: imaging features of 15 cases, and review of the literature. *Skeletal Radiol.* 2012;41:1525–1536.

Rozmaryn LM, Sadler AH, Dorfman HD. Intraosseous glomus tumor in ulna. A case report. *Clin Orthop Relat Res.* 1987;220:126–129.

Ruggieri P, Montalti M, Angelini A, Alberghini M, Mercuri M. Gorham-Staut disease: the experience of the Rizzoli Institute and review of the literature. *Skeletal Radiol.* 2011;40:1391–1397.

Settakorn J, Chalidapong P, Rangdaeng S, Arpornchayanon O, Chaiwun B. Primary intraosseous glomus tumor: a case report. *J Med Assoc Thai.* 2001;84:1641–1645.

Spieth ME, Greenspan A, Forrester DM, Ansari AN, Kimura RL, Gleason-Jordan I. Gorham's disease of the radius: radiographic, scintigraphic, and MRI findings with pathologic correlation. *Skeletal Radiol.* 1997;26:659–663.

Stewart DR, Sloan JL, Yao L, et al. Diagnosis, management, and complications of glomus tumors of the digits in neurofibromatosis type 1. *J Med Genet.* 2010;47:525–532.

Sung MS, Kim YS, Resnick D. Epithelioid hemangioma of bone. *Skeletal Radiol.* 2000;29:530–534.

Theumann NH, Goettmann S, Le Viet D, et al. Recurrent glomus tumors of fingertips: MR imaging evaluation. *Radiology.* 2002;223:143–151.

Urakawa H, Nakashima Y, Yamada Y, Tsushima M, Ohta T, Nishio T. Intraosseous glomus tumor of the ulna: a case report and a review of the literature. *Nagoya J Med Sci.* 2008;70:127–133.

van der Linden-van der Zwaag HMJ, Onvlee GJ. Massive osteolysis (Gorham's disease) affecting the femur. *Acta Orthop Belg.* 2006;72:261–268.

van der Mey AG, Maaswinkel-Mooy PD, Cornelisse CJ, Schmidt PH, van de Kamp JJ. Genomic imprinting in hereditary glomus tumours: evidence for new genetic theory. *Lancet.* 1989;2:1291–1294.

Vilanova JC, Barceló J, Smirniotopoulos JG, et al. Hemangioma from head to toe: MR imaging with pathologic correlation. *Radiographics.* 2004;24:367–385.

Waldron RT, Zeller JA. Diffuse skeletal hemangiomatosis with visceral involvement. *J Can Assoc Radiol.* 1969;20:119–123.

Wenger DE, Wold LE. Benign vascular lesions of bone: radiologic and pathologic features. *Skeletal Radiol.* 2000;29:63–74.

Wenger DE, Wold LE. Malignant vascular lesions of bone: radiologic and pathologic features. *Skeletal Radiol.* 2000;29:619–631.

Wold LE, Swee RG, Sim FH. Vascular lesions of bone. *Pathol Annu.* 1985;20(2):101–137.

Wunderbaldinger P, Paya K, Partik B, et al. CT and MRI imaging of generalized cystic lymphangiomatosis in pediatric patients. *AJR Am J Roentgenol.* 2000;174:827–832.

Yang DH, Goo HW. Generalized lymphangiomatosis: radiologic findings in three pediatric patients. *Korean J Radiol.* 2006;7:287–291.

CHAPTER 7

Miscellaneous Lesions

Several benign and malignant lesions that did not fit into the classification included in the previous chapters are discussed here. *Giant cell tumor*, a locally aggressive neoplasm, occurs almost exclusively after skeletal maturity, when the growth plates are obliterated. Less than 5% of these lesions are malignant, although no clear imaging criteria are established to render such diagnosis. *Simple bone cyst*, also known as unicameral bone cyst, is a tumor-like lesion of unknown cause, attributed to a local disturbance of bone growth. Although its pathogenesis is still debatable, the lesion appears to be reactive or developmental rather than to represent a true neoplasm. *Aneurysmal bone cyst* may arise *de novo* in bone, or it may be associated with various benign (e.g., giant cell tumor, osteoblastoma, chondroblastoma, chondromyxoid fibroma, fibrous dysplasia) or malignant (e.g., osteosarcoma, fibrosarcoma, chondrosarcoma) lesions. *Giant cell reparative granuloma*, also known as a solid variant of aneurysmal bone cyst, is a lesion very similar to ABC taking in consideration its morphology and biologic behavior. *Intraosseous lipoma* is a rare lesion; in fact, many so-called intraosseous lipomas on closer examination turned out to be merely the simple hyperplasia of normal fatty bone marrow. *Adamantinoma of long bones* is a malignant tumor characterized by the formation of epithelial cells surrounded by a spindle cell fibrous tissue. A close relationship of this tumor to osteofibrous dysplasia and fibrous dysplasia has been suggested by some investigators. Moreover, some pathologists, on the basis of clinical course and of molecular and immunohistochemical analysis, suggested that osteofibrous dysplasia may be a precursor lesion of adamantinoma. *Chordoma* is a tumor that arises from developmental embryonic remnants of the notochord, with predilection to the spinal axis. Primary *leiomyosarcoma of bone* is a very rare bone malignancy composed of spindle cells exhibiting smooth muscle differentiation. *Intraosseous liposarcoma* is an extraordinary rare tumor with only handful of cases described in the literature.

A. Benign Lesions
Giant Cell Tumor (GCT)
Simple Bone Cyst (SBC)
Aneurysmal Bone Cyst (ABC)
Giant Cell Reparative Granuloma (GCRG, Solid Variant of ABC)
Intraosseous Lipoma

B. Malignant Tumors
Adamantinoma of Long Bones
Chordoma
Leiomyosarcoma of Bone
Liposarcoma of Bone

A. BENIGN LESIONS

Giant Cell Tumor (GCT)

Definition:
- Benign but locally aggressive tumor composed of proliferating ovoid mononuclear stroma cells interspersed with evenly distributed osteoclast-like multinucleated giant cells.

Epidemiology:
- Represents about 5% of all primary bone tumors and 20% of benign primary bone tumors and is the sixth most common primary osseous neoplasm.
- Occurs almost invariably after skeletal maturity.
- The peak incidence is between ages 20 and 45, with mean age of 32.
- Female-to-male ratio of 2:1.

Sites of Involvement:
- Characteristically affects the articular ends of bone.
- Long bones are affected in 60% of cases.
- Preferential sites include the distal femur, proximal tibia, distal radius, proximal humerus, and sacrum.
- Less than 5% affects short tubular bones of the hands and feet.
- Very uncommonly the tumor is multifocal (usually associated with Paget disease).

Clinical Findings:
- Pain of increasing intensity associated with local swelling and tenderness in the affected areas.
- Limitation of motion in the adjacent joints.
- Pathologic fractures occur in 5% to 10% of patients.
- Less than 1% may undergo malignant transformation (mostly in older patients).
- Tumor may extend to soft tissue or metastasize to the lung (intravascular invasion).
- May arise in association with Goltz syndrome (focal dermal hypoplasia).

Imaging:
- Radiography shows eccentric lytic lesion with geographic type of bone destruction without sclerotic border extending into the articular end of bone, commonly without periosteal reaction (Figs. 7.1 and 7.2); lack of matrix mineralization; internal trabeculations may be present (Fig. 7.3); occasionally "soap-bubble" appearance; invasion of the cortex and soft-tissue mass may be seen (Fig. 7.4).
- Scintigraphy invariably shows increased uptake of the radiopharmaceutical agent (see Fig. 7.7B). In about 50% of cases, an abnormal pattern of uptake resembling a doughnut was observed.
- Computed tomography may outline the tumor extension and delineate better the cortical destruction (Figs. 7.5 to 7.7).
- Magnetic resonance imaging shows intermediate-to-low signal on T1-weighted sequences and high signal intensity on T2-weighting and other water-sensitive sequences. After intravenous administration of gadolinium, there is usually heterogeneous enhancement of the tumor (Figs. 7.7 to 7.10).

Pathology:
Gross (Macroscopy):
- Tumor tissue is usually soft and reddish brown, with occasional yellowish areas of xanthomatous change and firmer whitish areas representing fibrosis (Fig. 7.11).
- Cystic and hemorrhagic spaces may be seen mimicking aneurysmal bone cyst.

Histopathology:
- Tumor is composed of dual population of fibrocytic or monocytic round to oval in shape polygonal or elongated mononuclear stromal cells mixed with numerous evenly

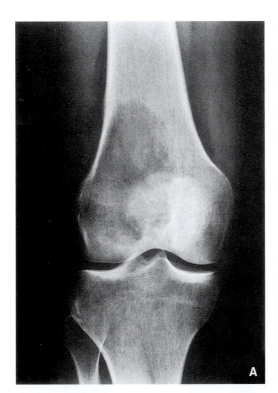 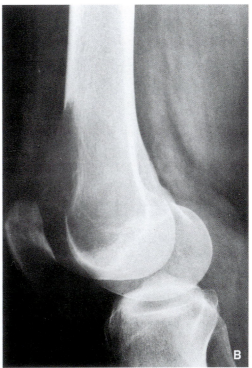

FIGURE 7.1 Radiography of giant cell tumor. (A) Anteroposterior and **(B)** lateral radiographs of the right knee of a 32-year-old man show a purely osteolytic lesion affecting the distal end of the femur. Note its narrow zone of transition, eccentric location, absence of reactive sclerosis, and the extension into the articular end of bone.

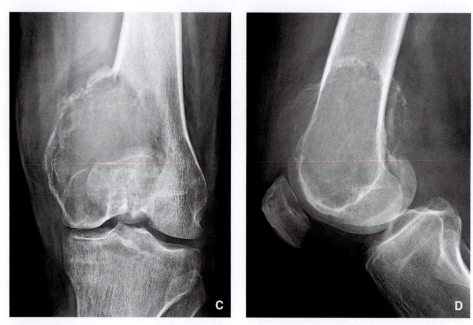

FIGURE 7.1 *(Continued).* **(C)** Anteroposterior and **(D)** lateral radiographs of the left knee of a 58-year-old man show eccentric osteolytic expansive lesion of the medial femoral condyle.

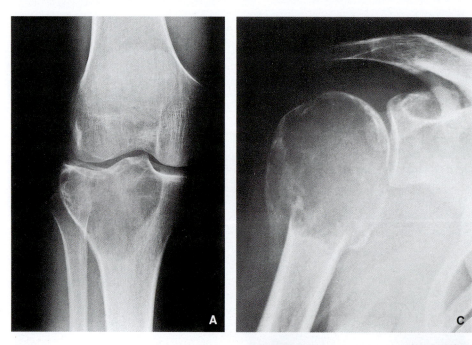

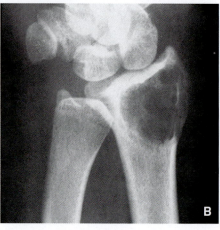

FIGURE 7.2 Radiography of giant cell tumor. (A) Anteroposterior radiograph of the right knee of a 30-year-old woman shows an osteolytic lesion eccentrically located in the proximal tibia, extending into the articular end of bone. **(B)** In another patient, a 25-year-old man, an eccentric osteolytic lesion extends into the articular end of distal radius. **(C)** Radiolucent lesion in a 27-year-old woman affects almost the entire proximal end of the right humerus. Observe a pathologic fracture at the distal extent of the tumor.

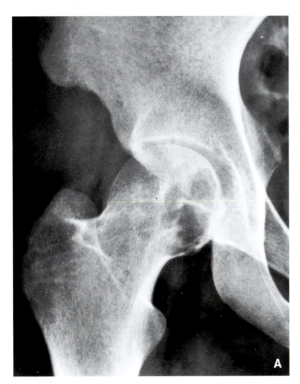
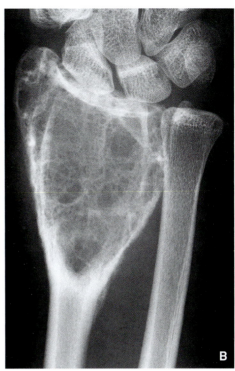

FIGURE 7.3 Radiography of giant cell tumor. (A) Anteroposterior radiograph of the right hip of a 27-year-old woman shows a radiolucent lesion with internal trabeculations in the femoral head. **(B)** Anteroposterior radiograph of the left wrist of a 36-year-old woman shows a trabeculated lesion in the distal radius.

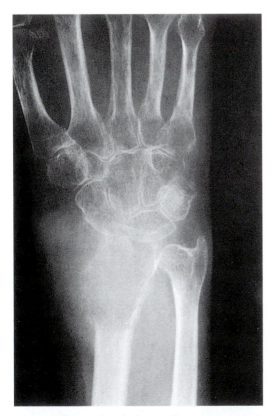

FIGURE 7.4 Radiography of giant cell tumor. Dorsovolar radiograph of the left wrist of a 56-year-old woman demonstrates an osteolytic lesion in the distal radius that has destroyed the cortex and extended into the soft tissues. Despite these aggressive features, the histopathologic examination revealed no malignancy.

- distributed, different in size, large osteoclast-like giant cells, which contain 20 to 100 nuclei (Figs. 7.12 and 7.13).
- The giant cells, unlike normal osteoclasts, do not possess a ruffled border and are not apposed to bone surfaces.
- It is generally accepted that the characteristic large osteoclast-like giant cells are not neoplastic.
- Mononuclear cells, arising from primitive mesenchymal stromal cells, represent the neoplastic component.
- Nuclei of the mononuclear stromal cells are very similar to those of the giant cells, having an open chromatin pattern and contain one or two small nucleoli.
- The cytoplasm is ill defined, and there is sparse intercellular collagen.
- Mitotic figures are invariably present, but no atypical mitoses are present.
- Fibrous histiocytoma-like storiform pattern may occasionally be seen.
- Secondary aneurysmal bone cyst changes may occur in 10% of cases.
- One-third of cases show presence of intravascular plugs, particularly at the periphery of the tumor.
- Areas of necrosis and hemorrhage, and occasional groups of foam cells and hemosiderin-laden macrophages may be present in large lesions.
- Small foci of reactive osteoid or bone formation may be seen, especially after a pathologic fracture of the tumor or prior biopsy.

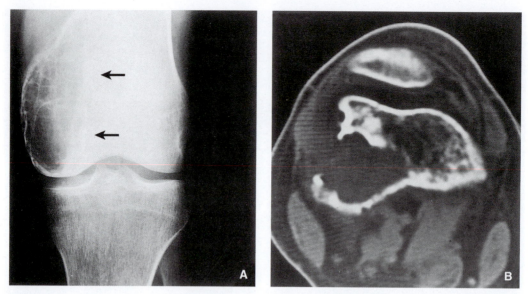

FIGURE 7.5 Radiography and computed tomography of giant cell tumor. (A) Anteroposterior radiograph of the left knee of a 33-year-old woman shows an osteolytic lesion in the medial femoral condyle (*arrows*). **(B)** Axial CT section through the tumor demonstrates destruction of the cortex and the presence of a soft-tissue mass.

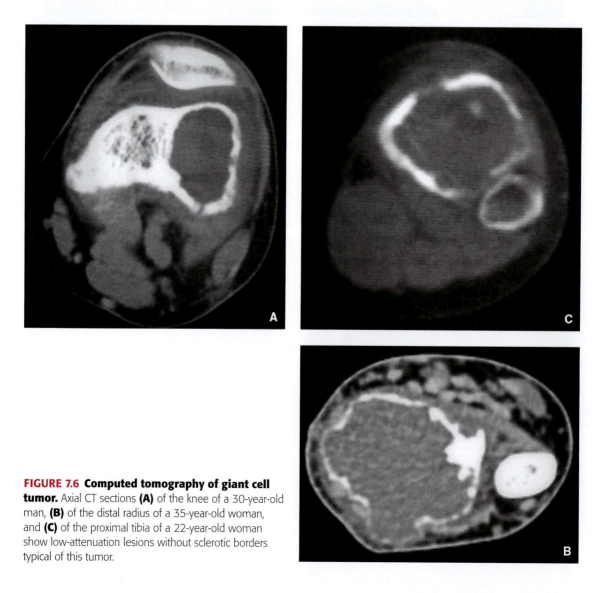

FIGURE 7.6 Computed tomography of giant cell tumor. Axial CT sections **(A)** of the knee of a 30-year-old man, **(B)** of the distal radius of a 35-year-old woman, and **(C)** of the proximal tibia of a 22-year-old woman show low-attenuation lesions without sclerotic borders typical of this tumor.

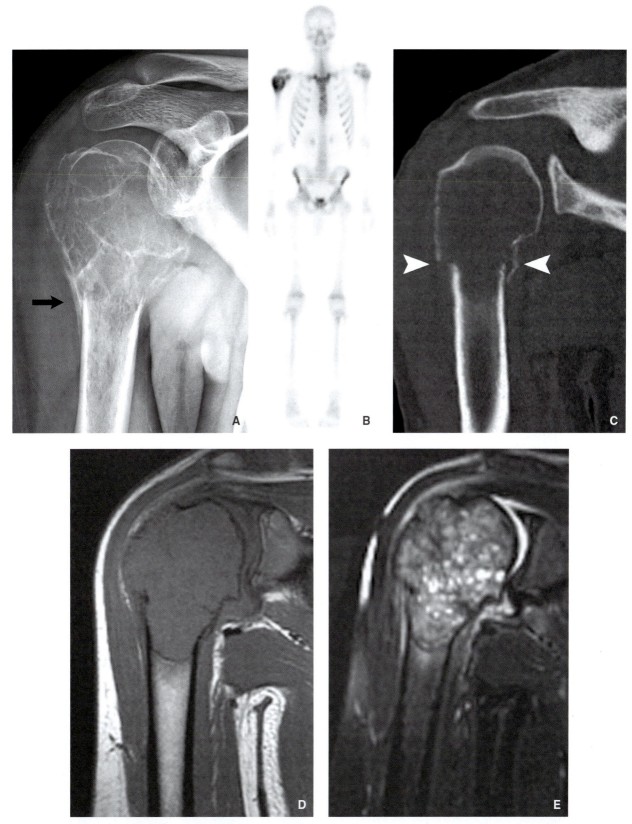

FIGURE 7.7 Radiography, scintigraphy, computed tomography, and magnetic resonance imaging of giant cell tumor.
(A) Anteroposterior radiograph of the right shoulder of a 19-year-old man shows an expansive radiolucent lesion of the proximal humerus with internal septations. Observe a pathologic fracture (*arrow*). **(B)** Total body radionuclide bone scan shows an increase uptake of the radiopharmaceutical tracer by the tumor. **(C)** Coronal reformatted CT image shows a pathologic fracture to better advantage (*arrowheads*). **(D)** Coronal T1-weighted MR image shows the lesion to be of homogeneous intermediate signal intensity. **(E)** Coronal T2-weighted fat-suppressed MRI shows heterogenous appearance of the tumor with foci of high signal intensity. Observe high-signal joint effusion.

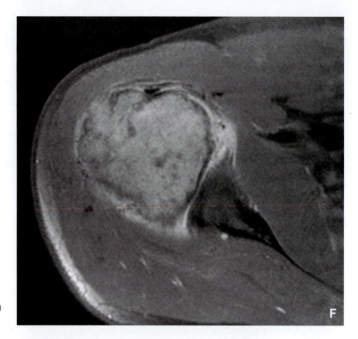

FIGURE 7.7 *(Continued).* **(F)** Axial T1-weighted fat-suppressed MR image obtained after intravenous administration of gadolinium shows heterogeneous enhancement of the tumor.

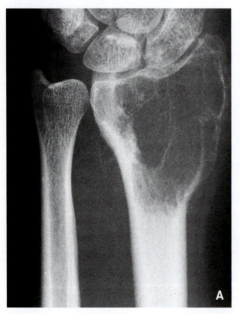
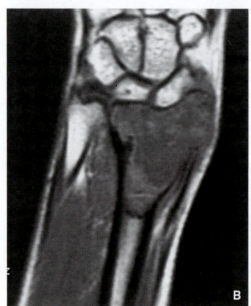
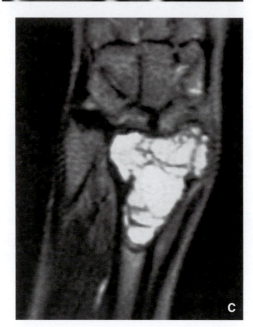

FIGURE 7.8 Radiography and magnetic resonance imaging of giant cell tumor. **(A)** Dorsovolar radiograph of the right wrist of a 36-year-old woman shows an osteolytic lesion of the distal radius. **(B)** Coronal T1-weighted MR image shows the tumor to be of intermediate-to-low signal intensity. **(C)** On coronal T2-weighted MRI, the lesion becomes bright, displaying low signal septations.

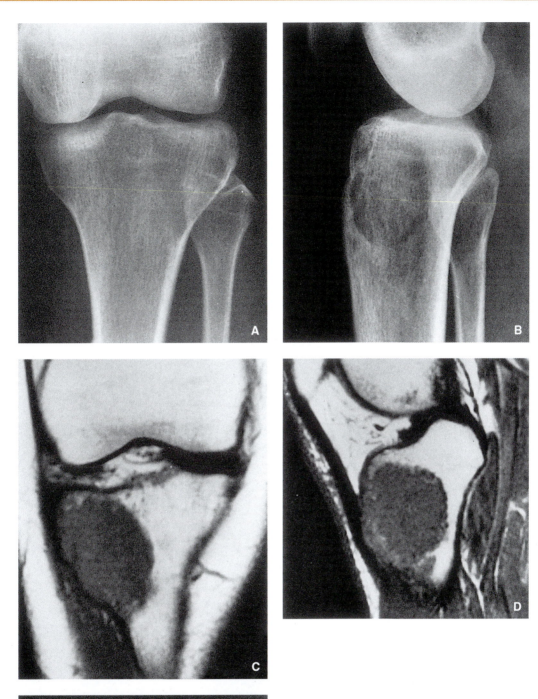
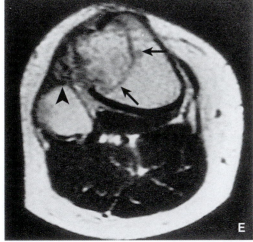

FIGURE 7.9 Radiography and magnetic resonance imaging of giant cell tumor.
(A) Anteroposterior and **(B)** lateral radiographs of the left knee of a 45-year-old woman show a radiolucent lesion in the proximal tibia. **(C)** Coronal and **(D)** sagittal T1-weighted MR images accurately outline the extent of the tumor, which displays an intermediate signal intensity. **(E)** Axial MRI reveals that the tumor (*arrows*) has penetrated the lateral cortex of the tibia and extends into the soft tissues (*arrowhead*).

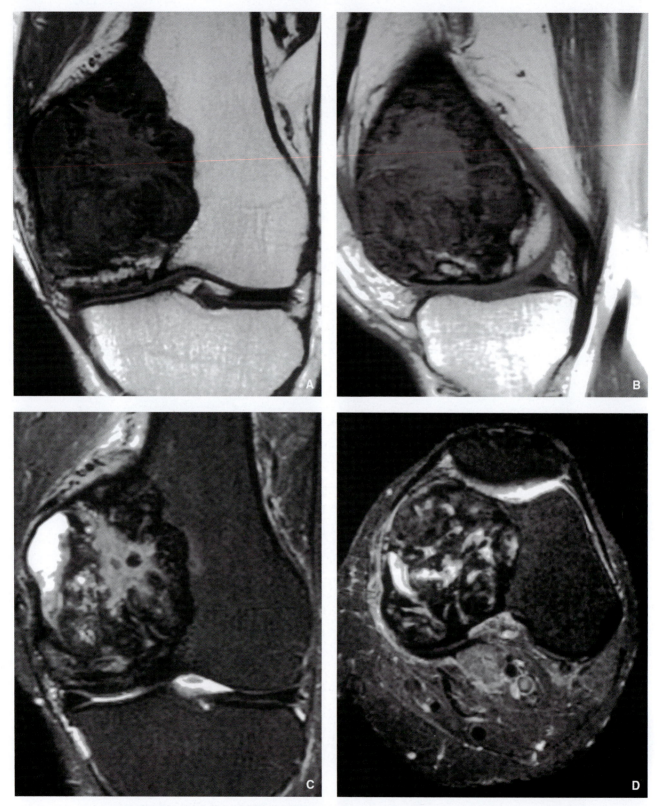

FIGURE 7.10 Magnetic resonance imaging of giant cell tumor. (A) Coronal and **(B)** sagittal T1-weighted MR images of the left knee of a 37-year-old woman show a low signal intensity lesion in the medial femoral condyle. The tumor extends to the articular end of bone. **(C)** Coronal and **(D)** axial T2-weighted MR images show that the tumor exhibits heterogeneous signal.

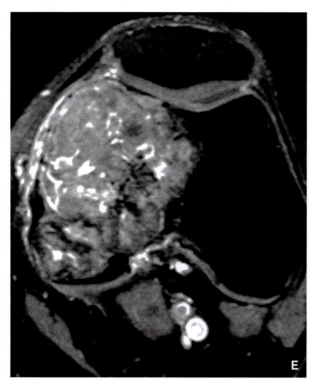

- Reactive woven bone formation can be present in old-standing tumors.
- Atypical mitotic figures and the presence of pleomorphic cells may indicate malignant transformation (Fig. 7.14).

Genetics:
- Telomeric associations (end-to-end fusions of apparently intact chromosomes) are the most frequent chromosomal aberration.
- Telomeres most commonly affected are 11p, 13p, 14p, 15p, 19q, 20q, and 21p.
- Some tumors showed rearrangement of chromosomes 16q22 and 17p13.
- Loss of heterozygosity (LOH) of 1p, 3p, 5q, 9q, 10q, and 19q has been reported.

Prognosis:
- Giant cell tumor is locally aggressive and occasionally produces distant metastases.
- Histopathologic features do not predict the extent of local aggression or local recurrence rate.
- Local recurrence occurs in approximately 25% of patients and is usually seen within 2 years.
- Pulmonary metastases may be seen in 2% of the patients on average 3 to 4 years after original diagnosis.

FIGURE 7.10 *(Continued).* **(E)** Axial T1-weighted fat-suppressed MRI obtained after intravenous administration of gadolinium shows significant enhancement of the tumor.

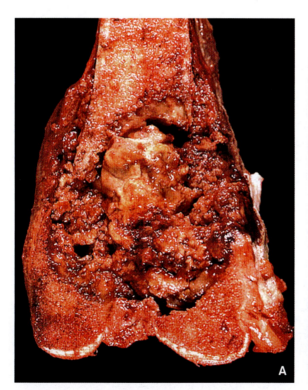
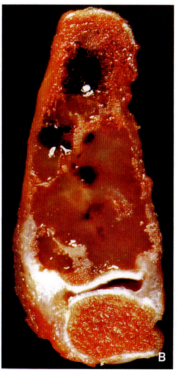

FIGURE 7.11 Gross specimen of giant cell tumor. (A) Coronal section of the resected surgical specimen of the distal femur shows a lobulated intramedullary tumor with hemorrhagic foci braking through the cortex and extending into the articular end of bone. **(B)** Coronal section of the surgical specimen of the first metacarpal bone shows pinkish-tan soft intramedullary mass exhibiting foci of hemorrhage. Observe extension of the tumor to the proximal end of bone and preservation of the first carpometacarpal joint. (B—from Bullough PG. *Atlas of Orthopedic Pathology with Clinical and Radiologic Correlations*. 2nd. ed. New York, NY: Gower Medical Publishing; 1992, p. 17.7, Fig. 17.17.)

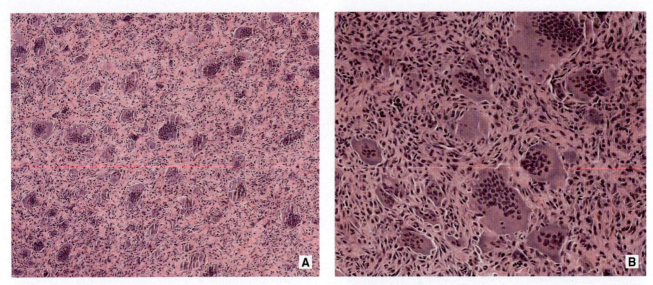

FIGURE 7.12 Histopathology of the giant cell tumor. (A) A low-power photomicrograph shows dual population of elongated mononuclear stromal cells mixed with numerous evenly distributed osteoclast-like giant cells exhibiting multiple nuclei (H&E, original magnification ×50). **(B)** High-power view shows the details of the large giant cells containing numerous nuclei (H&E, original magnification ×200).

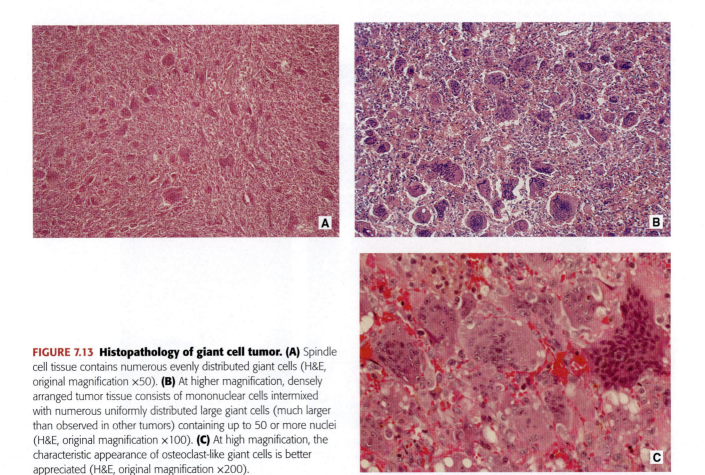

FIGURE 7.13 Histopathology of giant cell tumor. (A) Spindle cell tissue contains numerous evenly distributed giant cells (H&E, original magnification ×50). **(B)** At higher magnification, densely arranged tumor tissue consists of mononuclear cells intermixed with numerous uniformly distributed large giant cells (much larger than observed in other tumors) containing up to 50 or more nuclei (H&E, original magnification ×100). **(C)** At high magnification, the characteristic appearance of osteoclast-like giant cells is better appreciated (H&E, original magnification ×200).

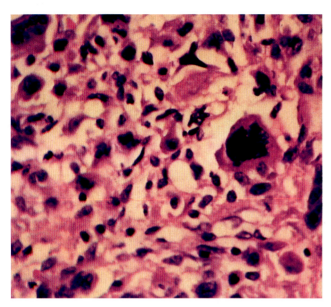

FIGURE 7.14 Histopathology of malignant giant cell tumor. Marked pleomorphism and nuclear atypia with sparse atypical giant cells scattered throughout the lesion are characteristic features of this malignancy. (From Bullough PG. *Atlas of Orthopedic Pathology with Clinical and Radiologic Correlations*. 2nd ed. New York, NY: Gower Medical Publishing; 1992, p. 17.8, Fig. 17.22.)

Differential Diagnosis:

- ***Aneurysmal bone cyst***
  Imaging studies show invariably presence of periosteal reaction in form of a well-defined buttress; sclerotic margin is a common feature; fluid–fluid levels on MR imaging is characteristic.
  Histopathology may show giant cells, but they are smaller than those of giant cell tumor and are in clusters rather than being evenly distributed; fibrous cell proliferation is often associated with strands of irregular islands of osteoid or bone.
- ***Intraosseous ganglion***
  Imaging may be similar to the giant cell tumor, since the intraosseous ganglion is radiolucent, eccentric, and located at the articular end of bone but, unlike GCT, invariably exhibits sclerotic margin; MRI shows no fluid–fluid levels.
  Histopathologic studies show lack of typical features of GCT, such as dual population of fibrocytic or monocytic mononuclear stromal cells and evenly distributed osteoclast-like giant cells.
- ***Fibrosarcoma***
  Imaging appearance of some lesions may be similar to the giant cell tumor; however, involvement of the articular end of bone is uncommon.
  Histopathology showing fascicles of spindle cells exhibiting characteristic "herringbone tweed" pattern is diagnostic.
- ***Plasmacytoma***
  Imaging appearance of some lesions may be similar to the giant cell tumor; however, the lesion is commonly central and not eccentric in location within the bone; involvement of the articular end of bone is unusual; the tumor affects much older population than giant cell tumor.
  Histopathology showing sheets of closely packed cells, which resemble normal plasma cells with eccentric nuclei; clustered chromatin with cartwheel pattern and prominent nucleoli; and abundant, dense basophilic cytoplasm, coupled with characteristic immunohistochemistry findings showing positivity for CD138, CD38, and MUM1, is diagnostic.
- ***Osteolytic metastasis***
  Imaging appearance of solitary metastatic lesion may be very similar to giant cell tumor; soft-tissue mass, however, is less common; generally, metastatic lesion does not extend into articular end of bone; metastases are present in much older population.
  Histopathology occasionally showing the origin of metastatic lesion, and immunohistochemistry studies (particularly application of cytokeratins), are diagnostic.
- ***Brown tumor of hyperparathyroidism***
  Solitary lytic bone lesion representing brown tumor of hyperparathyroidism may look on the imaging studies similar to the giant cell tumor; however, MRI shows often low signal intensity of the lesion, reflecting magnetic susceptibility to hemosiderin; other features of hyperparathyroidism including osteopenia, subperiosteal and chondral resorption, and soft-tissue calcifications are also helpful in the differential diagnosis.
  Histopathology showing clusters of multinucleated giant cells within fibroblastic and reactive stroma in addition to clumps of hemosiderin pigment is diagnostic.

Simple Bone Cyst (SBC)

Definition:
- Intramedullary, tumor-like lesion of unknown cause, attributed to local disturbance of bone growth, usually unilocular cyst filled with serous or serosanguineous fluid.

Epidemiology:
- Represents approximately 3% of all primary bone lesions.
- Eighty percent of patients are in the first two decades of life.
- Male-to-female ratio of 3:1.

Sites of Involvement:
- Any bone can be affected with most common locations of the proximal humerus followed by the proximal femur and proximal tibia.
- Metaphysis and proximal diaphysis are the most common sites in the long bone.

Clinical Findings:
- May be asymptomatic.
- The first symptom may be a pathologic fracture.
- Pain and local swelling.

Imaging:

- Radiography shows centrally located, well-circumscribed radiolucent lesion with sclerotic margins (Figs. 7.15 to 7.19) and absence of periosteal reaction (unless there has been a pathologic fracture); "fallen fragment" sign is a diagnostic feature (see Fig. 7.19).
- Magnetic resonance imaging shows intermediate signal intensity on T1-weighted sequences and homogenously high signal on T2-weighted and other water-sensitive sequences (Figs. 7.20 and 7.21).

Pathology:

Gross (Macroscopy):

- Well-demarcated cystic cavity with glistening membrane, and occasionally thin grayish-white fragments (Fig. 7.22).

Histopathology:

- Cyst's wall consists of a thin layer of fibrous tissue composed of scattered fibroblasts and collagen fibers, with occasionally a flattened single-cell lining (Fig. 7.23).
- Pathologic fractures may cause reactive changes and result in the presence of numerous reactive fibroblasts, osteoclast-type giant cells, hemosiderin deposits, and reactive woven bone.

Genetics:

- Clonal rearrangements involving chromosomes 4, 6, 8, 16, and 21.
- Translocation t(16;20)(p11.2;q13) has been described.

Prognosis:

- Recurrence after surgical treatment has been reported in about 10% to 20% of cases, especially in children.
- Growth arrest of the affected bone and avascular necrosis of the head of the femur after pathologic fracture have been reported.
- Spontaneous healing after pathologic fracture has been reported.

Differential Diagnosis:

- **Aneurysmal bone cyst**
  Imaging studies show eccentric location of the lesion and periosteal reaction in the form of a buttress; MRI shows fluid–fluid levels.

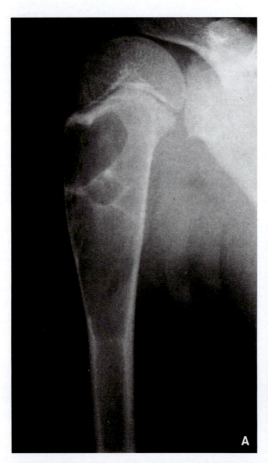 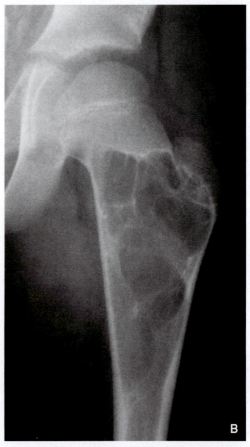

FIGURE 7.15 Radiography of simple bone cyst. (A) Anteroposterior radiograph of the right shoulder of a 6-year-old boy shows the radiolucent lesion centrally located in the metaphysis of the proximal humerus, extending into the diaphysis, exhibiting narrow zone of transition, geographic type of bone destruction, and pseudosepta. The cortex is slightly thinned out. Note the lack of periosteal reaction. **(B)** Anteroposterior radiograph of the left hip of an 11-year-old girl shows characteristic features of this lesion, very similar to those presented in part (A).

Histopathology shows solid areas containing giant cells and fibrous cell proliferation often associated with strands of irregular islands of osteoid or bone.
- **Nonossifying fibroma**
  Imaging studies show the lesion to be eccentric in location, commonly with lobulated, thick sclerotic border, and magnetic resonance imaging exhibits features of a solid, not cystic, lesion.
  Histopathology showing bland monomorphous spindle cells admixed with histiocytic cells commonly arranged in a swirling storiform pattern is diagnostic.
- **Monostotic fibrous dysplasia**
  Radiography shows characteristic rind sign; occasionally noted are focal calcifications.
  Magnetic resonance imaging exhibits features of a solid, not cystic, lesion.
  Histopathology showing metaplastic woven bone trabeculae resembling Chinese characters without osteoblastic activity is diagnostic.

Aneurysmal Bone Cyst (ABC)

Definition:
- Benign multiloculated, blood-filled cystic mass that is often expansive and locally destructive; may arise *de novo* in bone or may arise secondary within various benign and malignant osseous lesions.
- Primary aneurysmal bone cysts account for approximately 70% of all cases.
- Majority of secondary ABC arise in association with benign lesions, most commonly giant cell tumor of

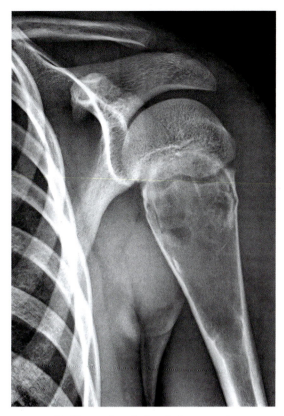

FIGURE 7.16 Radiography of simple bone cyst. Anteroposterior radiograph of the left shoulder of a 12-year-old boy shows a radiolucent lesion of the humeral diaphysis, extending into the metaphysis and abutting the growth plate. Observe a narrow zone of transition, thinning of the cortex, and lack of periosteal reaction.

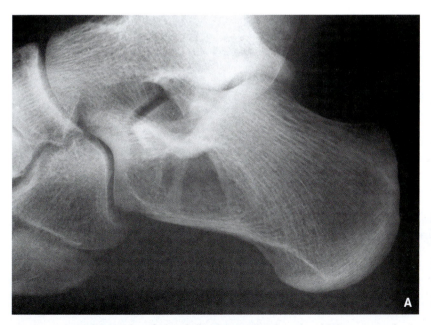 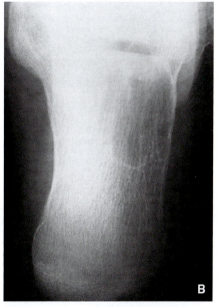

FIGURE 7.17 Radiography of simple bone cyst. (A) Lateral and **(B)** Harris-Beath views of the left hindfoot of a 32-year-old man demonstrate a radiolucent lesion in the calcaneus, exhibiting a thin sclerotic border. Typically, bone cysts occurring at this site are located in the anterolateral aspect of the bone.

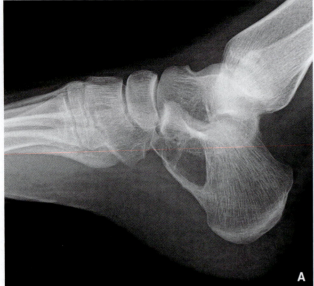
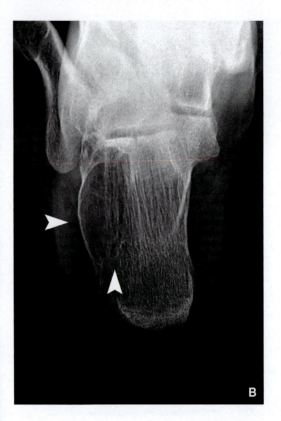
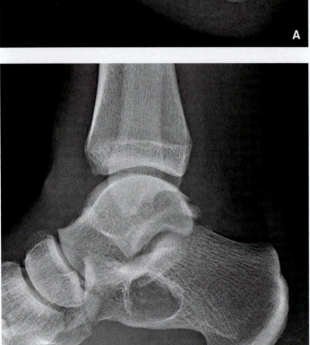

FIGURE 7.18 Radiography of simple bone cyst. **(A)** Lateral and **(B)** Harris-Beath views of the right hindfoot of a 35-year-old woman show a radiolucent lesion in the anterolateral aspect of the calcaneus (*arrowheads*). **(C)** A lateral radiograph of the hindfoot of a 20-year-old man shows a similar radiolucent lesion in the anterior calcaneus exhibiting a narrow zone of transition and a thin sclerotic border.

bone, chondroblastoma, osteoblastoma, chondromyxoid fibroma, and fibrous dysplasia, and less frequently, osteosarcoma or chondrosarcoma.

Epidemiology:
- Affects all age groups, but most common during the first two decades of life, 76% of cases occurring in patients younger than 20 years.
- No sex predilection.

Sites of Involvement:
- May affect any bone, but usually arises in the metaphysis of the long bones.
- Most common locations are the femur, tibia, humerus, and posterior elements (neural arch) of the vertebra.

Clinical Findings:
- Pain and local swelling.
- Occasionally, a pathologic fracture may be the first symptom.
- Neurologic symptoms if lesion is located in the spine.

Imaging:
- Radiography shows an eccentric, multicystic radiolucent lesion, commonly expansive, with buttress of periosteal reaction; narrow zone of transition and geographic type of bone destruction are characteristic features (Figs. 7.24 to 7.27); soft-tissue extension may be present (Fig. 7.28, see also Fig. 7.32).
- Skeletal scintigraphy shows increased uptake of radiopharmaceutical tracer (see Figs. 7.30 and 7.31).

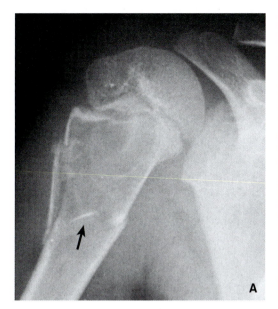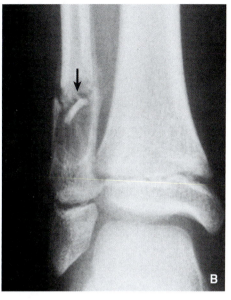

FIGURE 7.19 Radiography of simple bone cyst. (A) One of the most common complications of this lesion is a pathologic fracture, as seen here in the proximal humeral diaphysis of a 6-year-old boy. The presence of a "fallen fragment" sign (*arrow*) is a characteristic feature. **(B)** Anteroposterior radiograph of the right ankle of a 5-year-old boy shows a radiolucent lesion in the distal diaphysis of the fibula that underwent a pathologic fracture. A radiodense cortical fragment in the center of the lesion (*arrow*) represents the "fallen fragment" sign, identifying this lesion as a cystic structure.

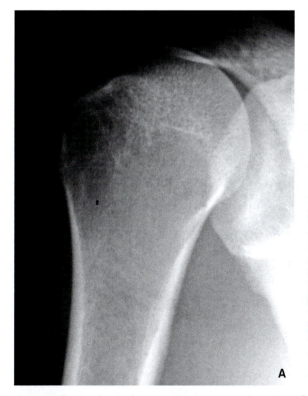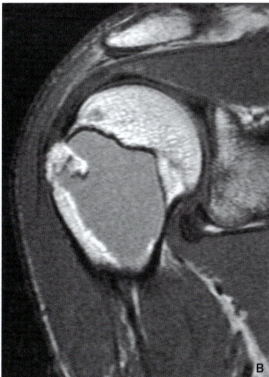

FIGURE 7.20 Radiography and magnetic resonance imaging of simple bone cyst. (A) Anteroposterior radiograph of the right shoulder of a 22-year-old man shows a radiolucent lesion with a narrow zone of transition in the proximal humeral shaft. **(B)** Coronal T1-weighted MRI shows the lesion to be of homogeneous intermediate signal intensity.

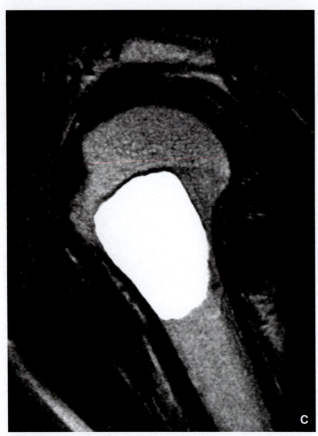

FIGURE 7.20 *(Continued).* **(C)** Sagittal T2-weighted MR image demonstrates homogeneous high signal intensity of the fluid-filled cyst.

- Computed tomography shows to better advantage the internal ridges and may demonstrate a shell of periosteal reaction surrounding the soft-tissue mass, not always well shown on the conventional radiography (Figs. 7.29 to 7.33).
- Magnetic resonance imaging shows cystic cavities exhibiting fluid–fluid levels (see Figs. 7.31E,F, 7.33C, 7.34E,F, and 7.35B). The wide range of signal intensities within the cyst on both T1- and T2-weighted images is probably due to settling of degraded blood products and reflects intracystic hemorrhages of different ages (Figs. 7.31 to 7.35).

Pathology:

Gross (Macroscopy):

- Well-defined sponge-like mass composed of multiple, blood-filled spaces separated by thin, tan-white septa; solid foci of various size may be present (Fig. 7.36).

Histopathology:

- Well circumscribed and composed of blood-filled cystic spaces lined by a single layer of flat undifferentiated cells (that react negatively with all endothelial markers), separated by fibrous septa, alternating with solid areas (Figs. 7.37 and 7.38).
- Fibrous septa are composed of uniform plump fibroblasts (which may show active mitoses without atypia),

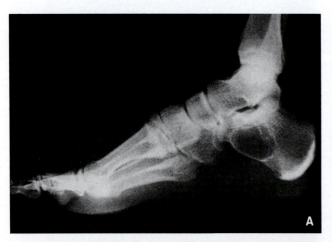
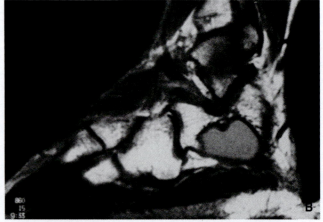

FIGURE 7.21 Radiography and magnetic resonance imaging of simple bone cyst. (A) Lateral radiograph of the right foot of an 18-year-old man shows a radiolucent lesion with thin sclerotic border within the calcaneus. **(B)** Sagittal T1-weighted MRI demonstrates homogeneous intermediate signal intensity within the lesion, rimmed by low signal intensity sclerotic margin.

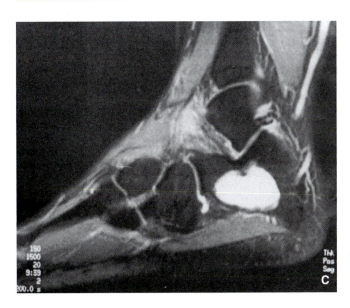

FIGURE 7.21 (Continued). (C) Sagittal STIR MRI shows the lesion exhibiting homogeneous high signal intensity consistent with fluid content.

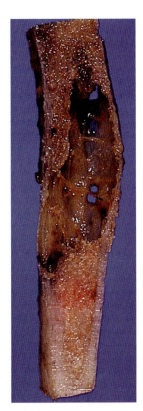

FIGURE 7.22 Gross specimen of simple bone cyst. Coronal section of resected segment of the humerus reveals a well-demarcated cystic cavity in the medullary portion of the bone. Note cortical thinning and glistening lining of the cyst. (From Bullough PG. *Atlas of Orthopedic Pathology with Clinical and Radiologic Correlations*. 2nd ed. New York, NY: Gower Medical Publishing; 1992, p. 15.4, Fig. 15.10.)

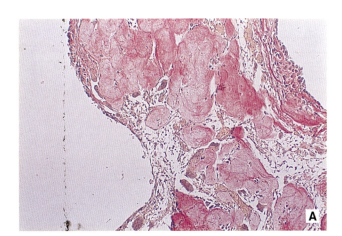

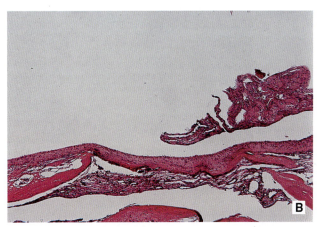

FIGURE 7.23 Histopathology of simple bone cyst. (A) The cyst cavity *(left)* is bordered by an undifferentiated flat cell layer. In the loose connective tissue of the cyst wall, there are extended areas of a "cloudy," loose collagen-positive material (van Gieson, original magnification ×25). **(B)** Flattened fibrous lining of the cyst contains a few bone trabeculae (H&E, original magnification ×25).

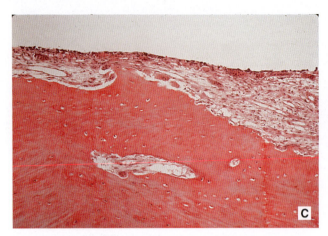
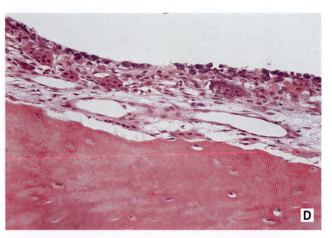

FIGURE 7.23 *(Continued).* **(C)** At higher magnification, observe within the fibrous lining several giant cells (H&E, original magnification ×100). **(D)** High-magnification photomicrograph shows more clearly the flat fibrous lining with scattered giant cells (H&E, original magnification ×250).

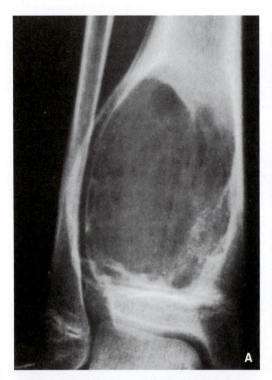
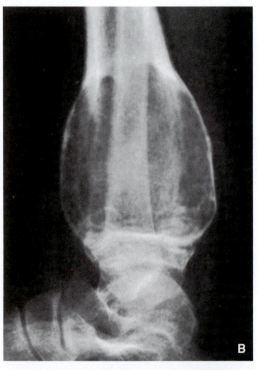

FIGURE 7.24 Radiography of aneurysmal bone cyst. (A) Anteroposterior and **(B)** lateral radiographs of the right lower leg of an 8-year-old girl show an expansive radiolucent lesion in the metaphysis of the distal tibia, abutting the growth plate and extending into the diaphysis. Observe its eccentric location in the bone and the solid buttress of periosteal reaction at the proximal aspect of the lesion.

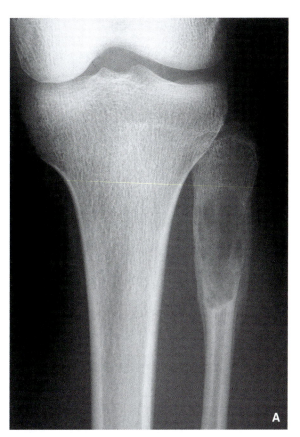 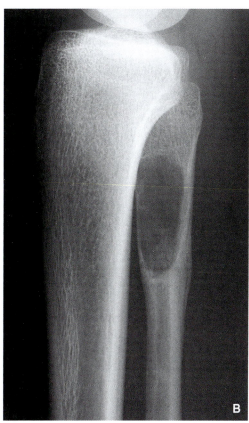

FIGURE 7.25 Radiography of aneurysmal bone cyst. (A) Anteroposterior and **(B)** lateral radiographs of the upper leg of a 17-year-old girl show a radiolucent lesion in the proximal fibula exhibiting a narrow zone of transition, a sclerotic border, and a well-organized periosteal reaction.

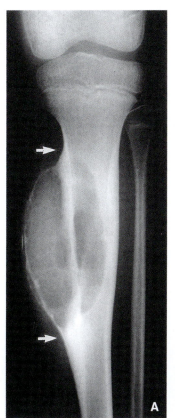 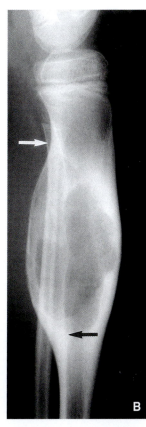

FIGURE 7.26 Radiography of aneurysmal bone cyst. (A) Anteroposterior and **(B)** lateral radiographs of the left upper leg of a 10-year-old girl show characteristic appearance of this lesion in the proximal tibia, including eccentric location, expansive character, and buttress of periosteal reaction proximally and distally (*arrows*).

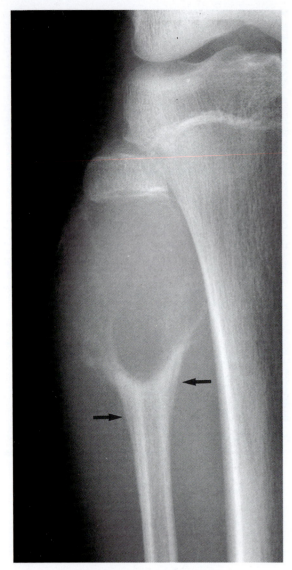

FIGURE 7.27 Radiography of aneurysmal bone cyst. A large, radiolucent expansive lesion in the proximal fibula of an 11-year-old girl reveals a buttress of periosteal reaction (*arrows*).

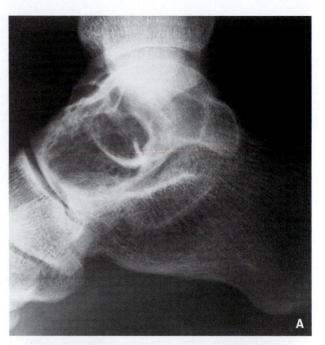

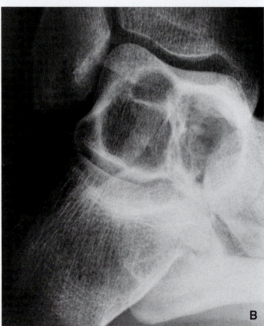

FIGURE 7.29 Radiography and computed tomography of aneurysmal bone cyst. (A) Anteroposterior and **(B)** oblique radiographs of the right ankle of a 24-year-old woman show a radiolucent, trabeculated lesion in the talus. Coronal CT sections through the tibiotalar joint.

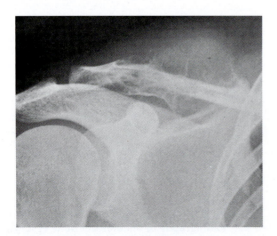

FIGURE 7.28 Radiography of aneurysmal bone cyst. Anteroposterior radiograph of the right shoulder of a 19-year-old woman shows an expansive, trabeculated lesion in the midportion of the clavicle. Note a soft-tissue extension.

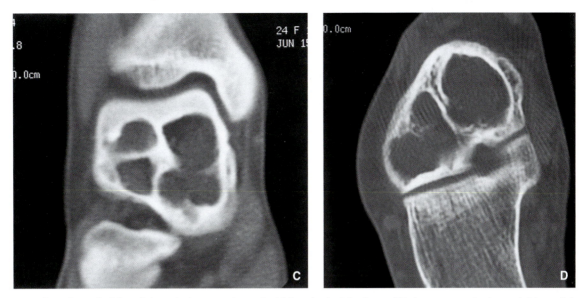

FIGURE 7.29 *(Continued).* **(C)** and through the posterior and middle subtalar joint facets **(D)** demonstrate the internal ridges of the lesion to better advantage.

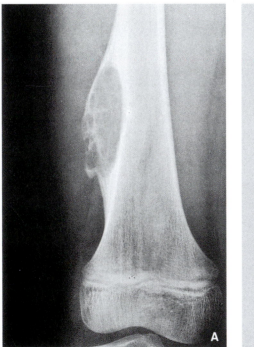

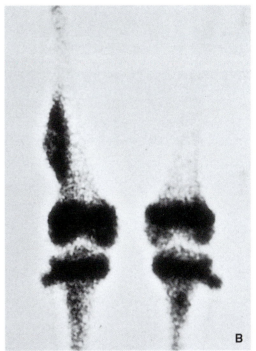

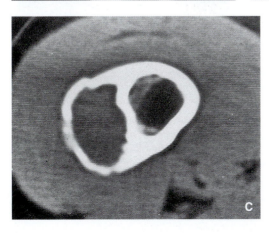

FIGURE 7.30 Radiography, scintigraphy, and computed tomography of aneurysmal bone cyst. (A) Anteroposterior radiograph of the right distal femur of an 8-year-old boy shows an eccentric, expansive radiolucent lesion in the femoral diaphysis. Observe a solid buttress of periosteal reaction at both ends of the lesion. **(B)** Radionuclide bone scan obtained after intravenous administration of 10 mCi (375 MBq) of technetium-99m–labeled methylene diphosphonate (MDP) shows increased uptake of radiopharmaceutical tracer by the lesion. **(C)** Axial CT section shows intracortical location of the lesion, which balloons out from the lateral aspect of the femur but is contained within an uninterrupted shell of periosteal new bone.

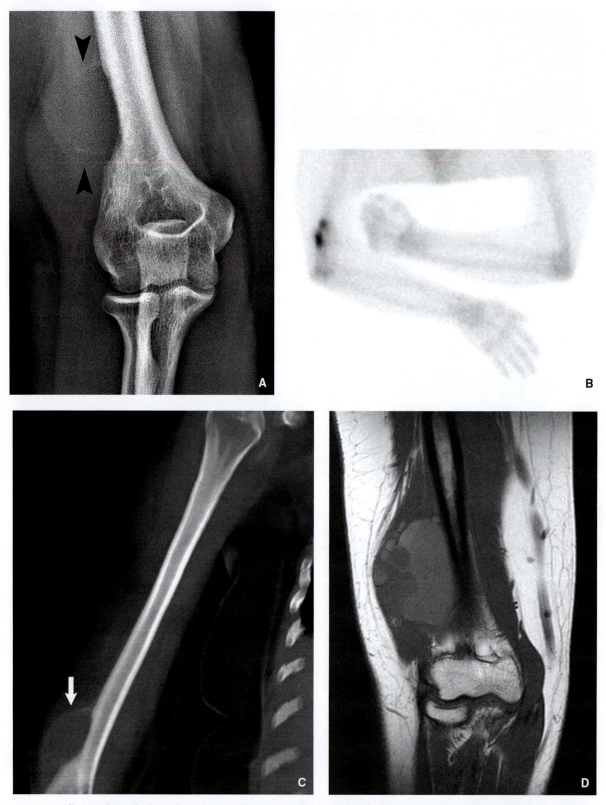

FIGURE 7.31 Radiography, scintigraphy, computed tomography, and magnetic resonance imaging of aneurysmal bone cyst. (A) Anteroposterior radiograph of the right elbow of a 21-year-old man shows an eccentric, expansive radiolucent lesion arising from the medial cortex of the distal humerus. Observe the soft-tissue extension (*arrowheads*). **(B)** Radionuclide bone scan shows increased uptake of the radiopharmaceutical tracer by the lesion. **(C)** 3D CT image reconstructed in maximum intensity projection (MIP) shows the soft-tissue mass contained by a thin shell of periosteal new bone (*arrow*). **(D)** Coronal T1-weighted MRI shows heterogeneous but predominantly intermediate signal intensity eccentric lesion extending into the soft tissues and compressing the high signal subcutaneous fat.

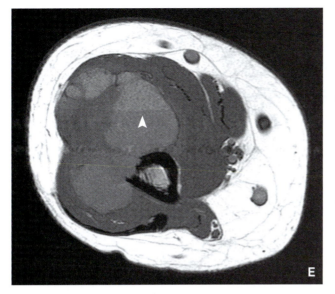
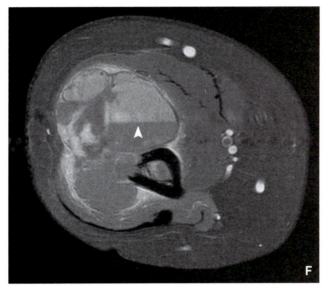
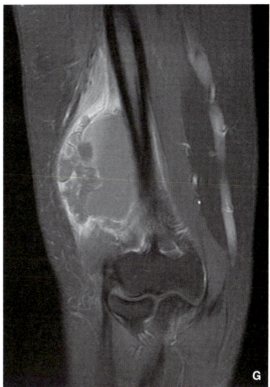

FIGURE 7.31 *(Continued).* **(E)** Axial T1-weighted and **(F)** T2-weighted MR images demonstrate fluid–fluid level within the lesion (*arrowhead*). **(G)** Coronal T1-weighted fat-suppressed contrast-enhanced MRI shows peripheral enhancement of the cyst.

multinucleated osteoclast-like giant cells, usually in clusters (sometimes they look like "jumping into swimming pool" of cystic spaces), and reactive woven bone rimmed by osteoblasts (Fig. 7.39).
- Solid tissue surrounding vascular spaces is composed of fibrous, richly vascular connective tissue (Figs. 7.40 and 7.41).
- Some of the reactive bone is basophilic and has been called "blue bone."
- Deposits of iron pigment are common findings.
- Atypical mitotic figures are absent (if, however, present, diagnosis of telangiectatic osteosarcoma should be contemplated).
- Necrotic areas are rare, unless there was a prior pathologic fracture.

Genetics:
- Rearrangements of the *USP6* (ubiquitin-specific peptidase 8/Tre-2) gene at chromosome 17q13.
- Clonal rearrangements of chromosome bands 16q22 and 17p13.
- Chromosome translocation t(16;17)(q22;p13).

Prognosis:
- Recurrence rate following curettage is variable (20% to 70%).

Differential Diagnosis:
- ***Simple bone cyst***
  Imaging studies show central location in bone and lack of "ballooning," periosteal reaction, or soft-tissue extension. If a pathologic fracture occurs, the "fallen fragment" sign is diagnostic.
  Histopathology shows thin layer of fibrous tissue composed of scattered fibroblasts and collagen fibers covering the cyst's wall; however, solid areas with significant number of giant cells are not present.

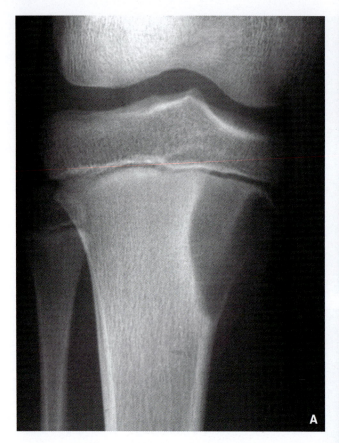
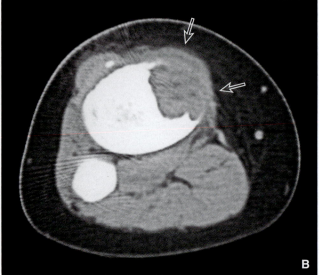
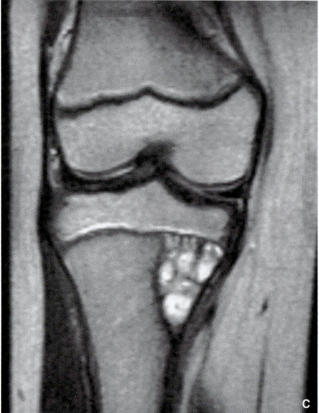

FIGURE 7.32 Radiography, computed tomography, and magnetic resonance imaging of aneurysmal bone cyst. **(A)** Anteroposterior radiograph of the right knee of a 9-year-old girl shows an eccentric radiolucent lesion in the medial tibial metaphysis abutting the growth plate. **(B)** Axial CT section shows a pathologic fracture of the tibia and extension of the lesion into the soft tissues (*arrows*). **(C)** Coronal T2-weighted MRI shows heterogeneous but predominantly high signal intensity of the lesion.

- *Giant cell tumor*
  Imaging studies show invariably closed growth plate and extension into the articular end of bone, commonly without periosteal reaction.
  Histopathology showing dual population of fibrocytic or monocytic mononuclear cells mixed with numerous evenly distributed large giant cells is diagnostic.
- *Chondromyxoid fibroma*
  Imaging findings, particularly radiography, may be very similar to those of ABC; however, MRI will demonstrate features of solid tumor, without characteristic for the cystic lesion feature of fluid–fluid levels.
  Histopathology showing lobulated appearance of the tumor tissue, and typical cartilaginous morphology is diagnostic.
- *Telangiectatic osteosarcoma*
  Imaging features may be indistinguishable from those of ABC, although the tumor usually shows more aggressive appearance.

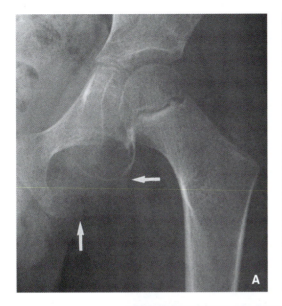
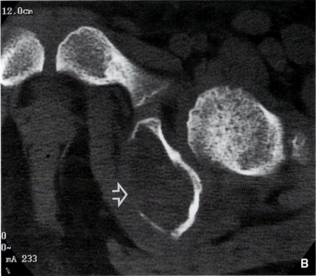
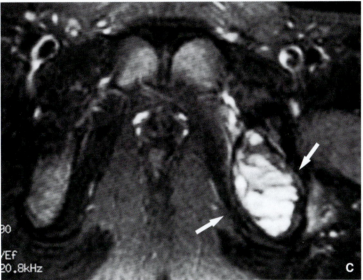

FIGURE 7.33 Radiography, computed tomography, and magnetic resonance imaging of aneurysmal bone cyst.
(A) Anteroposterior radiograph of the left hip of a 4-year-old girl shows an expansive radiolucent lesion destroying the ischial bone (*arrows*).
(B) Axial CT section demonstrates that the lesion broke through the medial cortex of the ischium (*open arrow*). **(C)** Axial T2-weighted MRI shows high signal intensity of the lesion (*arrows*) exhibiting multiple fluid–fluid levels.

Histopathology showing pleomorphic tumor tissue in close proximity to and bordering the blood-filled spaces, and presence of anaplastic cells is diagnostic.

Giant Cell Reparative Granuloma (GCRG, Solid Variant of ABC)

Definition:
- Nonneoplastic hemorrhagic process in bones, similar to aneurysmal bone cyst on the basis of morphology and biologic behavior.

Epidemiology:
- Most common in the second and third decades, with mean age of 18 years.
- Seventy-four percent of patients are younger than 30 years.
- Male-to-female ratio of 1:1.4.

Sites of Involvement:
- Short tubular bones of the hands and feet, followed by craniofacial bones; less common in the long bones such as the femur, tibia, and ulna.
- Multicentric presentation has been reported.

Clinical Findings:
- Usually asymptomatic condition.
- Sometimes painful swelling at the site of the lesion.

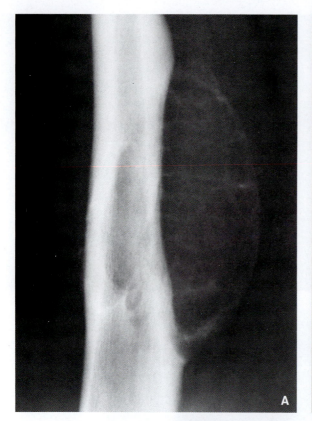
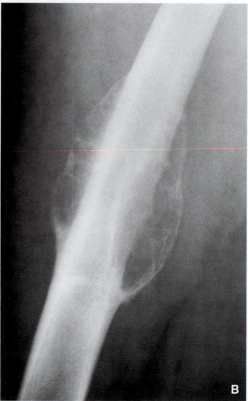
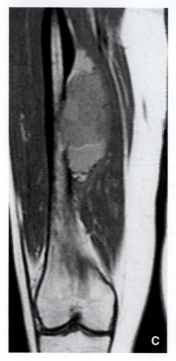
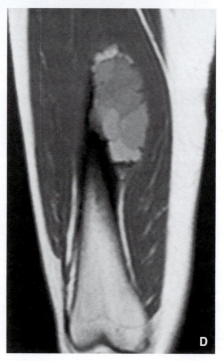

FIGURE 7.34 Radiography and magnetic resonance imaging of aneurysmal bone cyst. (A) Anteroposterior and **(B)** lateral radiographs of the midshaft of the right femur of a 15-year-old girl show an expansive lesion arising eccentrically from the medial aspect of the bone. Observe a thin shell of periosteal bone covering the lesion, and a buttress of periosteal reaction at the proximal and distal extent of the cyst. **(C,D)** Two coronal T1-weighted MR images show heterogeneity of the lesion and internal septations.

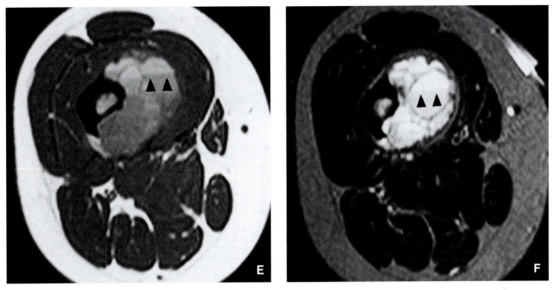

FIGURE 7.34 *(Continued).* **(E)** Axial T1-weighted and **(F)** axial T2-weighted MR images show characteristic for this lesion fluid–fluid level *(arrowheads)*.

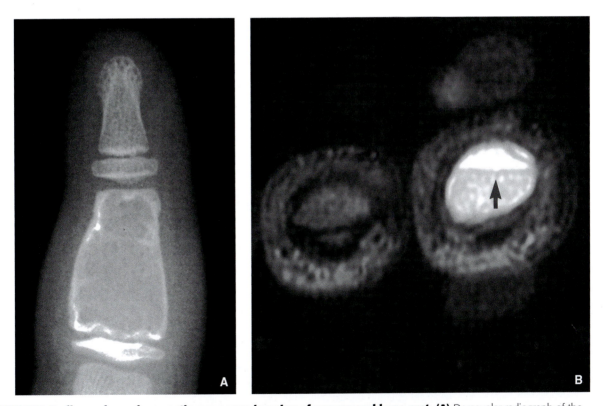

FIGURE 7.35 Radiography and magnetic resonance imaging of aneurysmal bone cyst. (A) Dorsovolar radiograph of the ring finger of a 6-year-old boy shows a radiolucent lesion with scalloped borders centrally located in the middle phalanx, resembling an enchondroma. **(B)** Axial T2-weighted fat-suppressed MRI shows a fluid–fluid level *(arrow)*, inconsistent with diagnosis of a solid tumor. Excision biopsy revealed an aneurysmal bone cyst.

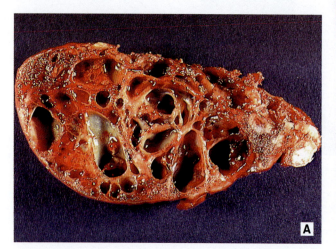
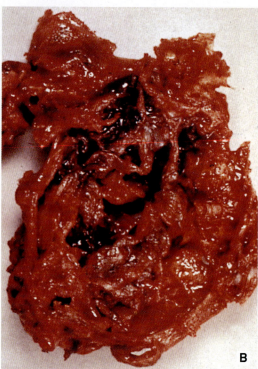

FIGURE 7.36 Gross specimen of aneurysmal bone cyst. (A) The tumor consists of a red spongy, honeycomb mass with cystic spaces of various sizes filled with blood and osseous tissue within some of the septated walls. (A—from Bullough PG. *Atlas of Orthopedic Pathology with Clinical and Radiologic Correlations*. 2nd ed. New York, NY: Gower Medical Publishing; 1992, p. 15.7, Fig. 15.18). **(B)** Surgical specimen removed from the neural arch of C2 shows a gritty osseous tumor with multiple blood-filled cystic spaces separated by fibrous septa.

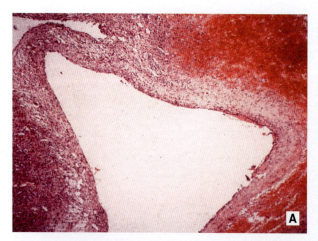
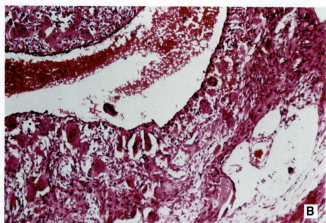

FIGURE 7.37 Histopathology of aneurysmal bone cyst. (A) Cystic spaces lined by flat undifferentiated cells are separated by solid tissue containing spindle cells (H&E, original magnification ×56). **(B)** On higher magnification, observe the vascular sinusoids, some filled with blood, separated by septa containing giant cells and spindle cells (H&E, original magnification ×100).

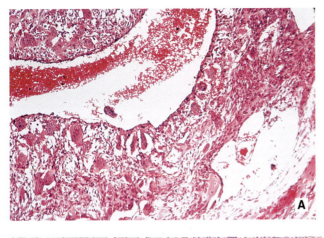
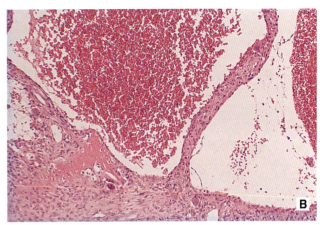
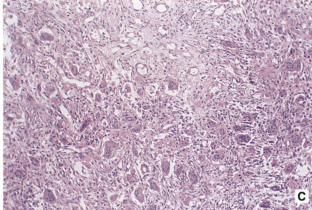

FIGURE 7.38 Histopathology of aneurysmal bone cyst.
(A) Blood-filled vascular spaces lined by flat undifferentiated cells are separated by narrow septa containing spindle fibroblasts. Newly formed osteoid is also present *(lower left)* (H&E, original magnification ×50). **(B)** In another area, vascular spaces are bordered by solid tissue containing spindle cells and giant cells (H&E, original magnification ×100). **(C)** Solid part of the lesion shows densely arranged capillaries and fairly large number of osteoclast-type giant cells grouped in clusters (H&E, original magnification ×50).

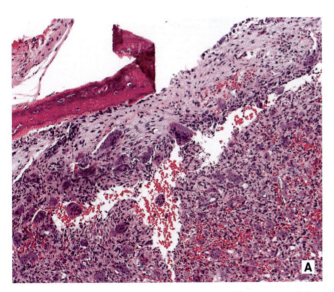
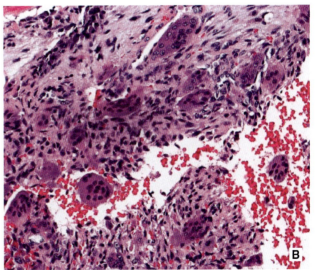

FIGURE 7.39 Histopathology of aneurysmal bone cyst. (A) Wall of the cystic space is composed of bland spindle cells and scattered osteoclast-type giant cells, some of them showing characteristic feature of "jumping into the swimming pool." In the left upper corner, note the reactive woven bone trabecula rimmed by the osteoblasts (H&E, original magnification ×100). **(B)** High-magnification photomicrograph shows plump fibroblasts and giant cells aggregating around and within the blood-filled spaces (H&E, original magnification ×200).

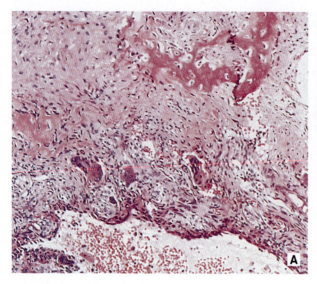
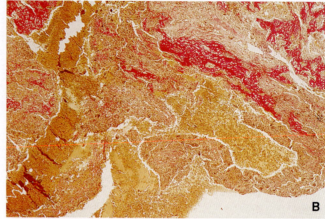
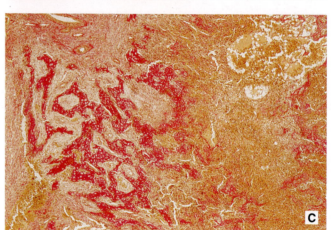

FIGURE 7.40 Histopathology of aneurysmal bone cyst.
(A) Cyst filled with blood *(bottom)* is lined by a seam of flat undifferentiated cells and randomly scattered small giant cells. Observe formation of considerable amount of primitive woven bone lined by osteoblasts *(top)* (H&E, original magnification ×40). **(B)** Typical lamellar structure *(lower right)* is surrounded by fresh blood. Fairly extended trabeculae of primitive woven bone *(red)* are seen close to the surface of the cyst *(upper right)* (van Gieson, original magnification ×12). **(C)** Solid areas of the lesion are made up of fibrous tissue with large amount of bone formation *(red)* and some cystic areas *(upper right corner)* (van Gieson, original magnification ×12).

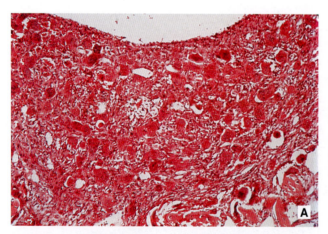
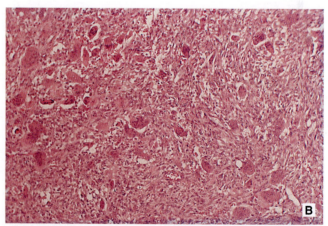

FIGURE 7.41 Histopathology of aneurysmal bone cyst. (A) Next to the cystic space *(top)* observe the solid part of the lesion displaying several giant cells but unevenly distributed within the fibrous tissue. Also present are foci of osteoid *(bottom right)* (H&E, original magnification ×100). **(B)** In another area, solid part of the tumor contains numerous giant cells of osteoclast type, similar to those of a giant cell tumor; however, they are much smaller and not uniformly distributed through the lesion (H&E, original magnification ×50).

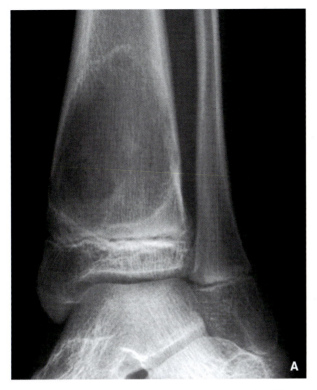
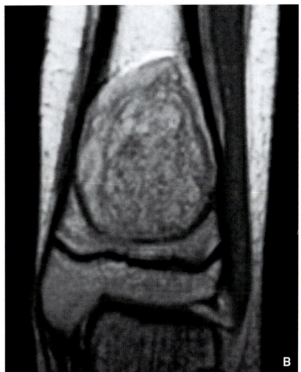
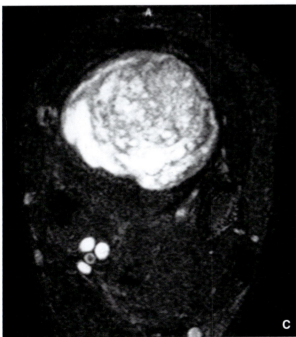

FIGURE 7.42 Radiography and magnetic resonance imaging of giant cell reparative granuloma.
(A) Oblique radiograph of the left ankle of an 11-year-old girl shows a sharply marginated radiolucent lesion in the distal metadiaphysis of the tibia. The cortex is thinned out, but there is no evidence of periosteal reaction. **(B)** Coronal T1-weighted MRI shows that the lesion exhibits heterogeneous but predominantly intermediate signal intensity, slightly higher than skeletal muscles. **(C)** On axial T2-weighted MR image, the lesion exhibits heterogeneous but predominantly high signal intensity.

Imaging:
- Radiography shows a radiolucent expansive commonly multiloculated lesion with internal trabeculations. It may or may not extend into the articular end of bone. The cortex is thin but usually intact. Limited matrix mineralization may be present (Fig. 7.42A).
- Magnetic resonance imaging shows the lesion to be solid without cystic changes, with signal intensity slightly higher than that of the muscles on T1-weighted images and heterogeneous but predominantly high on T2 weighting (Fig. 7.42B,C).

Histopathology:
- Mixture of collagen, plump bland fibroblasts, and multinucleated giant cells surrounding foci of hemorrhage (Fig. 7.43A).

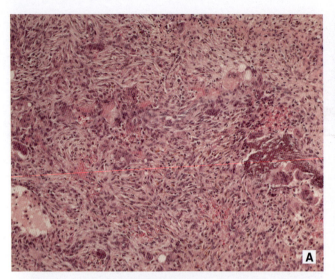 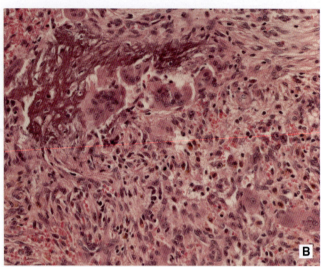

FIGURE 7.43 Histopathology of giant cell reparative granuloma. (A) Within a dense spindle cell stroma scattered are several multinucleated giant cells, accompanied by inflammatory cells and hemosiderin-laden macrophages. In addition, observe irregular islands of chondroosteoid *(right* and *center)* (H&E, original magnification ×100). **(B)** At higher magnification, note irregularly distributed giant cells in close proximity to chondroosteoid *(upper left)*. Inflammatory and spindle-shaped stromal cells are also present (H&E, original magnification ×200).

- Inflammatory and spindle-shaped stromal cells and foci of osteoid along the hemorrhagic areas are commonly present (Fig. 7.43B).

Differential Diagnosis:
- **Aneurysmal bone cyst**
  Although imaging features may show similarity to ABC, the periosteal reaction is more common, and MRI shows fluid–fluid levels.
  Histopathology of ABC shares many similar features with GCRG, particularly its solid part. However, it contains a significant number of blood-filled spaces.
- **Giant cell tumor**
  Imaging features of extension to the articular end of bone, lack of sclerotic border, and constant absence of mineralization should be helpful in differential diagnosis, particularly if soft-tissue component is present.
  Histopathology showing dual population of fibrocytic or monocytic mononuclear stromal cells mixed with evenly distributed large osteoclast-like giant cells is diagnostic.
- **Enchondroma**
  Imaging findings particularly in small tubular bones of the hands and feet may resemble GCRG; however, lack of periosteal reaction and absence of internal trabeculations, together with shallow endosteal scalloping and typical chondroid calcifications, are helpful diagnostic features.
  Histopathology showing chondroid differentiation of the lesion is diagnostic.

Intraosseous Lipoma

Definition:
- Benign lipomatous neoplasm of bone arising within the medullary cavity, cortex, or on the surface of bone.

Epidemiology:
- Rare lesion, representing less than 0.1% of primary bone tumors.
- Wide age range (second to eighth decades), but most patients are in their fifth decade of life.
- Male-to-female ratio of 4:3.
- Parosteal lipoma constitutes about 15% of cases and mostly develops in the fifth to sixth decades of life.

Sites of Involvement:
- Most commonly affects the intramedullary portions of long tubular bones, especially the femur (intertrochanteric region), tibia, fibula, and calcaneus.
- Infrequently seen in the pelvic bones, vertebrae, sacrum, skull, mandible, maxilla, and ribs.
- Parosteal lesions generally develop on the surface of the shafts of long tubular bones, especially the femur, humerus, and tibia.

Clinical Findings:
- May be asymptomatic, or produce aching pain or swelling.
- Rarely may present as a pathologic fracture.

Imaging:
- Radiography shows a radiolucent lesion with narrow zone of transition, occasionally with a thin sclerotic margin,

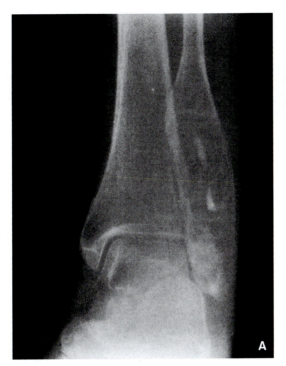
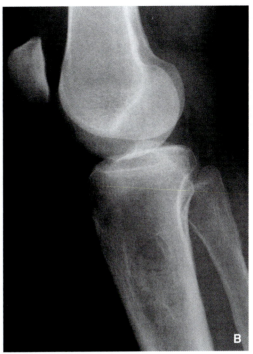

FIGURE 7.44 Radiography of intraosseous lipoma. **(A)** Anteroposterior radiograph of the left ankle shows a radiolucent lesion in the distal fibula exhibiting expansive character. Observe thinning of the cortex and central calcifications. **(B)** Lateral radiograph of the knee of another patient shows a radiolucent lesion with narrow zone of transition in the proximal tibia.

commonly with central ossification or calcification (Figs. 7.44 and 7.45).
- CT images show characteristic low-attenuation values of Hounsfield units compatible with fat (Fig. 7.46).
- Magnetic resonance imaging shows fat characteristics on all sequences and lack of enhancement on postcontrast images (Fig. 7.47).

Pathology:

Gross (Macroscopy):
- Usually presents as well-defined, soft, yellow mass with sizes ranging from 3 to 5 cm.
- The lesion may be enclosed by thin fibrous capsule (Fig. 7.48A).
- Surrounding bone is often sclerotic.
- Parosteal lipomas are usually 4 to 10 cm in greatest dimension, well defined, soft, and yellow, attached at the base to the cortex.
- Some lesions may contain gritty spicules of bone or firm nodules of cartilage at the base or scattered throughout the mass.

Histopathology:
- Lobules of mature adipose tissue containing mature lipocytes, which are slightly larger than nonneoplastic fat cells, in a background of fibroblasts.
- Lipocytes have a single large clear cytoplasmic vacuole that displaces the crescent-shaped nucleus to the periphery (Fig. 7.48C).
- Fat necrosis with foamy macrophages and fibrosis can be seen in some tumors.

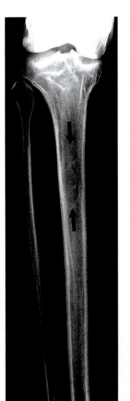
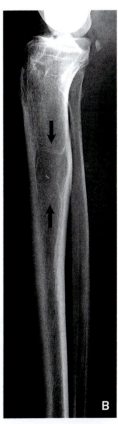

FIGURE 7.45 Radiography of intraosseous lipoma. **(A)** Anteroposterior and **(B)** lateral radiographs of the right leg of a 43-year-old man show a radiolucent lesion with narrow zone of transition within the proximal tibia (*arrows*), with internal foci of calcifications.

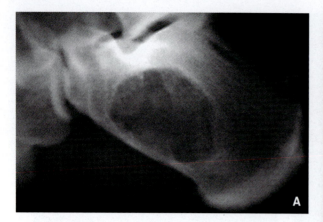
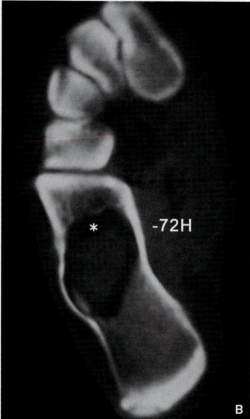

FIGURE 7.46 Radiography and computed tomography of intraosseous lipoma. (A) Lateral radiograph of the right hindfoot of a 40-year-old man shows a radiolucent lesion in the calcaneus. **(B)** CT image shows a lesion displaying low-attenuation values of minus 72 Hounsfield units, consistent with fat.

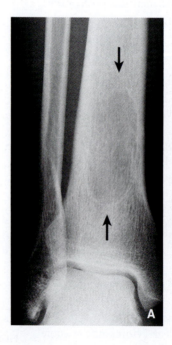
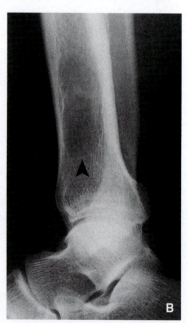

FIGURE 7.47 Radiography and magnetic resonance imaging of intraosseous lipoma. (A) Anteroposterior radiograph of the right ankle of a 42-year-old man shows a radiolucent lesion in the distal tibia exhibiting a thin sclerotic border (*arrows*). **(B)** On the lateral radiograph, there is suggestion of a faint calcification in the center of radiolucent lesion (*arrowhead*).

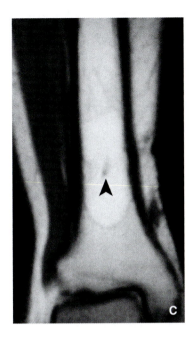
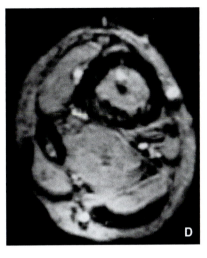

FIGURE 7.47 *(Continued).* (C) Coronal T1-weighted MRI demonstrates the lesion to be of high signal intensity paralleling that of the subcutaneous fat. A small focus of low signal within the lesion (*arrowhead*) represents calcification. **(D)** Axial T2-weighted MR image shows the lesion becoming now of intermediate signal intensity, again paralleling the signal of subcutaneous fat. Observe centrally placed focus of low signal calcification.

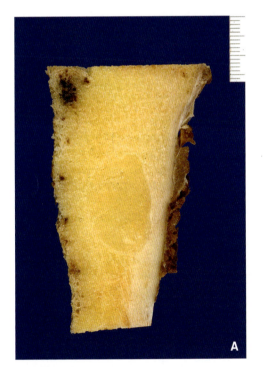
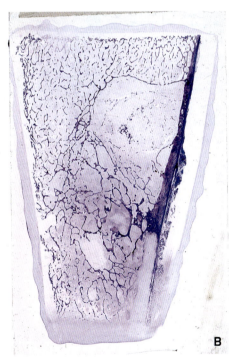
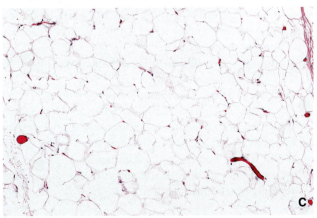

FIGURE 7.48 Gross specimen and histopathology of intraosseous lipoma. (A) Gross anatomic specimen of the tibia shows *oval, yellowish* lesion surrounded by thin fibrous capsule. **(B)** Whole-mount section shows replacement of trabecular bone by lipoma exhibiting central flocculent calcifications (*upper right*) (toluidine blue, original magnification ×1.5). **(C)** Under higher magnification, observe large lymphocytes with peripherally displaced crescent-shaped nuclei (H&E, original magnification ×100).

- Foci of calcifications or ossifications are commonly present (Fig. 7.48B).
- Ossifying lipomas show delicate trabeculae of woven and lamellar bone throughout the tumor.
- Parosteal lipoma consisting of well-defined mass of mature fat may contain hyaline cartilage, which undergoes endochondral ossification.

Immunohistochemistry:
- Neoplastic fat cells express positivity for vimentin and S-100 protein.

Genetics:
- Translocation t(3;12)(q28;q14) and its associated fusion transcript *HMGIC/LPP*, also present in lipoma of soft tissue, have been reported in parosteal tumors.

Prognosis:
- Excellent prognosis, almost never recurs after surgical intervention.

Differential Diagnosis:
- *Medullary bone infarct*
  Imaging features may be similar to those of intraosseous lipoma, particularly when the latter lesion exhibits ossifications or calcifications; however, the characteristic serpentine sclerotic margin separating the infracted from viable bone should be the diagnostic clue.
  Histopathology showing necrotic bone marrow tissue with foci of calcifications separated from the underlying viable bone by a zone of fibrosis and sclerosis, occasionally with surrounding areas of reparative changes, is diagnostic.
- *Simple bone cyst*
  Radiographic studies showing characteristic "fallen fragment" sign, and MRI showing fluid characteristics and lack of fat signal within the lesion, are diagnostic. If SBC is located in the calcaneus, it may look very similar to intraosseous lipoma of this bone; however, no calcifications or ossifications within the lesion are present.
  Histopathology of the lesion will show absence of lipocytes.
- *Pseudocyst of calcaneus*
  The radiolucent Ward triangle of calcaneus may look like intraosseous lipoma; however, no calcifications or ossifications are present.
- *Intraosseous liposarcoma*
  Imaging features show more aggressive appearance and not infrequently a soft-tissue mass.
  Histopathology of intraosseous liposarcoma varies depending upon the subtype. Well-differentiated tumor (lipoma-like liposarcoma) may exhibit similar morphology to intraosseous lipoma; however, some cells will show enlarged hyperchromatic nuclei, and some lipoblasts may contain cytoplasmic round vacuoles that scallop the nucleus. Myxoid liposarcoma consists of scattered lipoblasts and mildly atypical stellate and spindle in abundant myxoid stroma with fine arborizing vascular component. Pleomorphic liposarcoma shows spindle cells with prominent pleomorphism and hyperchromatism of the nuclei.

B. MALIGNANT TUMORS

Adamantinoma of Long Bones

Definition:
- Malignant biphasic tumor characterized by a variety of morphologic patterns, most commonly composed of epithelial cells, surrounded by a relatively bland spindle cell osteofibrous tissue.

Epidemiology:
- Constitutes about 0.4% of all primary bone tumors.
- Wide age range from 3 years up to 86 years, with a median age between 25 and 35 years.
- Younger patients usually present with osteofibrous dysplasia–like adamantinoma.
- Few cases of young children with classic adamantinoma have been reported.
- Slight predominance in males.

Sites of Involvement:
- Tibia, in particular the anterior aspect of metadiaphysis, is affected in 85% to 90% of cases.
- Multifocal involvement of the tibia was described, and in up to 10% of cases, concomitant involvement of the ipsilateral fibula was present.
- Rare involvement of the ulna and humerus was reported.

Clinical Findings:
- Localized swelling with or without pain.
- Physical examination reveals a firm, tender mass or swelling, usually firmly affixed to the underlying bone.

Imaging:
- Radiography shows well-delineated, elongated osteolytic defects of various sizes mixed with areas of sclerosis, occasionally having a soap-bubble appearance (Fig. 7.49A); a saw-toothed areas of cortical destruction are quite distinctive for this tumor (Fig. 7.49B); multiple satellite lesions may be present.
- Scintigraphy invariably demonstrates increased uptake of the radiopharmaceutical tracer (Fig. 7.50).
- Magnetic resonance imaging shows hypointense (compared to normal bone marrow) signal on T1-weighted sequences and hyperintense signal on T2 weighting. Postcontrast images may or may not show enhancement of the tumor. Some investigators reported intense and homogeneous static enhancement but lack of uniform dynamic enhancement pattern.

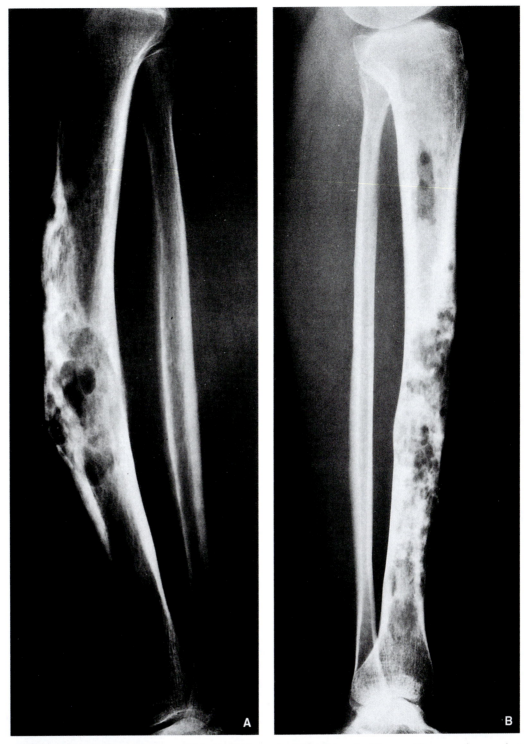

FIGURE 7.49 Radiography of adamantinoma. (A) Lateral radiograph of the left leg of a 64-year-old woman shows a destructive lesion in the midshaft of the tibia. The lesion is multiloculated with mixed osteolytic and sclerotic areas, creating a soap bubble appearance. **(B)** Lateral radiograph of the right leg of a 28-year-old woman shows multiple, confluent lytic lesions involving almost the entire tibia. The articular ends of the bone are spared. The anterior cortex exhibits a predominantly saw-tooth type of destruction.

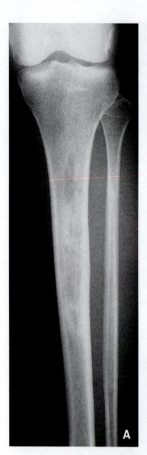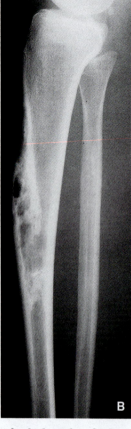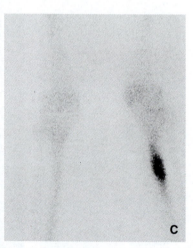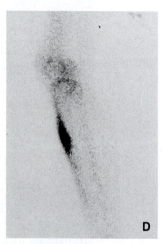

FIGURE 7.50 Radiography and scintigraphy of adamantinoma. (A) Anteroposterior radiograph of the left leg of a 46-year-old woman shows multiple radiolucent lesions in the midshaft of the tibia. The lateral cortex of the bone is slightly thickened. **(B)** Lateral radiograph shows a mixed sclerotic and lytic lesion predominantly affecting the anterior tibial cortex. **(C)** Frontal and **(D)** lateral images of radionuclide bone scan obtained after intravenous injection of 20 mCi (740 MBq) of ^{99m}Tc-labeled methylene diphosphonate (MDP) show markedly increased uptake of radiopharmaceutical tracer in the tumor.

Pathology:

Gross (Macroscopy):

- Usually presents as a cortical, well-demarcated, yellowish-gray, lobulated firm consistency tumor with peripheral sclerosis.
- Mostly single lesion but occasionally may be multifocal with normal cortical bone between the lesions (Fig. 7.51).
- Small lesions are usually within the cortex exhibiting white and gritty appearance.
- Larger lesions show more aggressive appearance with intramedullary extension and cortical breakthrough, occasionally accompanied by soft-tissue mass.
- Cystic changes within the tumor can be seen.

Histopathology:

- Biphasic architecture consisting of an epithelial component (islands of polyhedral cells in pavemented nests or in gland-like spaces exhibiting peripheral nuclear palisading) intimately admixed with osteofibrous component (composed of storiform-oriented spindle cells) in various proportions (Fig. 7.52).
- Four main morphologic patterns may be present: basaloid, tubular, spindle cell, and squamous.
- First two patterns (basaloid and tubular) are most common, but all patterns may be present in one lesion.
- Spindle cell pattern is more common in recurrent tumors and in metastases.
- In addition, an osteofibrous dysplasia–like pattern has been described, characterized by dominance of osteofibrous tissue with only small clusters or even single dispersed epithelial cells (Fig. 7.53).
- Both classic adamantinoma and osteofibrous dysplasia–like adamantinoma display a "zonal" architecture: in the former, the center of the tumor is dominated by epithelial component, whereas toward the periphery, the osteofibrous component prevails with increasing number of woven bone trabeculae, rimmed by osteoblasts, that are undergoing transformation to lamellar bone; in the latter, the zoning is reversed, the center being composed of

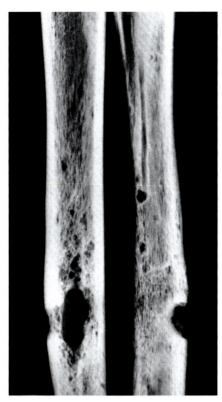

FIGURE 7.51 Radiography of the gross specimen of adamantinoma. Anteroposterior (*left*) and lateral (*right*) radiographs of the resected specimen of the tibial diaphysis of a 9-year-old boy show several various in size osteolytic lesions affecting the cortex and the medullary cavity. (From Bullough PG. *Atlas of Orthopedic Pathology with Clinical and Radiologic Correlations*. 2nd ed. New York, NY: Gower Medical Publishing; 1992, p. 17.22, Fig. 17.62.)

the fibrous tissue and scanty immature woven bone trabeculae, with only scattered epithelial elements more at the periphery.
- Myxoid change, foamy macrophages, mast cells, and multinucleated giant cells may be present.
- Low mitotic activity.

Immunohistochemistry:
- Fibrous tissue is positive for vimentin.
- Epithelial cells are positive for keratin, epithelial membrane antigen (EMA), vimentin, tumor protein p63 (encoded by *TP63* gene), and glycoprotein podoplanin.
- Coexpression of alpha-smooth muscle actin and cytokeratins in epithelial tumor cells has been reported.
- Epidermal growth factor/epidermal growth factor receptor (EGF/EGFR) expression is restricted only to epithelial component.
- Fibroblast growth factor 2/fibroblast growth factor receptor 1 (FGF2/FGFR1) is present in both components.

Genetics:
- Gain of chromosomes 7, 8, 12, 19, and 21.
- *TP53* gene aberrations and DNA aneuploidy are limited to the epithelial component of tumor.
- Some cases that exhibited histopathologic features of both adamantinoma and Ewing sarcoma (called also "atypical" adamantinoma or "Ewing-like" adamantinoma) revealed translocations t(11;22), not present in classic adamantinoma.

Prognosis:
- Recurrence after limited (intralesional or marginal) surgical intervention is high (up to 90%).
- The tumor may spread to the regional lymph nodes.
- Metastases (up to 29% of cases) have been recorded.

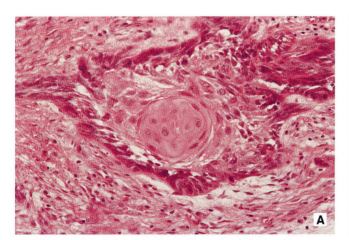
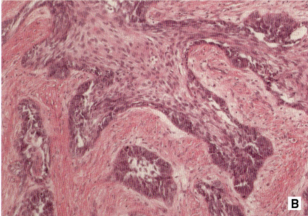

FIGURE 7.52 Histopathology of adamantinoma. (A) Admixed within a spindle cell fibrous stroma is an island of small epithelial cells containing area of squamous cell metaplasia (H&E, original magnification ×50). **(B)** In another field of view, noted are ameloblastoma-like areas with peripheral palisading of epithelial tumor cells (H&E, original magnification ×200).

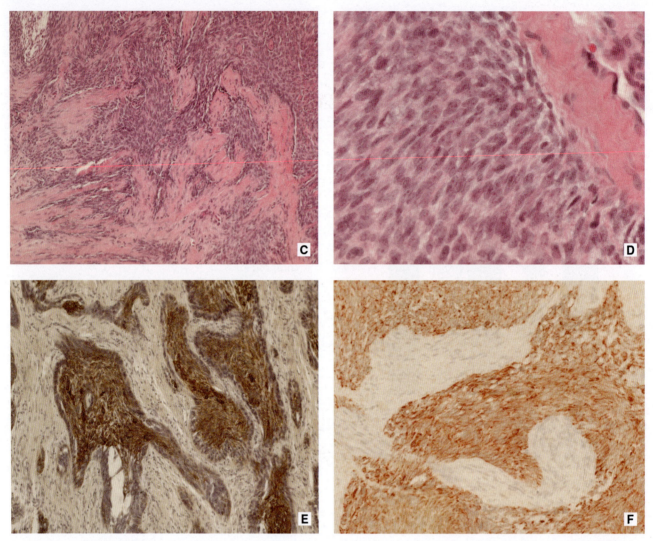

FIGURE 7.52 *(Continued).* **(C)** In another area, observe the spindle cell pattern of the tumor (H&E, original magnification ×200). **(D)** At high-power magnification, the tumor cells are densely packed and exhibit oval to spindle-shaped nuclei (H&E, original magnification ×400). **(E)** Immunohistochemistry stain shows that epithelial tumor cells are positive for cytokeratins (peroxidase–antiperoxidase method, original magnification ×200). **(F)** Densely packed spindle-shaped tumor cells are positive for cytokeratin 5 (PAP method, original magnification ×200).

Differential diagnosis:
- **Osteofibrous dysplasia**
  Imaging features may be similar to those of adamantinoma; however, there is no evidence of cortical destruction, and the lesion is seen in much younger patient population.
  Histopathology generally showing typical "dressed" osseous trabeculae with osteoblasts and lack of endothelial component should be diagnostic; however, diagnostic challenges may be encountered in so-called osteofibrous-like adamantinoma (see discussion above). The only feature differentiating the latter tumor from osteofibrous dysplasia are small clusters of epithelioid cells. Immunohistochemistry studies for keratins may provide further help in the differential diagnosis.

- **Fibrous dysplasia**
  Imaging findings of ground-glass appearance of the lesion, thinning of the cortex, rind sign, and lack of aggressive features, such as cortical destruction, are usually diagnostic.
  Histopathology showing metaplastic woven bone trabeculae resembling Chinese characters without osteoblastic activity is diagnostic.

- **Nonossifying fibroma**
  Less aggressive features on imaging studies, particularly lack of cortical destruction.
  Histopathology showing bland monomorphous spindle cells admixed with histiocytic cells commonly arranged in a swirling storiform pattern, and absence of epithelial component, is diagnostic.

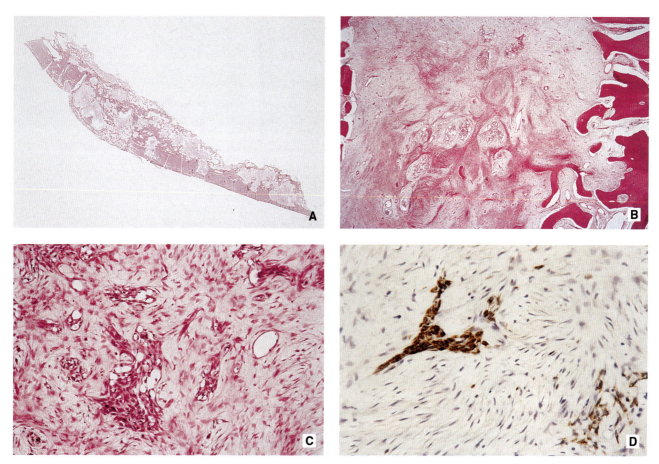

FIGURE 7.53 Histopathology of adamantinoma with osteofibrous dysplasia–like component. (A) Resected fragment of the anterior tibia shows irregular thickening of the cortex associated with metaplastic new bone formation (H&E, reduced scale). **(B)** Fibrous tissue of varying density contains an island of adamantinoma *(middle third)*. Metaplastic new bone formation is present *(lower right)*; observe also the inner aspect of cortical bone with sign of remodeling *(right)* (H&E, original magnification ×16). **(C)** At higher magnification, the tubular and solid structures of epithelial cells are more conspicuous. Some capillaries *(right middle* and *top)* are also present. Observe slight hyperchromatism and pleomorphism of the nuclei (H&E, original magnification ×200). **(D)** Immunohistochemistry shows positivity of epithelial cells *(brown)*, and a panepithelial marker displays groups and single positive cells *(lower right)* in the background of fibrous tissue [pancytokeratin antibody Lu5 peroxidase–antiperoxidase (PAS) method, original magnification ×100].

- *Osteomyelitis*
  Acute and chronic osteomyelitis, particularly affecting the tibia, may show similar imaging features to adamantinoma; however, periosteal reaction is invariably present. Clinical and laboratory findings are also helpful in differential diagnosis.
  Histopathology showing typical inflammatory changes and lack of epithelial component is diagnostic.

Chordoma

Definition:
- Malignant bone tumor that arises from developmental embryonic remnants of the notochord.

Epidemiology:
- Accounts for about 1% to 4% of all primary malignant bone tumors.
- Commonly is diagnosed the between fifth and seventh decades of life, with mean age of 56 years.
- Male-to-female ratio of 2:1.

Sites of Involvement:
- Most common locations are sacrococcygeal area, followed by spheno-occipital area (mainly clivus), and second cervical vertebra.
- Rare tumors in children and young adults are mostly seen in the cranial region.
- So-called chondroid chordomas occur exclusively at the base of the skull.

Clinical Findings:
- Skull-based tumor may cause headache, neck pain, diplopia, cranial nerve palsy, or endocrine dysfunction due to compression of the pituitary gland.
- Tumors of the spine and sacrum may present with chronic low back pain, bowel and bladder dysfunction, and paresthesia of the extremities.

Imaging:
- Radiography shows highly destructive, expansive, osteolytic lesion with irregular scalloped borders and

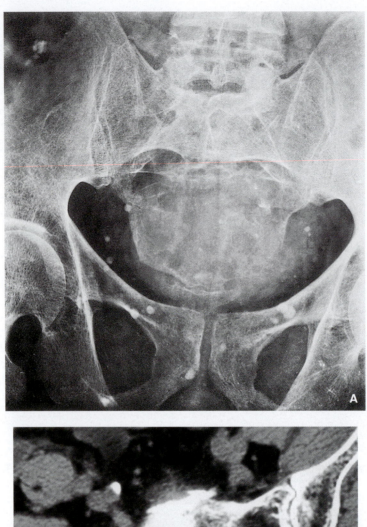
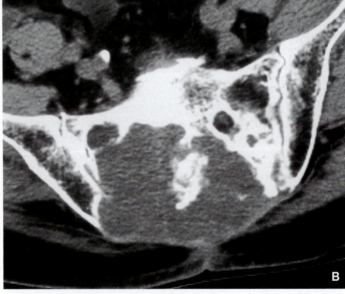

FIGURE 7.54 Radiography and computed tomography of chordoma. (A) Destructive osteolytic lesion located in the lower sacrum, with scalloped borders and amorphous calcifications within the tumor matrix, is present in this 60-year-old woman. **(B)** Axial CT section shows extensive bone destruction and a large soft-tissue mass.

occasionally matrix calcifications (Figs. 7.54A and 7.55A); sclerosis of the tumor edges may be observed, and a pathologic fracture is often present; soft-tissue mass is commonly present (Figs. 7.54B and 7.55D).
- 11C-methionine (MET) positron emission tomography (PET) shows high sensitivity (80%) for imaging of this tumor.
- Computed tomography better than radiography delineates the extent of bone destruction, soft-tissue mass, and growth within the spinal canal (Figs. 7.54B and 7.55B).
- Magnetic resonance imaging shows the tumor to be of intermediate-to-low signal intensity on T1-weighted images and high signal on T2-weighted and other water-sensitive sequences (Fig. 7.55C,D).

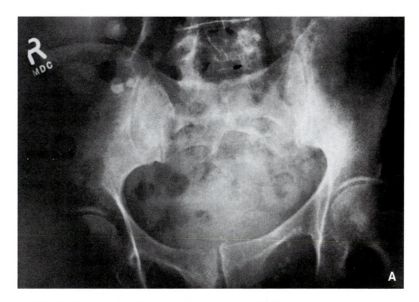
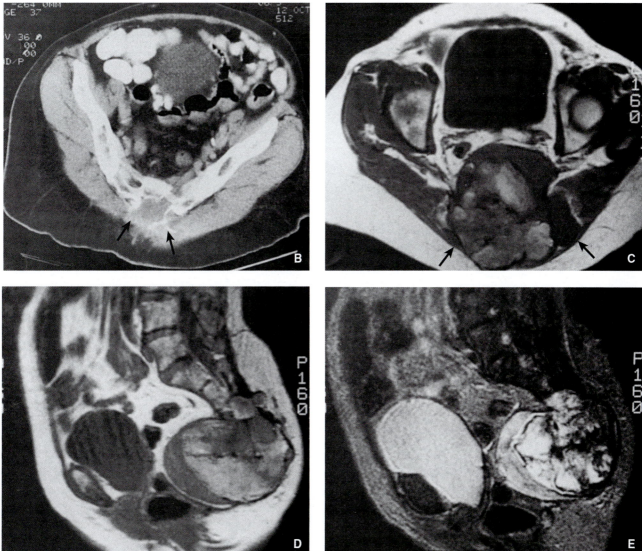

FIGURE 7.55 Radiography, computed tomography, and magnetic resonance imaging of chordoma. (A) Anteroposterior radiograph of the pelvis of a 68-year-old woman shows a destructive lesion in the middle and lower part of the sacrum associated with a soft-tissue mass. **(B)** Axial CT section demonstrates the low-attenuation tumor destroying the sacral bone (*arrows*). **(C)** Axial T1-weighted MR image shows a large heterogeneous tumor mass displaying predominantly intermediate signal intensity with scattered areas of high signal probably representing hemorrhage (*arrows*). **(D)** Sagittal T1-weighted MRI shows the extraosseous extension of the tumor. **(E)** Sagittal T2-weighted MRI shows the tumor exhibiting heterogeneous but predominantly high signal intensity.

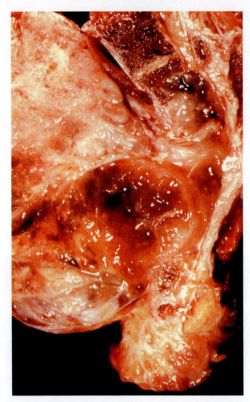

FIGURE 7.56 Gross specimen of chordoma. Sagittal section through the autopsy specimen of the lower lumbar vertebrae and sacrum shows a firm pink-gray-yellowish lobulated tumor destroying the sacral bone and L5 vertebra. A large fleshy soft-tissue mass is present anteriorly. Note prominent foci of hemorrhage. (From Bullough PG. *Atlas of Orthopedic Pathology with Clinical and Radiologic Correlations*. 2nd ed. New York, NY: Gower Medical Publishing; 1992, p. 16.28, Fig. 16.79.)

Pathology:
Gross (Macroscopy):
- Lobulated, dark-red hemorrhagic tumor, glistening, grayish tan to bluish white, mucogelatinous to friable, commonly extending into the soft tissues (Fig. 7.56).

Histopathology:
- Lobulated architecture with individual lobules separated by fibrous septa containing vascular channels and occasionally infiltrated by lymphocytes (Fig. 7.57A).
- Cord-like arrays and lobules of large polyhedral cells with a vacuolated "bubbly" cytoplasm and vesicular nuclei, referred to as physaliphorous cells (Fig. 7.57B,C).
- The vacuoles contain a mucinous substance with neutral mucopolysaccharides and a mixture of weakly sulfonated and carboxylated glycoprotein.
- Some cells are of the signet-ring type in which the nucleus is displaced to one side by one or two vacuoles.
- Abundant myxoid stroma is present.
- Mild-to-moderate nuclear atypia may be seen.
- Necrotic foci are frequently present.
- A rare type of dedifferentiated chordoma (sarcomatoid chordoma) represents a biphasic tumor composed of chordoma and high-grade sarcoma (undifferentiated pleomorphic sarcoma or osteosarcoma).

Immunohistochemistry:
- Positive for S-100 protein (Fig. 7.57D), cytokeratins, epithelial membrane antigen (EMA), and brachyury, a protein encoded by *T* gene (specificity above 90%).

Genetics:
- Partial or complete *PTEN* gene deficiency.
- Loss of chromosomes 3, 4, 10, and 13.
- Gains of chromosome arms 5q and 7q and chromosome 20.
- Hypodiploidy or diploidy with chromosome segments 1p31-pter, 3p21-pter, 3q21-qter, 9p24-pter, and 17q11-qter most often affected.
- Homozygous or heterozygous deletion of *CDKN2A* (p16) and *CDKN2B* (p15) loci on chromosome 9p21.
- Gain of brachyury 7q33 locus and the *EGFR7* (p12) locus is common.

Prognosis:
- Overall median survival is 7 years, but it depends on the site and size of tumor.
- Up to 40% of noncranial tumors metastasize.
- Chondroid chordomas have more indolent clinical course.
- Dedifferentiated tumors have worse prognosis.

Differential Diagnosis:
- **Chondrosarcoma**
  Imaging features, including presence of calcifications, may be very similar to those of chordoma; however, the chordoma is invariably midline in location, whereas chondrosarcoma may be eccentric.
  Histopathology showing typical chondroid differentiation of the tumor tissue is usually diagnostic, although myxoid chondrosarcoma with its lobar architecture, cord-like arrangement of cells, and myxoid matrix, so similar to chordoma, may create a challenge in differential diagnosis. Lack of physaliphorous cells and genetic feature of nonrandom t(9;22) (q22;q12) translation are the helpful hints to diagnose this tumor.
- **Plasmacytoma**
  Imaging features of absence of sclerotic margin and lack of calcifications as well as a normal or only slightly positive radionuclide bone scan are diagnostic.
  Histopathology showing typical sheets of atypical plasmacytoid cells is also diagnostic.
- **Metastasis**
  Imaging features occasionally may be similar to those of chordoma, but commonly in metastatic lesion, there is absence of sclerotic border and lack of calcifications.

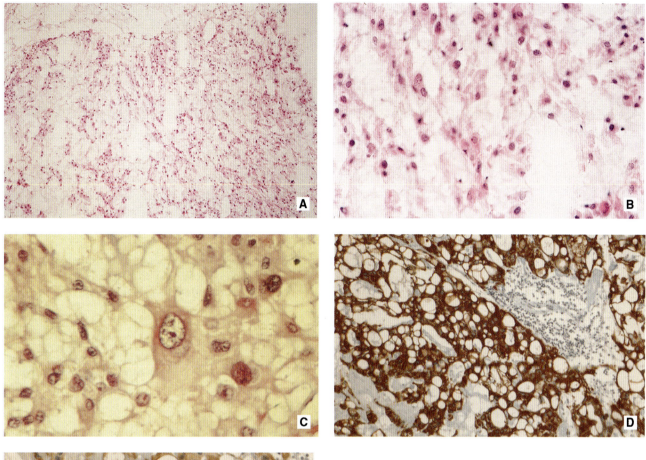
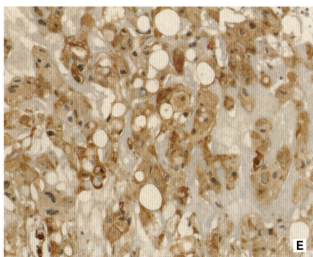

FIGURE 7.57 Histopathology of chordoma. (A) Cords and clusters of large polymorphous cells contain an eosinophilic cytoplasm and large roundish slightly pleomorphic nuclei. Between the cells observe faintly pale amorphous areas that represent mucus extruded by the cells (H&E, original magnification ×50). **(B)** At higher magnification, some of the large cells show vacuoles, giving rise to the typical physaliphorous appearance. The pleomorphism of the large dark nuclei is conspicuous (H&E, original magnification ×200). **(C)** High-magnification photomicrograph shows the large variegated and vacuolated physaliphorous cells characteristic of this tumor (H&E, original magnification ×400). **(D)** Tumor cells are positive for pancytokeratins (biotin–streptavidin peroxidase, original magnification ×200). **(E)** Tumor cells also react with S100 antibodies (biotin–streptavidin peroxidase, original magnification ×200).

Histopathology showing lack of physaliphorous cells and particularly immunohistochemical studies showing negativity for S100 protein are diagnostic.

Leiomyosarcoma of Bone

Definition:
- A primary malignant predominantly spindle cell neoplasm of bone showing smooth muscle differentiation.

Epidemiology:
- Wide age distribution 9 to 87 years old with mean age 44; occurrence before the age of 20 is uncommon.
- Male-to-female ratio of 2:1.

Sites of Involvement:
- Most lesions occur in the distal femur, proximal tibia, and proximal humerus.
- Other bones that may be affected include the pelvis, clavicle, ribs, and mandible.

Clinical Findings:
- Pain of variable duration and intensity, and occasionally soft-tissue mass.

Imaging:
- Radiography demonstrates either a lytic area of geographic type of bone destruction (Fig. 7.58A) or a radiolucent lesion with ill-defined borders, sometimes exhibiting moth-eaten or permeative type of bone destruction (Fig. 7.59A); periosteal reaction has been present in about 50% of reported cases.
- Computed tomography is helpful in delineating the full intraosseous and extraosseous extent of the tumor (Figs. 7.58B and 7.59B).
- MRI shows the lesion to be on T1-weighted sequences of intermediate signal intensity, isointense with the skeletal muscles, and hyperintense relative to the muscles on T2 weighting (Fig. 7.59C,D).

Pathology:
Gross (Macroscopy):
- Tumor size of wide range, averaging 6 cm.
- Gray to tan, creamy firm mass often with areas of necrosis or cystic degeneration.

Histopathology:
- Histopathologic appearance similar to leiomyosarcoma of soft tissue.
- Plump and pleomorphic spindle cells are arranged in bundles or fascicles (Fig. 7.60A).
- The tumor cells have eosinophilic (pyroninophilic) cytoplasm and elongated, cigar-shaped nuclei with blunted (depressed) ends caused by a clear vacuole (Fig. 7.60B).
- Mitotic figures are common (Fig. 7.60C).
- Areas of necrosis are present.
- High-grade tumors show prominent pleomorphism (Fig. 7.61).
- Rarely giant cells are present containing multiple hyperchromatic nuclei, prominent nucleoli, and indistinctive cytoplasmic borders.

Electron Microscopy:
- Fine filamentous actin fibrins are present in the cytoplasm.

Immunohistochemistry:
- Positivity for desmin, h-caldesmon (a protein combined with actin and tropomyosin that regulates cellular contraction), and smooth muscle actin (SMA).

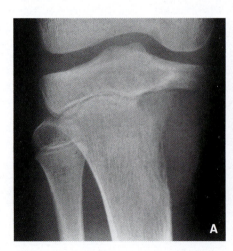
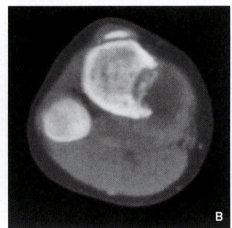

FIGURE 7.58 Radiography and computed tomography of leiomyosarcoma of bone. **(A)** Anteroposterior radiograph of the right knee of a 12-year-old boy shows an osteolytic lesion in the proximal metaphysis of the tibia destroying the medial cortex and extending into the soft tissues. **(B)** Axial CT section shows destruction of the medial aspect of the tibia and associated soft-tissue mass.

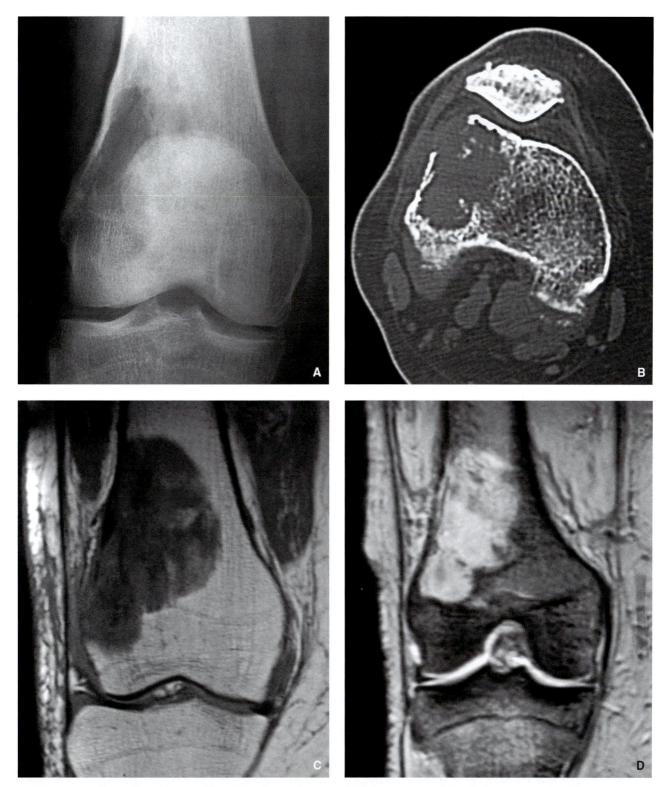

FIGURE 7.59 Radiography, computed tomography, and magnetic resonance imaging of leiomyosarcoma of bone.
(A) Anteroposterior radiograph of the right knee of a 66-year-old woman shows a lytic eccentric lesion in the lateral aspect of the distal femur. **(B)** Axial CT section shows destruction of the cortex of the lateral femoral condyle and soft-tissue extension of the tumor. **(C)** Coronal T1-weighed MRI shows the lesion to be isointense with the skeletal muscles. **(D)** Coronal T2-weighted MR image shows that the tumor exhibits heterogeneous but predominantly high signal intensity.

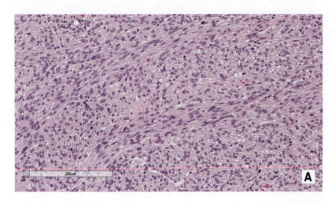
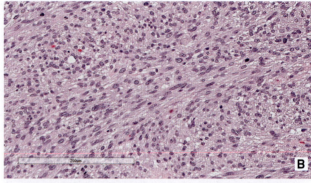
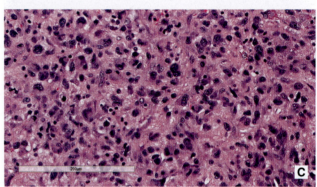

FIGURE 7.60 Histopathology of leiomyosarcoma of bone. (A) Numerous spindle cells exhibiting the smooth muscle features are arranged in the bundles and fascicles (H&E, original magnification ×100). **(B)** High-power magnification demonstrates characteristic elongated cigar-shaped nuclei of malignant cells (H&E, original magnification ×200). **(C)** In another field of view, observe the pleomorphism of the tumor cells and occasional mitoses (H&E, original magnification ×200).

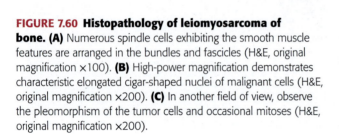
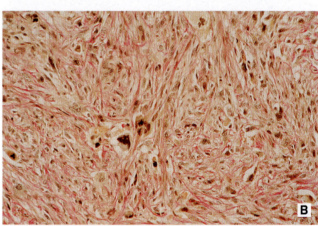
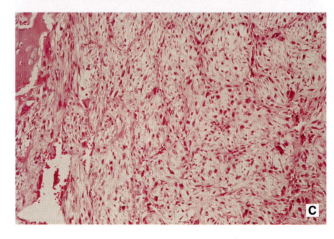

FIGURE 7.61 Histopathology of leiomyosarcoma of bone (same patient as shown in Fig 7.58). (A) Whole-mount section (H&E, original magnification ×1.5) shows that the tumor located in the metaphysis of the tibia destroyed the medial part of the growth plate and extended into the epiphysis, infiltrating the cancellous bone. **(B)** Irregular bundles of elongated spindle cells producing intracellular collagen *(red)* show marked pleomorphism of the nuclei. Some tumor giant cells are also present *(center)* (van Gieson, original magnification ×50). **(C)** In another field of view, observe pseudoepithelial clear cell aspect of the tumor (H&E, original magnification ×25).

Genetics:
- Genomic losses and absence of phosphorylated Rb (retinoblastoma protein encoded by gene *RB1* located on 13q14-q14.2).

Prognosis:
- Approximately 50% of patients develop metastases to the lungs within 5 years.

Differential Diagnosis:
- *Fibrosarcoma*
  Imaging features may be similar to those of leiomyosarcoma; however, occasionally, the characteristic feature of fibrosarcoma, in form of preservation of small sequestrum-like fragments of cortical bone and spongy trabeculae within the tumor mass, may be present facilitating the diagnosis.
  Histopathology showing fascicles of spindle cells exhibiting characteristic "herringbone tweed" pattern is diagnostic.
- *Lymphoma*
  Imaging features (including CT and MRI) of some tumors, particularly purely lytic, may be indistinguishable from those of leiomyosarcoma. Soft-tissue mass, however, is more commonly present in lymphoma, occasionally having characteristic feature of infiltrative appearance and involvement of more than just one compartment, rather than being round or oval displacing the adjacent anatomic structures.
  Histopathology showing aggregates of ovoid or rounded lymphoid cells with cleaved nuclei and prominent nucleoli, and immunohistochemistry showing positivity for CD45, CD20, and CD3 is diagnostic.
- *Osteolytic metastasis*
  Imaging features of solitary metastatic lesion may be similar to those of leiomyosarcoma, histopathologic features; however, particularly, immunohistochemistry (negativity for SMA) is diagnostic.

Liposarcoma of Bone

Definition:
- Malignant neoplasm that may arise within or on the surface of bone, whose phenotype recapitulates that of fat.

Epidemiology:
- Very rare tumor, constitutes less than 0.1% of all primary tumors of bone, with only sporadic cases reported in the literature.
- It may occur at all age groups but most often in adults.
- Men are affected slightly more commonly than are women.

Sites of Involvement:
- Tibia and femur are the preferential sites.

Clinical Features:
- Painful mass.
- Metastases to the lungs are common.

Imaging:
- Radiography shows predominantly osteolytic lesion, occasionally associated with a soft-tissue mass.
- Magnetic resonance imaging shows heterogeneous appearance with fat signal on both T1- and T2-weighted sequences.

Pathology:
Gross (Macroscopy):
- Large, yellow-to-tan-white in color, lobulated, soft-to-firm mass.
- Mucinous/myxoid changes within the mass may be present.

Histopathology:
- Histopathologic variants of liposarcoma reported in bone include well-differentiated lipoma-like, myxoid, and pleomorphic types.
- Well-differentiated lipoma-like liposarcoma consists of mature-appearing adipocytes and scattered tumor cells, some with enlarged hyperchromatic nuclei and some lipoblasts containing cytoplasmic round vacuoles that scallop the nucleus (Fig. 7.62).
- Myxoid liposarcoma consists of scattered lipoblasts and mildly atypical stellate and spindle cells in abundant myxoid stroma with finely arborizing vascular component.

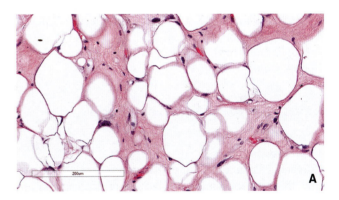
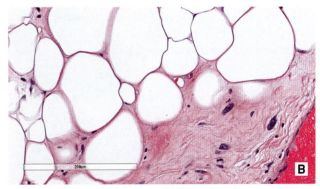

FIGURE 7.62 Histopathology of well-differentiated intraosseous liposarcoma. (A) A well-differentiated tumor is marked by large, mature, white fat cells and different in size adipocytes containing hyperchromatic nuclei (H&E, original magnification ×100). **(B)** On higher magnification, the details of the stromal tumor cells containing enlarged, varying in size, hyperchromatic nuclei are better appreciated (H&E, original magnification ×200).

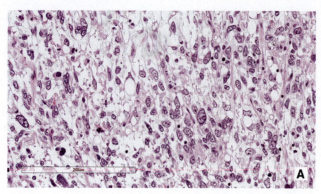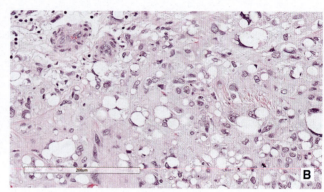

FIGURE 7.63 **Histopathology of pleomorphic intraosseous liposarcoma. (A)** Sheets of atypical pleomorphic cells with eosinophilic cytoplasm and hyperchromatic nuclei showing mitotic activity marked the higher grade of malignancy (H&E, original magnification ×200). **(B)** Foamy lipoblasts and signet ring cells are characteristic for this tumor (H&E, original magnification ×200).

- Pleomorphic liposarcoma shows proliferation of spindle cells with prominent pleomorphism and numerous atypical mitotic figures (Fig. 7.63A); characteristic foamy lipoblasts and signet ring cells may also be present (Fig. 7.63B).

Immunohistochemistry:
- Positive for human homologue of the murine double-minute type 2 (MDM2) and cyclin-dependent kinase 4 (CDK4).

Genetics:
- Amplification of 12q14.2-21.2 to include the *HMGA2* and *MDM2* gene regions.
- Amplification of 1q2.2-31.2 described in case of parosteal liposarcoma.

Prognosis:
- Pleomorphic variant has the worst prognosis.

Differential Diagnosis:
- ***Intraosseous lipoma***
  Imaging features including narrow zone of transition, thin sclerotic margin, and lack of soft-tissue mass are diagnostic.
  Histopathology showing typical benign lipocytes and absence of spindle cells, as well as lack of pleomorphism and hyperchromatism, is diagnostic.

REFERENCES

Abdelwahab IF, Hermann G, Kenan S, Klein MJ, Lewis MM. Case report 794. Primary leiomyosarcoma of the right femur. *Skeletal Radiol.* 1993;22:379–381.

Abdelwahab IF, Kenan S, Hermann G, Klein MJ, Lewis MM. Radiation-induced leiomyosarcoma. *Skeletal Radiol.* 1995;24:81–83.

Adler C-P. Case report 587. Adamantinoma of the tibia mimicking osteofibrous dysplasia. *Skeletal Radiol.* 1990;19:55–58.

Alles JU, Schulz A. Immunohistochemical markers (endothelial and histiocytic) and ultrastructure of primary aneurysmal bone cysts. *Hum Pathol.* 1986;17:39–45.

Alquacil-Garcia A, Alonso A, Pettigrew NM. Osteofibrous dysplasia (ossifying fibroma) of the tibia and fibula and adamantinoma. *Am J Clin Pathol.* 1984;82:470–474.

Althof PA, Ohmori K, Zhou M, et al. Cytogenetic and molecular cytogenetic findings in 43 aneurysmal bone cysts: aberrations of 17p mapped to 17p13.2 by fluorescence in situ hybridization. *Mod Pathol.* 2004;17:518–525.

Antonescu CR, Erlandson RA, Huvos AG. Primary leiomyosarcoma of bone: a clinicopathologic, immunohistochemical, and ultrastructural study of 33 patients and a literature review. *Am J Surg Pathol.* 1997;21:1281–1294.

Aoki J, Tanikawa H, Ishii K, et al. MR findings indicative of hemosiderin in giant-cell tumor of bone: frequency, cause, and diagnostic significance. *AJR Am J Roentgenol.* 1996;166:145–148.

Apaydin A, Ozkaynak C, Yihnaz S, et al. Aneurysmal bone cyst of metacarpal. *Skeletal Radiol.* 1996;25:76–78.

Athanasou NA, Bliss E, Gatter KC, Heryet A, Woods CG, McGee JO. An immunohistological study of giant-cell tumor of bone: evidence for an osteoclast origin of the giant cells. *J Pathol.* 1985;147:153–158.

Azzarelli A, Quagliuolo V, Cerasoli S, et al. Chordoma: natural history and treatment results in 33 cases. *J Surg Oncol.* 1988;37:185–191.

Bacchini P, Bertoni F, Ruggieri P, Campanacci M. Multicentric giant cell tumor of skeleton. *Skeletal Radiol.* 1995;24:371–374.

Backo M, Cindro L, Golouh R. Familial occurrence of infantile myofibromatosis. *Cancer.* 1992;69:1294–1299.

Baker ND, Greenspan A. Case report 172: pleomorphic liposarcoma, grade IV, of the soft tissue, arising in generalized plexiform neurofibromatosis. *Skeletal Radiol.* 1981;7:150–153.

Baker PL, Dockerty MD, Coventry MB. Adamantinoma (so-called) of the long bones. *J Bone Joint Surg Am.* 1954;36A:704–720.

Bancroft LW, Kransdorf MJ, Petersson JJ, O'Connor MI. Benign fatty tumors: classification, clinical course, imaging appearance, and treatment. *Skeletal Radiol.* 2006;35:719–733.

Baruffi MR, Neto JB, Barbieri CH, Casartelli C. Aneurysmal bone cyst with chromosomal changes involving 7q and 16p. *Cancer Genet Cytogenet.* 2001;129:177–180.

Beaugié JM, Mann CV, Butler ECB. Sacrococcygeal chordoma. *Br J Surg.* 1969;56:586–588.

Beltran J, Simon DC, Levy M, Herman L, Weis L, Mueller CF. Aneurysmal bone cysts: MR imaging at 1.5 T. *Radiology.* 1986;158:689–690.

Belza MG, Urich H. Chordoma and malignant fibrous histiocytoma. Evidence of transformation. *Cancer.* 1986;589:1082–1087.

Berlin O, Angervall L, Kindblom LG, Berlin IC, Stener B. Primary leiomyosarcoma of bone. A clinical, radiographic, pathologic-anatomic, and prognostic study of 16 cases. *Skeletal Radiol.* 1987;16:364–376.

Bertheussen KJ, Holck S, Schiodt T. Giant cell lesion of bone of the hand with particular emphasis on giant cell reparative granuloma. *J Hand Surg [Am]*. 1983;8:46–49.

Bertoni F, Present D, Enneking WF. Giant cell tumor of bone with pulmonary metastases. *J Bone Joint Surg Am*. 1985;67A:890–900.

Bertoni F, Present D, Sudanese A, Baldini N, Bacchini P, Campanacci M. Giant cell tumor of bone with pulmonary metastases: six case reports and a review of the literature. *Clin Orthop*. 1988;237:275–285.

Bertoni F, Bacchini P, Capanna R, et al. Solid variant of aneurysmal bone cyst. *Cancer*. 1993;71:729–734.

Bertoni F, Bacchini P, Staals EL. Malignancy in giant cell tumor. *Skeletal Radiol*. 2003;32:143–146.

Bhaduri A, Deshpande RB. Fibrocartilaginous mesenchymoma versus fibrocartilaginous dysplasia: are these a single entity? *Am J Surg Pathol*. 1995;19:1447–1448.

Biesecker JL, Marcove RC, Huvos AG, Mike V. Aneurysmal bone cysts. A clinicopathologic study of 66 cases. *Cancer*. 1970;26:615–625.

Binh MBN, Sastre-Garau X, Guillou L, et al. MDM2 and CDK4 immunostainings are useful adjuncts in diagnosing well-differentiated and dedifferentiated liposarcoma subtypes: a comparative analysis of 559 soft tissue neoplasms with genetic data. *Am J Surg Pathol*. 2005;29:1340–1347.

Blacksin MF, Ende N, Benevenia J. Magnetic resonance imaging of intraosseous lipomas: a radiologic-pathologic correlation. *Skeletal Radiol*. 1995;24:37–41.

Bonakdarpour A, Levy WM, Aegerter E. Primary and secondary aneurysmal bone cysts: a radiological study of 75 cases. *Radiology*. 1978;126:75–83.

Boseker EH, Bickel WH, Dahlin DC. A clinicopathologic study of simple unicameral bone cysts. *Surg Gynecol Obstet*. 1968;127:550–560.

Bridge JA, DeBoer J, Walker CW, et al. Translocation t(3;12)(q28;p14) in parosteal lipoma. *Genes Chromosomes Cancer*. 1995;73:1746–1752.

Bridge JA, Fidler ME, Neff JR, et al. Adamantinoma-like Ewing's sarcoma: genomic confirmation, phenotypic drift. *Am J Surg Pathol*. 1999;23:159–165.

Bullough PG. *Atlas of Orthopedic Pathology with Clinical and Radiologic Correlation*. 2nd ed. New York, NY: Gower; 1992:15.12–15.14.

Burmester GR, Winchester RJ, Dimitriu-Bona A, Klein M, Steiner G, Sissons HA. Delineation of four cell types comprising the giant cell tumor of bone. *J Clin Invest*. 1983;71:1633–1648.

Byers PD. A study of histological features distinguishing chordoma from chondrosarcoma. *Br J Cancer*. 1981;43:229–232.

Caluser CI, Scott AM, Schnieder J, et al. Value of lesion location and intensity of uptake in SPECT bone scintigraphy of the spine in patients with malignant tumors. *Radiology*. 1992;185(S):315.

Campanacci M. *Bone and Soft Tissue Tumors*. New York, NY: Springer Verlag; 1986:345–348.

Campanacci M, Giunti A, Olmi R. Giant-cell tumors of bone: a study of 209 cases with long-term follow-up in 130. *Ital J Orthop Traumatol*. 1975;1:249–277.

Campanacci M, Giunti A, Bertoni F, Laus M, Gitelis S. Adamantinoma of the long bones. The experience at the Istituto Ortopedico Rizzoli. *Am J Surg Pathol*. 1981;5:533–542.

Campanacci M, Capanna R, Picci P. Unicameral and aneurysmal bone cysts. *Clin Orthop*. 1986;204:25–36.

Campanacci M, Baldini N, Boriani S, Sudanese A. Giant cell tumor of bone. *J Bone Joint Surg Am*. 1987;69A:106–114.

Campbell RSD, Grainger AJ, Mangham DC, Beggs I, Teh J, Davies AM. Intraosseous lipoma: report of 35 new cases and a review of the literature. *Skeletal Radiol*. 2003;32:209–222.

Chu TA. Chondroid chordoma of the sacrococcygeal region. *Arch Pathol Lab Med*. 1987;111:861–864.

Chung EG, Enzinger FM. Infantile myofibromatosis. *Cancer*. 1981;48:1807–1818.

Clough JR, Price CH. Aneurysmal bone cyst: pathogenesis and long term results of treatment. *Clin Orthop*. 1973;97:52–63.

Cohen J. Etiology of simple bone cyst. *J Bone Joint Surg Am*. 1970;52A:1493–1497.

Cohen J. Unicameral bone cysts: a current synthesis of reported cases. *Orthop Clin North Am*. 1977;8:715–726.

Conway WF, Hayes CW. Miscellaneous lesions of bone. *Radiol Clin North Am*. 1993;31:339–358.

Czerniak B, Rojas-Corona RR, Dorfman HD. Morphologic diversity of long bone adamantinoma. The concept of differentiated (regressing) adamantinoma and its relationship to osteofibrous dysplasia. *Cancer*. 1989;64:2319–2334.

Dahlin DC. Giant cell tumor of bone: highlights of 407 cases. *AJR Am J Roentgenol*. 1985;144:955–960.

Dahlin DC. Giant cell bearing lesions of bone of the hands. *Hand Clin*. 1987;3:291–297.

Dahlin DC, MacCarty CS. Chordoma. A study of fifty-nine cases. *Cancer*. 1952;5:1170–1178.

Dahlin DC, McLeod RA. Aneurysmal bone cyst and other nonneoplastic conditions. *Skeletal Radiol*. 1982;8:243–250.

Dahlin DC, Unni KK. *Bone Tumors: General Aspects and Data on 8,542 Cases*. 4th ed. Springfield, PA: Charles C. Thomas; 1986:181–185, 193–336, 208–226, 379–393.

Dahlin DC, Cupps RE, Johnson EW Jr. Giant cell tumor: a study of 195 cases. *Cancer*. 1970;25:1061–1070.

Dahlin DC, Bertoni F, Beabout JW, Campanacci M. Fibrocartilaginous mesenchymoma with low grade malignancy. *Skeletal Radiol*. 1984;12:263–269.

Dickson BC, Gortzak Y, Bell RS, et al. P63 expression in adamantinoma. *Virchows Arch*. 2011;459:109–113.

Dumford K, Moore TE, Walker CW, Jaksha J. Multifocal, metachronous, giant cell tumor of the lower limb. *Skeletal Radiol*. 2003;32:147–150.

Duncan CP, Morton KS, Arthur JS. Giant cell tumor of bone: its aggressiveness and potential for malignant change. *Can J Surg*. 1983;26:475–476.

Fechner RE, Mills SE. *Atlas of Tumor Pathology. Tumors of the Bones and Joints*, 3rd series, fascicle 8. Washington, DC: Armed Forces Institute of Pathology; 1993:239–244.

Fechner RE, Mills SE. *Tumors of the Bones and Joints*. Washington, DC: Armed Forces Institute of Pathology; 1993:173–186, 203–209, 253–258.

Francis R, Lewis E. CT demonstration of giant cell tumor complicating Paget disease. *J Comput Assist Tomogr*. 1983;7:917–918.

Freeby JA, Reinus WR, Wilson AJ. Quantitative analysis of the plain radiographic appearance of aneurysmal bone cyst. *Invest Radiol*. 1995;30:433–439.

Ghert M, Simunovic N, Cowan RW, Colterjohn N, Singh G. Properties of the stromal cell in giant cell tumor of bone. *Clin Orthop Relat Res*. 2007;459:8–12.

Glass TA, Mills SE, Fechner RE, Dyer R, Martin R III, Armstrong P. Giant-cell reparative granuloma of the hands and feet. *Radiology*. 1983;149:65–68.

Goldenberg RR, Campbell CJ, Bonfiglio M. Giant-cell tumor of bone. An analysis of two hundred and eighteen cases. *J Bone Joint Surg Am*. 1970;52A:619–664.

Greenfield GB, Arrington JA. *Imaging of Bone Tumors*. Philadelphia, PA: JB Lippincott; 1995:217–218.

Greenspan A, Jundt G, Remagen W. *Differential Diagnosis in Orthopaedic Oncology*. 2nd ed. Philadelphia, PA: Lippincott Williams & Wilkins; 2007:387–431.

Grote HJ, Braun M, Kalinski T, et al. Spontaneous malignant transformation of conventional giant cell tumor. *Skeletal Radiol*. 2004;33:169–175.

Hazelbag HM, Taminiau LH, Fleuren GJ, Hogendoorn PC. Adamantinoma of the long bones. A clinicopathological study of thirty-two patients with emphasis on histological subtype, precursor lesion, and biological behavior. *J Bone Joint Surg Am*. 1994;74A:1482–1499.

Hazelbag HM, Fleuren GJ, Cornelisse CJ, van den Broek LJ, Hogendoorn PC. DNA aberrations in the epithelial cell component of adamantinoma of long bones. *Am J Pathol*. 1995;147:1770–1779.

Higinbotham NL, Phillips RF, Farr HW, Hustu HO. Chordoma. Thirty-five-year study at Memorial Hospital. *Cancer*. 1967;20:1841–1850.

Hoch B, Hermann G, Klein MJ, Abdelwahab IF, Springfield D. Giant cell tumor complicating Paget disease of long bone. *Skeletal Radiol*. 2007;36:973–978.

Hong WS, Sung MS, Kim J-H, et al. Giant cell tumor with secondary aneurysmal bone cyst: A unique presentation with an ossified extraosseous soft tissue mass. *Skeletal Radiol.* 2013;42:1605–1610.

Hudson TM. Fluid levels in aneurysmal bone cysts: a CT feature. *AJR Am J Roentgenol.* 1984;141:1001–1004.

Hudson TM. Scintigraphy of aneurysmal bone cysts. *AJR Am J Roentgenol.* 1984;142:761–765.

Hudson TM. *Radiologic Pathologic Correlation of Musculoskeletal Lesions.* Baltimore, MD: Williams & Wilkins; 1987:209–237, 249–252, 261–265, 287–303, 359–397, 421–440.

Hudson TM, Schiebler M, Springfield DS, Enneking WF, Hawkins IF Jr, Spanier SS. Radiology of giant cell tumors of bone: computed tomography, arthrotomography, and scintigraphy. *Skeletal Radiol.* 1984;11:85–95.

Hudson TM, Hamlin DJ, Fitzimmons JR. Magnetic resonance imaging of fluid levels in an aneurysmal bone cyst and in anticoagulated human blood. *Skeletal Radiol.* 1985;13:267–270.

Hutter RVP, Worcester JN Jr, Francis KC, Foote FW Jr, Stewart FW. Benign and malignant giant cell tumors of bone. A clinicopathological analysis of the natural history of the disease. *Cancer.* 1962;15:653–690.

Huvos AG. *Bone Tumors: Diagnosis, Treatment, and Prognosis.* 2nd ed. Philadelphia, PA: WB Saunders; 1991:599–624, 695–711, 713–743.

Huvos AG, Marcove RC. Adamantinoma of long bones: a clinicopathological study of fourteen cases with vascular origin suggested. *J Bone Joint Surg Am.* 1975;57A:148–154.

Ilaslan H, Sundaram M, Unni KK. Solid variant of aneurysmal bone cysts in long tubular bones: giant cell reparative granuloma. *AJR Am J Roentgenol.* 2003;180:1681–1687.

Ishida T, Iijima T, Kikuchi F, et al. A clinicopathological and immunohistochemical study of osteofibrous dysplasia, differentiated adamantinoma, and adamantinoma of long bones. *Skeletal Radiol.* 1992;21:493–502.

Jaffe HL. Aneurysmal bone cyst. *Bull Hosp Joint Dis.* 1950;11:3–13.

Jaffe HL. Giant-cell reparative granuloma, traumatic bone cyst, and fibrous (fibroosseous) dysplasia of the jawbones. *Oral Surg.* 1953;6:159–175.

Jaffe HL. *Tumors and Tumorous Conditions of the Bones and Joints.* Philadelphia, PA: Lea & Febiger; 1958.

Jaffe HL, Lichtenstein L. Solitary unicameral bone cyst with emphasis on the roentgen picture, the pathologic appearance, and the pathogenesis. *Arch Surg.* 1942;44:1004–1025.

Jaffe HL, Lichtenstein L, Perris RB. Giant cell tumor of bone. Its pathologic appearance, grading, supposed variants and treatment. *Arch Pathol.* 1940;30:993–1031.

Jain D, Jain VK, Vasishta RK, Rajan P, Kumar Y. Adamantinoma: a clinicopathological review and update. *Diagn Pathol.* 2008;3:8–15.

Jambhekar NA, Rekhi B, Thorat K, Dikshit R, Agrawal M, Puri A. Revisiting chordoma with brachyury, a "new age" marker: analysis of a validation study on 51 cases. *Arch Pathol Lab Med.* 2010;134:1181–1187.

Jordanov MI. The "rising bubble" sign: a new aid in the diagnosis of unicameral bone cysts. *Skeletal Radiol.* 2009;38:597–600.

Jundt G, Moll C, Nidecker A, Schilt R, Remagen W. Primary leiomyosarcoma of bone: report of eight cases. *Hum Pathol.* 1994;25:1205–1212.

Jundt G, Remberger K, Roessner A, Schulz A, Bohndorf K. Adamantinoma of long bones. A histopathological and immunohistochemical study of 23 cases. *Pathol Res Pract.* 1995;191:112–120.

Junghanns H. Lipomas (fatty marrow areas) in the vertebral column. In: *Handbuch de Speziellen Pathologischen Anatomic und Histologic, Tome IX/4.* Berlin, Germany: Springer-Verlag; 1939:333–334.

Kanamori M, Antonescu CR, Scott M, et al. Extra copies of chromosomes 7, 8, 12, 19, and 21 are recurrent in adamantinoma. *J Mol Diagn.* 2001;3:16–21.

Kaplan PA, Murphy M, Greenway G, Resnick D, Sartoris DJ, Harms S. Fluid-fluid levels in giant cell tumors of bone: report of two cases. *Computed Tomogr.* 1987;11:151–155.

Kashima T, Dongre A, Flanagan AM, Hogendoorn PC, Taylor R, Athanasou NA. Podoplanin expression in adamantinoma of long bones and osteofibrous dysplasia. *Virchows Arch.* 2011;459:41–46.

Keats TE. *Atlas of Normal Roentgen Variants That May Simulate Disease.* 5th ed. St. Louis, MO: Mosby Year Book; 1992:637–648.

Keeney GL, Unni KK, Beabout JW, Pritchard DJ. Adamantinoma of long bones. A clinicopathologic study of 85 cases. *Cancer.* 1989;64:730–737.

Kenan S, Lewis MM, Abdelwahab IF, Hermann G, Klein MJ. Case report 652: primary intraosseous low grade myxoid sarcoma of the scapula (myxoid liposarcoma). *Skeletal Radiol.* 1991;20:73–75.

Kitsoulis P, Charchanti A, Paraskevas G, Marini A, Karatzias G, et al. Adamantinoma (review article). *Acta Orthop Belg.* 2007;73:425–431.

Knapp RH, Wick MR, Scheithauer BW, Unni KK. Adamantinoma of bone. An electron microscopic and immunohistochemical study. *Virchows Arch A Pathol Anat Histopathol.* 1982;398:75–86.

Kohler A, Zimmer EA. *Borderlands of Normal and Early Pathologic Findings in Skeletal Radiography.* 13th ed. Revised by Schmidt H, Freyschmidt J. Stuttgart, Germany: Thieme Verlag; 1993:797–814.

Kordos J, Makai F, Galbavy S, Paukovic J, Svec A. Primary intraosseous liposarcoma—case report. *Acta Chir Orthop Traumatol Cech.* 1998;65:184–186.

Kransdorf MJ, Sweet DE. Aneurysmal bone cyst: concept, controversy, clinical presentation, and imaging. *AJR Am J Roentgenol.* 1995;164:573–580.

Kransdorf MJ, Sweet DE, Buetow PC, Giudici MA, Moser RP Jr. Giant cell tumor in skeletally immature patients. *Radiology.* 1992;184:233–237.

Kricun ME. Tumors of the foot. In: Kricun ME, ed. *Imaging of Bone Tumors.* Philadelphia, PA: WB Saunders; 1993:221–225.

Kyriakos M, Hardy D. Malignant transformation of aneurysmal bone cyst, with an analysis of the literature. *Cancer.* 1991;68:1770–1780.

Larizza L, Mortini P, Riva P. Update on the cytogenetics and molecular genetics of chordoma. *Hered Cancer Clin Pract.* 2005;3:29–41.

Lee MY, Jee W-H, Jung CK, et al. Giant cell tumor of soft tissue: a case report with emphasis on MR imaging. *Skeletal Radiol* 2015;44:1039–1043.

Levy WM, Miller AS, Bonakdarpour A, Aegerter E. Aneurysmal bone cyst secondary to other osseous lesions. Report of 57 cases. *Am J Clin Pathol.* 1975;63:1–8.

Lichtenstein L. Aneurysmal bone cyst. A pathological entity commonly mistaken for giant cell tumor and occasionally for hemangioma and osteogenic sarcoma. *Cancer.* 1950;3:279–289.

Lichtenstein L. Aneurysmal bone cyst. Observations on fifty cases. *J Bone Joint Surg Am.* 1957;39A:873–882.

Llombart-Bosch A, Ortuno-Pacheco G. Ultrastructural findings supporting the angioblastic nature of the so-called adamantinoma of the tibia. *Histopathology.* 1978;2:189–200.

Lmejjati M, Loqa C, Haddi M, Hakkou M, banAli SA. Primary liposarcoma of the lumbar spine. *Joint Bone Spine.* 2008;75:482–485.

Lomasney LM, Basu A, Demos TC, Laskin W. Fibrous dysplasia complicated by aneurysmal bone cyst formation affecting multiple cervical vertebrae. *Skeletal Radiol.* 2003;32:533–536.

Lorenzo JC, Dorfman HD. Giant-cell reparative granuloma of short tubular bones of the hands and feet. *Am J Surg Pathol.* 1980;4:551–563.

Macarenco RS, Erickson-Johnson M, Wang X, Jenkins RB, Nascimento AG, Oliveira AM. Cytogenetic and molecular genetic findings in dedifferentiated liposarcoma with neural-like whirling pattern and metaplastic bone formation. *Cancer Genet Cytogenet.* 2006;171:126–129.

Macmull S, Atkinson HDE, Saso S, Tirabosco R, O'Donnell P, Skinner JA. Primary intra-osseous liposarcoma of the femur: a case report. *J Orthop Surg.* 2009;17:374–378.

Markel SF. Ossifying fibroma of long bone. Its distinction from fibrous dysplasia and its association with adamantinoma of long bone. *Am J Clin Pathol.* 1978;69:91–97.

Martinez V, Sissons HA. Aneurysmal bone cyst. A review of 123 cases including primary lesions and those secondary to other bone pathology. *Cancer.* 1988;61:2291–2304.

Marui T, Yamamoto T, Yoshihara H, Kurosaka M, Mizuno K, Akamatsu T. De novo malignant transformation of giant cell tumor of bone. *Skeletal Radiol.* 2001;30:104–108.

Matcuk GR, Patel DB, Schein AJ, et al. Giant cell tumor: rapid recurrence after cessation of long-term denosumab therapy. *Skeletal Radiol* 2015;44:1027–1031.

May DA, Good RB, Smith DK, Parsons TW. MR imaging of musculoskeletal tumors and tumor mimickers with intravenous gadolinium: experience with 242 patients. *Skeletal Radiol.* 1997;26:2–15.

McDonald DJ, Sim FH, McLeod RA, Dahlin DC. Giant cell tumor of bone. *J Bone Joint Surg Am.* 1986;68A:235–242.

McGlynn FJ, Mickelson MR, El-Khoury GY. The fallen fragment sign in unicameral bone cyst. *Clin Orthop.* 1981;156:157–159.

McGrath J. Giant-cell tumour of bone: an analysis of fifty-two cases. *J Bone Joint Surg [Br].* 1972;54B:216–229.

Meis JM, Dorfman HD, Nathanson SD, Haggar AM, Wu KK. Primary malignant giant cell tumor of bone: dedifferentiated giant cell tumor. *Mod Pathol.* 1989;2:541–546.

Milgram JW. Intraosseous lipoma: radiologic and pathologic manifestations. *Radiology.* 1988;167:155–160.

Milgram JW. Intraosseous lipomas. A clinicopathological study of 66 cases. *Clin Orthop.* 1988;231:277–302.

Morton KS. The pathogenesis of unicameral bone cyst. *Can J Surg.* 1964;7:140–150.

Mulder JD, Kroon HM, SchCtte HE, Taconis WK. *Radiologic Atlas of Bone Tumors.* Amsterdam, the Netherlands: Elsevier; 1993:241–254, 267–274, 507–516, 557–590, 607–625.

Murphey MD, Nomikos GC, Flemming DJ, Gannon FH, Temple HT, Kransdorf MJ. From the archives of the AFIP. Imaging of giant cell tumor and giant cell reparative granuloma of bone: radiologic-pathologic correlation. *Radiographics.* 2001;21:1283–1309.

Murray RO, Jacobson HG. *The Radiology of Bone Diseases.* 2nd ed. New York, NY: Churchill Livingstone; 1977:585.

Myers JL, Arocho J, Bernreuter W, Dunham W, Mazur MT. Leiomyosarcoma of bone. A clinicopathologic, immunohistochemical, and ultrastructural study of five cases. *Cancer.* 1991;67:1051–1056.

Nascimento AG, Huvos AG, Marcove RC. Primary malignant giant cell tumor of bone: a study of eight cases and review of the literature. *Cancer.* 1979;44:1393–1402.

Nikitakis NG, Lopes MA, Pazoki AE, Ord RA, Sauk JJ. MDM2+/CDK4+/p53+ oral liposarcoma: case report and review of the literature. *Surg Oral Med Oral Pathol Oral Radiol Endod.* 2001;92:194–201.

Norman A, Schiffman M. Simple bone cyst: factors of age dependency. *Radiology.* 1977;124:779–782.

Norman A, Steiner GC. Radiographic and morphological features of cyst formation in idiopathic bone infarction. *Radiology.* 1983;146:335–338.

Oda Y, Tsuneyoshi M, Shinohara N. Solid variant of aneurysmal bone cyst (extragnatic giant cell reparative granuloma) in the axial skeleton and long bones: a study of its morphologic spectrum and distinction from allied giant cell lesions. *Cancer.* 1992;70:2642–2649.

Oliveira AM, Hsi BL, Weremowicz S, et al. USP6 (Tre2) fusion oncogenes in aneurysmal bone cyst. *Cancer Res.* 2004;64:1920–1923.

Oliveira AM, Perez-Atayde AR, Dal Cin P, et al. Aneurysmal bone cyst variant translocations upregulate USP6 transcription by promoter swapping with the ZNF9, COL1A1, TRAP150, and OMD genes. *Oncogene.* 2005;24:3419–3426.

Panchwagh Y, Puri A, Agarwal M, Chinoy R, Jambhekar N. Case report: metastatic adamantinoma of the tibia—an unusual presentation. *Skeletal Radiol.* 2006;35:190–193.

Pardo-Mindan FJ, Ayala H, Joly M, Gimeno E, Vázquez JJ. Primary liposarcoma of bone: light and electron microscopic study. *Cancer.* 1981;48:274–280.

Patel K, French C, Khaniwala SS, Rohrer M, Kademani D. Intraosseous leiomyosarcoma of the mandible: a case report. *J Oral Maxillofac Surg.* 2013;71:1209–1216.

Peimer CA, Schiller AL, Mankin HJ, Smith RJ. Multicentric giant cell tumor of bone. *J Bone Joint Surg Am.* 1980;62A:652–656.

Picci P, Manfrini M, Zucchi V, et al. Giant cell tumor bone in skeletally immature patients. *J Bone Joint Surg Am.* 1983;65A:486–490.

Picci P, Baldini N, Sudanese A, Boriani S, Campanacci M. Giant cell reparative granuloma and other giant cell lesions of the bones of the hand and feet. *Skeletal Radiol.* 1986;15:415–421.

Potter HG, Schneider R, Ghelman B, Healey JH, Lane JM. Multiple giant cell tumors and Paget disease of bone: radiographic and clinical correlations. *Radiology.* 1991;180:261–264.

Presneau N, Shalaby A, Ye H, et al. Role of the transcription factor T (brachyury) in the pathogenesis of sporadic chordoma: a genetic and functional-based study. *J Pathol.* 2011;223:327–335

Ratner V, Dorfman HD. Giant-cell reparative granuloma of the hand and foot bones. *Clin Orthop.* 1990;260:251–258.

Remagen W, Lampérth BE, Jundt G, Schildt R. Das sogenannte osteolytische Dreieck de Calcaneus. Radiologische und pathoanatomische Befunde. *Osteologie.* 1994;3:275–283.

Resnick D, Niwayama J. *Diagnosis of Bone and Joint Disorders.* Philadelphia, PA: WB Saunders; 1988:3782–3786.

Resnick D, Niwayama G. Skeletal metastases. In: Resnick D, ed. *Diagnosis of Bone and Joint Disorders.* 3rd ed. Philadelphia, PA: WB Saunders; 1995:3991–4065.

Resnick D, Kyriakos M, Greenway GD. Tumors and tumor-like lesions of bone: imaging and pathology of specific lesions. In: Resnick D, ed. *Diagnosis of Bone and Joint Disorders.* 3rd ed. Philadelphia, PA: WB Saunders; 1995:3628–3938.

Reynolds J. The fallen fragment sign in the diagnosis of unicameral bone cysts. *Radiology.* 1969;92:949–953.

Richkind KE, Mortimer E, Mowery-Rushton P, et al. Translocation (16:20) (p11.2q13) sole cytogenetic abnormality in a unicameral bone cyst. *Cancer Genet Cytogenet.* 2002;137:153–155.

Rock MG, Beabout JW, Unni KK, Sim FH. Adamantinoma. *Orthopedics.* 1983;6:472–477.

Rock MG, Pritchard DJ, Unni KK. Metastases from histologically benign giant-cell tumor of bone. *J Bone Joint Surg Am.* 1984;66A:269–274.

Rock MG, Sim FH, Unni KK, et al. Secondary malignant giant-cell tumor of bone. Clinicopathological assessment of nineteen patients. *J Bone Joint Surg Am.* 1986;68A:1073–1079.

Rosai J. Adamantinoma of the tibia: electron microscopic evidence of its epithelial origin. *Am J Clin Pathol.* 1969;51:786–792.

Rosai J, Pinkus GS. Immunohistochemical demonstration of epithelial differentiation in adamantinoma of the tibia. *Am J Surg Pathol.* 1982;6:427–434.

Salerno M, Avnet S, Alberghini M, Giunit A, Baldini N. Histogenetic characterization of giant cell tumor of bone. *Clin Orthop Relat Res.* 2008;466:2081–2088.

Sanerkin NG. Primary leiomyosarcoma of the bone and its comparison with fibrosarcoma. *Cancer.* 1979;44:1375–1387.

Sanerkin NG. Malignancy, aggressiveness and recurrence in giant cell tumor of bone. *Cancer.* 1980;46:1641–1649.

Sanerkin NG, Mott MG, Roylance J. An unusual intraosseous lesion with fibromyxoid elements: solid variant of aneurysmal bone cyst. *Cancer.* 1983;51:2278–2286.

Sangoi AR, Karamchandani J, Lane B, et al. Specificity of brachyury in the distinction of chordoma from clear cell renal carcinoma and germ cell tumors: a study of 305 cases. *Mod Pathol.* 2011;24:425–429.

Sarita-Reyes CD, Greco MA, Steiner GC. Mesenchymal-epithelial differentiation of adamantinoma of long bones: an immunohistochemical and ultrastructural study. *Ultrastruct Pathol.* 2012;36:23–30.

Schajowicz F. *Tumors and Tumorlike Lesions of Bone: Pathology, Radiology, and Treatment.* 2nd ed. Berlin, Germany: Springer-Verlag; 1994: 257–299, 301–367, 468–481, 552–566.

Schajowicz F, Santini-Araujo E. Adamantinoma of the tibia masked by fibrous dysplasia. Report of three cases. *Clin Orthop.* 1989;238: 294–301.

Schajowicz F, Slullitel J. Giant cell tumor associated with Paget's disease of bone. *J Bone Joint Surg Am.* 1966;48A:1340–1349.

Schneider HM, Wunderlich T, Puls P. The primary liposarcoma of bone. *Arch Orthop Trauma Surg.* 1980;96:235–239.

Schoedel K, Shankman S, Desai P. Intracortical and subperiosteal aneurysmal bone cysts: a report of three cases. *Skeletal Radiol.* 1996;25:455–459.

Sciot R, Dorfman H, Brys P, et al. Cytogenetic-morphologic correlations in aneurysmal bone cyst, giant cell tumor of bone and combined lesions. A report from the CHAMP study group. *Mod Pathol.* 2000;13:1206–2010.

Selzer G, Raffaele D, Revach M, Cvibah TJ, Fried A. Goltz syndrome with multiple giant-cell tumor-like lesions in bones: a case report. *Ann Intern Med.* 1974;80:714–716.

Shankman S, Greenspan A, Klein MJ, Lewis MM. Giant cell tumor of the ischium. A report of two cases and review of the literature. *Skeletal Radiol.* 1988;17:46–51.

Shao L, Mardis N, Nopper A, Jarka D, Singh V. Giant cell tumor of bone in a child with Goltz syndrome. *Pediatr Dev Pathol.* 2013;16:308–311.

Sim FH, Dahlin DC, Beabout JW. Multicentric giant cell tumors of bone. *J Bone Joint Surg Am.* 1977;59A:1052–1060.

Skubitz KM, Cheng EY, Clohisy DR, Thompson RC, Skubitz AP. Gene expression in giant-cell tumors. *J Lab Clin Med.* 2004;144:193–200.

Smith RW, Smith CF. Solitary unicameral bone cyst of the calcaneus. A review of 20 cases. *J Bone Joint Surg Am.* 1974;56A:49–56.

Smith LT, Mayerson J, Nowak NJ, et al. 20q11.1 amplification in giant-cell tumor of bone: array CGH, FISH, and association with outcome. *Genes Chromosomes Cancer.* 2006;45:957–966.

Soper JR, De Silva M. Infantile myofibromatosis: a radiological review. *Pediatr Radiol.* 1993;23:189–194.

Spjut HJ, Dorfman HD, Fechner RE, Ackerman LV. *Atlas of Tumor Pathology. Tumors of Bone and Cartilage.* 2nd series, fascicle 5. Washington, DC: Armed Forces Institute of Pathology; 1971:347–390.

Spjut HJ, Dorfman HD, Fechner RE, Ackerman LV. *Tumors of Bone and Cartilage.* Washington, DC: Armed Forces Institute of Pathology; 1971.

Springfield DS, Rosenberg AE, Mankin HJ, Mindell ER. Relationship between osteofibrous dysplasia and adamantinoma. *Clin Orthop.* 1994;309:234–244.

Stacy GS, Peabody TD, Dixon LB. Pictorial essay. Mimics on radiography of giant cell tumor of bone. *AJR Am J Roentgenol.* 2003;181:1583–1589.

Stanton RP, Abdel-Mota'al MM. Growth arrest resulting from unicameral bone cyst. *J Pediatr Orthop.* 1998;18:198–201.

Steiner GC, Ghosh L, Dorfman HD. Ultrastructure of giant cell tumor of bone. *Hum Pathol.* 1972;3:569–586.

Stout AP, Lattes R. Tumors of the soft tissues. In: *Atlas of Tumor Pathology.* 2nd fascicle, series 1. Washington, DC: Armed Forces Institute of Pathology; 1967.

Struhl S, Edelson C, Pritzker H, Seimon LP, Dorfman HD. Solitary (unicameral) bone cyst. The fallen fragment sign revisited. *Skeletal Radiol.* 1989;18:261–265.

Sundaram M, McLeod RA. MR imaging of tumor and tumorlike lesions of bone and soft tissue. *AJR Am J Roentgenol.* 1990;155:817–824.

Sundaram M, Akduman I, White LM, McDonald DJ, Kandel R, Janney C. Primary leiomyosarcoma of bone. *AJR Am J Roentgenol.* 1999;172:771–776.

Sung MS, Lee GK, Kang HS. Sacrococcygeal chordoma: MR imaging in 30 patients. *Skeletal Radiol.* 2005;34:87–94.

Sweet DE, Vinh TN, Devaney K. Cortical osteofibrous dysplasia of long bone and its relationship to adamantinoma. A clinicopathologic study of 30 cases. *Am J Surg Pathol.* 1992;16:282–290.

Szuhai K, Ijszenga M, Knijnenburg J, et al. Does parosteal liposarcoma differ from other atypical lipomatous tumors/well-differentiated liposarcomas? A molecular cytogenetic study using combined multicolor COBRA-FISH karyotyping and array-based comparative genomic hybridization. *Cancer Genet Cytogenet.* 2007;176:115–120.

Tanaka H, Yasui N, Kuriskaki E, Shimomura Y. The Golz syndrome associated with giant cell tumour of bone. A case report. *Int Orthop.* 1990;14:179–181.

Taybi H, Lachman RS. *Radiology of Syndromes, Metabolic Disorders, and Skeletal Dysplasias.* 4th ed. St. Louis, MO: CV Mosby, 1996:580–581.

Tsai JC, Dalinka MK, Fallon MD, Zlatkin MB, Kressel HY. Fluid-fluid level: a nonspecific finding in tumors of bone and soft tissue. *Radiology.* 1990;175:779–782.

Tubbs WS, Brown LR, Beabout JW, Rock MG, Unni KK. Benign giant-cell tumor of bone with pulmonary metastases: clinical findings and radiologic appearance of metastases in 13 cases. *AJR Am J Roentgenol.* 1992;158:331–334.

Ueda Y, Roessner A, Bosse A, Edel G, Böcker W, Wuisman P. Juvenile intracortical adamantinoma of the tibia with predominant osteofibrous dysplasia-like features. *Pathol Res Pract.* 1991;187:1039–1043.

Unni KK. *Dublin's Bone Tumors: General Aspects and Data on 11,087 Cases.* 5th ed. New York, NY: Lippincott-Raven Publishers; 1996.

Unni KK, Dahlin DC, Beabout JW, Ivins JC. Adamantinoma of long bones. *Cancer.* 1974;34:1796–1805.

Van der Woude HJ, Hazelbag HM, Bloem JL, Taminiau AH, Hogendoorn PC. MRI of adamantinoma of long bones in correlation with histopathology. *AJR Am J Roentgenol.* 2004;183:1737–1744.

Verelst SJ, Hans J, Hanselmann RG, Wirbel RJ. Genetic instability in primary leiomyosarcoma of bone. *Hum Pathol.* 2004;35:1404–1412.

Vergel De Dios AM, Bond JR, Shives TC, McLeod RA, Unni KK. Aneurysmal bone cyst. A clinicopathologic study of 238 cases. *Cancer.* 1992;69:2921–2931.

Vester H, Wegener B, Weiler C, Baur-Melnyk A, Jansson V, Dürr HR. First report of a solid variant of aneurysmal bone cyst in the os sacrum. *Skeletal Radiol.* 2010;39:73–77.

Watanabe K, Kusakabe T, Hoshi N, Saito A, Suzuki T. h-Caldesmon in leiomyosarcoma and tumors with smooth muscle cell-like differentiation: its specific expression in the smooth muscle cell tumor. *Hum Pathol.* 1999;30:392–396.

Weisel A, Hecht HL. Development of a unicameral bone cyst. *J Bone Joint Surg Am.* 1980;62A:664–666.

Weiss SW. Ultrastructure of the so-called "chordoid sarcoma." Evidence supporting cartilaginous differentiation. *Cancer.* 1976;37:300–306.

Weiss SW, Dorfman HD. Adamantinoma of long bone. An analysis of nine new cases with emphasis on metastasizing lesions and fibrous dysplasia-like changes. *Hum Pathol.* 1977;8:141–153.

Wilner D. *Radiology of Bone Tumors and Allied Disorders.* Philadelphia, PA: WB Saunders; 1982:387.

Wippold FJ III, Koeller KK, Smirniotopoulos JG. Clinical and imaging features of cervical chordoma. *AJR Am J Roentgenol.* 1999;172:1423–1426.

Wold LE, Swee RG. Giant cell tumor of the small bones of the hands and feet. *Semin Diagn Pathol.* 1984;1:173–184.

Wold LE, Dobyns JH, Swee RG, Dahlin DC. Giant cell reaction (giant cell reparative granuloma) of the small bones of the hands and feet. *Am J Surg Pathol.* 1986;10:491–496.

Wyatt-Ashmead J, Bao L, Eilert RE, Gibbs P, Glancy G, McGavran L. Primary aneurysmal bone cysts: 16q22 and/or 17p13 chromosome abnormalities. *Pediatr Dev Pathol.* 2001;4:418–419.

Ye Y, Pringle LM, Lau AW, et al. TRE17/USP6 oncogene translocated in aneurysmal bone cyst induces matrix metalloproteinase production via activation of NF-kappaB. *Oncogene.* 2010;29:3619–3629.

Yochum TR, Rowe LJ. Tumor and tumor-like processes. In: Yochum TR, Rowe LJ, eds. *Essentials of Skeletal Radiology.* Vol. 2. Baltimore, MD: Williams & Wilkins; 1987:699–919.

Yoneyama T, Winter WG, Milsow L. Tibial adamantinoma: its histogenesis from ultrastructural studies. *Cancer.* 1977;40:1138–1142.

Zehr RJ, Recht MP, Bauer TW. Adamantinoma. *Skeletal Radiol.* 1995;24:553–555

CHAPTER 8
Tumors and Tumor-like Lesions of the Joints

Synovial (osteo)chondromatosis (also known as synovial chondromatosis or synovial chondrometaplasia) is an uncommon benign disorder marked by the metaplastic proliferation of multiple cartilaginous nodules in the synovial membrane of the joints, bursae, or tendon sheaths. This condition was discussed in Chapter 3 under the heading of benign cartilage-forming (chondrogenic) lesions. *Pigmented villonodular synovitis (PVNS)*, also known as diffuse-type tenosynovial giant cell tumor, is a locally destructive fibrohistiocytic proliferation, characterized by many villous and nodular synovial protrusions, which affects the joints, bursae, and tendon sheaths. This condition can be diffuse or localized. When the entire synovium of the joint is affected, the condition is referred to as diffuse PVNS. When a discrete intra-articular mass is present, the condition is called localized PVNS. When the process affects the tendon sheaths, it is called localized giant cell tumor of the tendon sheaths, nodular tenosynovitis, or according to the recent World Health Organization (WHO) classification, tenosynovial giant cell tumor. *Synovial hemangioma*, a rare benign lesion whose pathogenesis is still unclear (although some investigators suggest it is a form of vascular malformation), commonly affects the knee joint, although the other articulations such as the elbow, wrist, and ankle may also be the site of this disorder. *Lipoma arborescens*, also known as villous lipomatous proliferation of the synovial membranes, is a rare intra-articular disorder characterized by a nonneoplastic lipomatous proliferation of the synovium. The term "arborescens" describes the characteristic tree-like morphology of the lesion, which resembles a frond-like mass. *Synovial sarcoma* (also known as synovioma) is an uncommon malignant mesenchymal neoplasm, that despite its name, does not arise from the synovium. It occurs mainly in para-articular regions close to the joint capsules, bursae, and tendon sheaths. *Synovial chondrosarcoma* is a rare tumor that originates from the synovial membrane. It may arise as a primary synovial tumor or it may develop as a malignant transformation of synovial (osteo)chondromatosis.

A. Benign Joint Lesions
Synovial (Osteo)Chondromatosis
Pigmented Villonodular Synovitis (PVNS, Diffuse-Type Tenosynovial Giant Cell Tumor)
Localized Pigmented Nodular Tenosynovitis (Giant Cell Tumor of the Tendon Sheath, Localized Tenosynovial Giant Cell Tumor)
Synovial Hemangioma
Lipoma Arborescens
Juxta-Articular Myxoma

B. Malignant Joint Tumors
Synovial Sarcoma
Synovial Chondrosarcoma

A. BENIGN JOINT LESIONS

Synovial (Osteo)Chondromatosis

This condition marked by the metaplastic proliferation of multiple cartilaginous nodules in the synovial membrane was discussed in Chapter 3.

Pigmented Villonodular Synovitis (PVNS, Diffuse-Type Tenosynovial Giant Cell Tumor)

Definition:
- Locally destructive fibrohistiocytic proliferation characterized by multiple villous and nodular synovial protrusions composed of synovial-like mononuclear cells admixed with multinucleated giant cells, foam cells, siderophages, and inflammatory cells.

Epidemiology:
- Young and middle-aged individuals are most commonly affected, with peak incidence in the third and fourth decades.
- Male-to-female ratio of 1:2.

Sites of Involvement:
- Most common site is the knee joint (75%); less frequently affected are the hip (15%), ankle, wrist, elbow, and shoulder joints.

Clinical Findings:
- Slowly progressing process that manifests by mild pain, joint swelling, and limitation of movements in the affected joint.
- Duration of symptoms may range from 6 months to as long as 25 years.

Imaging:
- Radiography shows soft-tissue density within the joint greater than expected with joint effusion; occasionally, lobulated soft-tissue mass can be present (Fig. 8.1).
- Marginal, well-defined erosions of subchondral bone with sclerotic margin on both sides of the joint may be present in about 15% to 50% of cases (see Fig. 8.1). Occasional narrowing of the joint space.
- Contrast arthrography demonstrates multiple lobulated masses with villous projections that appear as filling defects in the contrast-filled joint (Fig. 8.2).
- Magnetic resonance imaging features depend on the proportions of hemosiderin, fat, and fibrovascular elements. Generally, high amount of hemosiderin deposition results in low signal intensity of the lesion on both T1- and T2-weighted images. However, most of the intra-articular masses will exhibit a combination of high signal intensity areas representing fluid and congested synovium, interspersed with areas of intermediate-to-low signal intensity secondary to random distribution of hemosiderin in synovium (Figs. 8.3 and 8.4). Low signal intensity on gradient-echo sequences is characteristic. Postcontrast studies show significant enhancement of the lesion.

Pathology:
Gross (Macroscopy):
- Tan-colored or reddish-brown synovial mass, firm or sponge-like, with hypertrophic villi (Fig. 8.5).

Histopathology:
- Proliferating collagen-producing polyhedral cells with scattered multinucleated giant cells usually around hemorrhagic foci are commonly present (Fig. 8.6A,B).
- Iron deposits and aggregates of foam cells may be present, usually at the periphery of the lesion (Fig. 8.6C).
- Dense infiltration of small ovoid or spindle-shaped mononuclear histiocyte-like cells with pale eosinophilic cytoplasm and small ovoid or angulated nuclei commonly displaying longitudinal grooves, accompanied by plasma cells and lymphocytes may be present (Fig. 8.7).
- Larger mononuclear cells with kidney-shaped or lobulated nuclei, abundant eosinophilic cytoplasm with peripheral rim of hemosiderin granules, and occasionally with paranuclear eosinophilic filamentous inclusions (Fig. 8.8).
- Mitotic figures are not uncommon.
- Variable amount of hemosiderin can be present.
- Stroma shows variable degree of fibrosis and hyalinization (Fig. 8.9).
- Blood-filled pseudoalveolar spaces may be present.
- Extremely rare malignant variant with necrotic areas, significantly increased mitotic rate (more than 20 mitoses/HPF), and spindling of mononuclear cells in myxoid stroma.

Immunohistochemistry:
- Positivity for CD68, CD163, CD45, and some cases for CD34.

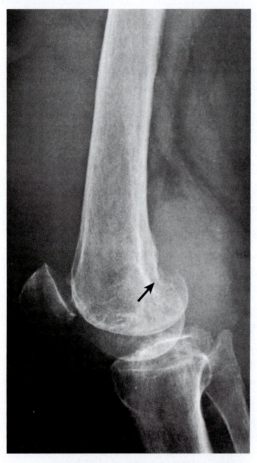

FIGURE 8.1 Radiography of pigmented villonodular synovitis. Lateral radiograph of the knee of a 58-year-old man shows large suprapatellar joint effusion and a dense, lumpy soft-tissue mass eroding the posterior aspect of the lateral femoral condyle (*arrow*). Observe that the density of the posterior mass is greater than that of a suprapatellar fluid.

Chapter 8 • Tumors and Tumor-like Lesions of the Joints   **355**

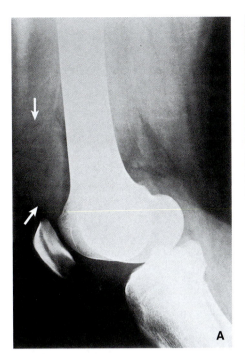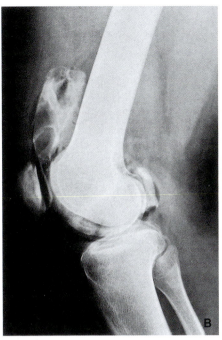

FIGURE 8.2 Radiography and contrast arthrography of pigmented villonodular synovitis. (A) Lateral radiograph of the knee of a 25-year-old woman shows what appears to be a suprapatellar joint effusion (*arrows*). The density of the fluid, however, is increased, and there is some lobulation present. **(B)** Contrast arthrogram of the knee shows lobulated filling defects in the suprapatellar bursa, representing lumpy synovial masses. Joint aspiration yielded thick bloody fluid. Subsequent arthroscopic surgery confirmed the diagnosis of PVNS.

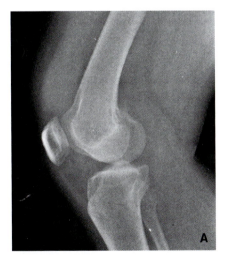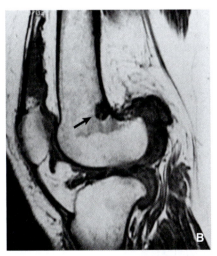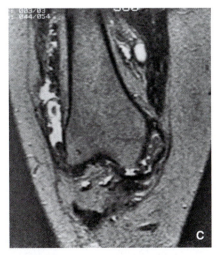

FIGURE 8.3 Radiography and magnetic resonance imaging of pigmented villonodular synovitis. (A) Lateral radiograph of the knee of a 22-year-old woman shows fullness in the suprapatellar bursa. In addition, there is increased density in the region of the popliteal fossa and subtle erosion of the posterior aspect of the distal femur. **(B)** Sagittal T1-weighted MRI shows a lobulated mass in the suprapatellar bursa extending into the knee joint and invading the infrapatellar Hoffa fat pad. Observe also the lobulated mass in the posterior aspect of joint capsule, extending toward the posterior tibia. These masses exhibit an intermediate-to-low signal intensity. The erosion at the posterior aspect of the distal femur (supracondylar) is clearly demonstrated by an area of low signal intensity (*arrow*). **(C)** Coronal T2-weighted MRI shows areas of high signal intensity that represent fluid and congested synovium, interspersed with foci of low signal intensity, characteristic of hemosiderin deposits.

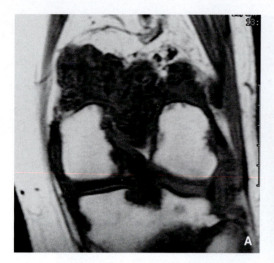
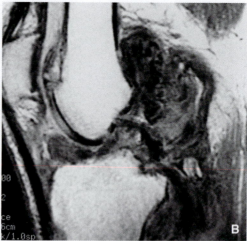
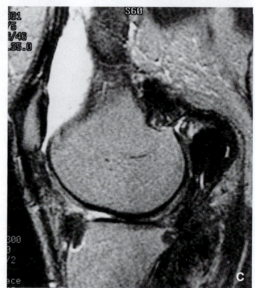

FIGURE 8.4 Magnetic resonance imaging of pigmented villonodular synovitis. (A) Coronal and **(B)** sagittal T1-weighted MR images of the left knee of a 40-year-old man show lobulated low signal intensity masses mainly located in the popliteal region. **(C)** Sagittal T2-weighted MR image demonstrates high signal intensity fluid in the suprapatellar bursa. The lobulated masses remain of low signal intensity.

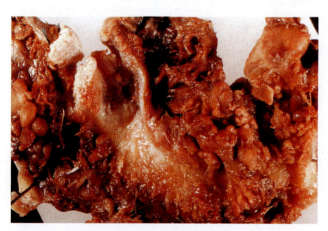

FIGURE 8.5 Gross specimen of pigmented villonodular synovitis. Photograph of the surgical specimen of the knee synovium shows plump papillary projections of the lesion. The *reddish-brown* staining is due to hemosiderin deposition. (From Bullough P. *Atlas of Orthopedic Pathology with Clinical and Radiologic Correlations*. 2nd ed. New York, NY: Gower Medical Publishing; 1992, p.17.27, Fig. 17.76.)

Genetics:
- The translocation t(1;2)(p11;q37) with *COL6A3-CSF1* gene fusion.
- Rearrangements of the 1p11-13 regions.

Prognosis:
- Common recurrence (about 18% to 46%).

Differential Diagnosis:
- *Synovial (osteo)chondromatosis*
  Radiography usually will show several small uniform in size osteochondral bodies within the joint. MRI will show lack of hemosiderin deposition paramagnetic features.
  Histopathology showing the presence of calcified or noncalcified intra-articular chondro-osseous bodies is diagnostic.

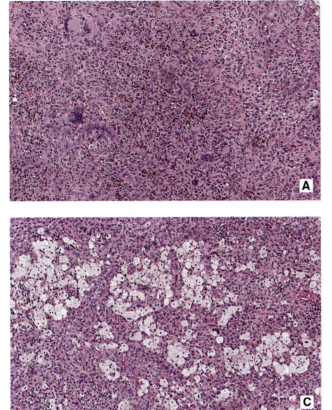
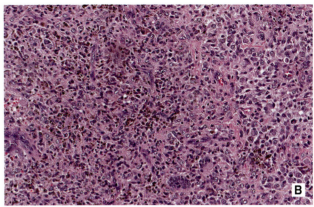

FIGURE 8.6 Histopathology of pigmented villonodular synovitis. (A) Tumor tissue is composed of admixture of small histiocyte-like cells and irregularly distributed osteoclast-like giant cells (H&E, original magnification ×100). **(B)** On higher magnification, observe, in addition to giant cells and small histiocytoid cells, the presence of large dendritic cells with abundant cytoplasm and deposits of hemosiderin (*brown foci*) (H&E, original magnification ×200). **(C)** On the periphery of the lesion, note the sheets of foamy cells (H&E, original magnification ×200).

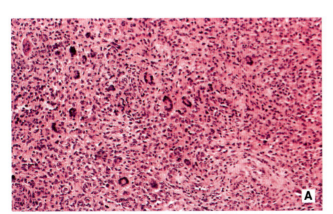
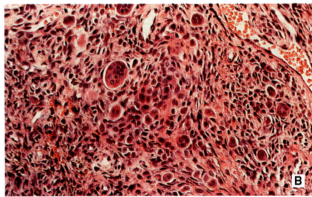

FIGURE 8.7 Histopathology of pigmented villonodular synovitis. (A) Low-power photomicrograph shows subsynovial nodular accumulation of mononuclear cells with interspersed giant cells exhibiting peripherally located nuclei (H&E, original magnification ×4). **(B)** Under higher magnification, observe large histiocytic cells, spindle-shaped fibroblasts, scattered giant cells, and foci of hemorrhage (H&E, original magnification ×25). (From Bullough P. *Atlas of Orthopedic Pathology with Clinical and Radiologic Correlations*. 2nd ed. New York, NY: Gower Medical Publishing; 1992, p. 17.27, Fig. 17.78.)

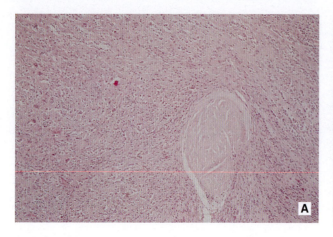
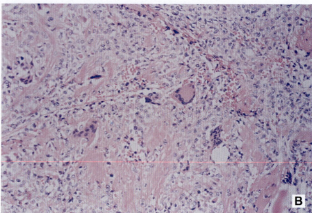
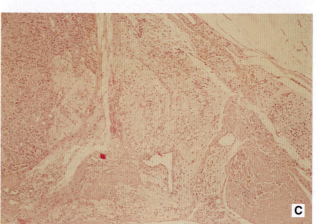

FIGURE 8.8 Histopathology of pigmented villonodular synovitis. (A) Extended strands of roundish histiocytic cells and scattered giant cells have formed bundles of condensed collagen *(center and upper right)*. In other areas *(lower right)*, the cells are more spindled (H&E, original magnification ×25). **(B)** At larger magnification, observe accumulation of mononuclear cells and intersperse giant cells that exhibit peripherally arranged nuclei *(center)*. Condensed collagen fibers resemble bone matrix *(bottom)* (H&E, original magnification ×50). **(C)** In another field of view, there are extended areas of lipid-laden macrophages and scattered hemosiderin-containing macrophages (H&E, original magnification ×25).

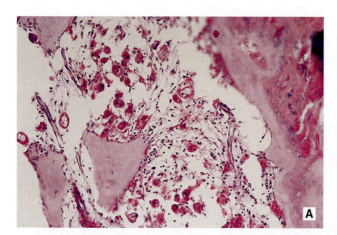
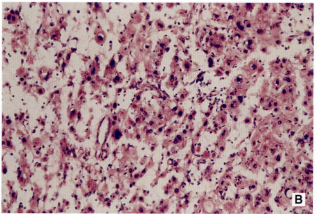

FIGURE 8.9 Histopathology of pigmented villonodular synovitis. (A) Cancellous bone from articular end of the tibia shows infiltration by large roundish cells exhibiting some pleomorphism and nuclear hyperchromatism (H&E, original magnification ×100). **(B)** The tissue obtained from the interior of the knee joint shows typical appearance of PVNS (H&E, original magnification ×100).

- *Lipoma arborescens*
  MRI features of fat signal intensity on all sequences are diagnostic.
  Histopathology showing features of hyperplasia of subsynovial fat, formation of mature fat cells, and presence of proliferative villous projections is diagnostic.
- *Synovial hemangioma*
  Imaging features, and particularly MR images showing intra-articular masses of high signal intensity on both T1-weighted and T2-weighted sequences, with low signal fibrofatty septa, are diagnostic.
  Histopathology showing vascular morphology of the lesion, particularly arborizing vascular channels of different sizes is diagnostic.
- *Hemophilic arthropathy*
  Imaging studies will show typical changes of joint arthropathy with narrowing of the joint space, articular erosions, epiphyseal overgrowth, and hemarthrosis.
  Histopathology showing copious iron deposition and markedly hyperplastic synovium usually limited to the synovial lining cells, together with characteristic clinical features, is diagnostic.

Localized Pigmented Nodular Tenosynovitis (Giant Cell Tumor of the Tendon Sheath, Localized Tenosynovial Giant Cell Tumor)

Definition:
- Well-circumscribed lesion that affects a small area of synovium or the tendon sheath, most commonly occurring in the digits, consisting of mononuclear cells mixed with variable number of multinucleated giant cells, foamy macrophages, and chronic inflammatory cells.

Epidemiology:
- May occur at any age but usually between 30 and 50 years.
- Slight female predominance.

Sites of Involvement:
- Predominantly affecting the digits of the hand (85%).
- Less common in the wrist, ankle, foot, or knee.

Clinical Findings:
- Painless swelling or mass.
- May gradually develop even for several years.

Imaging:
- Radiography shows localized well-circumscribed dense soft-tissue mass often associated with osseous erosion (Fig. 8.10).
- Magnetic resonance imaging shows in most cases low signal intensity on both T1- and T2-weighted sequences, with strong homogeneous enhancement after administration of gadolinium.

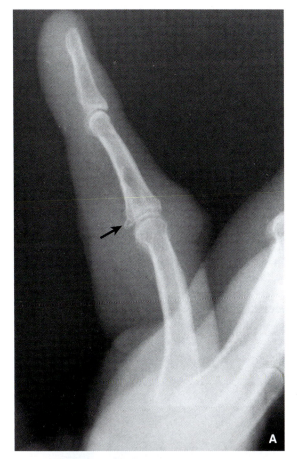

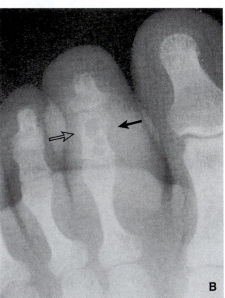

FIGURE 8.10 Radiography of giant cell tumor of the tendon sheath. (A) Lateral radiograph of the index finger of a 58-year-old man shows a soft-tissue mass at the site of the proximal interphalangeal joint. A small erosion is present at the base of the middle phalanx (*arrow*). **(B)** Anteroposterior radiograph of the toes of the middle-aged man shows a soft-tissue swelling of the second toe associated with several osteolytic defects in the middle phalanx (*arrows*).

Pathology:

Gross (Macroscopy):

- Most lesions are small, up to 4 cm.
- Well-circumscribed and lobulated tumor, white-tan to gray in color with yellowish and brown foci, partially encased by a fibrous capsule, may invade the bone or joint (Fig. 8.11).

Histopathology:

- Tissue is composed of different proportions of small, round, or spindle-shaped mononuclear cells with pale cytoplasm and round or kidney-shaped commonly grooved nuclei, osteoclast-like multinucleated giant cells, foamy macrophages, and siderophages (Fig. 8.12).
- Giant cells contain a variable number of nuclei (from a few to more than 50) and are commonly distributed at the periphery of the tumor (Fig. 8.13).
- Larger epithelioid cells with glassy cytoplasm and rounded vesicular nuclei may be present.
- Xanthoma cells associated with cholesterol clefts may be seen at the periphery of the tumor.
- Hemosiderin deposits are almost always present.
- Stroma may shows variable degree of hyalinization and may occasionally exhibit osteoid-like appearance (Fig. 8.13B).
- Mitotic activity usually averages 3 to 5 mitoses per 10 HPF but may reach up to 20/10 HPF.

Immunohistochemistry:

- Mononuclear cells expressed positivity for CD68 and CD163.
- Multinucleated giant cells are positive for CD68 and CD45.

Genetics:

- Same translocation as in diffuse type of tenosynovial giant cell tumor.

Prognosis:

- Low percentage of local recurrence after surgical intervention.

Differential Diagnosis:

- **Enchondroma**
  Imaging features of radiolucent lesion within the phalanges or metacarpals/metatarsals may occasionally mimic the erosive changes of GCT of the

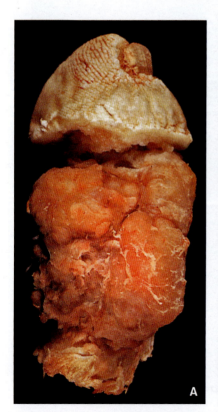
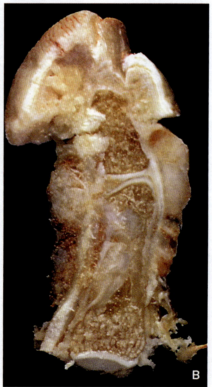
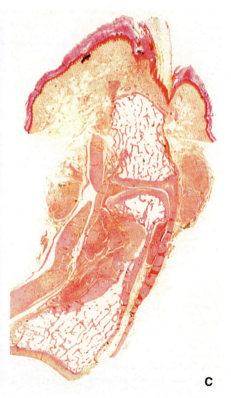

FIGURE 8.11 Gross specimen and histopathology of giant cell tumor of the tendon sheath (same patient as presented in Fig. 8.10B). (A) Photograph of the amputated second toe shows a tan tumor encasing the middle phalanx. **(B)** Sagittal section through the specimen shown in part (A) demonstrates soft-tissue tumor extending around and involving the distal interphalangeal joint. The lesion also invades the medullary cavity of the middle phalanx. **(C)** Whole-mount sagittal section through the second toe shows the tumor in the soft tissue, bone, and joint space. The *pink* foci within the tumor tissue represent areas of collagination (phloxine and tartrazine, original magnification ×1). (From Bullough P. *Atlas of Orthopedic Pathology with Clinical and Radiologic Correlations*. 2nd ed. New York, NY: Gower Medical Publishing; 1992, p. 17.25, Figs. 17.70, 17.71, and 17.72).

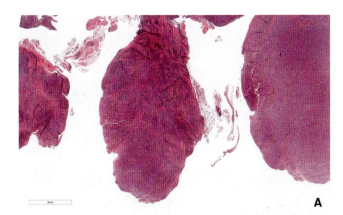 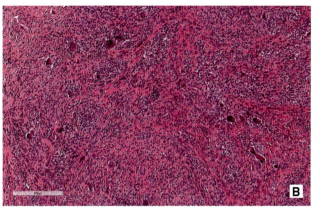

FIGURE 8.12 Histopathology of giant cell tumor of the tendon sheath. (A) Well-circumscribed and lobulated histiocytic in character mass is partially covered by a fibrous capsule (H&E, original magnification ×40). **(B)** Small round and spindle-shaped mononuclear cells are mixed with osteoclast-like giant cells (H&E, original magnification ×100).

tendon sheaths, but presence of typical chondroid calcifications and lack of soft-tissue swelling/mass is diagnostic.

Histopathology showing typical hyaline cartilage morphology of the lesion without atypia is diagnostic.

- *Soft-tissue chondroma*

  Imaging features of soft-tissue mass with typical chondroid calcifications and lack of erosive changes are diagnostic.

  Histopathology showing typical cartilaginous morphology of the lesion is diagnostic.

- *Gout*

  Radiographic features of tophaceous gout affecting the fingers or toes may occasionally mimic the appearance of GCT of the tendon sheath, but mineralization in the juxta-articular tophi and characteristic erosions exhibiting overhanging edges are diagnostic. In addition, in doubtful cases, dual-energy color-coded CT showing characteristic features of gouty tophi is diagnostic as well.

  Examination of synovial fluid showing typical monosodium urate crystals is diagnostic.

- *Synovial sarcoma*

  Imaging features of a large soft-tissue mass, commonly with foci of mineralization, associated with destructive changes of the adjacent bone, and in particular, MRI showing characteristic triple signal intensity sign, are diagnostic.

  Histopathology showing typical biphasic (spindle and epithelioid components) or monophasic (predominantly spindle component) morphology with clearly malignant cells is diagnostic.

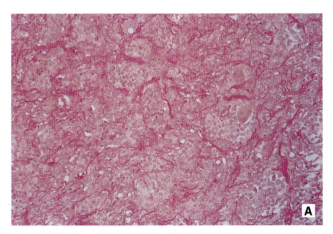 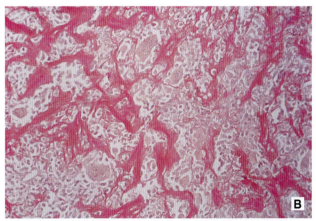

FIGURE 8.13 Histopathology of giant cell tumor of the tendon sheath. (A) Observe predominantly histiocytic character of the tumor. The collagen septa are less conspicuous (van Gieson, original magnification ×50). **(B)** In another field of view, sclerotic bundles of collagen fibers resembling osteoid predominate (*red structures*), surrounded by clusters of fairly large histiocytes and giant cells (van Gieson, original magnification ×50).

Synovial Hemangioma

Definition:
- Benign proliferation of blood vessels arising in a synovium-lined surface, including the joints, bursae, and tendon sheaths.

Epidemiology:
- Very rare lesion, occurring most commonly in children and adolescents.
- Predilection for males.

Sites of Involvement:
- Most common site is the knee joint, followed by the elbow, wrist, and ankle.

Clinical Findings:
- Slowly growing lesion often associated with swelling, joint effusion, and limitation of movement in the joint.
- Recurrent pain is a common symptom.
- Recurrent hemarthrosis may be encountered.

Imaging:
- Radiography may only show a joint effusion, occasionally associated with marginal erosions of bone (Fig. 8.14).
- Computed tomography also may demonstrate joint effusion and marginal erosions (Fig. 8.15).
- Magnetic resonance imaging shows soft-tissue mass of intermediate signal intensity on T1-weighted sequences, appearing isointense with or slightly brighter than muscle but less bright than fat. T2 weighting will demonstrate a high signal intensity mass (Fig. 8.16) with thin, serpentine low-intensity septa (Figs. 8.17 and 8.18). Occasionally, fluid–fluid levels will be present, particularly in cavernous type of the lesions (Fig. 8.19). Postcontrast studies show significant enhancement of the lesion.

Pathology:
Gross (Macroscopy):
- Vascular, lobulated, soft, brown, doughty mass exhibiting different size of vessels, with overlying villous synovium often stained mahogany-brown by hemosiderin (Fig. 8.20).

Histopathology:
- Morphology similar to cavernous hemangioma with dilated thin-walled arborizing vascular channels of different sizes (Fig. 8.21A).
- Vascular channels are located underneath the hyperplastic synovial membrane in the myxoid or fibrotic stroma (Fig. 8.21B).
- Some cases may have the appearance of either a capillary or arteriovenous hemangioma.
- Hemosiderin deposition can be seen.
- Some cases may show villous hyperplasia of the synovium.

Prognosis:
- Small lesions can be removed completely without risk of local recurrence.

Differential Diagnosis:
- **Pigmented villonodular synovitis**
  Radiographic features may mimic those of intra-articular hemangioma; however, MRI showing on T2-weighted sequences intra-articular masses exhibiting a combination of high signal intensity areas representing fluid and congested synovium, interspersed with areas of intermediate-to-low signal intensity secondary to random distribution of hemosiderin in synovium is very helpful in differential diagnosis. In addition, low signal intensity on T1- and T2-weighted images particularly on gradient-echo sequences due to hemosiderin deposition is characteristic.
  Histopathology showing dense infiltration of mononuclear histiocytes accompanied by plasma cells, lymphocytes, and variable number of resorptive giant cells, coupled with a characteristic villi made up of collagen and reticulin fibers, is diagnostic.
- **Synovial (osteo)chondromatosis**
  Radiography may show numerous small and more or less uniform in size and shape osteochondral bodies. MRI demonstrating high signal intensity fluid within the joint together with signal-void or low signal intensity calcifications is diagnostic.
  Histopathology showing many highly cellular intra-articular osteocartilaginous bodies is diagnostic.

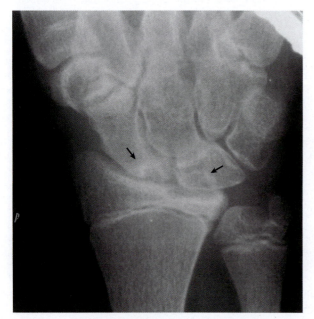

FIGURE 8.14 Radiography of synovial hemangioma. Dorsovolar radiograph of the left wrist of a 15-year-old boy shows narrowing of the radiocarpal joint, irregular articular surfaces of the trapezioscaphoid and fifth carpometacarpal joints, and erosions of the scaphoid and lunate bones (*arrows*).

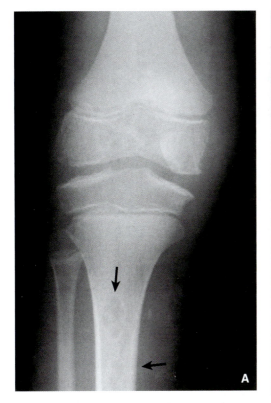
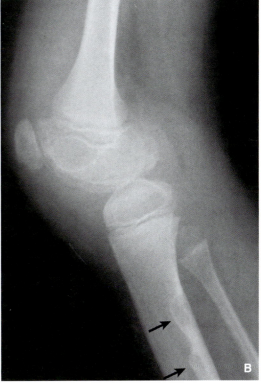
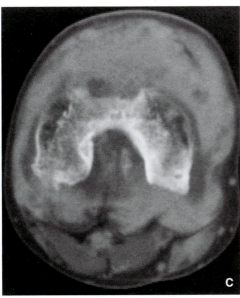

FIGURE 8.15 Radiography and computed tomography of synovial hemangioma.
(A) Anteroposterior and **(B)** lateral radiographs of the right knee of a 7-year-old boy show articular erosions at the femorotibial joint compartments. Soft-tissue masses are present anteriorly and posteriorly. An incidental finding is a nonossifying fibroma in the posterior tibial diaphysis (*arrows*). **(C)** Axial CT section through the knee shows marginal erosions of the femoral condyles. Heterogeneous masses are seen anteriorly and posteriorly with hypodense areas representing fat.

- *Lipoma arborescens*
  Radiographic features may be very similar to those of intra-articular hemangioma; however, MRI is very characteristic, demonstrating frond-like masses arising from the synovium that exhibit fat characteristics on all imaging sequences.
  Histopathology showing hyperplasia of subsynovial fat, formation of mature fat cells, and the presence of proliferative villous projections is diagnostic.

- *Hemophilic arthropathy*
  Radiography demonstrates typical changes of joint arthropathy, including periarticular osteoporosis, joint space narrowing, destruction of articular surface, and epiphyseal overgrowth. In the knee joint, it demonstrates widening of the intercondylar notch and squaring of the patella. Osseous pseudotumors may be also visualized. MRI shows hemarthrosis and deposit of hemosiderin along the intra-articular ligaments and tendons.

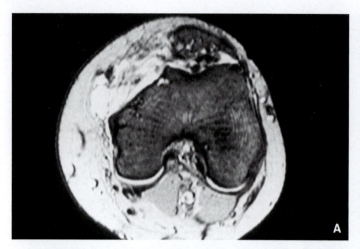
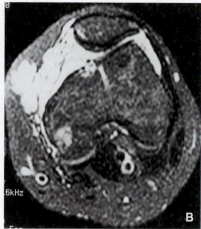

FIGURE 8.16 Magnetic resonance imaging of synovial hemangioma. (A) Axial T2*-weighted (MPGR) and **(B)** axial fast spin echo (FSE) fat-suppressed MR images of the left knee of a 16-year-old girl show a large intra-articular lesion exhibiting high signal intensity.

Histopathology shows copius iron deposition and markedly hyperplastic synovium usually limited to the synovial lining cells.

■ *Inflammatory arthritis*

Radiographic features include periarticular osteoporosis, joint space narrowing, and articular erosions. MRI shows typical inflammatory changes of the synovium and joint effusion.

Histopathology showing proliferation of synovial lining cells and the aggregates of infiltrating inflammatory cells, consisting of a mixture of T and B lymphocytes, macrophages, and polyclonal plasma cells, is diagnostic.

Lipoma Arborescens

Definition:
■ Intra-articular disorder characterized by nonneoplastic lipomatous proliferation of the synovial membrane.

Epidemiology:
■ Rare condition, consisting of less than 1% of all lipomatous lesions.
■ Most of the patients are between the fourth and fifth decades.
■ More prevalent in males.

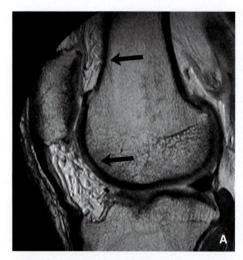
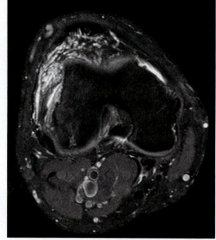
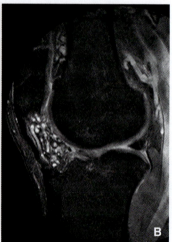

FIGURE 8.17 Magnetic resonance imaging of synovial hemangioma. (A) Sagittal T1-weighted MRI of the right knee of a 34-year-old man shows lace-like pattern of several vascular channels within the femoropatellar joint compartment and in the Hoffa fat pat (*arrows*) exhibiting high signal intensity. **(B)** Axial (*left*) and sagittal (*right*) T2-weighted MR images confirm the presence of hemangioma within the synovial membrane. Note the vascular structures exhibiting high signal intensity, separated by low signal linear structures representing fibrofatty septa.

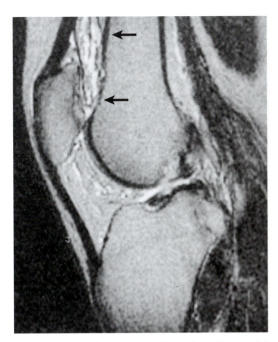

FIGURE 8.18 Magnetic resonance imaging of synovial hemangioma. Sagittal T2-weighted MR image of the knee of a 47-year-old woman demonstrates thin, low-intensity fibrofatty septa within a vascular lesion (*arrows*).

Sites of Involvement:

- Most common site is a knee joint, less frequently the shoulder, hip, elbow, and ankle joints.
- Occasionally more than one joint is affected.

Clinical Findings:

- Long-standing, slowly progressing swelling of the affected joint.
- Pain and limited motion within the joint.

Imaging:

- Radiography shows soft-tissue density within the joint resembling joint effusion.
- Magnetic resonance imaging shows characteristic frond-like masses arising from synovium exhibiting fat signal (bright on T1 and intermediate on T2 weighting) on all sequences (Figs. 8.22 and 8.23). Lack of significant enhancement on postcontrast studies.

Pathology:

Gross (Macroscopy):

- Yellowish-white mass with villous proliferation.

Histopathology:

- Hyperplasia of subsynovial fat tissue with morphology similar to soft-tissue lipoma (Fig. 8.24).
- Occasionally chondroid metaplasia.

Prognosis:

- Cured by synovectomy; recurrences are uncommon.

Differential Diagnosis:

- **Pigmented villonodular synovitis**
  Imaging features including marginal erosions with sclerotic margin and typical MRI appearance consisting of low signal intensity of the lesion on both

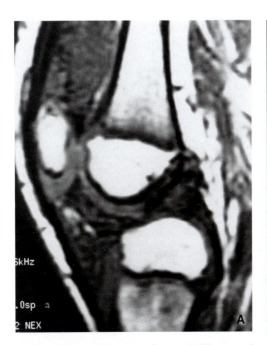 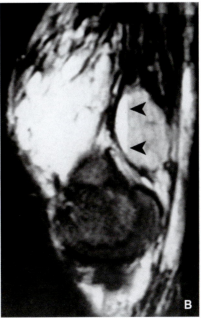

FIGURE 8.19 Magnetic resonance imaging of synovial hemangioma. (A) Sagittal T1-weighted MRI of a 9-year-old boy shows isointense with the muscles masses within the suprapatellar bursa and infrapatellar Hoffa fat pad. **(B)** Sagittal T2-weighted fat-suppressed MR image shows the masses becoming very bright. The fluid–fluid level seen in the popliteal region (*arrowheads*) is typical for the cavernous type of this lesion.

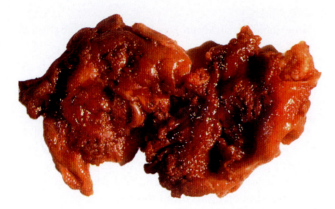

FIGURE 8.20 Gross specimen of synovial hemangioma. Surgical specimen removed from the knee joint of the patient with synovial hemangioma shows strawberry-like appearance of the synovial lining and marked hemosiderin staining of the tissue. (From Bullough P. *Atlas of Orthopedic Pathology with Clinical and Radiologic Correlations*. 2nd ed. New York, NY: Gower Medical Publishing; 1992, p. 15.14, Fig. 15.36.)

T1- and T2-weighted sequences due to hemosiderin deposition, coupled with lack of fat characteristics, are diagnostic.

Histopathology showing proliferation of small histiocyte-like cells with some larger cells and scattered multinucleated giant cells coupled with hemorrhagic foci and focal areas of hemosiderin deposition is diagnostic.

- *Synovial hemangioma*
  MRI showing on T1-weighted sequences a soft-tissue mass of intermediate signal intensity, but brighter than muscles, becoming bright on T2 weighting with thin, serpentine low-intensity septa, coupled with fluid–fluid levels, is characteristic.
  Histopathology showing dilated thin-walled arborizing vascular channels of different sizes, and foci of hemosiderin deposition is diagnostic.

- *Synovial (osteo)chondromatosis*
  Radiography may show numerous small, uniform in size and shape joint bodies. MRI demonstrating high signal intensity fluid within the joint together with signal-void or low signal intensity calcifications is diagnostic. Histopathology showing many highly cellular intra-articular osteocartilaginous bodies is diagnostic.

- *Hemophilic arthropathy*
  Imaging studies showing typical changes of joint arthropathy, with articular erosions, and epiphyseal overgrowth, coupled with MRI showing hemarthrosis and characteristic for hemosiderin deposits paramagnetic imaging features, particularly well demonstrated on gradient echo sequences, are diagnostic. Histopathology shows copious iron deposition and markedly hyperplastic synovium usually limited to the synovial lining cells. Lack of distinct submembranous mononuclear cells and giant cells proliferation is also a diagnostic feature.

Juxta-Articular Myxoma

Definition:
- Rare, benign soft-tissue lesion arising close to the large joints, histologically resembling intramuscular myxoma.

Epidemiology:
- Age range from 16 to 83 years, with median age of 43 years.
- More commonly in men.

Sites of Involvement:
- Most common site is around the knee joint.
- Less common locations include the elbow, shoulder, ankle, and hip.

Clinical Findings:
- Palpable and painful mass.
- Symptoms may range from weeks to years.

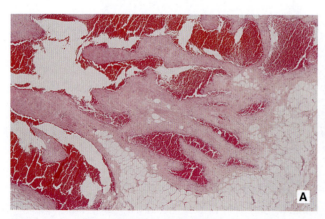 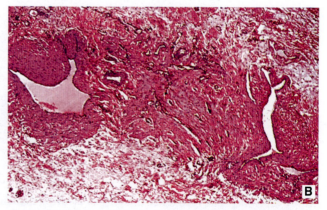

FIGURE 8.21 Histopathology of synovial hemangioma. (A) The lesion consists of a network of connected blood-filled spaces within the loose connective tissue of the synovium (H&E, original magnification ×12.5). **(B)** Observe prominent vascular spaces, copious hemosiderin deposition, and hyperplastic reactive synovial tissue (H&E, original magnification ×10). (**B**—from Bullough P. *Atlas of Orthopedic Pathology with Clinical and Radiologic Correlations*. 2nd ed. New York, NY: Gower Medical Publishing; 1992, p. 15.14, Fig. 15.37.)

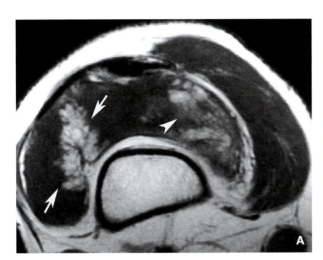
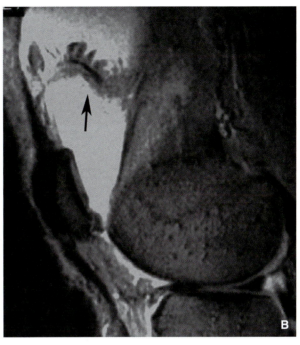

FIGURE 8.22 Magnetic resonance imaging of lipoma arborescens. (A) Axial T1-weighted MR image shows an intra-articular "tree-like" lipomatous mass in the fluid-distended suprapatellar bursa of the knee joint (*arrows*). In addition, observe lipomatous growth in the medial aspect of suprapatellar recess (*arrowhead*). **(B)** Sagittal T2-weighted MRI demonstrates the tree-like lesion showing fat characteristics (*arrow*).

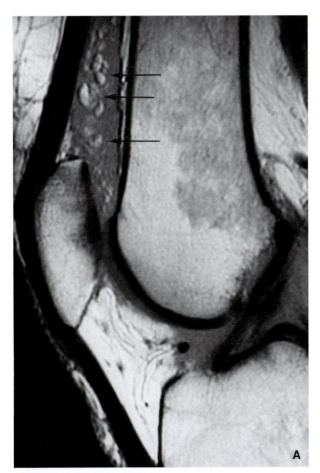
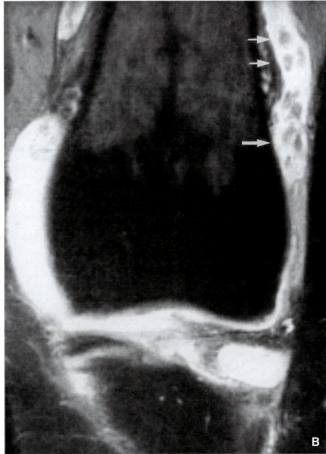

FIGURE 8.23 Magnetic resonance imaging of lipoma arborescens. (A) Sagittal proton density–weighted MRI of the left knee of a 54-year-old woman shows numerous small masses within the suprapatellar bursa exhibiting signal intensity consistent with fat (*arrows*). **(B)** Coronal T2-weighted fat-suppressed MR image demonstrates high signal intensity joint effusion and intermediate signal intensity fatty proliferations (*arrows*).

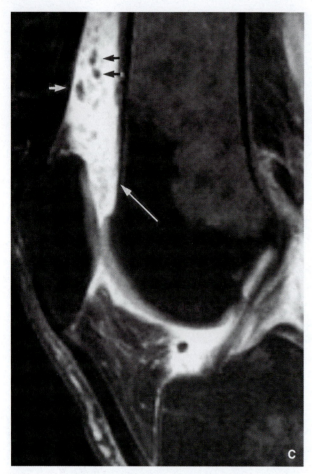

FIGURE 8.23 *(Continued).* **(C)** Sagittal T2-weighted MR image shows bright joint effusion (long arrow) and hypertrophic synovial villi (short arrows) exhibiting signal consistent with fat.

Imaging:
- Radiographic features are not specific.
- MRI shows the mass being either isointense or slightly brighter than muscles on T1-weighted sequences and of homogenously high signal intensity on T2 weighting. After administration of gadolinium, the mass shows heterogeneous enhancement.

Pathology:

Gross (Macroscopy):
- Slimy and gelatinous mass with common cystic changes
- Size typically range from 0.6 to 12 cm (mean 3.8 cm).

Histopathology:
- Tissue resembles cellular form of intramuscular myxoma and is composed of bland-appearing spindle cells embedded in a hypovascular myxoid matrix (Fig. 8.25A).
- Increased cellularity may be present, but mitotic figures are absent or very rare.
- Cystic or ganglion-like spaces lined by layer of delicate fibrin or thick collagen are often present (Fig. 8.25B).
- Margins of the lesion are ill defined and often infiltrate the adjacent tissues.
- Areas of hemorrhage, hemosiderin deposition, and chronic inflammation may be seen, particularly in recurrent lesions.

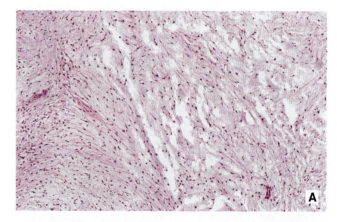

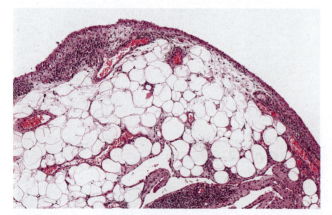

FIGURE 8.24 **Histopathology of lipoma arborescens.** Synovial villi are distended by mature adipocytes located in subsynovial connective tissue (H&E, original magnification ×50).

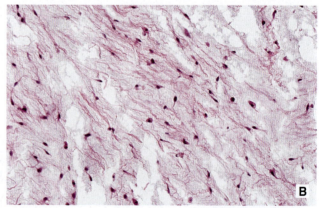

FIGURE 8.25 **Histopathology of juxta-articular myxoma.** **(A)** Bland-appearing spindle cells are embedded in hypovascular myxoid stroma (H&E, original magnification ×50). **(B)** High-power photomicrograph shows various in size cystic spaces between the sheets of spindle cells (H&E, original magnification ×200).

Immunohistochemistry:
- Positive for CD34, vimentin, and actin.

Genetics:
- Lack mutations of the *GNAS1* gene, in contrast to intramuscular myxomas.

Prognosis:
- Local recurrence after surgical intervention reported in 34% of cases.

Differential Diagnosis (Around the Knee Joint):
- **Meniscal and parameniscal cyst**
  Usually associated with a meniscal tear. Both cysts show connection with the joint space. MRI shows increased signal intensity on T2-weighted sequences but not as high as synovial fluid. There is lack of enhancement on postcontrast studies.
  Histopathology shows a parameniscal cyst to be lined by a true epithelium, a feature not present in a meniscal cyst.
- **Periarticular ganglion**
  Imaging features may resemble juxta-articular myxoma, but MRI may show high signal intensity on T1-weighted sequences due to high proteinaceous content or hemorrhage. In addition, on T2 weighting commonly demonstrated are low signal intensity septa. Postcontrast studies show either rim enhancement or rarely, diffuse enhancement of the ganglionic cyst.
  Histopathology shows lack of epithelial lining and, in some cases, myxoid changes.
- **Localized extra-articular pigmented villonodular synovitis**
  Focal nodular form usually affects the anterior aspect of the knee joint. MRI shows low signal intensity on both T1- and T2-weighted sequences due to hemosiderin deposit.
  Histopathology showing dense infiltration of mononuclear histiocytes accompanied by plasma cells, lymphocytes, and variable number of giant cells, and focal areas of hemosiderin deposition, is diagnostic.

B. MALIGNANT JOINT TUMORS

Synovial Sarcoma

Definition:
- Malignant mesenchymal spindle cell neoplasm exhibiting variable epithelial differentiation.

Epidemiology:
- Accounts for 5% to 10% of soft-tissue sarcomas.
- Predominantly tumor of young adults, between 16 and 35 years.
- Ninety percent of cases occur before age of 50 years.
- Males are affected more commonly than are females.

Sites of Involvement:
- Lower extremities account for about 83% of all cases, usually periarticular in location.
- Most common around the knee and foot.

Clinical Findings:
- Soft-tissue swelling or mass near the joint accompanied by progressive pain.
- Usually slow-growing tumor with indolent course, but metastases to the lungs and soft tissues have been reported.

Imaging:
- Radiographic features include soft-tissue mass in close proximity to the joint, occasionally causing bone erosion; soft-tissue amorphous calcifications are present in about 25% to 30% of cases (Figs. 8.26 and 8.27).
- Scintigraphy shows increased uptake of the radiopharmaceutical agent (Fig. 8.28A–C).
- Magnetic resonance imaging shows heterogeneous tumor with infiltrative margins on T1-weighted sequences, displaying high signal on T2 weighting and other water-sensitive sequences (Figs. 8.28D,E and 8.29). Some tumors show high signal intensity on both T1- and T2-weighted images secondary to hemorrhage within the mass. Characteristic is so-called triple signal intensity sign, with mixed low, intermediate, and high signal intensities areas on T2 weighting (Figs. 8.30 and 8.31). Postcontrast studies show diffuse enhancement of the tumor (Fig. 8.31E,F).

Pathology:

Gross (Macroscopy):
- Tan or gray commonly multinodular soft mass (3 to 10 cm in diameter), occasionally multicystic, sometimes with areas of hemorrhage and necrosis (Fig. 8.32).

Histopathology:
- There are several subtypes of the tumor: biphasic (fibrous and epithelial), monophasic, poorly differentiated, purely glandular, and calcifying variants.
- The biphasic type shows distinct spindle-cell and epithelial components arranged in gland-like or nest-like patterns (Fig. 8.33). Spindle cells are small and fairly uniform with ovoid, pale-staining nuclei.
- The monophasic type is composed of interdigitating fascicles and ball-like structures formed by the spindle cells (Fig. 8.34).
- The poorly differentiated type shows high cellularity with atypical cells, numerous mitotic figures, and often foci of necrosis.
- The glandular form exhibits predominantly gland-like pattern identical to adenocarcinoma and only minute foci of spindle cells.
- The calcifying type shows spindle cell elements and calcifications localized to areas of hyalinization (Fig. 8.35).

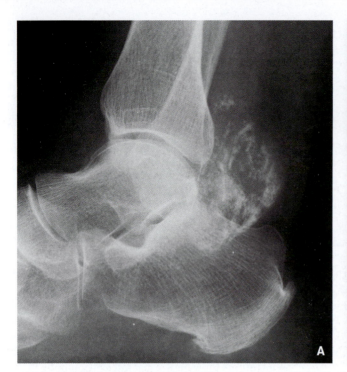
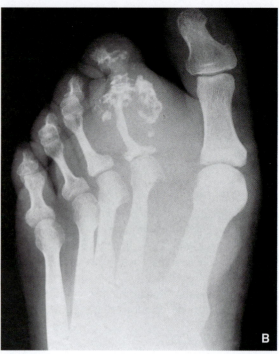

FIGURE 8.26 Radiography of synovial sarcoma. (A) Lateral radiograph of the left ankle of a 71-year-old woman shows a large calcified mass located in the soft tissues anteriorly to the Achilles tendon not affecting the adjacent bones. **(B)** Dorsoplantar radiograph of the right foot of a 55-year-old woman shows a large mass with coarse calcifications, eroding the proximal phalanx of the second toe.

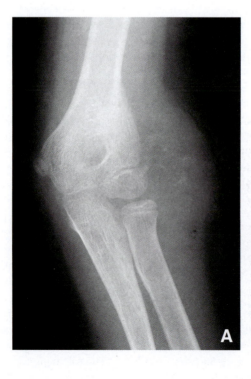
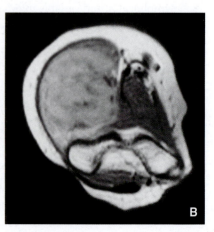

FIGURE 8.27 Radiography and magnetic resonance imaging of synovial sarcoma. (A) Oblique radiograph of the left elbow of an 8-year-old girl shows a soft-tissue mass ubbutting the elbow joint and exhibiting fine calcifications. **(B)** Axial T1-weighted MRI shows a soft-tissue mass exhibiting intermediate signal intensity, with foci of low signal representing calcifications.

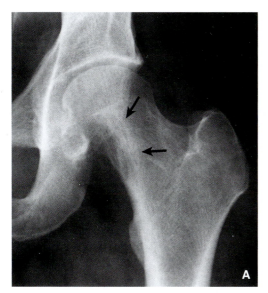
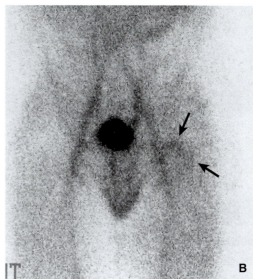
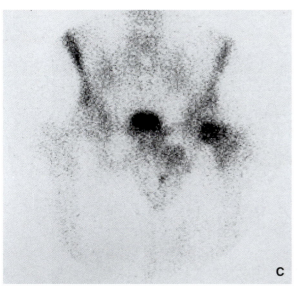
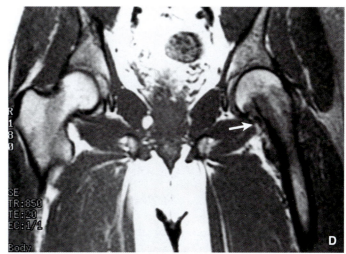
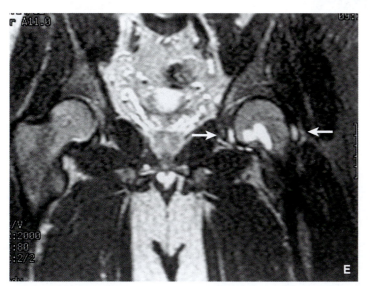

FIGURE 8.28 Radiography, scintigraphy, and magnetic resonance imaging of synovial sarcoma.
(A) Anteroposterior radiograph of the left hip of a 37-year-old man shows an osteolytic lesion in the femoral neck bordered laterally by a sclerotic margin (*arrows*).
(B) Radionuclide bone scan (blood pool stage) demonstrates increased vascularity to the left hip joint (*arrows*).
(C) Delayed scintigraphic image shows increased uptake of the radiopharmaceutical agent in the femoral head and neck and around the hip joint. **(D)** Coronal T1-weighted MRI shows a low signal intensity lesion affecting the medial aspect of the femoral neck (*arrow*). **(E)** Coronal T2-weighted MR image demonstrates increased signal at the junction of femoral head and neck and in the medial and lateral aspects of the hip joint (*arrows*).

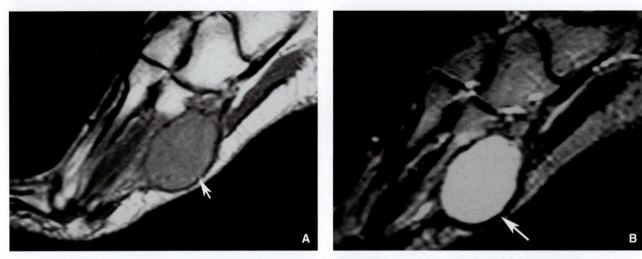

FIGURE 8.29 Magnetic resonance imaging of synovial sarcoma. (A) Sagittal T1-weighted MR image of the left foot of a young man shows well-circumscribed hypointense tumor with low signal intensity capsule located in the plantar aspect of the foot (*arrow*). **(B)** Sagittal T2-weighted MRI shows uniformly high signal intensity of the tumor (*arrow*).

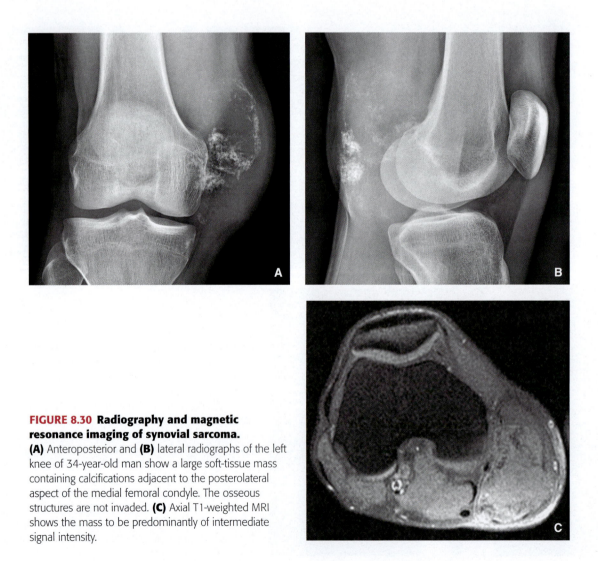

FIGURE 8.30 Radiography and magnetic resonance imaging of synovial sarcoma.
(A) Anteroposterior and **(B)** lateral radiographs of the left knee of 34-year-old man show a large soft-tissue mass containing calcifications adjacent to the posterolateral aspect of the medial femoral condyle. The osseous structures are not invaded. **(C)** Axial T1-weighted MRI shows the mass to be predominantly of intermediate signal intensity.

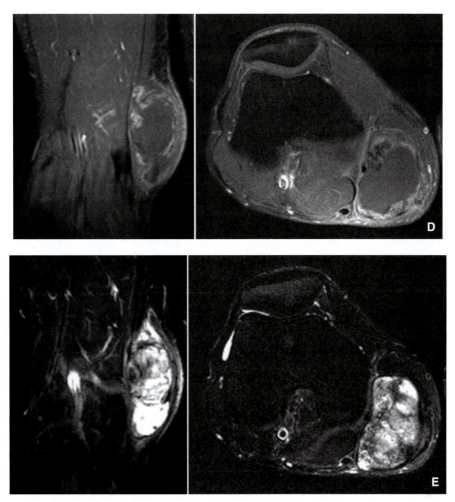

FIGURE 8.30 *(Continued).* **(D)** Coronal *(left)* and axial *(right)* T1-weighted MR images obtained after intravenous administration of gadolinium show peripheral enhancement of the tumor. **(E)** Coronal *(left)* and axial *(right)* T2-weighted MR images demonstrate heterogeneous tumor exhibiting mixture of high, intermediate, and low signal intensities (triple signal intensity sign) characteristic of synovial sarcoma.

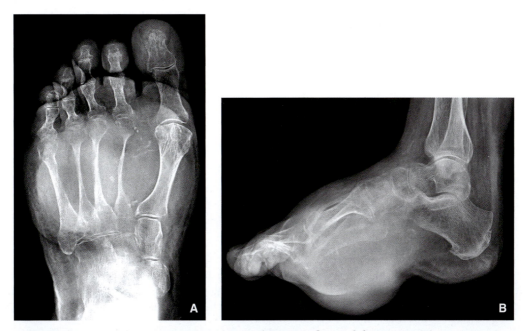

FIGURE 8.31 **Radiography, magnetic resonance imaging, and PET–CT of synovial sarcoma. (A)** Anteroposterior and **(B)** lateral radiographs of the right foot of a 57-year-old woman show a large soft-tissue mass containing calcifications, mainly affecting the plantar aspect of the foot. Note erosions of the second, third, and fourth metatarsal bones.

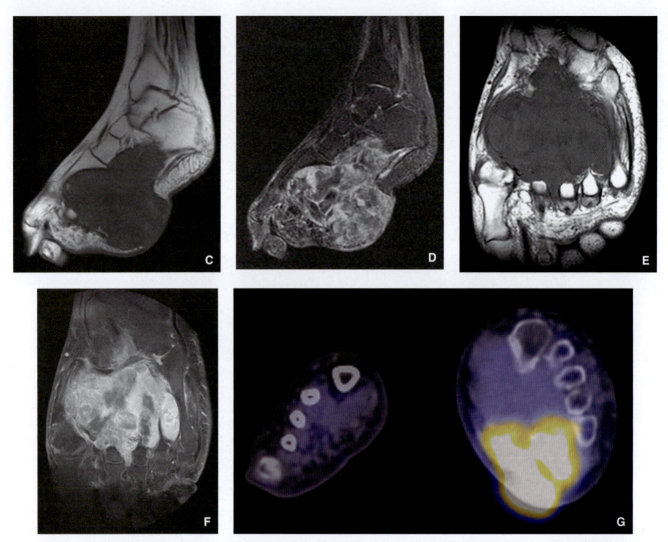

FIGURE 8.31 *(Continued).* (C) Sagittal T1-weighted MRI shows the mass to be of intermediate-to-low signal intensity. **(D)** Sagittal inversion recovery (IR) MR image shows the heterogeneous mass exhibiting mixture of high, intermediate, and low signal intensities (triple signal intensity sign). **(E)** Axial (long axis) T1-weighted MR image and **(F)** one obtained after intravenous administration of gadolinium demonstrate heterogeneous enhancement of the tumor. **(G)** Axial fused PET-CT image of both feet reveals a large hypermetabolic tumor in the soft tissues of the left foot.

Immunohistochemistry:
- Strong positivity for cytokeratins 7, 8, 14, and 19, and epithelial membrane antigen (EMA) in the epithelial areas (see Fig. 8.34C).
- Positivity for cytokeratin, EMA, and vimentin in the spindle cell elements.
- Positivity for CD99 and BCL2 (see Fig. 8.34D), and negativity for CD34.
- Positivity for transducin-like enhancer protein 1 (TLE 1) encoded by the *TLE1* gene in all subtypes.

Genetics:
- Translocation involving chromosomes X and 18 [t(X;18)(p11;q11)] giving rise to a fusion transcript of the *SYT* gene on chromosome 18 and the *SSX* gene on the chromosome X (see Fig. 8.34E).
- SS18-SSX1 fusion in about 75% of cases, and SS18-SSX2 fusion in about 33% of cases.

Prognosis:
- Best prognosis in tumors smaller than 5 cm.
- Better prognosis in children.
- Local recurrence after surgical resection is greater than 50%.

Differential Diagnosis:
- *Soft-tissue chondroma*
  Imaging features of soft-tissue mass containing typical chondroid calcifications and lack of erosive changes

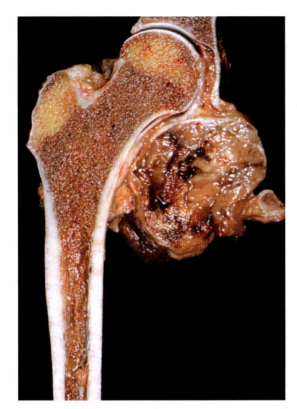

FIGURE 8.32 Gross specimen of synovial sarcoma. Coronal section of the specimen of the right hip joint and proximal femur shows a large well-circumscribed tan-yellowish juxta-articular soft-tissue mass displaying foci of hemorrhage. (From Bullough P. *Atlas of Orthopedic Pathology with Clinical and Radiologic Correlations*. 2nd ed. New York, NY: Gower Medical Publishing; 1992, p. 17.23, Fig.17.63.)

of the adjacent osseous structures, and MRI findings without triple intensity signal sign are diagnostic. Histopathology showing typical benign cartilaginous morphology of the lesion is diagnostic.

- **Myositis ossificans**
  Imaging features of zonal phenomenon and lack of osseous invasion coupled with regression of the lesion with time are diagnostic.
  Histopathology showing trabecular bone and fibrous marrow, and immature bone in the center of the lesion with proliferating osteoblasts and fibroblasts but mature bone on the periphery, is diagnostic.

- **Tumoral calcinosis**
  Imaging features comprise well-circumscribed mineralized subcutaneous soft-tissue mass, without aggressive features.
  Histopathology reveals milky, gritty whitish material and admixture of apatite crystals associated with histiocytic response and foreign body giant cells but absence of malignant cells.

- **Gout**
  Radiography shows characteristic articular and para-articular erosions with overhanging edges. Dual-energy color-coded CT showing characteristic features of gouty tophi is diagnostic.

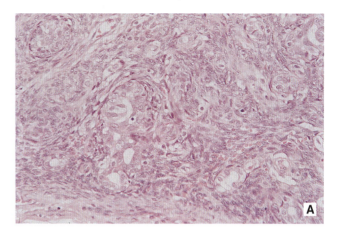
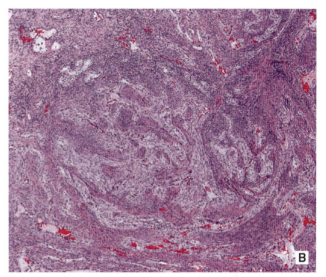
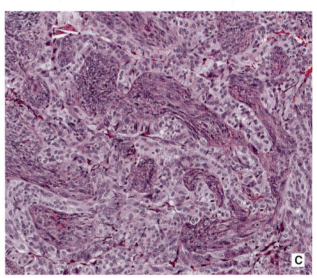

FIGURE 8.33 Histopathology of synovial sarcoma. **(A)** Typical biphasic appearance of the tumor with gland-like spaces *(left and below)* side-by-side with spindle cell sarcomatous areas (H&E, original magnification ×80). **(B)** Spindle and epithelioid cells in some areas are arranged in gland-like pattern, in other areas in nest-like pattern (H&E, original magnification ×100). **(C)** On higher-magnification photomicrograph, this biphasic arrangement is better appreciated (H&E, original magnification ×200).

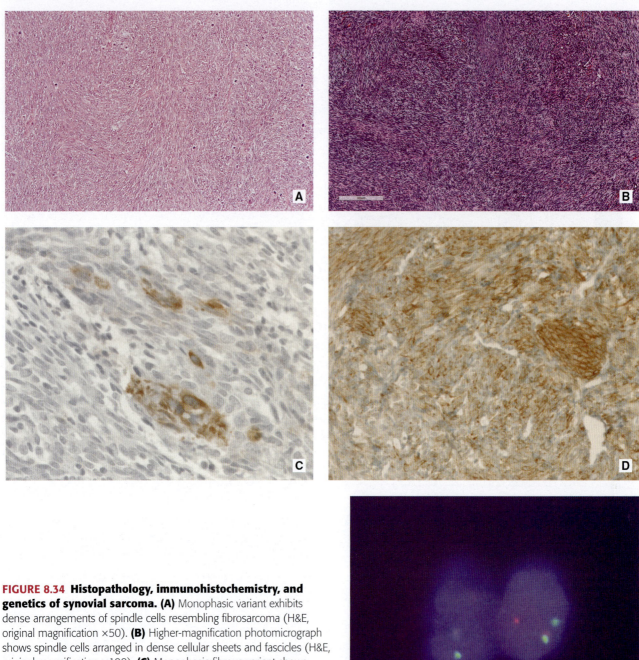

FIGURE 8.34 Histopathology, immunohistochemistry, and genetics of synovial sarcoma. (A) Monophasic variant exhibits dense arrangements of spindle cells resembling fibrosarcoma (H&E, original magnification ×50). **(B)** Higher-magnification photomicrograph shows spindle cells arranged in dense cellular sheets and fascicles (H&E, original magnification ×100). **(C)** Monophasic fibrous variant shows focal positivity for epithelial membrane antigen (EMA) (biotin–avidin peroxidase, original magnification ×400). **(D)** In addition to positivity for CD99 and cytokeratins (not shown here), synovial sarcoma is also positive for BCL2 (biotin–avidin peroxidase, original magnification ×200). **(E)** Using a double-labeled fluorescent break-apart probe for the SYT-gene, *red* and *green* signal splitting indicates gene rearrangement (FISH, original magnification ×1,000).

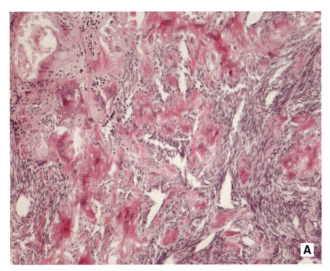
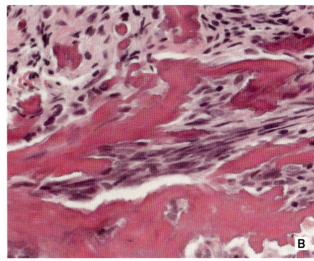

FIGURE 8.35 **Histopathology of synovial sarcoma. (A)** Calcifying type of the tumor exhibits extensive mineralization (H&E, original magnification ×100). **(B)** At high magnification, observe uniformity of the spindle cells with only mild pleomorphism surrounding areas of mineralization (H&E, original magnification ×400).

Examination of synovial fluid showing typical monosodium urate crystals is diagnostic.

- *Soft-tissue osteosarcoma*

  Imaging features of soft-tissue mass with amorphous calcifications and ossifications may resemble synovial sarcoma. MRI findings, however, similar to those of conventional osteosarcoma and lack of triple signal intensity sign characteristic for synovial sarcoma, are usually diagnostic.

  Histopathology showing malignant cells forming osteoid or bone is diagnostic.

- *Soft-tissue chondrosarcoma*

  Imaging features of soft-tissue mass with foci of calcifications may be very similar to synovial sarcoma. However, MRI will demonstrates lack of typical triple signal intensity sign seen in the latter tumor.

  Histopathology showing malignant cartilage formation by the tumor cells with permeation and entrapment of osseous trabeculae is diagnostic.

Synovial Chondrosarcoma

This is a rare tumor that originates from the synovial membrane. It may arise as a primary malignancy or it may developed as a malignant transformation of synovial (osteo)chondromatosis. This entity was discussed in Chapter 3.

REFERENCES

Abdelwahab IF, Kenan S, Hermann G, Lewis MM, Klein MJ. Intramuscular myxoma: magnetic resonance features. *Br J Radiol.* 1992;65:485–490.

Abdelwahab IF, Kenan S, Steiner GC, Abdul-Quader M. True bursal pigmented villonodular synovitis. *Skeletal Radiol.* 2002;31:354–358.

Abrahams TG, Pavlov H, Bansal M, Bullough P. Concentric joint space narrowing of the hip associated with hemosiderotic synovitis (HS) including pigmented villonodular synovitis (PVNS). *Skeletal Radiol.* 1988;17:37–45.

Ackerman LV. Extra-osseous localized non-neoplastic bone and cartilage formation (so-called myositis ossificans). Clinical and pathological confusion with malignant neoplasms. *J Bone Joint Surg Am.* 1958;40A:279–298.

Adams ME, Saifuddin A. Characterisation of intra-articular soft tissue tumours and tumour-like lesions. *Eur Radiol.* 2007;17:950–958.

Aglietti P, Di Muria GV, Salvati EA, Stringa G. Pigmented villonodular synovitis of the hip joint (review of the literature and report of personal case material). *Ital J Orthop Traumatol.* 1983;9:487–496.

Al-Shraim MM. Intra-articular lipoma arborescens of the knee joint. *Ann Saudi Med.* 2011;31:194–196.

Antonescu CR, Kawai A, Leung DH, et al. Strong association of SYT-SSX fusion type and morphologic epithelial differentiation in synovial sarcoma. *Diagn Mol Pathol.* 2000;9:1–8.

Arkun R, Memis A, Akalin T, Ustun EE, Sabah D, Kandiloglu G. Liposarcoma of soft tissue: MRI findings with pathologic correlation. *Skeletal Radiol.* 1997;26:167–172.

Armstrong SJ, Watt I. Lipoma arborescens of the knee. *Br J Radiol.* 1989;62:178–180.

Atmore WG, Dahlin DC, Ghormley RK. Pigmented villonodular synovitis: a clinical and pathologic study. *Minn Med.* 1956;39:196–202.

Azouz D, Tekaya R, Hamdi W, et al. Lipoma arborescens of the knee. *J Clin Rheumatol.* 2008;14:370–372.

Babar SA, Sandison A, Mitchell AW. Synovial and tenosynovial lipoma arborescens of the ankle in an adult: a case report. *Skeletal Radiol.* 2008;37:75–77.

Baker ND, Klein JD, Weidner N, Weissman BN, Brick GW. Pigmented villonodular synovitis containing coarse calcifications. *AJR Am J Roentgenol.* 1989;153:1228–1230.

Balsara ZN, Staiken BF, Martinez AJ. MR image of localized giant cell tumor of the tendon sheath involving the knee. *J Comput Assist Tomogr.* 1989;13:159–162.

Bejia I, Younes M, Moussa A, Said M, Touzi M, Bergaoui N. Lipoma arborescens affecting multiple joints. *Skeletal Radiol.* 2005;34:536–538.

Bertoni F, Unni KK, Beabout JW, Sim FH. Chondrosarcomas of the synovium. *Cancer.* 1991;67:155–162.

Bertoni F, Unni KK, Beabout JW, Sim FH. Malignant giant cell tumor of the tendon sheaths and joints (malignant pigmented villonodular synovitis). *Am J Surg Pathol.* 1997;21:153–163.

Besette PR, Cooley PA, Johnson RP, Czarnecki DJ. Gadolinium-enhanced MRI of pigmented villonodular synovitis of the knee. *J Comput Assist Tomogr.* 1992;16:992–994.

Bixby SD, Hettmer S, Taylor GA, Voss SD. Synovial sarcoma in children: imaging features and common benign mimics. *AJR Am J Roentgenol.* 2010;195:1026–1032.

Blacksin MF, Ghelman B, Freiberger RH, Salvata E. Synovial chondromatosis of the hip: evaluation with air computed arthrotomography. *Clin Imaging.* 1990;14:315–318.

Bravo SM, Winalski CS, Weissman BN. Pigmented villonodular synovitis. *Radiol Clin North Am.* 1996;34:311–326.

Brodsky AE. Synovial hemangioma of the knee joint. *Bull Hosp Jt Dis Orthop Inst.* 1956;17:58–69.

Bullough PG. *Atlas of Orthopaedic Pathology with Clinical and Radiologic Correlations.* 2nd ed. New York, NY: Gower; 1992:17.25–17.28.

Burnstein MI, Fisher DR, Yandow DR, Hafez GR, De Smet AA. Case report 502. Intra-articular synovial chondromatosis of shoulder with extra-articular extension. *Skeletal Radiol.* 1988;17:458–461.

Cadman NL, Soule EH, Kelly PJ. Synovial sarcoma: an analysis of 134 tumors. *Cancer.* 1965;18:613–627.

Campanacci M. *Bone and Soft-tissue Tumors.* New York, NY: Springer-Verlag; 1990:998–1012.

Chen DY, Lan JL, Chou SJ. Treatment of pigmented villonodular synovitis with yttrium-90: changes in immunologic features. Tc-99m uptake measurements, and MR imaging of one case. *Clin Rheumatol.* 1992;11:280–285.

Coll JP, Ragsdale BC, Daughters TC. Best cases from the AFIP: Lipoma arborescens of the knees in a patient with rheumatoid arthritis. *Radiographics.* 2011;31:333–337.

Cotten A, Flipo R-M, Chastanet P, Desvigne-Noulet MC, Duquesnoy B, Delcambre B. Pigmented villonodular synovitis of the hip: review of radiographic features in 58 patients. *Skeletal Radiol.* 1995;24:1–6.

Cotten A, Flipo RM, Herbaux B, Gougeon F, Lecomte-Houcke M, Chastanet P. Synovial haemangioma of the knee: a frequently misdiagnosed lesion. *Skeletal Radiol.* 1995;24:257–261.

Crotty JM, Monu JUV, Pope TL Jr. Synovial osteochondromatosis. *Radiol Clin North Am.* 1996;34:327–342.

Cupp JS, Miller MA, Montgomery KD, et al. Translocation and expression of CSF1 in pigmented villonodular synovitis, tenosynovial giant cell tumor, rheumatoid arthritis and other reactive synovitides. *Am J Surg Pathol.* 2007;31:970–976.

Daluiski A, Seeger LL, Doberneck SA, Finerman GA, Eckardt JJ. A case of juxta-articular myxoma of the knee. *Skeletal Radiol.* 1995;24:389–391.

De Beuckeleer L, De Schepper A, De Belder F, et al. Magnetic resonance imaging of localized giant cell tumour of the tendon sheath (MRI of localized GCTTS). *Eur Radiol.* 1997;7:198–201.

De St. Aubain Sommerhausen N, Dal Cin P. Giant cell tumour of tendon sheath. In: Fletcher CDM, Unni KK, Mertens F, eds. *World Health Organization Classification of Tumours. Pathology and Genetics. Tumours of Soft Tissue and Bone.* Lyon, France: IARC Press; 2002:110–111.

De St. Aubain Sommerhausen N, Dal Cin P. Diffuse-type giant cell tumour. In: Fletcher CDM, Unni KK, Mertens F, eds. *World Health Organization Classification of Tumours. Pathology and Genetics. Tumours of Soft Tissue and Bone.* Lyon, France: IARC Press; 2002:112–114.

Devaney K, Vinh TN, Sweet DE. Synovial hemangioma: report of 20 cases with differential diagnostic considerations. *Hum Pathol.* 1993;24:737–745.

Dorwart RH, Genant HK, Johnston WH, Morris JM. Pigmented villonodular synovitis of synovial joints: clinical, pathologic, and radiologic features. *AJR Am J Roentgenol.* 1984;143:877–885.

Doyle AJ, Miller MV, French JG. Lipoma arborescens in the bicipital bursa of the elbow: MRI findings in two cases. *Skeletal Radiol.* 2002;31:656–660.

Dunn EJ, McGavran MH, Nelson P, Greer RB III. Synovial chondrosarcoma. Report of a case. *J Bone Joint Surg Am.* 1974;56A:811–813.

Enzinger FM, Weiss SW. Benign tumors and tumor-like lesions of synovial tissue. In: *Soft Tissue Tumors.* St. Louis, MO: CV Mosby; 1988:638–658.

Enzinger FM, Weiss SW. *Soft Tissue Tumors.* 3rd ed. St. Louis, MO: CV Mosby; 1995:749–751, 757–786.

Eustace SE, Harrison M, Srinivasen U, Stack J. Magnetic resonance imaging in pigmented villonodular synovitis. *Can Assoc Radiol J.* 1994;45:283–286.

Evans HL. Synovial sarcoma: a study of 23 biphasic and 17 probably monophasic examples. *Pathol Annu.* 1980;15:309–313.

Feller JF, Rishi M, Hughes EC. Lipoma arborescens of the knee: MR demonstration. *AJR Am J Roentgenol.* 1994;163:162–164.

Fletcher AG Jr, Horn RC Jr. Giant-cell tumor of tendon sheath origin: a consideration of bone involvement and report of 2 cases with extensive bone destruction. *Ann Surg.* 1951;133:374–385.

Foo WC, Cruise MV, Wick MR, Homick JL. Immunohistochemical staining for TLE1 distinguishes synovial sarcoma from histologic mimics. *Am J Clin Pathol.* 2011;135:839–844.

Georgen TG, Resnick D, Niwayama G. Localized nodular synovitis of the knee: a report of two cases with abnormal arthrograms. *AJR Am J Roentgenol.* 1976;126:647–650.

Goldman RL, Lichtenstein L. Synovial chondrosarcoma. *Cancer.* 1964;17:1233–1240.

Greenspan A, Azouz EM, Matthews J II, Décarie J-C. Synovial hemangioma: imaging features in eight histologically proved cases, review of the literature, and differential diagnosis. *Skeletal Radiol.* 1995;24:583–590.

Grieten M, Buckwalter KA, Cardinal E, Rougraff B. Case report 873. Lipoma arborescens (villous lipomatous proliferation of the synovial membrane). *Skeletal Radiol.* 1994;23:652–655.

Haldar M, Randall RL, Capecchi MR. Synovial sarcoma: from genetics to genetic-based animal modeling. *Clin Orthop Relat Res.* 2008;466:2156–2167.

Hallel T, Lew S, Bansal M. Villous lipomatous proliferation of the synovial membrane (lipoma arborescens). *J Bone Joint Surg Am.* 1988;70A:264–270.

Hamilton A, Davis RI, Hayes D, Mollan RA. Chondrosarcoma developing in synovial chondromatosis. A case report. *J Bone Joint Surg [Br].* 1987;69B:137–140.

Hermann G, Abdelwahab IF, Klein MJ, et al. Synovial chondromatosis. *Skeletal Radiol* 1995;24:298–300.

Hermann G, Klein MJ, Abdelwahab IF, Kenan S. Synovial chondrosarcoma arising in synovial chondromatosis of the right hip. *Skeletal Radiol.* 1997;26:366–369.

Hisoaka M, Matsuyama A, Shimajiri S, et al. Ossifying synovial sarcoma. *Pathol Res Pract.* 2009;205:195–198.

Huang G-S, Lee C-H, Chan WP, Chen CY, Yu JS, Resnick D. Localized nodular synovitis of the knee: MR imaging appearance and clinical correlates in 21 patients. *AJR Am J Roentgenol.* 2003;181:539–543.

Hughes TH, Sartoris DJ, Schweitzer ME, Resnick DL. Pigmented villonodular synovitis: MRI characteristics. *Skeletal Radiol.* 1995;24:7–12.

Ishida T, Iijima T, Moriyama S, Nakamura C, Kitagawa T, Machinami R. Intra-articular calcifying synovial sarcoma mimicking synovial chondromatosis. *Skeletal Radiol.* 1996;25:766–769.

Jaffe HL, Lichtenstein L, Sutro CJ. Pigmented villonodular synovitis, bursitis and tenosynovitis. *Arch Pathol Lab Med.* 1941;31:731–765.

Jelinek JS, Kransdorf MJ, Utz JA, et al. Imaging of pigmented villonodular synovitis with emphasis on MR imaging. *AJR Am J Roentgenol.* 1989;152:337–342.

Jelinek JS, Kransdorf MJ, Shmookler BM, Aboulafia AA, Malawer MM. Giant cell tumor of the tendon sheath: MR findings in nine cases. *AJR Am J Roentgenol.* 1994;162:919–922.

Jones FE, Soule EM, Coventry MB. Fibrous xanthoma of synovium (giant-cell tumor of tendon sheath, pigmented nodular synovitis). A study of 118 cases. *J Bone Joint Surg Am.* 1969;51A:76–86.

Jones BC, Sundaram M, Kransdorf MJ. Synovial sarcoma: MR imaging findings in 34 patients. *AJR Am J Roentgenol.* 1993;161:827–830.

Kaiser TE, Ivins JC, Unni KK. Malignant transformation of extra-articular synovial chondromatosis: report of a case. *Skeletal Radiol.* 1980;5:223–226.

Kakkar N, Vasishta RK, Anand H. Pathological case of the month. Synovial lipomatosis. *Arch Pediatr Adolesc Med.* 1999;153:203–204.

Kalil RK, Unni KK. Malignancy in pigmented villonodular synovitis. *Skeletal Radiol.* 1998;27:392–395.

Kallas KM, Vaughan L, Haghighi P, Resnick D. Pigmented villonodular synovitis of the hip presenting as retroperitoneal mass. *Skeletal Radiol.* 2001;30:469–474.

Karantanas AH, Mitsionis GI, Skopelitou AS. PVNS of the knee simulating lipoma arborescens on MR imaging. *CMIG Extra Cases.* 2004;28:23–26.

Karasick D, Karasick S. Giant cell tumor of tendon sheath: spectrum of radiologic findings. *Skeletal Radiol.* 1992;21:219–224.

Kawai A, Woodruff J, Healey JH, Brennan MF, Antonescu CR, Ladanyi M. SYT-SSX gene fusion as a determinant of morphology and prognosis in synovial sarcoma. *N Engl J Med.* 1998;338:153–160.

Khan S, Neumann CH, Steinbach LS, Harrington KD. MRI of giant cell tumor of tendon sheath of the hand: a report of three cases. *Eur Radiol.* 1995;5:467–470.

Khan AM, Cannon S, Levack B. Primary intra-articular liposarcoma of the knee. *J Knee Surg.* 2003;16:107–109.

Kindblom LG, Gunterberg B. Pigmented villonodular synovitis involving bone. Case report. *J Bone Joint Surg Am.* 1978;60A:830–832.

King JW, Spjut HJ, Fechner RE, Vanderpool DW. Synovial chondrosarcoma of the knee joint. *J Bone Joint Surg Am.* 1967;49A:1389–1396.

Kloen P, Keel SB, Chandler HP, Geiger RH, Zarins B, Rosenberg AE. Lipoma arborescens of the knee. *J Bone Joint Surg [Br].* 1998;80-B:298–301.

Krall RA, Kostinovsky M, Patchefsky AS. Synovial sarcoma: a clinical, pathological, and ultrastructural study of 26 cases supporting the recognition of monophasic variant. *Am J Surg Pathol.* 1981;5:137–151.

Ladanyi M, Antonescu CR, Leung DH, et al. Impact of SYT-SSX fusion type on the clinical behavior of synovial sarcoma. A multi-institutional retrospective study of 243 patients. *Cancer Res.* 2002;62:135–140.

Laorr A, Peterfy CG, Tirman PF, Rabassa AE. Lipoma arborescens of the shoulder: magnetic resonance imaging findings. *Can Assoc Radiol J.* 1995;46:311–313.

Lin J, Jacobson JA, Jamadar DA, Ellis JH. Pigmented villonodular synovitis and related lesions: the spectrum of imaging findings. *AJR Am J Roentgenol.* 1999;172:191–197.

Llauger J, Monill JM, Palmer J, Clotet M. Synovial hemangioma of the knee: MRI findings in two cases. *Skeletal Radiol.* 1995;24:579–581.

Llauger J, Palmer J, Rosón N, Cremades R, Bagué S. Pigmented villonodular synovitis and giant cell tumors of the tendon sheath: radiologic and pathologic features. *AJR Am J Roentgenol.* 1999;172:1087–1091.

Mahajan H, Lorigan JG, Shirkhoda A. Synovial sarcoma: MR imaging. *Magn Reson Imaging.* 1989;7:211–216.

McMaster PE. Pigmented villonodular synovitis with invasion of bone. Report of six cases. *J Bone Joint Surg Am.* 1960;42A:1170–1183.

Meis JM, Enzinger FM. Juxta-articular myxoma: a clinical and pathological study of 65 cases. *Hum Pathol* 1992;23:639–646.

Miettinen M, Virtanen I. Synovial sarcoma—a misnomer. *Am J Pathol.* 1984;117:18–25.

Morton MJ, Berquist TH, McLeod RA, Unni KK, Sim FH. MR imaging of synovial sarcoma. *AJR Am J Roentgenol.* 1991;156:337–340.

Mullins F, Berard CW, Eisenberg SH. Chondrosarcoma following synovial chondromatosis. A case study. *Cancer.* 1965;18:1180–1188.

Murphey MD, Gibson MS, Jennings BT, Crespo-Rodríguez AM, Fanburg-Smith J, Gajewski DA. From the archives of the AFIP: Imaging of synovial sarcoma with radiologic-pathologic correlation. *Radiographics.* 2006;26:1543–1565.

Murphey MD, Vidal JA, Fanburg-Smith JC, Gajewski DA. Imaging of synovial chondromatosis with radiologic-pathologic correlation. *Radiographics.* 2007;27:1465–1488.

Myers BW, Masi AT. Pigmented villonodular synovitis and tenosynovitis, a clinical epidemiologic study of 166 cases and literature review. *Medicine.* 1980;59:224–238.

Nassar WAM, Bassiony AA, Elghazaly HA. Treatment of diffuse pigmented villonodular synovitis of the knee with combined surgical and radio-synovectomy. *Hospital Spec Surg J.* 2009;5:19–23.

Norman A, Steiner GC. Bone erosion in synovial chondromatosis. *Radiology.* 1986;161:749–752.

O'Sullivan PJ, Harris AC, Munk PL. Radiological features of synovial cell sarcoma. *Br J Radiol* 2008;81:346–356.

Okamoto S, Hisaoka M, Meis-Kindblom JM, Kindblom LG, Hashimoto H. Juxta-articular myxoma and intramuscular myxoma are two distinct entities. Activating Gs alpha mutation at Arg 201 codon does not occur in juxta-articular myxoma. *Virchows Arch.* 2002;440:12–15.

Ontell F, Greenspan A. Chondrosarcoma complicating synovial chondromatosis: findings with magnetic resonance imaging. *Can Assoc Radiol J.* 1994;45:318–323.

Ottaviani S, Ayral X, Dougados M, Gossec L. Pigmented villonodular synovitis: a retrospective single-center study of 122 cases and review of the literature. *Semin Arthritis Rheum.* 2011;40:539–546.

Parsonage S, Mehr A, Davies MD. Lipoma arborescense: a definitive MR imaging diagnosis. *Osteol Közlem.* 2001;9:80–82.

Peh WCG, Shek TWH, Davies AM, Wong JW, Chien EP. Osteochondroma and secondary synovial osteochondromatosis. *Skeletal Radiol.* 1999;28:169–174.

Perry BE, McQueen DA, Lin JJ. Synovial chondromatosis with malignant degeneration to chondrosarcoma. Report of a case. *J Bone Joint Surg Am.* 1988;70A:1259–1261.

Rao AS, Vigorita VJ. Pigmented villonodular synovitis (giant-cell tumor of the tendon sheath and synovial membrane). A review of eighty-one cases. *J Bone Joint Surg Am.* 1984;66A:76–94.

Resnick D, Oliphant M. Hemophilia-like arthropathy of the knee associated with cutaneous and synovial hemangiomas. *Radiology.* 1975;114:323–326.

Rosenthal DI, Aronow S, Murray WT. Iron content of pigmented villonodular synovitis detected by computed tomography. *Radiology.* 1979;133:409–411.

Rubin BP. Tenosynovial giant cell tumor and pigmented villonodular synovitis: a proposal for unification of these clinically distinct but histologically and genetically identical lesions. *Skeletal Radiol.* 2007;36:267–268.

Rybak LD, Khaldi L, Wittig J, Steiner GC. Primary synovial chondrosarcoma of the hip joint in a 45-year-old male: case report and literature review. *Skeletal Radiol.* 2011;40:1375–1381.

Ryu KN, Jaovisidha S, Schweitzer M, Motta AO, Resnick D. MR imaging of lipoma aborescens of the knee joint. *AJR Am J Roentgenol.* 1996;167:1229–1232.

Sánchez Reyes JM, Alcaraz Mexia M, Quiñones Tapia D, Aramburu JA. Extensively calcified synovial sarcoma. *Skeletal Radiol.* 1997;26:671–673.

Schajowicz F. Synovial chondromatosis. In: *Tumors and Tumorlike Lesions of Bones and Joints.* New York, NY: Springer-Verlag; 1981:541–545.

Senocak E, Gurel K, Gurel S, et al. Lipoma arborescens of the suprapatellar bursa and extensor digitorum longus tendon sheath: report of 2 cases. *J Ultrasound Med.* 2007;26:1427–1433.

Shaerf DA, Mann B, Alorjani M, Aston W, Saifuddin A. High-grade intra-articular liposarcoma of the knee. *Skeletal Radiol.* 2011;40:363–365.

Sheldon PJ, Forrester DM, Learch TJ. Imaging of intraarticular masses. *Radiographics.* 2005;25:105–119.

Sherry JB, Anderson W. The natural history of pigmented villonodular synovitis of tendon sheath. *J Bone Joint Surg Am.* 1956;37A:1005–1011.

Siva C, Brasington R, Tony W, Sotelo A, Atkinson J. Synovial lipomatosis (lipoma arborescens) affecting multiple joints in a patient with congenital short bowel syndrome. *J Rheumatol.* 2002;29:1088–1092.

Soler T, Rodriguez E, Bargiela A, Da Riba M. Lipoma arborescens of the knee: MR characteristics in 13 joints. *J Comput Assist Tomogr.* 1998;22:605–609.

Sommerhausen NSA, Fletcher CDM. Diffuse-type giant cell tumor. Clinicopathologic and immunohistochemical analysis of 50 cases with extraarticular disease. *Am J Surg Pathol.* 2000;24:479–492.

Soule EH. Synovial sarcoma. *Am J Surg Pathol.* 1986;10:78–82.

Strickland B, Mackenzie DH. Bone involvement in synovial sarcoma. *J Faculty Radiol.* 1959;10:64–72.

Sultan I, Rodriguez-Galindo C, Saab R, Yasir S, Casanova M, Ferrari A. Comparing children and adults with synovial sarcoma in the Surveillance, Epidemiology, and End Results program, 1983 to 2005. An analysis of 1268 patients. *Cancer.* 2009;115:3537–3547.

Terry J, Saito T, Subramanian S, et al. TLE1 as a diagnostic immunohistochemical marker for synovial sarcoma emerging from gene expression profiling studies. *Am J Surg Pathol.* 2007;31:240–246.

Ushijima M, Hashimoto H, Tsuneyoshi M, Enjoji M. Giant cell tumor of the tendon sheath (nodular tenosynovitis). A study of 207 cases to compare the large joint group with the common digit group. *Cancer.* 1986;57:875–884.

van Rijswijk CSP, Hogendoorn PCW, Taminiau AHM, Bloem JL. Synovial sarcoma: dynamic contrast-enhanced MR imaging features. *Skeletal Radiol.* 2001;30:25–30.

Varela-Duran J, Enzinger FM. Calcifying synovial sarcoma. *Cancer.* 1982;50:345–352.

Vergara-Lluri ME, Stohr BA, Puligandla B, Brenholz P, Horvai AE. A novel sarcoma with dual differentiation: clinicopathologic and molecular characterization of a combined synovial sarcoma and extraskeletal myxoid chondrosarcoma. *Am J Surg Pathol.* 2012;36:1093–1098.

White EA, Omid R, Mateuk GR, et al. Lipoma arborescens of the biceps tendon sheath. *Skeletal Radiol.* 2013;42:1461–1464.

Wilkerson BW, Crim JR, Hung M, Layfield LJ. Characterization of synovial sarcoma calcification. *AJR Am J Roentgenol.* 2012;199:W730-W734.

Winnepenninckx V, De Vos R, Debiec-Rychter M, et al. Calcifying/ossifying synovial sarcoma shows t(x;18) with SSX2 involvement and mitochondrial calcifications. *Histopathology.* 2001;38:141–145.

Wittkop B, Davies AM, Mangham DC. Primary synovial chondromatosis and synovial chondrosarcoma: a pictorial review. *Eur Radiol.* 2002;12:2112–2119.

Wright PH, Sim FH, Soule EH, Taylor WF. Synovial sarcoma. *J Bone Joint Surg Am* 1982;64A:112–122.

CHAPTER 9

Osseous Metastases

Skeletal metastases are the most common variety of bone tumors, particularly in the elderly patients. Some malignant tumors demonstrate a far greater predilection for osseous involvement than do others. Cancers of the breast, prostate, lung, and kidney account for about 80% of all metastatic lesions to bone. In men, carcinoma of the prostate accounts for about 60% and carcinoma of the lung for about 25% of all bone metastases. In women, carcinoma of the breast is responsible for about 70% of all metastatic lesions, the remaining 30% being mainly due to carcinoma of the thyroid, uterus, and kidneys. Other primary tumors responsible for bone metastases include carcinomas of the stomach, colon, urinary bladder, melanoma, and some neurogenic tumors. Some sarcomas, such as osteosarcoma and Ewing sarcoma, may also occasionally metastasize to the osseous structures. In children aged 5 years and younger, neuroblastoma is usually the primary tumor responsible for metastatic disease.

Metastases can be solitary or multiple, and they can be further subdivided into purely lytic, purely sclerotic, or mixed lesions. Osteolytic metastases are the most common, representing about 75% of all metastatic lesions. The primary source is usually a carcinoma of the kidney, lung, breast, gastrointestinal tract, and thyroid (Fig. 9.1). Osteoblastic metastases represent approximately 15% of all metastatic lesions. In men, they are caused mainly by primary carcinoma of the prostate or a seminoma. In women, the primary source is usually carcinoma of the breast, uterus, or ovary. In both genders, sclerotic metastases may originate from carcinoid tumors, urinary bladder tumors (particularly transitional cell carcinoma), certain neurogenic tumors (such as medulloblastoma), and osteosarcoma (Fig. 9.2). Mixed metastases (osteoblastic and osteolytic) represent approximately 10% of all metastatic lesions. Any primary tumor may give rise to mixed metastases, the most common primaries being breast and lung carcinomas. Cortical metastases are very rare, the primary tumor being almost invariably in the lungs. Acrometastases (metastatic lesions affecting the distal phalanges) are extremely unusual, and if present, the primary tumor is usually in the lung and less likely in the breast or kidney.

Histopathologically metastatic carcinomas are sometimes easier to diagnose than are some primary bone tumors because of their epithelial pattern. Occasionally, a metastatic lesion may exhibit a characteristic morphologic pattern that strongly suggests a source of primary tumor, such as the clear cells of hypernephroma, follicular or giant cell carcinoma of the thyroid, or the pigment production of melanoma. Moreover, some neoplasms are associated with the production of enzymes or antigens, which can be detected after the decalcification procedure. It is possible, for example, to perform a prostate-specific antigen (PSA) study or a prostate-specific acid phosphatase by immunohistochemistry to identify the primary tumor site in the prostate. The other studies may demonstrate nuclear transcription factors such as homeobox gene CDX2 (occurring in gastrointestinal carcinomas) or thyroid transcription termination factor I, TTFI (occurring in lung and thyroid cancers), or to analyze the pattern of cytokeratin (CK) filaments (e.g., presence of CK20 and absence of CK7 in GI but not in lung cancers), supplemented by additional immunoreactions of cytokeratins, classification determinant (CD) endothelial markers CD20, CD99, and neuron-specific enolase (NSE) for the differentiation of small round blue cell tumors, all leading to identification of unknown primary tumor.

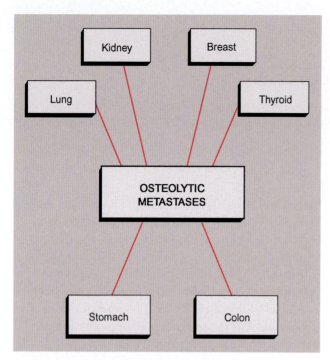

FIGURE 9.1 Origin of osteolytic metastases.

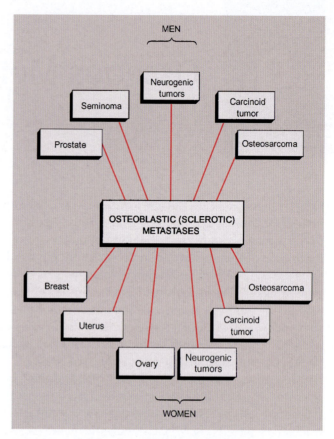

FIGURE 9.2 Origin of osteoblastic metastases.

SKELETAL METASTASES

Definition:
- The spread of the cancer cells from the initial site of the tumor to the bones.

Epidemiology:
- Metastases are relatively rare in patients younger than 40 years, most common after the sixth decade.
- Both genders are equally affected.

Sites of Involvement:
- Axial skeleton (skull, spine, pelvis).
- Proximal segments of the limb bones.
- Extremely rare distal to the elbows and distal to the knees.

Clinical Findings:
- The majority of metastases are asymptomatic, at least in the early stages.
- In advanced cases, pain is the primary symptom, rarely a pathologic fracture.

Imaging:
- Radiographic features of skeletal metastases generally are not specific; solitary metastatic lesion may look just like a primary bone tumor (Figs. 9.3 to 9.6); however, periosteal reaction and soft-tissue mass are uncommon. Bubbly, highly expansive (blow-out) metastatic lesions usually originate from a primary carcinoma of the kidney or thyroid (Fig. 9.7). Metastases located in the cortical bone (so-called "cookie bite" or "cookie cutter" lesions) are characteristic for primary bronchogenic carcinoma (Figs. 9.8 and 9.9). Multicentric osteoblastic metastases in form of round sclerotic foci or diffuse increase in bone density are often seen in primary carcinoma of the prostate gland (Fig. 9.10A,B) or the breast (Fig. 9.10C). Multifocal osteolytic or even mixed metastases may look like multiple myeloma (Fig. 9.11).
- Scintigraphy is the most sensitive modality to detect metastatic lesions in the skeletal system (Figs. 9.12 and 9.13). In addition, it is an effective modality in differentiating multifocal osteolytic metastases (almost invariably exhibiting positive findings on radionuclide bone scan in form of increased uptake of the radiotracer) from multiple myeloma (which usually displays a normal bone scan).
- PET and PET–CT are very sensitive in demonstrating all metastatic lesions (Figs. 9.14 to 9.16).
- Magnetic resonance imaging shows variety of signal intensity, depending whether the metastasis is lytic, sclerotic, or mixed (Figs. 9.17 and 9.18). Occasionally, this modality is useful in determining the origin of the metastatic lesion, such as a "flow-void" sign apparently characteristic for metastatic renal carcinoma. Postcontrast studies show significant enhancement of highly vascularized metastatic lesions.

Pathology:
Gross (Macroscopy):
- Gross appearance of the metastatic tumor depends upon the type—whether it is osteolytic or sclerotic variant.

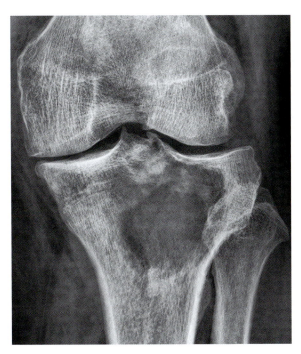

FIGURE 9.3 Radiography of osteolytic metastasis.
A 45-year-old man presented with a solitary osteolytic lesion in the left proximal tibia, originally misinterpreted as a giant cell tumor. An extensive clinical workup and excision biopsy lead to the diagnosis of metastasis from renal cell carcinoma.

The first type will present as a soft, hemorrhagic mass, whereas the second type will exhibit firm in consistency, white-grayish lesion.

Histopathology:

- Many metastatic lesions exhibit a desmoplastic fibrotic reaction and the presence of woven or mature bone trabeculae with intertrabecular fibrosis (Figs. 9.19 to 9.21).
- Poorly differentiated epithelial carcinoma cells or gland-forming adenocarcinoma may indicate primary carcinoma in the colon (Fig. 9.22).
- Metastatic melanoma may show variety of morphologic features with prominent pleomorphism and atypia. Identification of melanin pigment within the tumor cells is also a helpful diagnostic feature (Fig. 9.23).
- Metastatic follicular carcinoma from the thyroid resembles the normal microscopic pattern of the thyroid gland. Foci of papillary formation and follicular elements with cells containing clear nuclei with pseudoinclusions may be present.
- Presence of glycoproteins such as gross cystic disease fluid protein (GCDFP15) in the cells from metastatic breast carcinoma is a helpful diagnostic feature.
- Metastasis from renal cell carcinoma may show clear cells.
- Metastatic sarcomas show poorly differentiated spindle cells with prominent pleomorphism.

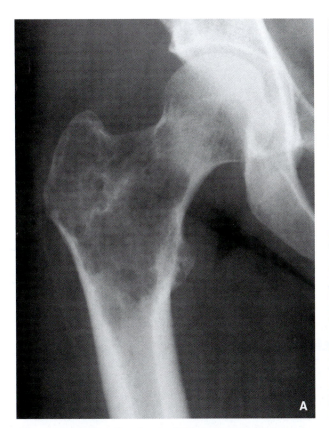
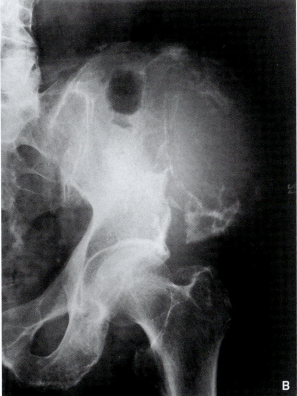

FIGURE 9.4 Radiography of osteolytic metastasis. (A) Anteroposterior radiograph of the right hip of a 52-year-old woman shows a large lytic lesion in the intertrochanteric region of the femur, proved to be a metastasis from carcinoma of the colon. **(B)** Anteroposterior radiograph of the left hemipelvis of an 83-year-old man shows an osteolytic lesion in the ilium, proved to be a metastasis from the thyroid carcinoma.

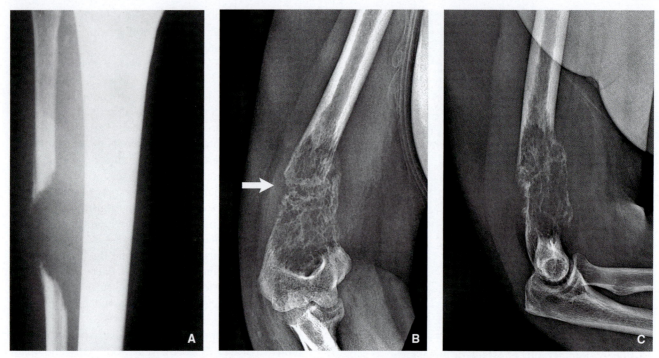

FIGURE 9.5 **Radiography of osteolytic metastasis. (A)** Anteroposterior radiograph of the right leg of a 41-year-old woman with renal cell carcinoma shows a lytic lesion in the fibula, breaking through the cortex and extending into the soft tissues. **(B)** Anteroposterior and **(C)** lateral radiographs of the right elbow of a 44-year-old woman with soft-tissue leiomyosarcoma of the buttock show lytic metastasis to the distal humerus. Note associated pathologic fracture (*arrow*).

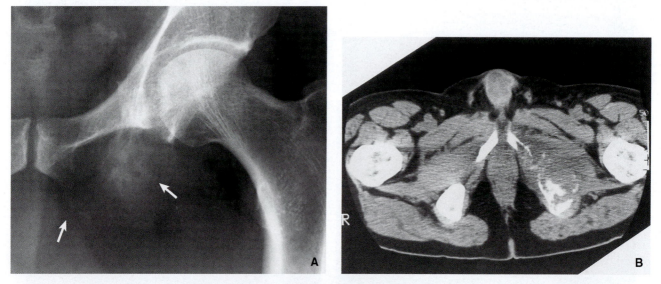

FIGURE 9.6 **Radiography and computed tomography of osteolytic metastasis. (A)** Anteroposterior radiograph of the left hip of a 50-year-old man with renal cell carcinoma shows an osteolytic lesion almost completely destroying the ischium (*arrows*). **(B)** Axial CT section demonstrates the extent of bone destruction and a soft-tissue extension.

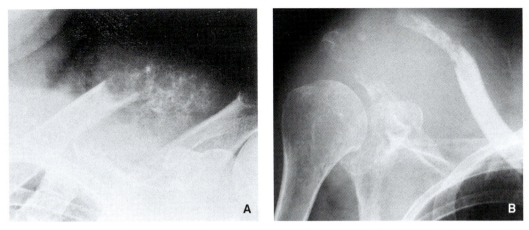

FIGURE 9.7 Radiography of osteolytic metastases. (A) Blown-out osteolytic metastasis in the acromial end of the left clavicle of a 52-year-old man with renal cell carcinoma (hypernephroma). **(B)** Blown-out osteolytic metastases in the acromial end of the right clavicle, acromion, and glenoid, associated with a soft-tissue mass of a 59-year-old woman with renal cell carcinoma.

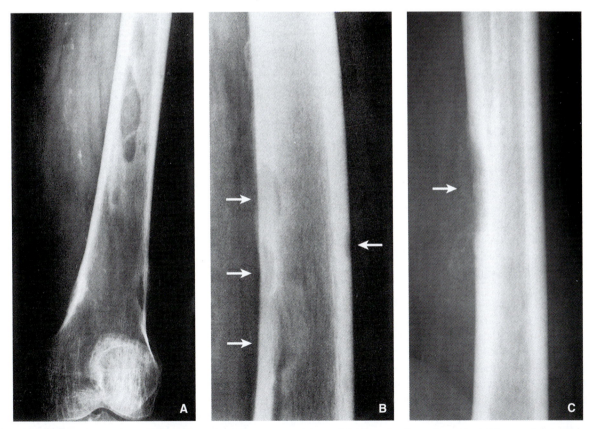

FIGURE 9.8 Radiography of cortical metastases. (A) Anteroposterior and **(B)** lateral radiographs of the left femur of an 82-year-old man with bronchogenic carcinoma show characteristic cookie bite appearance of the lesion (*arrows*). **(C)** Osteolytic cortical metastasis to the femur (*arrow*) of a 62-year-old man with bronchogenic carcinoma.

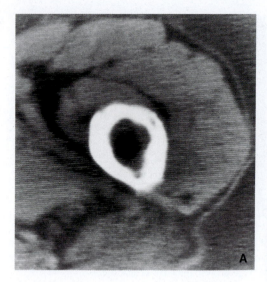
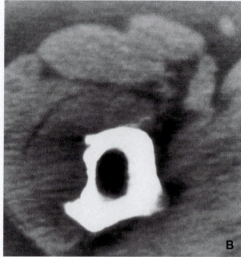
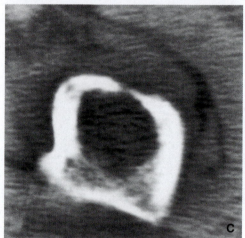

FIGURE 9.9 Computed tomography of cortical metastasis. (A) Cortical metastasis in the left femur of a 70-year-old man. **(B)** Cortical metastasis in the right femur of a 46-year-old woman. **(C)** Cortical metastasis in the right femur of a 72-year-old woman.

Immunohistochemistry:
- Positive findings of epithelial membrane antigen (EMA) or keratin are strongly suggestive of metastatic carcinoma.
- Keratins will highlight carcinoma cells interspersed between the bone trabeculae (Fig. 9.24).
- Metastatic carcinoma from the prostate shows positivity for PSA (Fig. 9.25).
- Metastatic adenocarcinomas of intestinal origin will react to CDX2 (see Fig. 9.22B).
- Particular combinations of CK7 and CK20 can be useful for the preliminary differentiation of the origin of primary carcinomas, as follows:
  - $CK7^+/CK20^+$—carcinoma of bile duct and primary mucous tumors of ovary, upper gastrointestinal tract, urinary bladder, and endocervix;
  - $CK7^+/CK20^-$—breast carcinoma, endometrial carcinomas, carcinoma of esophagus, lung carcinoma, salivary carcinoma, thyroid carcinoma, and mesothelioma;
  - $CK7^-/CK20^+$—carcinoma of colon, primary carcinoma of adrenal cortex, and prostate carcinoma.
- Metastatic small cell lung carcinomas will show positivity for NSE.
- Metastatic melanomas will show positivity for the following markers: S-100 protein, vimentin, antikeratins, melanoma antigen recognized by T cells 1 (MART-1), and human melanoma black 45 (HMB-45). These findings coupled with strong reaction of the tumor cells with anti–melanin A are diagnostic (see Fig. 9.23B).
- Angiosarcomas will show positivity for CD34, CD31, and factor VIII.
- Mesenchymal sarcomas will be positive for vimentin.

Genetics:
- Some genetic mutations may be helpful to distinguish subtype and origin of the metastatic tumors, for example, translocation t(X;18)(p11.2; q11.2) characteristic for synovial sarcoma, translocation t(1;13)(p36;q14) characteristic for alveolar rhabdomyosarcoma, translocation t(17;22)(q22;q13) characteristic for dermatofibrosarcoma protuberans (giant cell fibroblastoma), or translocation t(12;22)(q13;q12) characteristic for clear cell sarcoma (malignant melanoma of soft parts).

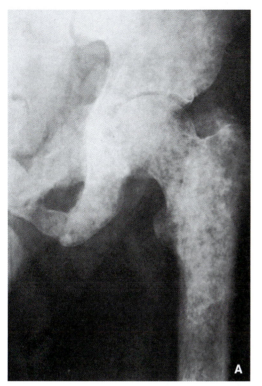
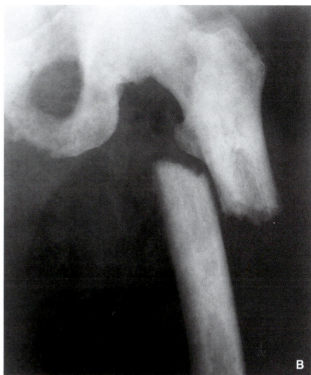
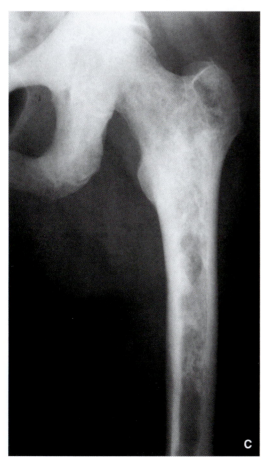

FIGURE 9.10 Radiography of osteoblastic metastases.
(A) Anteroposterior radiograph of the left hip of a 55-year-old man with carcinoma of the prostate shows multiple sclerotic foci scattered through the ilium, pubis, ischium, and proximal femur. **(B)** Anteroposterior radiograph of the left hip of a 68-year-old man with prostate carcinoma shows diffuse osteoblastic metastases affecting the femur and pelvic bones, associated with a pathologic fracture. **(C)** Anteroposterior radiograph of the proximal left femur of a 57-year-old woman with carcinoma of the breast shows numerous sclerotic lesions.

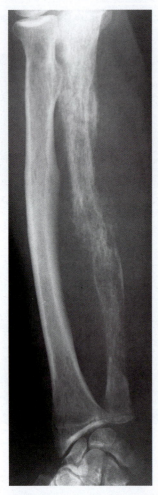

FIGURE 9.11 Radiography of mixed metastases. Anteroposterior radiograph of the forearm of a 66-year-old woman with breast carcinoma shows combination of lytic and sclerotic lesions in the ulna.

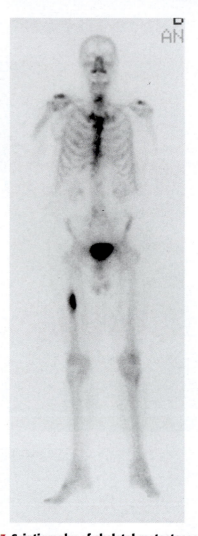

FIGURE 9.13 Scintigraphy of skeletal metastases. A total body radionuclide bone scan obtained in a 55-year-old man with bronchogenic carcinoma demonstrates metastatic lesions in the sternum, the cervical and thoracic spine, and the right femur.

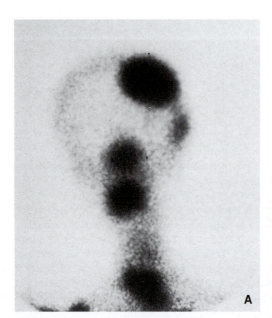
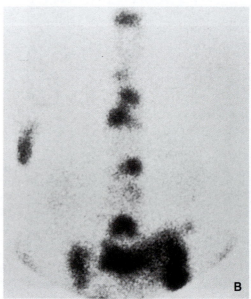

FIGURE 9.12 Scintigraphy of skeletal metastases. Radionuclide bone scan performed after intravenous injection of 15 mCi (555 MBq) of technetium-99m methylene diphosphonate (MDP) in a 68-year-old woman with breast carcinoma shows increased uptake of the radiopharmaceutical tracer in **(A)** the skull and cervical spine and **(B)** the lumbar spine and pelvic bones, localizing multiple metastatic lesions.

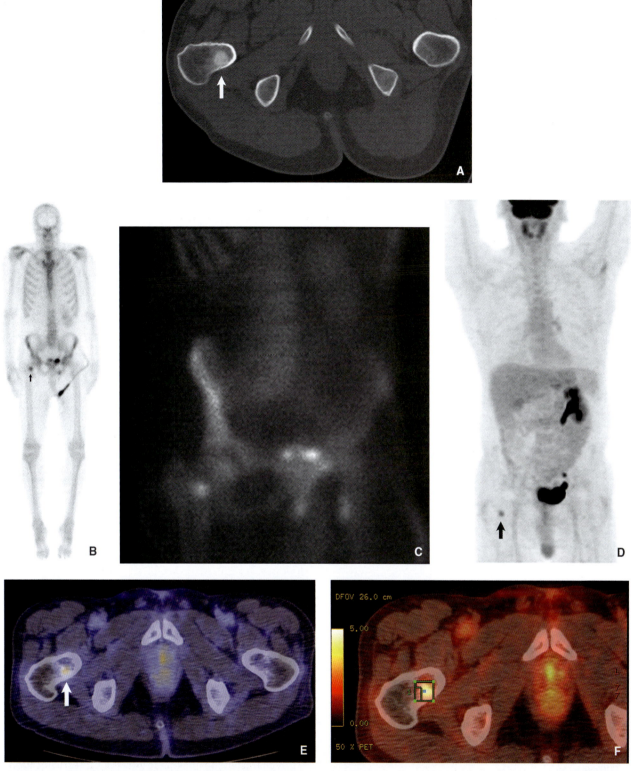

FIGURE 9.14 Computed tomography, scintigraphy, FDG PET, and PET-CT of sclerotic metastasis. (A) Axial CT image through the proximal femora of a 60-year-old man with transitional cell carcinoma of the urinary bladder shows a low-attenuation sclerotic lesion in the right femoral neck (*arrow*). **(B)** Total body radionuclide bone scan and **(C)** coned-down oblique scintigraphic image of the pelvis show solitary focus of increased activity of the radiopharmaceutical tracer in the right femoral neck (*arrow*). **(D)** Total body FDG PET scan shows a hypermetabolic focus in the right femoral neck (*arrow*), confirming the presence of the metastatic lesion, further documented on **(E,F)** two axial PET-CT–fused images (*arrow*).

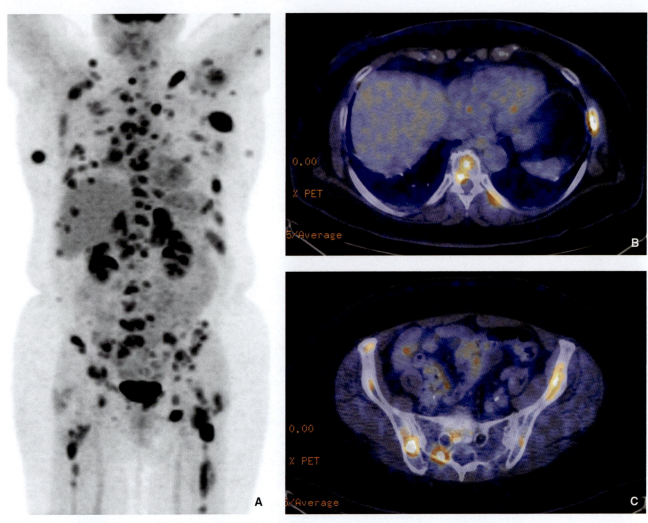

FIGURE 9.15 FDG positron emission tomography and PET-CT of skeletal metastases. (A) Whole-body PET scan of a 60-year-old woman with advanced adenocarcinoma of the breast shows numerous hypermetabolic foci in the bones, lymph nodes, and internal organs, representing diffuse metastatic disease. Axial fused FDG PET-CT images obtained at the level of the chest **(B)** and abdomen **(C)** demonstrate hypermetabolic metastases in the vertebra, ribs, iliac bones, and sacrum.

Differential Diagnosis:
Solitary Osteolytic Metastasis:

- **Plasmacytoma**
  Imaging features of solitary lesion may be undistinguishable from metastasis. Radionuclide bone scan, however, almost always will be normal or only slightly positive.
  Histopathology showing sheets of atypical plasmacytoid cells containing round nuclei with dense, coarse chromatin that has a typical cartwheel-like distribution is diagnostic.
- **Fibrosarcoma**
  Imaging features of osteolytic metastasis may be identical to fibrosarcoma or malignant fibrous histiocytoma, and one must rely on clinical and histopathologic findings.
  Histopathology showing interwoven bundles of spindle cells with pleomorphism and hyperchromatism producing characteristic herringbone pattern is diagnostic.
- **Lymphoma**
  Imaging features of a solitary focus of osteolytic variant of lymphoma may be identical to metastatic lesion; however, the patients are usually younger.
  Histopathology showing diffuse growth pattern of aggregates of malignant round or ovoid lymphoid cells containing large, sometimes indented (cleaved) or horseshoe-shaped nuclei with prominent nucleoli is diagnostic.
- **Giant cell tumor**
  Occurs in younger population of patients, and exhibits characteristic imaging features of eccentric location, internal trabeculations, and extension into the articular end of bone.
  Histopathology showing a dual population of fibrocytic or monocytic mononuclear stromal cells and large giant cells that are uniformly distributed throughout the tumor is diagnostic.

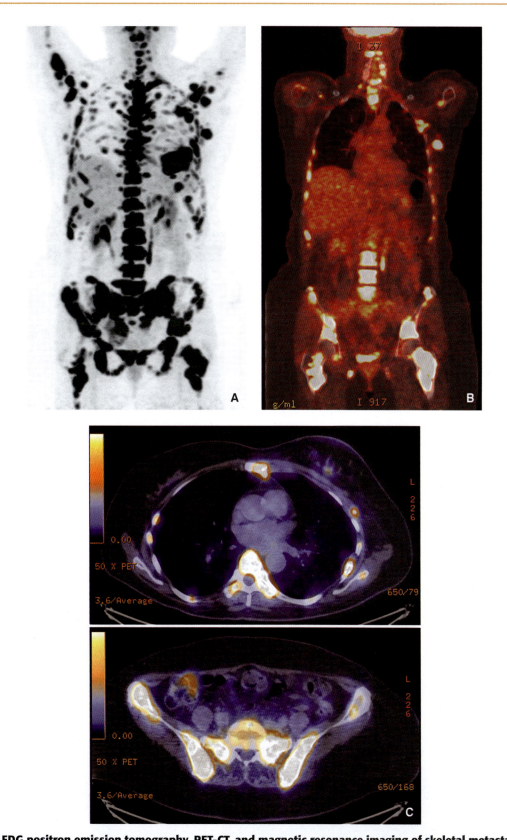

FIGURE 9.16 FDG positron emission tomography, PET-CT, and magnetic resonance imaging of skeletal metastases.
(A) Whole-body PET scan and **(B)** coronal reformatted postcontrast PET-CT of a 57-year-old woman with adenocarcinoma of the breast show several hypermetabolic foci within the osseous structures consistent with metastatic process. **(C)** Axial fused FDG PET-CT images obtained at the level of the chest *(top)* and pelvis *(bottom)* demonstrate hypermetabolic lesions in the vertebrae, ribs, sternum, pelvic bones, and sacrum.

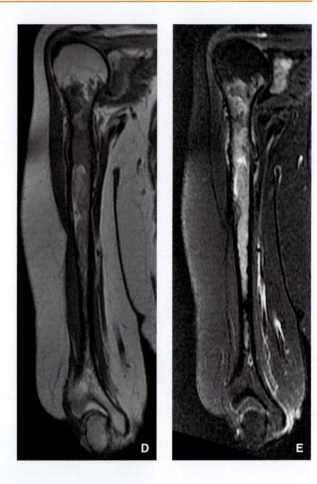

FIGURE 9.16 *(Continued).* **(D)** Coronal T1-weighted and **(E)** coronal STIR MR images show diffuse involvement of the bone marrow of the right humerus.

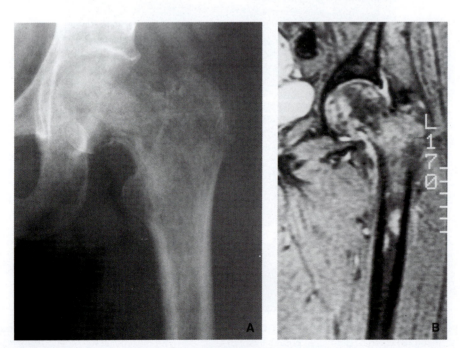

FIGURE 9.17 Radiography and magnetic resonance imaging of mixed metastasis. (A) Anteroposterior radiograph of the left hip of a 60-year-old woman with breast carcinoma shows diffuse mixed lytic and sclerotic metastasis affecting the proximal femur. **(B)** Coronal T2*-weighted MPGR MR image demonstrates heterogeneous but predominantly high signal intensity of the lesion. The uninvolved bone marrow remains of low signal intensity.

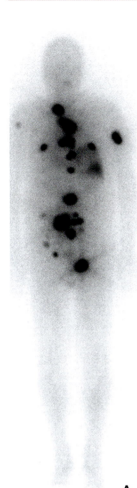
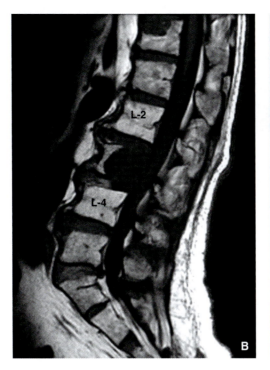
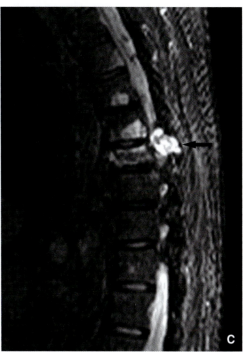

FIGURE 9.18 Scintigraphy and magnetic resonance imaging of skeletal metastases. (A) Total body radionuclide bone scan of a 70-year-old man with follicular thyroid carcinoma, performed after oral administration of 155 mCi 131-I sodium iodide, shows multiple skeletal metastases. **(B)** Sagittal T1-weighted MRI demonstrates the involvement of T12 and L3 vertebral bodies. **(C)** Sagittal STIR MR image shows extension of metastatic tumor into the spinal canal (*arrow*).

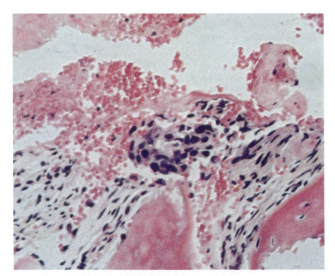

FIGURE 9.19 Histopathology of skeletal metastasis. A photomicrograph of a needle biopsy specimen was obtained from a sclerotic vertebral body suspected to be metastatic. There is evidence of reactive bone formation as well as fibrous scarring. In addition, conglomerate of atypical cells is present, strongly suggestive of a tumor; however, the definite diagnosis as to the origin of the lesion is not possible (H&E, original magnification ×400).

- **Brown tumor of hyperparathyroidism**

    Imaging features of a solitary brown tumor may resemble metastatic lesion; however, other characteristic findings of hyperparathyroidism such as subperiosteal and chondral resorption, rugger-jersey spine, or soft-tissue calcifications may also be present.

    Histopathology of brown tumor that is composed of reactive stromal cells in which multinucleated giant cells are arranged in clusters, and the large aggregates of hemosiderin pigment, is diagnostic.

Solitary Osteoblastic Metastasis:

- **Enostosis (Bone island)**

    Radiographic features, including so-called thorny radiation or "pseudopodia" (rough border of the lesion) representing thickened bone trabeculae that radiate in streaks from the lesion, aligned with the axes of surrounding uninvolved host bone trabeculae, and blending with them in a feathered or brush-like fashion, are diagnostic. In addition, majority of bone islands will exhibit normal skeletal scintigraphy.

    Histopathology showing a focus of a compact bone structure within cancellous bone with prominent

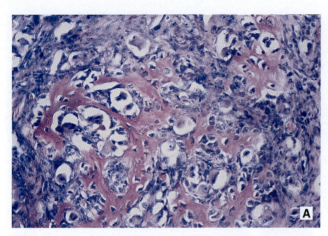
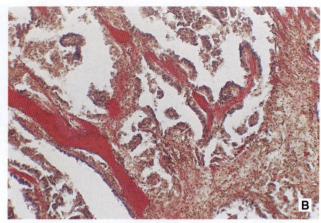

FIGURE 9.20 Histopathology of skeletal metastasis. (A) Metastatic lesion from a well-differentiated papillary carcinoma of the thyroid exhibits, in addition to glandular cells, formation of reactive bone (*pinkish foci*) (Giemsa, original magnification ×50). **(B)** Another field of view shows metaplastic formation of woven bone trabeculae (van Gieson, original magnification ×50).

cement lines and occasionally haversian systems of nutrient canals is also diagnostic.

- *Osteoblastoma*
  Usually occurs in much younger population than do metastases, and imaging studies generally shows some degree of fluffy radiopacities within the lesion and prominent periosteal reaction.
  Histopathology showing substantial amount of osteoid production by osteoblasts is diagnostic.
- *Calcifying enchondroma*
  Imaging studies show typical "popcorn"-like chondroid calcifications and lack of aggressive features. Larger lesions exhibit shallow scalloping of the endocortex.

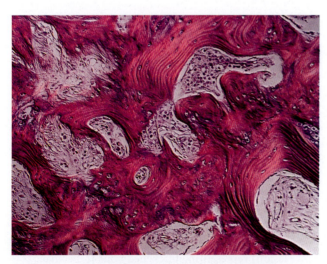

FIGURE 9.21 Histopathology of skeletal metastasis. Osteoblastic metastasis from carcinoma of the prostate exhibits woven bone trabeculae produced in response to the tumor invasion, firmly adherent to the surface of the normal lamellar bone. The spaces in between are filled with fibrous tissue and malignant cells (H&E, original magnification ×4). (From Bullough P. *Atlas of Orthopedic Pathology*. 2nd ed. New York, NY: Gower Medical Publishing; 1992, p. 17.84, Fig. 17.29.)

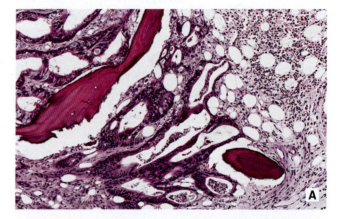
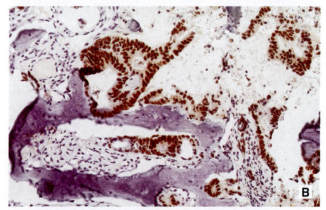

FIGURE 9.22 Histopathology and immunohistochemistry of skeletal metastasis. (A) Metastatic colon carcinoma is forming glandular structures and infiltrates bone marrow between the bone trabeculae (H&E, original magnification ×200). **(B)** Specific stain CDX2 for colon cancer highlights the tumor cells forming glandular structures (*brown color*) and invading bone trabeculae (*purple color*) (original magnification ×200).

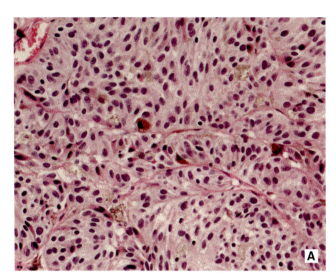 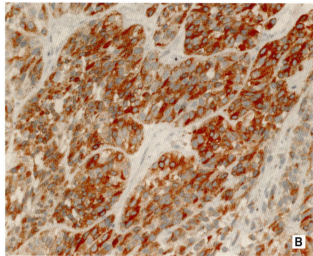

FIGURE 9.23 **Histopathology and immunohistochemistry of skeletal metastasis.** **(A)** Metastasis from melanoma exhibits melanin pigment within some malignant cells (H&E, original magnification ×200). **(B)** Immunohistochemistry shows strong reaction of tumor cells with anti–melanin A (biotin–avidin peroxidase, original magnification ×200).

Histopathology showing lobules of hyaline cartilage of variable cellularity, and cells located in the lacunae containing small, dark-stained nuclei, coupled with intercellular uniformly translucent matrix, is diagnostic.

- *Lymphoma*

  Imaging features of a solitary lesion may resemble metastatic lesion. If, however, the soft-tissue mass is disproportionally larger than is the bone lesion, diagnosis of lymphoma rather than metastasis should be made.

  Histopathology showing diffuse growth pattern of aggregates of malignant rounded or ovoid lymphoid cells containing large, sometimes indented (cleaved) or horseshoe-shaped nuclei with prominent nucleoli is diagnostic.

- *Erdheim-Chester disease*

  Imaging features may resemble metastatic lesion, although cortical thickening should be a helpful hint in the differential diagnosis.

  Histopathology showing diffuse infiltration of bone marrow by foamy histiocytes, lymphocytes, plasma cells, and Touton giant cells, associated with dense fibrosis, is diagnostic.

Multifocal Osteolytic Metastases:

- *Multiple myeloma*

  Imaging features of small, usually uniform in size "punched-out" lesions, endosteal scalloping, and generally normal radionuclide bone scan are diagnostic.

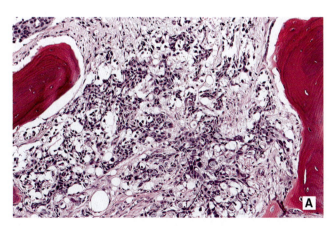 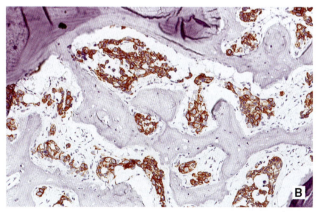

FIGURE 9.24 **Immunohistochemistry of skeletal metastasis.** **(A)** Metastatic bladder carcinoma shows poorly differentiated cells invading bone marrow between the bone trabeculae (H&E, original magnification ×200). **(B)** Tumor cells infiltrating marrow spaces between bone trabeculae (*light pinkish color*) are highlighted by cytokeratin 20 (*brown color*) (CK20, original magnification ×200).

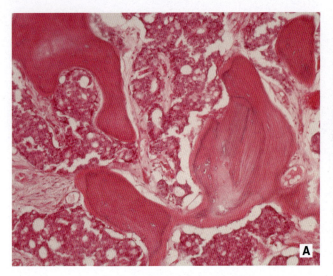
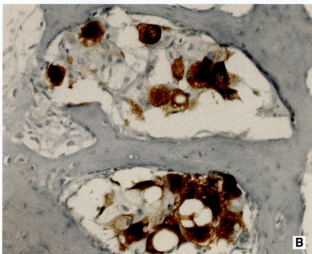
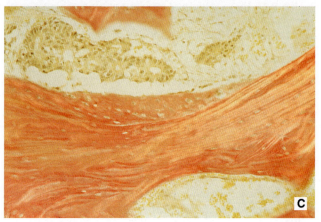

FIGURE 9.25 Histopathology and immunohistochemistry of skeletal metastasis. (A) Osteoblastic metastasis from a moderately differentiated adenocarcinoma of the prostate shows tumor-filled marrow spaces and thickened trabeculae (H&E, original magnification ×100). **(B)** In another field of view, the trabecula of lamellar bone with attached cell-rich layer of new woven bone on the upper surface and rim of osteoblasts on the lower surface is seen. In the marrow space *(top)*, tumor cells of adenocarcinoma of the prostate are present (van Gieson, original magnification ×200). **(C)** Tumor cells react with an antibody against prostate-specific antigen (PSA) (biotin-streptavidin peroxidase, original magnification ×200).

Histopathology showing sheets of atypical plasmacytoid cells containing round nuclei with a dense, coarse chromatin that has a typical cartwheel-like distribution is diagnostic.

- **Brown tumors of hyperparathyroidism**
  Multiple brown tumors may look on imaging studies similar to metastases; however, MRI often shows low signal intensity within the lesions reflecting magnetic susceptibility to hemosiderin.
  Histopathology showing clusters of multinucleated giant cells with fibroblastic and reactive stroma coupled with clumps of hemosiderin pigment is diagnostic.

- **Langerhans cell histiocytosis**
  Although imaging features may be similar to osteolytic metastases, the condition occurs in much younger patients. "Hole-in-hole" appearance of some of the lesions is characteristic.
  Histopathology showing typical Langerhans cells, and EM identification of Birbeck granules, is diagnostic.

- **Gaucher disease**
  Imaging features of reactive periostitis, Erlenmeyer flask deformity, intramedullary bone infarcts, and osteonecrotic changes are characteristic for this disorder.
  Histopathology showing infiltration of the bone marrow spaces by large macrophages (Gaucher cells) possessing round to ovoid nuclei and abundant striped cytoplasm that has a characteristic "crumpled tissue paper" appearance is diagnostic.

- **Diffuse osteoporosis**
  Imaging studies will show lack of discrete osteolytic lesions, and radionuclide bone scan will be normal. PET scan will show lack of hypermetabolic foci.
  Histopathology showing lack of malignant cells is diagnostic.

Multifocal Osteoblastic Metastases:

- **Osteopoikilosis (Osteopathia condensans disseminata)**
  Radiographic features of this disorder, which is characterized by multiple bone islands symmetrically distributed and clustered near the articular ends of a bone, are identical to those of a single bone island. Also, this condition exhibits normal radionuclide bone scan.
  Histopathology identical to that of a single bone island (see above) is diagnostic.

- **Mastocytosis**
  Radiographic features may be very similar to metastatic disease, although the sclerotic lesions, in addition to involve the axial skeleton, are usually grouped at the ends of the long bones.

Histopathology showing mast cells hyperplasia characterized by diffuse increase in mature, round, or spindle-shaped metachromatic mast cells is diagnostic. In addition, immunohistochemistry using antibodies against mast cell–associated antigens such as immunoexpression of tryptase or CD117 is also a very helpful diagnostic tool.

- ***Osteosarcomatosis (Multicentric osteosarcoma)***
Imaging features of multicentric osteosarcoma are identical with appearance of skeletal metastases from primary osteosarcoma elsewhere in the bones. Likewise, the histopathologic findings in both conditions are identical. However, if multiple bones are affected in the absence of pulmonary metastases, and in particular, if osseous lesions are present in the bones rarely affected by metastatic disease (such as those distal to the knees and elbows), multicentric osteosarcoma should be strongly considered.

REFERENCES

Abrams HL. Skeletal metastases in carcinoma. *Radiology.* 1950;55:534–538.

Abrams HL, Spiro R, Goldstein N. Metastases in carcinoma. Analysis of 1000 autopsied cases. *Cancer.* 1950;3:74–85.

Algra PR, Bloem JL, Tissing H, Falke TH, Arndt JW, Verboom LJ. Detection of vertebral metastases: comparison between MR imaging and bone scintigraphy. *Radiographics.* 1991;11:219–232.

Algra PR, Heimans JJ, Valk J, Nauta JJ, Lachniet M, Van Kooten B. Do metastases in vertebrae begin in the body or the pedicles? Imaging study in 45 patients. *AJR Am J Roentgenol.* 1992;158:1275–1279.

Ardran GM. Bone destruction not demonstrable by radiography. *Br J Radiol.* 1951;24:107–109.

Avrahami E, Tadmor R, Dally O, Hadar H. Early MR demonstration of spinal metastases in patients with normal radiographs and CT and radionuclide bone scans. *J Comput Assist Tomogr.* 1989;13:598–602.

Berrettoni B, Carter JR. Mechanisms of cancer metastasis to bone. *J Bone Joint Surg Am.* 1986;68A:308–312.

Bloom RA, Libson E, Husband JE, Stoker DJ. The periosteal sunburst reaction to bone metastases. A literature review and report of 20 additional cases. *Skeletal Radiol.* 1987;16:629–634.

Brown B, Laorr A, Greenspan A, Stadalnik R. Negative bone scintigraphy with diffuse osteoblastic breast carcinoma metastases. *Clin Nucl Med.* 1994;19:194–196.

Bushnell DL, Kahn D, Huston B, Bevering CG. Utility of SPECT imaging for determination of vertebral metastases in patients with known primary tumors. *Skeletal Radiol.* 1995;24:13

Choi J-A, Lee KH, Jun WS, Yi MG, Lee S, Kang HS. Osseous metastasis from renal cell carcinoma: "flow-void" sign at MR imaging. *Radiology.* 2003;228:629–634.

Citrin DL, Bessent RG, Greig WR. A comparison of the sensitivity and accuracy of the 99m Tc-phosphate bone scan and skeletal radiograph in the diagnosis of bone metastases. *Clin Radiol.* 1977;28:107–117.

Coerkamp EG, Kroon HM. Cortical bone metastases. *Radiology.* 1988;169:525–528.

Daldrup-Link HE, Franzius C, Link TM, et al. Whole-body MR imaging for detection of bone metastases in children and young adults: comparison with skeletal scintigraphy and FDG PET. *AJR Am J Roentgenol.* 2001;177:229–236.

Delbeke D, Powers TA, Sandler MP. Negative scintigraphy with positive magnetic resonance imaging in bone metastases. *Skeletal Radiol.* 1990;19:113–116.

Deutsch A, Resnick D. Eccentric cortical metastases to the skeleton from bronchogenic carcinoma. *Radiology.* 1980;137:49–52.

Deutsch A, Resnick D, Niwayama G. Case report 145. Bilateral, almost symmetrical skeletal metastases (both femora) from bronchogenic carcinoma. *Skeletal Radiol.* 1981;6:144–148.

Esscher T, Bergh J, Steinholtz L, Nöu E, Nilsson K, Påhlman S. Neuron-specific enolase in small-cell carcinoma of the lung: the value of combined immunocytochemistry and serum determination. *Anticancer Res.* 1989;9:1717–1720.

Evison G, Pizey N, Roylance J. Bone formation associated with osseous metastases from bladder carcinoma. *Clin Radiol.* 1981;32:303–309.

Galasko CSB. Mechanisms of lytic and blastic metastatic disease of bone. *Clin Orthop.* 1982;69:20–27.

Geurts van Kessel A, de Bruijn D, Hermsen L, et al. Masked t(X;18)(p11;q11) in biphasic synovial sarcoma revealed by FISH and RT-PCR. *Genes Chromos Cancer.* 1998;23:198–201.

Ghandur-Mnaymneh L, Broder LE, Mnaymneh WA. Lobular carcinoma of the breast metastatic to bone with unusual clinical, radiologic, and pathologic features mimicking osteopoikilosis. *Cancer.* 1984;53:1801–1803.

Gleason BC, Nascimento AF. HMB-45 and Melan-A are useful in the differential diagnosis between granular cell tumor and malignant melanoma. *Am J Dermatopathol.* 2007;29:22–27.

Gold RI, Seeger LL, Bassett LW, Steckel RJ. An integrated approach to the evaluation of metastatic bone disease. *Radiol Clin North Am.* 1990;28:471–483.

Greenspan A, Norman A. Osteolytic cortical destruction: an unusual pattern of skeletal metastases. *Skeletal Radiol.* 1988;17:402–406.

Greenspan A, Stadalnik RC. Bone island: scintigraphic findings and their clinical application. *Can Assoc Radiol J.* 1995;46:368–379.

Greenspan A, Klein MJ, Lewis MM. Case report 272. Skeletal cortical metastases in the left femur arising from bronchogenic carcinoma. *Skeletal Radiol.* 1984;11:297–301.

Greenspan A, Klein MJ, Lewis MM. Case report 284. Osteolytic cortical metastasis in the femur from bronchogenic carcinoma. *Skeletal Radiol.* 1984;12:146–150.

Greenspan A, Gerscovich EO, Szabo RM, Matthews JG II. Condensing osteitis of the clavicle: a rare but frequently misdiagnosed condition. *AJR Am J Roentgenol.* 1991;156:1011–1015.

Gunawan B, Fuzesi L, Granzen B, et al. Clinical aspect of alveolar rhabdomyosarcoma with translocation t(1;13)(p36;q14) and hypotetraploidy. *Pathol Oncol Res.* 1999;5:211–213.

Gutzeit A, Doert A, Froehlich JM, et al. Comparison of diffusion-weighted whole body MRI and skeletal scintigraphy for the detection of bone metastases in patients with prostate or breast carcinoma. *Skeletal Radiol.* 2010;39:333–343.

Hamada M, Morishita F, Mori Y. Bladder tumor presenting multiple osteoblastic bone metastases. *Gan No Rinsho.* 1986;32:945–948.

Harding M, McAllister J, Hulks G, et al. Neuron specific enolase (NSE) in small cell lung cancer: a tumour marker of prognostic significance? *Br J Cancer.* 1990;61:605–607.

Healey JH, Turnbull AD, Miedema B, Lane JM. Acrometastases. A study of twenty-nine patients with osseous involvement of the hands and feet. *J Bone Joint Surg Am.* 1986;68A:743–746.

Hendrix RW, Rogers LF, Davis TM Jr. Cortical bone metastases. *Radiology.* 1991;181:409–413.

Hove B, Gyldensted C. Spiculated vertebral metastases from prostatic carcinoma. *Neuroradiology.* 1990;32:337–339.

Ilievska Poposka B, Spirovski M, Trajkov D, Stefanovski T, Atanasova S, Metodieva M. Neuron specific enolase—selective marker for small-cell lung cancer. *Radiol Oncol.* 2004;38:21–26.

Jacobson HG, Poppel MH, Shapiro JH, Grossberger S. The vertebral pedicle sign: a roentgen finding to differentiate metastatic carcinoma from multiple myeloma. *AJR Am J Roentgenol.* 1958;80:817–821.

Kattapuram SV, Khurana JS, Scott JA, el-Khoury GY. Negative scintigraphy with positive magnetic resonance imaging in bone metastases. *Skeletal Radiol.* 1990;19:113–116.

Lehrer HZ, Maxfield WS, Nice CM. The periosteal sunburst pattern in metastatic bone tumors. *AJR Am J Roentgenol.* 1970;108:154–161.

Mazziotta RM, Borczuk AC, Powell CA, Mansukhani M. CDX2 immunostaining as a gastrointestinal marker: expression in lung carcinoma is a potential pitfall. *Appl Immunohistochem Mol Morphol.* 2005;13:55–60.

Moskaluk CA, Zhang H, Powell SM, Cerilli LA, Hampton GM, Frierson HF Jr. Cdx2 protein expression in normal and malignant human tissues: an immunohistochemical survey using tissue microarrays. *Mod Pathol.* 2003;16:913–919.

Mulvey RB. Peripheral bone metastases. *AJR Am J Roentgenol.* 1964;91:155–160.

Napoli LD, Hansen HH, Muggia FM, Twigg HL. The incidence of osseous involvement in lung cancer, with special reference to the development of osteoblastic changes. *Radiology.* 1973;108:17–21.

Norman A, Ulin R. A comparative study of periosteal new-bone response in metastatic bone tumors (solitary) and primary bone sarcomas. *Radiology.* 1969;92:705–708.

Ontell FK, Greenspan A. Blastic osseous metastases in ovarian carcinoma. *Can Assoc Radiol J.* 1995;46:231–234.

Panebianco AC, Kaupp HA. Bilateral thumb metastasis from breast carcinoma. *Arch Surg.* 1968;96:216–218.

Pittas AG, Adler M, Fazzani M, et al. Bone metastases from thyroid carcinoma: clinical characteristics and prognostic variables in one hundred forty-six patients. *Thyroid.* 2000;10:261–268.

Powell JM. Metastatic carcinoid of bone. Report of two cases and review of the literature. *Clin Orthop.* 1988;230:266–272.

Schajowicz F, Velan O, Santini Araujo E, et al. Metastases of carcinoma in pagetic bone. *Clin Orthop.* 1988;228:290–296.

Shih WJ, Riley C, Magoun S, Ryo UY. Paget's disease mimicking skeletal metastases in a patient with coexisting prostatic carcinoma. *Eur J Nucl Med.* 1988;15:422–423.

Shipley JM, Clark J, Crew AJ, et al. The t(X;18)(p11.2;q11.2) translocation found in human synovial sarcomas involves two distinct loci on the X chromosome. *Oncogene.* 1994;9:1447–1453.

Sim FH, Frassica FJ. Metastatic bone disease. In: Unni KK, ed. *Bone Tumors.* New York, NY: Churchill Livingstone; 1988:226.

Söderlund V. Radiological diagnosis of skeletal metastases. *Eur Radiol.* 1996;6:587–595.

Thrall JH, Ellis BI. Skeletal metastases. *Radiol Clin North Am.* 1987;25:1155–1170.

Trias A, Fery A. Cortical circulation of long bones. *J Bone Joint Surg Am.* 1979;61A:1052–1059.

Vilar JL, Lezena AH, Pedrosa CS. Spiculated periosteal reaction in metastatic lesions in bone. *Skeletal Radiol.* 1979;3:230–233.

Werling RW, Yaziji H, Bacchi CE, Gown AM. CDX2, a highly sensitive and specific marker of adenocarcinomas of intestinal origin: an immunohistochemical survey of 476 primary and metastatic carcinomas. *Am J Surg Pathol.* 2003;27:303–310.

Wong HH, Chu P. Immunohistochemical features of the gastrointestinal tract tumors. *J Gastrointest Oncol.* 2012;3:262–284.

Zubovitis J, Buzney E, Yu L, Duncan LM. HMB-45, S-100, NK1/C3, and MART-1 in metastatic melanoma. *Hum Pathol.* 2004;35:217–223.

CHAPTER 10

Mock-Board Review Questions

QUESTIONS

Question 1
A 22-year-old man presented with nocturnal pain in the left groin. The anteroposterior radiograph of the left hip and histopathologic section of the lesion removed from the medial cortex of the femur are shown below. What is your diagnosis?

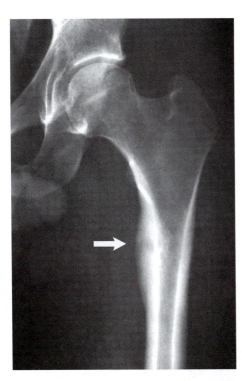

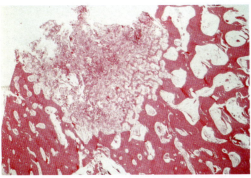

A) Osteoid osteoma.
B) Chondroblastoma.
C) Osteofibrous dysplasia.
D) Osteosarcoma.
E) Ewing sarcoma.

Question 2
Association of Ollier disease and hemangiomas is known as:

A) von Recklinghausen disease of bone.
B) Li-Fraumeni syndrome.
C) Maffucci syndrome.
D) Hereditary multiple exostoses.
E) Gardner syndrome.

Question 3
Which of the following is associated with high risk of osteosarcoma?

A) Germ-line mutation of p53.
B) Translocation t(X;18).
C) Translocation t(12;16).
D) 1p rearrangements.
E) Nonrandom translocation t(9;22).

Question 4
Which one of the following should NOT be included in the differential diagnosis of Ewing sarcoma?

A) Lymphoma.
B) Metastatic neuroblastoma.
C) Mesenchymal chondrosarcoma.
D) Leiomyosarcoma of bone.
E) Metastatic embryonal rhabdomyosarcoma.

Question 5
Which one of the following osteosarcomas has a better prognosis?

A) Paget osteosarcoma.
B) Periosteal osteosarcoma.
C) Parosteal osteosarcoma.
D) Telangiectatic osteosarcoma.
E) Small cell osteosarcoma.

399

Question 6

Adamantinoma of long bones is associated with the following features EXCEPT one:

A) The most common histopathologic variants are basaloid, spindle, squamous, and tubular.
B) The epithelial component expresses positivity for cytokeratins 8 and 18.
C) Younger age of the patients is associated with better prognosis.
D) An osteofibrous dysplasia–like type is the least common histopathologic variant.
E) Pain at presentation is associated with less favorable prognosis.

Question 7

A 14-year-old girl injured her right knee in a fall. The radiograph demonstrated a lesion in the proximal diaphysis of fibula (*arrow*). An open biopsy was performed. Based on the radiographic presentation and histopathologic section, what is your diagnosis?

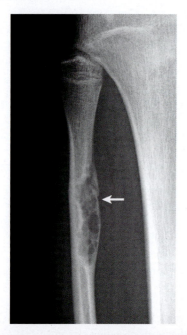

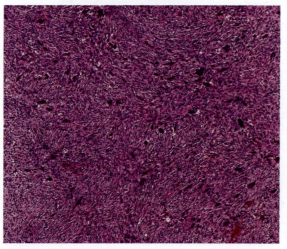

A) Giant cell tumor (GCT)
B) Nonossifying fibroma (NOF)
C) Aneurysmal bone cyst (ABC)
D) Chondroblastoma
E) Giant cell–rich osteosarcoma

Question 8

An 8-year-old boy presented with pain in his left lower thigh knee for past 3 months. Based on the submitted radiograph and histopathologic section, what is the most likely diagnosis?

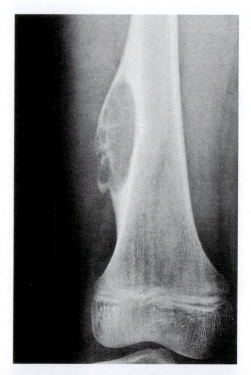

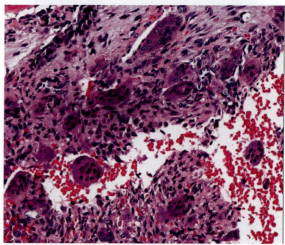

A) Nonossifying fibroma (NOF).
B) Aneurysmal bone cyst (ABC).
C) Simple bone cyst (SBC).
D) Giant cell tumor (GCT).
E) Telangiectatic osteosarcoma.

Question 9
An 8-year-old boy presented with proximal tibia epiphyseal lesion. Given the histopathologic section, what is the most likely diagnosis?

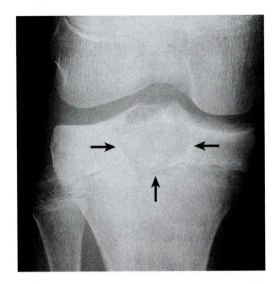

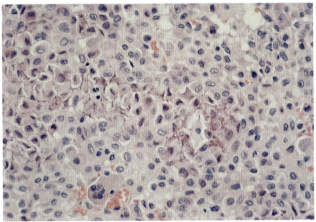

A) Giant cell tumor (GCT).
B) Nonossifying fibroma (NOF).
C) Osteosarcoma.
D) Chondroblastoma.
E) Aneurysmal bone cyst (ABC).

Question 10
Which one of the following is NOT a feature of an osteochondroma?

A) It usually stops growing after skeletal maturity.
B) The cortex of the host bone merges without interruption with the cortex of osteochondroma.
C) The cancellous portion of the lesion is continuous with the medullary cavity of the adjacent diaphysis.
D) Malignant transformation of a solitary lesion approaches 5%.
E) Malignant transformation before age of 20 is uncommon.

Question 11
Concerning giant cell tumor, which one of the following statements is NOT true?

A) It may metastasize to the lung.
B) It is eccentric in location.
C) It extends into the articular end of bone.
D) It has invariably a sclerotic margin.
E) Distal radius is a common location.

Question 12
An adult patient presented with long-standing deformity of the right lower extremity. Two coronal MR images, including T2-weighted fat-suppressed and T1-weighted fat-suppressed obtained after intravenous administration of gadolinium, show osseous and soft-tissue abnormalities. Which one of the following is the most likely diagnosis?

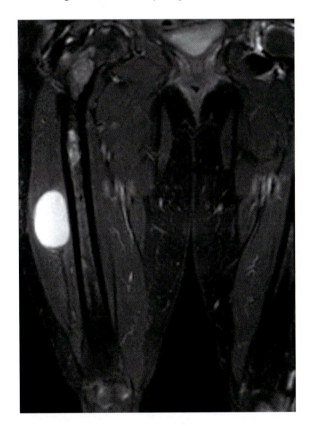

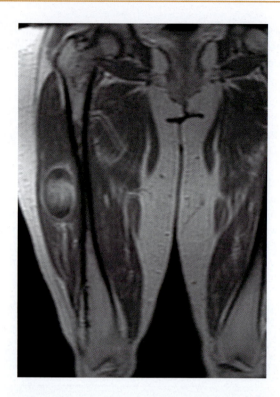

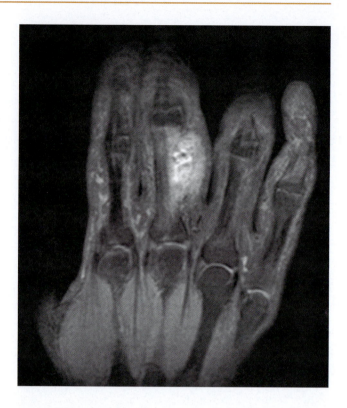

A) Osteosarcoma of the proximal femur with soft-tissue metastasis.
B) Mazabraud syndrome.
C) Jaffe-Campanacci syndrome.
D) Rothmund-Thomson syndrome.
E) Werner syndrome.

A) Ewing sarcoma.
B) Angiosarcoma.
C) Hemangioma.
D) Langerhans cell histiocytosis.
E) Enchondroma.

Question 13
You are shown a radiograph and a coronal T2-weighted MRI of the hand of a 36-year-old woman. Which one of the following is the most likely diagnosis?

Question 14
A 76-year-old woman presented with a severe headache. She gives a history of right breast lumpectomy 3 years ago. Based on the lateral radiograph of the skull and axial CT section of the skull, what is your diagnosis?

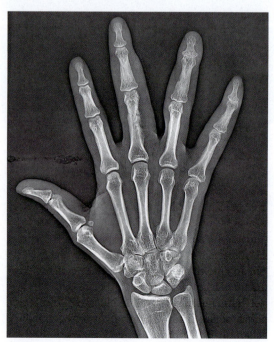

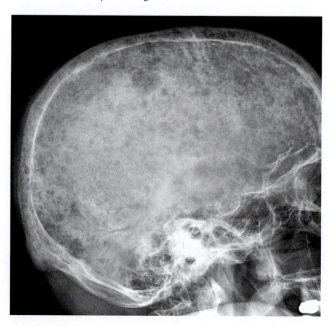

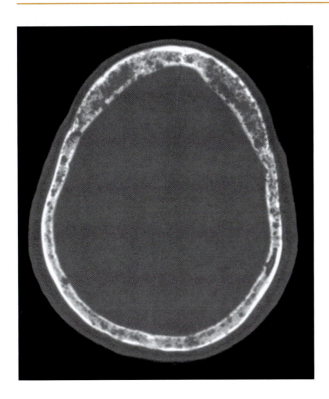

A) Osteolytic metastases.
B) Hyperparathyroidism.
C) Fibrous dysplasia.
D) Paget disease.
E) Multiple myeloma.

Question 15
Concerning multiple myeloma, which one of the following statements is NOT true?

A) The skeletal scintigraphy shows invariably increased uptake of the radiopharmaceutical tracer.
B) By immunohistochemistry, the tumor cells show monoclonal expression of lambda light chains.
C) Patients with POEMS syndrome do not have an increased incidence of amyloidosis and rarely have Bence Jones proteinuria.
D) Endosteal scalloping is a characteristic feature of myeloma affecting long tubular bones.
E) A well-differentiated tumors may exhibit almost normal-appearing plasma cells.

Question 16
Concerning polyostotic fibrous dysplasia, which one of the following statements is correct?

A) Histopathology shows woven bone trabeculae surrounded by active osteoblasts.
B) A "shepherd's crook" deformity of the femur is often the result of multiple pathologic fractures.
C) Skull lesions are seen primarily at the calvaria.
D) Postcontrast MR images show lack of enhancement.
E) McCune-Albright syndrome is caused by gains of chromosomes 1q, 3q, 9q, 11q, and 15q.

Question 17
A 35-year-old woman presented with hand deformities. The most likely diagnosis is:

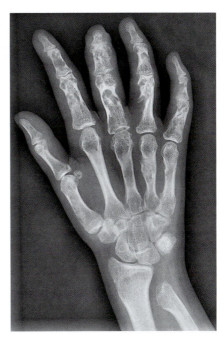

A) Polyostotic fibrous dysplasia.
B) Multiple osteochondromas.
C) Ollier disease.
D) Maffucci syndrome.
E) Neurofibromatosis.

Question 18
A 19-year-old man presented with pain and mass around the left knee. Based on the radiographs and MRI, what is the most likely diagnosis?

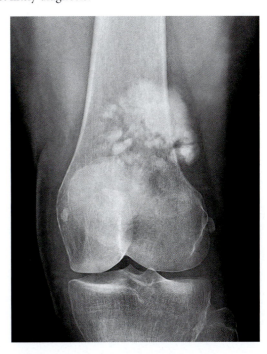

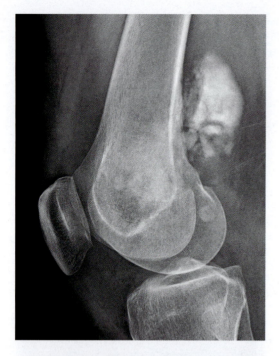

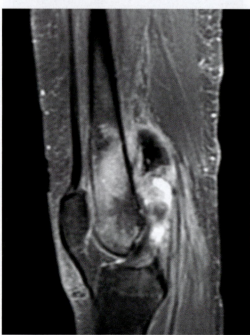

A) Chondrosarcoma.
B) Conventional osteosarcoma.
C) Parosteal osteosarcoma.
D) Periosteal osteosarcoma.
E) Melorheostosis.

Question 19
The following features are characteristic for this lesion EXCEPT:

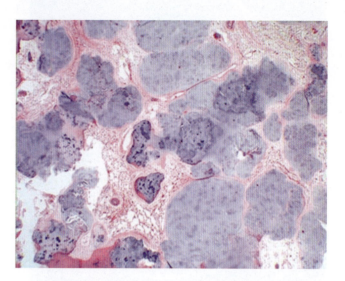

A) Erosion of adjacent bones is a common radiographic finding.
B) Cartilage nodules show small oval or spindled cells.
C) The lesion most commonly arises in the synovium of the joints, bursae, or tendon sheaths.
D) Complete synovectomy is a treatment option.
E) Clinical symptoms include pain, swelling, and stiffness of the joints.

Question 20
Which of the following statements concerning this lesion is FALSE?

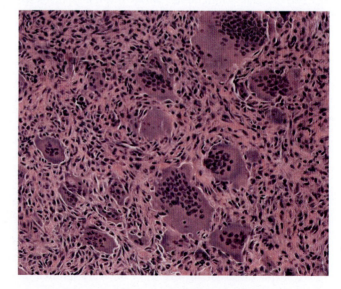

A) The preferential location in the long bone is metaphysis.
B) Most common locations in the skeleton are the distal radius, proximal tibia, distal femur, and proximal humerus.
C) Osteolytic lesion with narrow zone of transition and geographic type of bone destruction are the characteristic radiographic features.
D) It can metastasize to the lung.
E) Most common chromosomal aberration is telomeric associations involving chromosomes 11p, 13p, 14p, 15p, 19q, 20q, and 21p.

Question 21
Which of the following osseous lesion is associated with Jaffe-Campanacci syndrome?

A) Osteochondroma.
B) Osteoid osteoma.
C) Nonossifying fibroma.
D) Osteoblastoma.
E) Fibrous dysplasia.

Question 22
Which clinical scenario would be most consistent with osteofibrous dysplasia of bone?

A) A 25-year-old woman with swelling of the jaw.
B) A 10-year-old girl with lesion in the distal femur.
C) A 15-year-old boy with lesion in the distal finger.
D) A 65-year-old woman with lesion in the proximal tibia.
E) A 2-year-old boy with cortical lesion in the tibia.

Question 23
Which statement is FALSE regarding mesenchymal chondrosarcoma?

A) Small round tumor cells with low-grade cartilaginous component is characteristic.
B) Cytogenetic studies for t(11;22) are critical to distinguish this tumor from Ewing/PNET sarcoma family.
C) It has indolent behavior with low metastatic rate.
D) Most often involve bones of the jaw and ribs in young adults.
E) Small round tumor cells express positivity for immunohistochemistry stain CD99.

Question 24
Which of the following features are characteristic for clear cell chondrosarcoma?

A) Imaging studies may resemble chondroblastoma.
B) Reactive bone formation may be observed.
C) Large cells with clear or slightly eosinophilic cytoplasm and small nuclei are characteristic.
D) Clear cells of the tumor are positive for S-100 protein.
E) All of the above.

Question 25
Which of the following lesions histologically resembles an osteoblastoma?

A) Osteochondroma.
B) Osteoid osteoma.
C) Chondroblastoma.
D) Aneurysmal bone cyst.
E) Fracture callus.

Question 26
A 13-year-old girl presented with pain in the leg after being kicked during a soccer game. Based on the submitted radiograph and the histopathologic section, what is the most likely diagnosis?

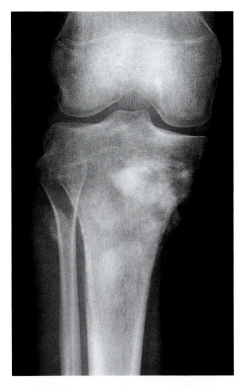

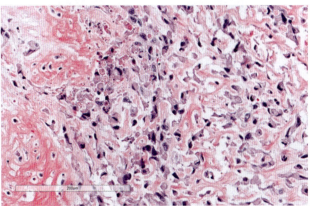

A) Osteoblastoma.
B) Osteoid osteoma.
C) Giant cell–rich osteosarcoma.
D) Conventional osteosarcoma.
E) Healing fracture of the proximal tibia.

Question 27

Concerning lipoma arborescens, which of the following statements is (are) true?

A) The lesion is more prevalent in males, usually in the fourth and fifth decades.
B) Imaging features are not characteristic, and only biopsy is diagnostic.
C) MRI shows high signal intensity on T1-weighted sequences.
D) A and C.
E) All of the above.

Question 28

Concerning synovial (osteo)chondromatosis, which of the following statements is (are) true?

A) The knee is a preferential site.
B) Joint effusion is a common clinical finding.
C) Histopathology shows pleomorphic cartilaginous cells arranged in clusters, exhibiting dark nuclei.
D) A and C.
E) All of the above.

Question 29

A 65-year-old man presented with pain in the thigh. Based on the submitted radiograph, CT, and histopathologic section, what is the most likely diagnosis?

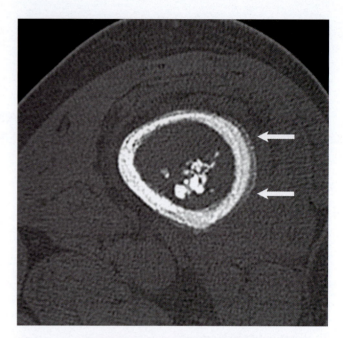

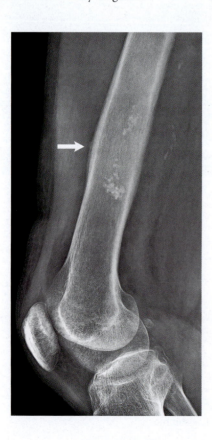

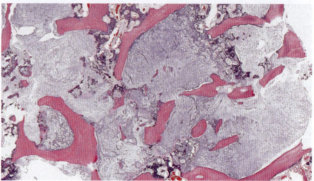

A) Enchondroma.
B) Conventional chondrosarcoma.
C) Medullary bone infarct.
D) Chondromyxoid fibroma.
E) Chondroblastoma.

Question 30

Which one of the following statements concerning chondromyxoid fibroma is NOT true?

A) The radiography shows typical chondroid calcifications.
B) Narrow zone of transition and geographic type of bone destruction are the characteristic imaging features.
C) Tibia is a preferential site of the lesion.
D) Histopathology shows lobulated areas of spindle-shaped or stellate cells distributed within abundant myxoid stroma.
E) Imaging appearance may be similar to an aneurysmal bone cyst.

Question 31
Based on the submitted histopathologic section, what is the most likely diagnosis?

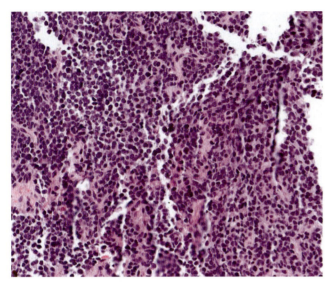

A) Langerhans cell histiocytosis.
B) Ewing sarcoma.
C) Large B-cell lymphoma.
D) Mesenchymal chondrosarcoma.
E) Multiple myeloma.

Question 32
Concerning multiple myeloma, which of the following statements is (are) true?

A) Most of the time the scintigraphy is normal.
B) Sclerosing variant is the part of POEMS syndrome.
C) Endosteal scalloping is a common radiographic feature.
D) By immunohistochemistry, the tumor cells show a monoclonal expression of lambda light chains.
E) All statements are true.

Question 33
Which of the following statements is inconsistent with diagnosis of periosteal osteosarcoma?

A) Cartilaginous matrix is a major component of the tumor.
B) It is more aggressive than parosteal osteosarcoma.
C) Belongs to the group of surface tumors.
D) The majority of the tumors affect the tibia and the femur.
E) MRI shows characteristic fluid–fluid levels.

Question 34
Which of the following lesions does not contain giant cells?

A) Giant cell tumor.
B) Nonossifying fibroma.
C) Hemangioma.
D) Aneurysmal bone cyst.
E) Brown tumor of hyperparathyroidism.

Question 35
Regarding this lesion, which one of the following statements is FALSE?

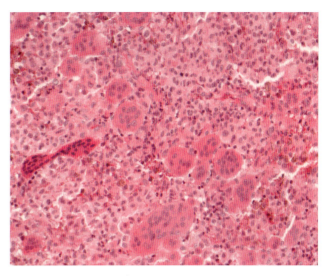

A) Lamellated periosteal reaction is a common finding.
B) Imaging features may resemble osteomyelitis.
C) The neoplastic cells are positive for CD45 and CD68.
D) "Floating teeth" is a characteristic feature.
E) Electron microscopy shows characteristic Birbeck granules.

Question 36
Which one of the following lesions generally does not produce periosteal reaction?

A) Chondromyxoid fibroma.
B) Aneurysmal bone cyst.
C) Langerhans cell histiocytosis.
D) Osteoblastoma.
E) Simple bone cyst.

Question 37
Which one of the following lesions generally does not exhibit matrix mineralization?

A) Osteoid osteoma.
B) Giant cell tumor.
C) Chondroblastoma.
D) Enchondroma.
E) Clear cell chondrosarcoma.

Question 38
Concerning desmoplastic fibroma, which of the following statements is FALSE?

A) It shows always a narrow zone of transition.
B) It is a locally aggressive lesion.
C) Histopathology shows densely collagenized hypocellular stroma containing spindle-shaped fibroblasts.
D) Honeycomb pattern of bone destruction is commonly observed.
E) Histopathologically, the lesion may resemble periosteal desmoid.

Question 39
Which one of the following lesions may be associated with a soft-tissue mass?

A) Aneurysmal bone cyst.
B) Simple bone cyst.
C) Giant cell tumor.
D) A and C only.
E) All of the above.

Question 40
Based on the submitted radiograph and histopathologic section, what is the most likely diagnosis?

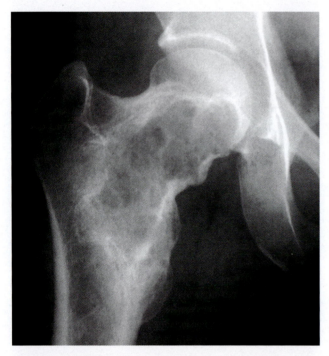

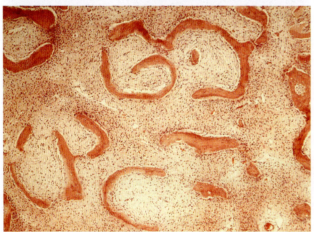

A) Osteofibrous dysplasia.
B) Fibrous dysplasia.
C) Fibrosarcoma.
D) Desmoplastic fibroma.
E) Giant cell tumor.

Question 41
Concerning osteofibrous dysplasia, which one of the following statements is true?

A) Cytogenetic studies revealed trisomies for chromosomes 7, 8, 12, and 22.
B) Bone trabeculae show appositional activity by polarized osteoblasts.
C) Anterior aspect of the tibia is a preferential location.
D) It may exhibit similar imaging and histopathologic features to the adamantinoma of the long bones.
E) All statements are correct.

Question 42
Regarding polyostotic fibrous dysplasia, which one of the following statements is NOT true?

A) It may be associated with hyperparathyroidism.
B) Massive formation of cartilage may be observed.
C) Osteoblastic activity is a characteristic feature.
D) Skull lesions affect primarily the base.
E) It may be part of Mazabraud syndrome.

Question 43
Concerning synovial sarcoma, which one of the following statements is FALSE?

A) It arises from the synovial membrane of the joint.
B) A translocation involving chromosomes X and 18 [t(X;18)(p11;q11)] is a common feature.
C) MRI shows fluid–fluid levels in 18% of patients.
D) It shows positivity for CD99 and cytokeratins.
E) The tumor occurs usually before the age of 50.

Question 44
Regarding fibrosarcoma, which of the following statements is true?

A) Radiography shows a sclerotic lesion associated with periosteal reaction.
B) Histopathology shows characteristic herringbone tweed pattern of arrangement of the malignant cells.
C) The spindle cells have normochromatic nuclei with decreased ratio of nucleus to cytoplasm.
D) Fluid–fluid levels on MRI are commonly encountered.
E) It is a common lesion in the pediatric age.

Question 45
A 45-year-old man injured his ankle. Based on this lateral radiograph, what is the most likely diagnosis?

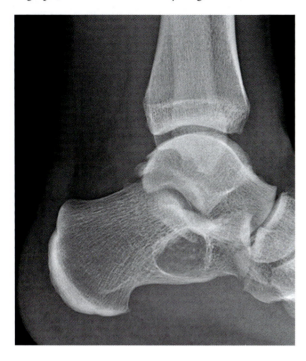

A) Posttraumatic cyst.
B) Intraosseous lipoma.
C) Intraosseous ganglion.
D) Simple bone cyst.
E) Aneurysmal bone cyst.

Question 46
A 35-year-old woman presented with right shoulder pain of 4 months' duration. Based on the submitted radiograph and histopathologic section, what is the most likely diagnosis?

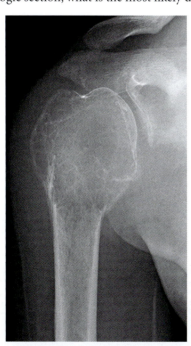

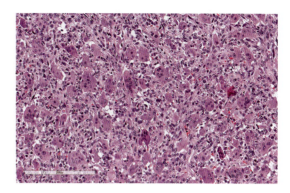

A) Simple bone cyst.
B) Aneurysmal bone cyst.
C) Giant cell tumor.
D) Plasmacytoma.
E) Metastasis from renal cell carcinoma.

Question 47
Regarding simple bone cyst, which one of the following statements is FALSE?

A) A "fallen fragment" sign is a characteristic radiographic feature.
B) Most of the lesions occur in the proximal humerus and proximal femur.
C) About 65% of the cysts occur in teenagers.
D) In the calcaneus, it is located within the Ward triangle.
E) Periosteal reaction is a common feature.

Question 48
One of the following lesions DOES NOT affect the spine:

A) Osteoid osteoma.
B) Osteoblastoma.
C) Hemangioma.
D) Osteofibrous dysplasia.
E) Aneurysmal bone cyst.

Question 49
Concerning Hodgkin lymphoma, all of the following statements are true EXCEPT one:

A) "Ivory vertebra" is a common finding.
B) Reed-Sternberg cells are positive for CD30.
C) Postcontrast MRI shows enhancement of the lesion.
D) Skeletal scintigraphy shows absence of uptake of the radiopharmaceutical tracer.
E) Fibrous stroma with mixed cellular infiltrate of small round cells and large histiocytes is characteristic for this lesion.

Question 50
All of the following conditions should be included in the differential diagnosis of osteoid osteoma, EXCEPT for which one?

A) Stress fracture.
B) Osteoblastoma.
C) Brodie abscess.
D) Enostosis.
E) Parosteal osteosarcoma.

Question 51
Which one of the following lesions histopathologically resembles an osteoblastoma?

A) Osteochondroma.
B) Osteoid osteoma.
C) Chondroblastoma.
D) Aneurysmal bone cyst.
E) Fracture callus.

Question 52
Which one of these patients most likely has a metastatic lesion?

A) A 32-year-old woman with permeative lesion in the proximal femur exhibiting an interrupted periosteal reaction.
B) A 72-year-old man with osteolytic lesion in the proximal right humerus exhibiting a narrow zone of transition.
C) A 75-year-old woman with osteolytic lesion in the proximal left humerus exhibiting a wide zone of transition, an interrupted periosteal reaction, and a large soft-tissue mass.
D) A 68-year-old man with punched-out lesions in the skull.
E) An 8-year-old girl with osteolytic lesion in the left tibia, exhibiting wide zone of transition and lamellated type of periosteal reaction.

Question 53
A 39-year-old man presented with a large mass in the popliteal region of the knee of several months' duration. He experienced only mild discomfort but noticed a slow increase in the size of the mass. Based on the submitted radiograph and histopathologic section, what is the most likely diagnosis?

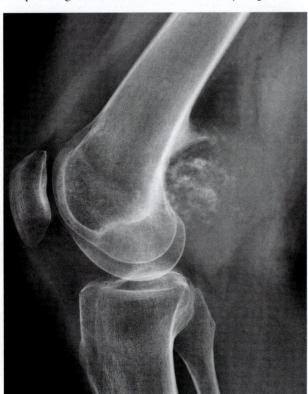

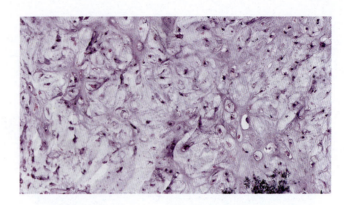

A) Parosteal osteosarcoma.
B) Periosteal chondroma.
C) Periosteal chondrosarcoma.
D) Conventional chondrosarcoma.
E) Tumoral calcinosis.

Question 54
Which one of the following features is characteristic for clear cell chondrosarcoma?

A) Commonly epiphyseal lesion.
B) Clear cytoplasm.
C) Woven bone.
D) Clear cells are positive for S-100 protein.
E) All of the above.

Question 55
What is the characteristic neoplastic cell of a chordoma?

A) Chondrocyte.
B) Myocyte.
C) Neuroglia.
D) Osteoblast.
E) Physaliphorous cell.

Question 56
An 82-year-old man presented with lower back pain. Radiographic examination demonstrated "missing" pedicle of L4 vertebra, without additional abnormalities. What is the most likely diagnosis?

A) Metastasis.
B) Congenital absence of the pedicle.
C) Aneurysmal bone cyst.
D) Osteoblastoma.
E) Plasmacytoma.

Question 57
What description is most consistent with a malignant bone tumor?

A) Radiolucent lesion with geographic type of bone destruction and a narrow zone of transition.
B) Radiolucent lesion with moth-eaten bone destruction, without periosteal reaction.

C) Radiolucent lesion with geographic type of bone destruction and a soft-tissue mass.
D) Radiolucent lesion with geographic type of bone destruction, narrow zone of transition, and a solid buttress of periosteal reaction.
E) Sclerotic lesion with a rough border, exhibiting thorny radiations and a positive radionuclide bone scan.

Question 58
Which one of the following markers is most specific for the diagnosis of chordoma?

A) S-100 protein.
B) Cytokeratins.
C) Brachyury.
D) CEA.
E) EMA.

Question 59
A 72-year-old woman presented with pain in the upper left arm. Based on the submitted radiograph and histopathologic section, what is the most likely diagnosis?

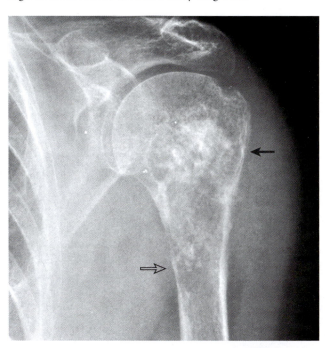

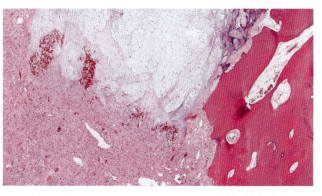

A) Mesenchymal chondrosarcoma.
B) Dedifferentiated chondrosarcoma.
C) Undifferentiated pleomorphic sarcoma.
D) Enchondromatosis.
E) Chondroblastic osteosarcoma.

Question 60
Which one of the following statements concerning chordoma is NOT true?

A) Cord-like arrays and lobules of large polyhedral cells with a vacuolated "bubbly" cytoplasm is a characteristic feature.
B) Loss of chromosomes 3, 4, 10, and 13 has been reported.
C) Partial or complete *PTEN* gene deficiency.
D) Clivus is one of the preferential sites.
E) Occurs only at sites in which notochordal remnants are normally present.

Question 61
A 42-year-old woman injured her right shoulder in a skiing accident. Based on the submitted radiograph, what is the most likely diagnosis?

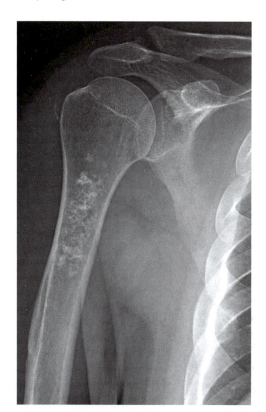

A) Medullary bone infarct.
B) Conventional chondrosarcoma.
C) Clear cell chondrosarcoma.
D) Chondromyxoid fibroma.
E) Enchondroma.

Question 62
Concerning chondromyxoid fibroma, all the following statements are correct EXCEPT which one?

A) Chondroid calcifications are a common feature.
B) Eccentric location within the bone.
C) It may resemble an aneurysmal bone cyst.
D) Periosteal reaction is a common finding in a long bone.
E) Giant cells are a part of histopathologic presentation.

Question 63
A 45-year-old man was admitted to the hospital with severe back pain. Radiography demonstrated a sclerotic L2 vertebra. An open biopsy was performed. Based on the submitted histopathologic section, what is the most likely diagnosis?

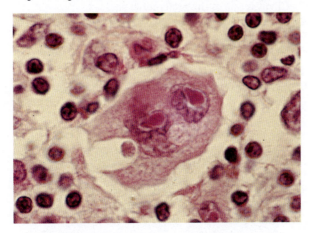

A) Plasmacytoma.
B) Hodgkin lymphoma.
C) Large B-cell lymphoma.
D) Langerhans cell histiocytosis.
E) Metastasis from thyroid carcinoma.

Question 64
All of the following tumors may metastasize to the lungs, EXCEPT for which one?

A) Telangiectatic osteosarcoma.
B) Giant cell tumor.
C) Parosteal osteosarcoma.
D) Chondroblastoma.
E) Synovial sarcoma.

Question 65
Based on the submitted MRI and histopathologic section, what is the most likely diagnosis?

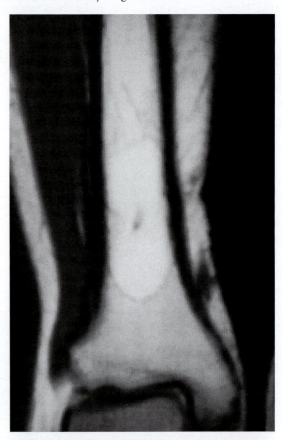

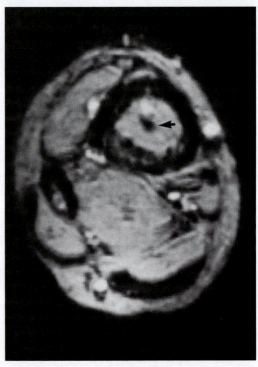

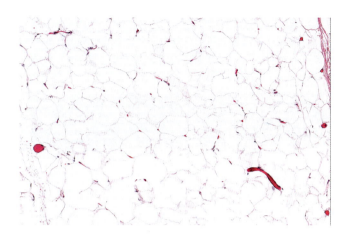

A) Intramedullary bone infarction.
B) Liposarcoma of bone.
C) Intraosseous lipoma.
D) Intraosseous ganglion.
E) Langerhans cell histiocytosis.

Question 66
Regarding liposarcoma of bone, which one of the following statements is FALSE?

A) Presents as a painful mass.
B) Histopathologic variants include well-differentiated, myxoid, and pleomorphic.
C) Majority of the patients are children.
D) It is a tumor of long tubular bones.
E) Behavior of the tumor correlates with histopathologic grade.

Question 67
A 68-year-old woman presented with a progressively enlarging soft-tissue mass in the popliteal region of her right knee. Based on CT and histopathologic section, what is the most likely diagnosis?

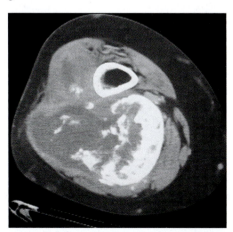

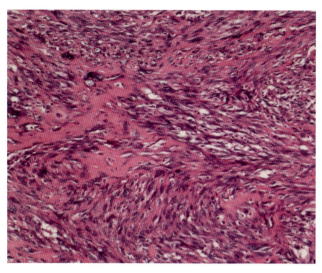

A) Myositis ossificans.
B) Periosteal chondroma.
C) Soft-tissue chondrosarcoma.
D) Soft-tissue osteosarcoma.
E) None of the above.

Question 68
No history given. Based on MRI and histopathologic section, what is the most likely diagnosis?

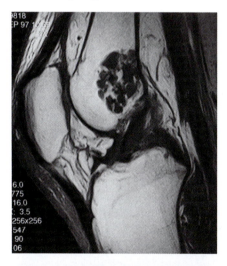

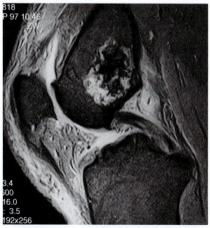

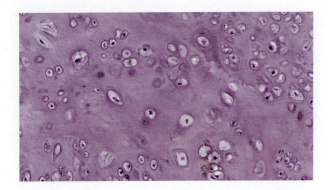

A) Enchondroma.
B) Low-grade chondrosarcoma.
C) Chondromyxoid fibroma.
D) Periosteal chondroma.
E) Chondroblastoma.

Question 69
Regarding chondroblastoma, all of the following statements are true, EXCEPT for which one?

A) Imaging studies may resemble features of clear cell chondrosarcoma.
B) It is an epiphyseal lesion.
C) It may metastasize to the lungs.
D) Most tumors are DNA diploid.
E) Osteoclast-like giant cells are not a part of histopathologic spectrum.

Question 70
Regarding periosteal chondroma, which of the following statements is NOT true?

A) Preferential sites include the proximal humerus, femur, and tibia.
B) Unlike an enchondroma, majority of the cases are seen in the sixth and seventh decades of life.
C) Bone erosion is commonly present.
D) The tumor tissue is more cellular than enchondroma.
E) Imaging features of some lesions may mimic osteochondromas and aneurysmal bone cysts.

Question 71
Concerning telangiectatic osteosarcoma, which of the following statements is (are) true?

A) It represents one of the most aggressive type of osteosarcomas.
B) Most of these tumors arise in the femur or tibia.
C) Imaging and histopathologic features may resemble those of aneurysmal bone cyst.
D) A and C only.
E) All statements are correct.

Question 72
A 14-year-old boy on MRI studies was diagnosed as having a bone tumor. Based on the histopathologic section, what is the most likely diagnosis?

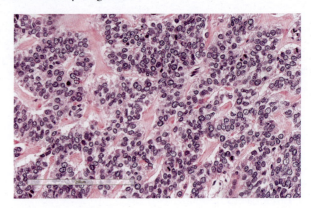

A) Osteoblastoma.
B) Fibrous dysplasia.
C) Small cell osteosarcoma.
D) Telangiectatic osteosarcoma.
E) Periosteal osteosarcoma.

Question 73
A 55-year-old woman presented with left knee pain after a fall. The radiograph was obtained followed by CT. The radionuclide bone scan (not shown here) demonstrated a moderate uptake of the radiopharmaceutical tracer. What should be done next?

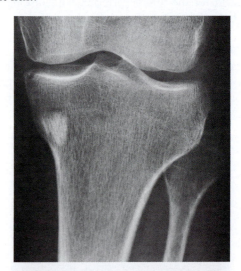

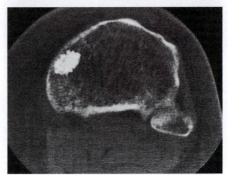

A) Perform MRI for better characterization of the lesion.
B) The lesion looks like osteosarcoma; therefore, an open biopsy should be performed.
C) The lesion looks like a metastatic tumor; therefore, an extensive clinical workup has to be done to look for the primary source.
D) The lesion looks like an osteoma; therefore, a clinical workup should be done to exclude Gardner syndrome.
E) The lesion shows characteristic features of a bone island; therefore, nothing invasive should be contemplated; however, to repeat radiographs in about 6 months is a prudent action.

Question 74

Which of the following lesions SHOULD NOT be biopsied? Choose all that are pertinent.

A)

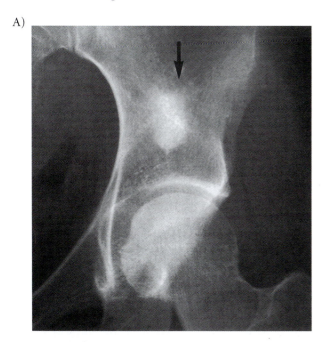

B)

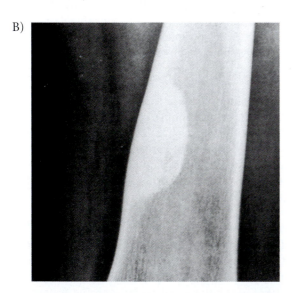

C)

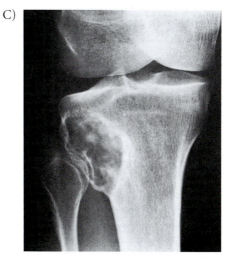

D)

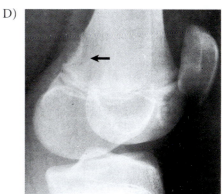

E)

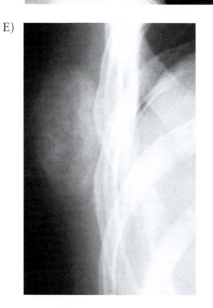

Question 75

Which one of the following conditions is responsible for most osteosarcomas seen in patients older than 50 years?

A) Fibrous dysplasia.
B) Prior radiation.
C) Paget disease.
D) Chronic draining sinus tract of osteomyelitis.
E) Intramedullary bone infarct.

ANSWERS

Answer to question 1: A
The radiograph shows a radiolucent lesion (*arrow*) within the medial femoral cortex exhibiting narrow zone of transition and surrounded by sclerotic area. There is associated well-organized periosteal reaction. Histopathologic section shows sharply circumscribed lesion containing bone trabeculae within vascularized connective tissue, lined by the plump osteoblasts and surrounded by sclerotic bone. Both, imaging characteristics and histopathologic features, are consistent with **osteoid osteoma**. (B) *Chondroblastoma* usually is present in the immature skeleton and is invariably located in the epiphysis. Histopathology shows chondroid matrix and not osteoblasts. (C) *Osteofibrous dysplasia* predominantly occurs in childhood (more than 60% of the patients are younger than 12 years old) and affects the cortex of the tibia (not femur). Histopathology shows characteristic immature woven bone trabeculae with peripherally displayed lamellar bone, lined by osteoblasts ("dressed trabeculae"). (D) *Osteosarcoma* and (E) *Ewing sarcoma* are predominantly intramedullary tumors, exhibiting more aggressive imaging characteristics. Histopathology shows malignant cells.

Answer to question 2: C
Maffucci syndrome is characterized by multiple enchondromas (Ollier disease) and cavernous hemangiomas located in the skin and soft tissues. This syndrome carries a greater risk of chondrosarcoma as well as nonskeletal malignancies, particularly of the ovaries and brain. (A) *von Recklinghausen disease of bone*, also known as osteitis fibrosa cystica generalisata, refers to severe bone disorder of primary hyperparathyroidism, characterized by increased osteoblastic activity, osteoclastic resorption, peritrabecular fibrosis, and brown tumors. (B) *Li-Fraumeni syndrome* caused by inherited mutation of p53 is associated with greater risk of sarcomas (particularly osteosarcoma) and other malignancies, such as breast cancer, brain tumors, and leukemias. (D) *Hereditary multiple exostoses*, also known as diaphyseal aclasis, is an autosomal dominant disorder characterized by the presence of multiple osteochondromas, particularly at the knee, hip, ankle, and shoulder joints. (E) *Gardner syndrome*, an autosomal dominant disorder, consists of a combination of multiple osteomas, intestinal polyposis, skin fibromatosis, and epidermal sebaceous cysts.

Answer to question 3: A
Mutation of p53 (Li-Fraumeni syndrome) is associated with greater risk of sarcomas, particularly 500-fold greater risk of osteosarcoma. (B) *Translocation t(X;18)* is characteristic of synovial sarcoma. (C) *Translocation t(12;16)* is characteristic of myxoid liposarcoma. (D) *1p rearrangements* are characteristic for conventional chondrosarcoma. (E) *Translocation t(9;22)* is characteristic for myxoid chondrosarcoma.

Answer to question 4: D
(A) *Lymphoma*, (B) *metastatic neuroblastoma*, (C) *mesenchymal chondrosarcoma*, and (E) *embryonal rhabdomyosarcoma* show similar morphologic features to Ewing sarcoma, all characterized by small round blue tumor cells. **Leiomyosarcoma of bone**, on the other hand, is composed of bundles of fascicles of spindle cells.

Answer to question 5: C
Parosteal osteosarcoma is low-grade (grade 1) sarcoma. (B) *Periosteal osteosarcoma* is a grade 2, and (A) *Paget osteosarcoma*, (D) *telangiectatic osteosarcoma*, and (E) *small cell osteosarcoma* are high-grade (grade 3) sarcomas.

Answer to question 6: B
The epithelial component of adamantinoma expresses positivity for cytokeratins 14 and 19. CK8 and CK18 are expressed in epithelioid component of synovial sarcoma. The statements (A), (C), (D), and (E) are all correct.

Answer to question 7: B
The radiograph shows well-defined eccentric radiolucent lesion with sclerotic lobulated border, exhibiting no evidence of periosteal reaction (*arrow*), all imaging features of **nonossifying fibroma**. Histopathology shows fibrous stroma displaying a storiform arrangement, and several scattered giant cells, confirming the radiologic diagnosis. (A) *Giant cell tumor* almost always occurs in skeletally mature patients and extends into the articular end of bone. Generally, it does not exhibit a sclerotic border. Histopathology shows mononuclear cells intermixed with numerous uniformly distributed giant cells. (C) *Aneurysmal bone cyst* characteristically shows expansive features and well-organized periosteal reaction in the form of a buttress. Histopathology shows multiple blood-filled spaces alternating with more solid areas. (D) *Chondroblastoma* is an epiphyseal lesion, exhibiting chondroid calcifications. Histopathology shows nodules of fairly mature cartilaginous matrix surrounded by a highly cellular tissue composed of round and polygonal chondroblast-like cells, and matrix calcifications having a spatial arrangement that resembles the hexagonal configuration of chicken wire. (E) *Giant cell–rich osteosarcoma* exhibits aggressive imaging features with poorly defined borders showing wide zone of transition. Histopathology is similar to that of a giant cell tumor; however, tumor bone or tumor osteoid is present in the vicinity of malignant cells.

Answer to question 8: B
The radiograph shows an eccentric radiolucent lesion with narrow zone of transition and geographic type of bone destruction, exhibiting a noninterrupted periosteal reaction in form of a buttress, all typical imaging features of

aneurysmal bone cyst (ABC). Histopathology shows plump fibroblasts and giant cells aggregating around and within the blood-filled spaces, some of them showing characteristic feature of "jumping into the swimming pool", confirming the radiologic diagnosis. (**A**) *Nonossifying fibroma* exhibits no expansive imaging features and lack of periosteal reaction. Histopathology shows predominantly bland monomorphous spindle cells admixed with histiocytic cells frequently arranged in a swirling storiform pattern and occasionally scattered giant cells. (**C**) *Simple bone cyst* shows almost invariably central location and lack of periosteal reaction, unless there is a pathologic fracture present. Histopathology shows walls of the cyst covered by a flattened single-cell lining. (**D**) *Giant cell tumor*, although occasionally may exhibit expansive imaging features, generally shows lack of sclerotic border and lack of buttress type of periosteal reaction, characteristic features of ABC. Histopathology shows mononuclear cells intermixed with numerous uniformly distributed giant cells. (**E**) *Telangiectatic osteosarcoma*, although occasionally similar in appearance to ABC, shows more aggressive imaging features associated with a soft-tissue mass. Interrupted periosteal reaction in form of lamellar, sunburst, or Codman triangle is commonly present. Histopathology shows malignant cells forming tumor bone or tumor osteoid.

Answer to question 9: D

The radiograph shows a radiolucent lesion with fine matrix calcifications, exhibiting a narrow zone of transition and thin sclerotic border, located in the epiphysis of the proximal tibia and abutting the growth plate, all characteristic features of **chondroblastoma**. Histopathology showing polygonal chondroblasts with indistinct outlines and uniformly shaped nuclei, scattered giant cells, and fine "chicken-wire" calcifications confirm this diagnosis. (**A**) *Giant cell tumor*, although also occurring in the end of bone, invariably is seen in the mature skeleton, after the growth plate has been obliterated. In addition, it never exhibits matrix mineralization. Histopathology shows numerous large giant cells uniformly distributed throughout the lesion. (**B**) *Nonossifying fibroma* is a diaphyseal lesion, never occurring in the epiphysis and shows no evidence of matrix calcifications. Histopathology shows whorled pattern of fibrous tissue containing giant cells, hemosiderin, and lipid-laden histiocytes. (**C**) *Osteosarcoma* generally shows a metaphyseal or diaphyseal location and exhibits more aggressive imaging features commonly with sclerotic foci representing tumor-bone formation. Soft-tissue mass is a typical feature. Histopathology shows malignant cells forming tumor osteoid and tumor bone and invasion of marrow spaces and bone trabeculae. (**E**) *Aneurysmal bone cyst* is located in the diaphysis or metaphysis, show blown-up imaging features, and lack of mineralization. It also exhibits a well-organized periosteal reaction. Histopathology shows blood-filled vascular spaces bordered by solid areas containing spindle cells and giant cells with occasional foci of osteoid.

Answer to question 10: D

Malignant transformation of a solitary osteochondroma is extremely rare and was reported in less than 1% of cases. The statements (**A**), (**B**), (**C**), and (**E**) are all correct.

Answer to question 11: D

Giant cell tumor commonly exhibits **lack of sclerotic border**. The statements (**A**), (**B**), (**C**), and (**E**) are all correct.

Answer to question 12: B

MR images show a signal abnormality in the right proximal femur extending into the middle of the shaft. In the intertrochanteric region, there are at least two lesions with sclerotic border. In the soft tissue, there is a well-circumscribed lesion showing homogeneous high signal intensity on T2-weighted sequences and rim enhancement on the postcontrast study. All lesions show absence of aggressive features. These findings combined with the clinical history of long-standing deformity are consistent with polyostotic fibrous dysplasia and soft-tissue myxoma, features of **Mazabraud syndrome**. (**A**) *Osteosarcoma* will show more aggressive imaging features, and it extremely rare metastasizes to the soft tissue. Besides, metastatic soft-tissue lesion will not exhibit homogeneous high signal on T2 weighting, but rather heterogeneity with some evidence of bone formation. (**C**) *Jaffe-Campanacci syndrome* consists of coexistence of nonossifying fibromas and neurofibromatosis, associated with formation of café-au-lait spots on the skin. (**D**) *Rothmund-Thomson syndrome*, also known as congenital poikiloderma, is a hereditary disorder characterized by erythematous and maculopapular skin lesions with areas of hyperpigmentation and coexistence of conventional osteosarcoma. (**E**) *Werner syndrome*, also known as adult progeria, is characterized by premature aging, scleroderma-like skin changes, and coexistence of osteosarcomas.

Answer to question 13: C

Radiograph shows a several small radiolucent channels traversing the medullary portion and the cortex of the proximal phalanx of the middle finger associated with a soft-tissue prominence. Coronal T2-weighted fat-suppressed MRI shows high signal intensity lesion affecting both the bone and soft tissue. Low signal intensity foci represent the phleboliths. From the given choices, the most likely diagnosis is an intraosseous **hemangioma** with soft-tissue extension. (**A**) *Ewing sarcoma* is a malignant tumor predominantly affecting the long and flat bones, and involvement of the short tubular bone, although reported in the literature, is extremely rare. (**B**) The possibility of *angiosarcoma* should be considered in the differential diagnosis; however, majority of the reported cases were affecting long bones and bones of the pelvis. Involvement of the short tubular bone is unlikely. In addition, the imaging features of angiosarcoma are more aggressive than presented in this case. (**D**) *Langerhans cell histiocytosis* is a condition predominantly affecting children, with peak incidence between the ages of 5 and 10 years.

The sites of involvement include the axial skeleton and the long bones. Periosteal reaction is usually lamellated. Phleboliths are not the part of presentation. (**E**) Although the short tubular bones are the common sites of *enchondroma*, this benign cartilaginous lesion does not extend into the soft tissues, unless it is multifocal such as in Ollier disease.

Answer to question 14: E

Lateral radiograph of the skull shows numerous various-in-size punched-out lesions, characteristic of **multiple myeloma**. CT section shows predominant involvement of the diploë, also typical feature for myeloma. (**A**) *Osteolytic metastases* to the skull commonly present as a larger areas of destruction. In contrast to myeloma, the inner and outer tables are also affected. (**B**) Skull abnormalities seen in *hyperparathyroidism* consist of osteopenia, which gives a characteristic granular appearance of the bones of the vault, referred to as "salt and pepper" appearance, not the punched-out lesions. (**C**) *Fibrous dysplasia* affects predominantly the base of the skull in form of areas of sclerosis. (**D**) Osteolytic phase of *Paget disease* in the skull is known as osteoporosis circumscripta, appearing as a large area of geographic bone destruction. Mixed and cool phases of the disease affecting the skull manifest as areas of ill-defined focal densities resembling cotton balls.

Answer to question 15: A

One of the characteristic features of multiple myeloma, in contrast to metastatic disease, is essentially **normal radionuclide bone scan**. The remaining statements (**B**), (**C**), (**D**), and (**E**) are all correct.

Answer to question 16: B

One of the characteristic features of polyostotic fibrous dysplasia affecting the femur is so-called **shepherd's crook deformity**, which is commonly the result of multiple pathologic fractures. (**A**) Histopathology of fibrous dysplasia shows immature woven bone trabeculae *without osteoblastic rimming*, so-called naked trabeculae. (**C**) Skull lesions in fibrous dysplasia are seen predominantly *at the base of the skull* in form of increased sclerosis. (**D**) Postcontrast MRI shows invariably *enhancement of the lesions* of fibrous dysplasia. (**E**) *Gains of chromosomes 1q, 3q, 9q, 11q, and 15q* are characteristic features of multiple myeloma, not polyostotic fibrous dysplasia. McCune-Albright syndrome, which is the association of polyostotic fibrous dysplasia with endocrine disturbances (such as premature sexual development, gigantism or acromegaly, hyperparathyroidism, and Cushing syndrome) and skin pigmentation (cafe-au-lait spots), is caused by somatic mutations in the *GNAS1* gene located in chromosome 20q13.

Answer to question 17: C

The radiograph of the hand shows multiple sharply marginated radiolucent lesions within the metacarpals and phalanges, some within the cortex, typical for enchondromas. In addition, there is growth stunting of the distal ulna. The combination of these findings is characteristic for **Ollier disease**. (**A**) *Polyostotic fibrous dysplasia* exhibits thinning of the cortex associated with smoky or ground-glass appearance of the medullary portion of bones, without sharply marginated radiolucent lesions typical for enchondromatosis. In addition, overgrowth of the bone rather than growth stunting is occasionally present. (**B**) The most important identifying features of *osteochondromas* are that the cortex of the lesion merges without interruption with the cortex of the host bone and that the cancellous portion of the lesion is continuous with the medullary cavity of the adjacent diaphysis, findings not present in the case under consideration. (**D**) *Maffucci syndrome* consists of association of Ollier disease with soft-tissue hemangiomas. The radiography will invariably demonstrate phleboliths, which appear as round calcific foci, not present on the submitted radiograph. (**E**) *Neurofibromatosis* may be associated with osseous deformities, characteristic pit-like cortical erosions, and soft-tissue masses, features not present in the case under consideration.

Answer to question 18: B

Anteroposterior and lateral radiographs show ill-defined sclerotic lesion in the medullary portion of the left distal femur associated with a large, dense soft-tissue mass. Sagittal T1-weighted fat-suppressed MR image obtained after intravenous administration of gadolinium shows significant enhancement of both medullary tumor and soft-tissue mass. Nonenhanced area represents tumor bone formation. The imaging features are typical for **conventional osteosarcoma**. (**A**) *Chondrosarcoma*, although may present as a sclerotic lesion, most of the time exhibits characteristic chondroid calcifications in the form of stippling, flocculent densities, or rings and arcs ("o"s and "c"s). In addition, there is invariably present a deep endosteal scalloping and cortical thickening, absent in the case under consideration. (**C**) *Parosteal osteosarcoma* is a surface lesion, usually exhibiting well-defined sclerotic mass outside of the cortex, which is slightly less dense on the periphery. It may possess an incomplete cleft between the tumor and underlying cortex. (**D**) *Periosteal osteosarcoma* is also a surface lesion, displaying ill-defined heterogeneous ossifications with calcified spiculations interspersed with areas of radiolucencies representing uncalcified matrix. (**E**) *Melorheostosis*, a form of sclerosing dysplasia, may occasionally mimic osteosarcoma, although the surface ossifications, in contrast to osteosarcoma, are well defined, resembling wax dripping on one side of the candle.

Answer to question 19: B

Histopathologic section shows typical appearance of synovial (osteo)chondromatosis. Several cartilaginous nodules are seen covered by a thin layer of synovium. Although the nodules are highly cellular, there is no evidence of spindle cells. All other statements (**A**), (**C**), (**D**), and (**E**) are correct.

Answer to question 20: A
Histopathologic section shows the classic features of the giant cell tumor: fibrocytic and monocytic stromal cells and large giant cells containing numerous nuclei. The preferential location of this tumor is the articular end of bone in skeletally mature patient and not in the metaphysis. The remaining statements (**B**), (**C**), (**D**), and (**E**) are all correct.

Answer to question 21: C
Jaffe-Campanacci syndrome consists of association of multiple nonossifying fibromas with neurofibromatosis.

Answer to question 22: E
Osteofibrous dysplasia, also known as Kempson-Campanacci lesion, characteristically affects children, with about 60% of the affected patients being younger than 5 years. The preferential site is the anterior cortex of the tibia.

Answer to question 23: C
Mesenchymal chondrosarcoma is an aggressive tumor with common distant metastases. The remaining statements (**A**), (**B**), (**D**), and (**E**) are all correct.

Answer to question 24: E
All statements concerning clear cell chondrosarcoma are true.

Answer to question 25: B
Histopathologically, osteoid osteoma and osteoblastoma exhibit similar features. Both lesions show irregular woven bone trabeculae with various degrees of mineralization, osteoblasts and giant cells, ectatic blood vessels, and reactive periosteal shell of new bone. The difference is in size: osteoid osteoma exhibits limited growth potential and size less than 2 cm, whereas osteoblastoma is commonly greater than 2 cm in size.

Answer to question 26: D
Anteroposterior radiograph of the right knee shows fluffy sclerotic densities in the metaphysis and proximal diaphysis of the tibia representing tumor bone formation, associated with velvet-type periosteal reaction. Similar densities are seen within the soft-tissue mass at the site of the proximal fibula. These are the typical imaging features of **conventional osteosarcoma**. The diagnosis is confirmed by the histopathologic section, showing markedly pleomorphic osteoblastic tumor cells with hyperchromatic nuclei forming lace-like osteoid. (**A**) Imaging features of *osteoblastoma* occasionally may mimic those of osteosarcoma; however, the lesion exhibits more focally confined densities, and the periosteal reaction is solid, not interrupted as in the case under consideration. Histopathology shows large but benign osteoblasts forming immature woven bone trabeculae. (**B**) *Osteoid osteoma* shows resemblance to osteoblastoma but exhibits completely different imaging features than osteosarcoma. The size of the lesion is usually less than 2 cm, and periosteal reaction is of solid type. Moreover, the lesion does not produce the soft-tissue mass. Histopathology shows a well-defined nidus composed of osteoid and trabeculae of immature woven bone, surrounded by sclerotic reactive bone. (**C**) Imaging features of *giant cell–rich osteosarcoma* may be indistinguishable from that of conventional osteosarcoma; however, histopathology shows striking resemblance to giant cell tumor with numerous osteoclast-like giant cells and scant osteoid formation, unlike the histopathologic section under consideration. (**E**) Callus formation of *healing fracture* shows more organized pattern on imaging studies, and there is no soft-tissue mass present. Furthermore, histopathology shows lack of malignant cells and lack of tumor bone or tumor osteoid.

Answer to question 27: D
Lipoma arborescent is a rare intra-articular disorder characterized by a nonneoplastic lipomatous proliferation of the synovium resembling a frond-like mass. It is more prevalent in males and usually diagnosed in the fourth and fifth decades of life. MRI features are characteristic and diagnostic for this disorder, showing fat signal intensity on all imaging sequences.

Answer to question 28: E
Synovial (osteo)chondromatosis is marked by the metaplastic proliferation of multiple cartilaginous nodules in the synovial membrane of the joints, bursae, or tendon sheaths. The knee joint is a preferential site of involvement. Joint effusion, tenderness, limited motion in the joint, and a soft-tissue mass are common clinical findings. Histopathology shows numerous highly cellular cartilaginous nodules. The cells with plump and dark nuclei are arranged in clusters and show moderate pleomorphism.

Answer to question 29: B
Lateral radiograph of the distal femur shows intramedullary lesion with wide zone of transition and chondroid calcifications. In addition, noted is focal cortical thickening and periosteal reaction (*arrows*). These findings are also demonstrated on the axial CT section through the tumor. The histopathology shows pleomorphic tumor with hyperchromatic nuclei permeating the bone trabeculae. The imaging findings and histopathology are characteristic for **conventional intramedullary chondrosarcoma**. (**A**) Although *enchondroma* also may display chondroid calcifications, generally there is no periosteal reaction, unless the pathologic fracture has occurred. Also, the cortex is not thickened; to the contrary, most of the time noted is thinning of the cortex. (**C**) *Medullary bone infarction* also exhibits calcifications, but in contrast to the chondroid tumors, the calcifications are coarser, and peripheral serpentine sclerotic fibro-osseous wall is commonly observed. Moreover, the cortex is not thickened. (**D**) *Chondromyxoid fibroma* exhibits narrow zone of transition and lack of visible calcifications. (**E**) *Chondroblastoma* is

a tumor of immature skeleton, invariably located within an epiphysis. It exhibits narrow zone of transition and lack of periosteal reaction at the site of the lesion.

Answer to question 30: A
Chondromyxoid fibroma is the only cartilaginous lesion that does not show visible calcifications on radiography. The remaining statements (**B**), (**C**), (**D**), and (**E**) are all correct.

Answer to question 31: B
The histopathologic section shows uniformly arranged small round cells exhibiting indistinguished borders, with darkly stained round nuclei, and scanty eosinophilic cytoplasm, highly characteristic for Ewing sarcoma. (**A**) *Langerhans cell histiocytosis* generally shows large pale histiocytes (Langerhans cells) and giant cells, as well as numerous eosinophilic granulocytes. The nuclei exhibit characteristic longitudinal grooves. (**C**) *Large B-cell lymphoma* exhibits pleomorphic round cells with well-defined cytoplasmic outline and enlarged, occasionally cleaved nuclei with nucleoli. (**D**) *Mesenchymal chondrosarcoma* on histopathologic examination shows two components: small, round uniform-sized cells of mesenchymal tissue with round or ovoid nuclei, which resemble Ewing sarcoma, and chondroblastic tissue with small spindle cells. (**E**) *Multiple myeloma* shows plasma cells with eccentric nuclei and basophilic cytoplasm.

Answer to question 32: E
All statements concerning **multiple myeloma** are true.

Answer to question 33: E
Fluid–fluid levels seen on MRI are characteristic features of telangiectatic osteosarcoma and not **periosteal osteosarcoma**. All remaining statements are correct.

Answer to question 34: C
All listed lesions except of **hemangioma** contain giant cells.

Answer to question 35: C
The histopathologic section shows densely arranged large pale histiocytes (Langerhans cells) as well as giant cells and eosinophilic granulocytes, characteristic of **Langerhans cell histiocytosis**. The tumor cells are positive for S-100 protein and CD1a but not for CD45 and CD68. The remaining statements concerning Langerhans cell histiocytosis are all correct.

Answer to question 36: E
All listed lesions except of a **simple bone cyst** are associated with a periosteal reaction.

Answer to question 37: B
Giant cell tumor invariably does not exhibit any matrix mineralization. In contrast, *osteoid osteoma* may show mineralization of the nidus, and *chondroblastoma*, *enchondroma*, and *clear cell chondrosarcoma* all show chondroid calcifications.

Answer to question 38: A
Desmoplastic fibroma is a locally aggressive lesion characterized by formation of abundant collagen fibers by the tumor cells. Radiographically, it exhibits the expansive features, usually with nonsclerotic but sharply defined borders, although occasionally a wide zone of transition is present. The remaining statements are all correct.

Answer to question 39: D
Aneurysmal bone cyst and **giant cell tumor**, although both the benign lesions, may be occasionally associated with a soft-tissue mass. To the contrary, a *simple bone cyst* never exhibits a soft-tissue extension.

Answer to question 40: B
The anteroposterior radiograph of the right hip shows a radiolucent lesion with narrow zone of transition and sclerotic border (rind sign) within the femoral neck. There is no evidence of a periosteal reaction. The histopathologic section shows irregularly shaped immature woven bone trabeculae resembling Chinese characters, with conspicuous absence of osteoblastic rimming (so-called naked trabeculae), diagnostic of **fibrous dysplasia**. (**A**) *Osteofibrous dysplasia* affects predominantly the tibia, and histopathology, in contrast to fibrous dysplasia, shows prominent osteoblastic rimming of the bone trabeculae ("dressed" trabeculae). (**C**) *Fibrosarcoma* is an aggressive tumor showing permeative or moth-eaten type of bone destruction and periosteal reaction. Histopathology shows pleomorphic spindle cells arranged in long fascicles forming characteristic "herringbone tweed" pattern. (**D**) *Desmoplastic fibroma*, although may exhibit a narrow zone of transition, usually have a nonsclerotic border. The histopathology shows densely collagenized hypocellular stroma that contains spindle-shaped fibroblasts. (**E**) *Giant cell tumor* invariably extends into the articular end of bone and shows lack of sclerotic border. Histopathology shows characteristic dual population of stromal cells (fibrocytic or monocytic) and of giant cells uniformly distributed throughout the lesion.

Answer to question 41: E
All statements concerning **osteofibrous dysplasia** are correct.

Answer to question 42: C
In contrast to osteofibrous dysplasia, the characteristic histopathologic feature of **fibrous dysplasia** is the presence of immature woven bone trabeculae without osteoblastic activity ("naked" trabeculae). The remaining statements are all true.

Answer to question 43: A
Synovial sarcoma is an uncommon malignant mesenchymal neoplasm. Despite its name, it does not arise from synovium. It occurs mainly in para-articular regions close to joint capsule, bursae, and tendon sheets. The remaining statements are all true.

Answer to question 44: B
The characteristic histopathologic feature of **fibrosarcoma** is "herringbone tweed" pattern of arrangement of the malignant pleomorphic spindle cells. (**A**) Radiography shows an osteolytic lesion with wide zone of transition and no evidence of sclerosis. (**C**) The spindle cells show hyperchromatic nuclei with increased ratio of nucleus to cytoplasm. (**D**) Fluid–fluid levels on MRI are not the feature of fibrosarcoma. (**E**) Fibrosarcoma usually occurs in the third to sixth decade of life, and only a few cases have been reported in children.

Answer to question 45: D
The lateral radiograph of the ankle shows a radiolucent lesion with narrow zone of transition and geographic type of bone destruction, located within the Ward triangle of the calcaneus. It has all characteristic features of a **simple bone cyst** and typical location in this portion of calcaneus. (**A**) *Posttraumatic cyst* is uncommon lesion, and usually appears as the result of a fracture about 2 months after injury. These lesions were reported in children, the radius being the usual site. (**B**) *Intraosseous lipoma* has a very similar imaging feature as a simple bone cyst; however, it shows invariably a central mineralization (ossifications or calcifications). (**C**) *Intraosseous ganglion* is commonly located in a long tubular bone, close to the joint. (**E**) The calcaneus is an unusual site of *aneurysmal bone cyst*. Moreover, this lesion commonly shows expansive features and periosteal reaction.

Answer to question 46: C
The radiograph of the right shoulder shows a radiolucent lesion affecting proximal humerus and extending into the articular end of the bone. There is evidence of a prior pathologic fracture at the proximal part with associated well-organized periosteal reaction. No obvious soft-tissue mass is present. There is absence of mineralization. The histopathologic section shows numerous osteoclast-like giant cells uniformly scattered among round and spindle-shaped mononuclear tumor cells. The most likely diagnosis in the patient of this age is a **giant cell tumor**. (**A**) Although a proximal humerus is a common site of the *simple bone cyst*, these lesions invariably are metaphyseal or diaphyseal in location and do not extend into the subchondral part of bone, as giant cell tumor does. Moreover, majority of these lesions occur in children. (**B**) Imaging features of *aneurysmal bone cyst* may mimic those of a giant cell tumor; however, similarly to the simple bone cyst, these lesions occur predominantly in children and young adults. Furthermore, solid buttress of periosteal reaction is a common feature in the long tubular bones. (**D**) *Plasmacytoma* usually presents as a radiolucent lesion and at times may affect the articular end of a long bone. The tumor, however, usually is seen in much older group of patients, commonly between the fifth and seventh decades. (**E**) *Lytic metastases from renal cell carcinoma* may mimic the appearance of a giant cell tumor; however, involvement of the articular end of bone is unusual.

Answer to question 47: E
Simple bone cyst typically shows **no periosteal reaction**, unless a pathologic fracture has occurred. The remaining statements are all true.

Answer to question 48: D
All of the listed conditions may affect the spine, except for **osteofibrous dysplasia**, which commonly affects the tibia.

Answer to question 49: D
Hodgkin lymphoma invariably shows **increased uptake** of the radiopharmaceutical tracer. The remaining statements are all correct.

Answer to question 50: E
Parosteal osteosarcoma has characteristic imaging features, most notably a homogenously sclerotic ivory mass attached to the cortex of a long or flat bone. Conversely, all the other listed conditions may occasionally mimic the features of osteoid osteoma. (**A**) *Stress fracture* may be mistaken for cortical osteoid osteoma, although linear radiolucency runs perpendicular or at angle to the cortex, whereas the radiolucent nidus of osteoid osteoma is round or oblong. (**B**) *Osteoblastoma* may look exactly like osteoid osteoma, except for its size: while the nidus of osteoid osteoma measures usually 1.5 cm or less, the lesion of osteoblastoma is commonly 2.0 cm or larger. (**C**) *Brodie abscess* may mimic medullary osteoid osteoma, the important differential feature being the commonly present serpentine radiolucent tract extending from the abscess. (**D**) *Enostosis*, also known as a bone island, may mimic medullary osteoid osteoma. The important diagnostic feature of the former lesion includes distinctive radiating streaks (thorny radiation, pseudopodia) forming a rough border.

Answer to question 51: B
Histopathologically, **osteoid osteoma** and osteoblastoma show very similar features. Both lesions show irregular woven bone with various degrees of mineralization, osteoblasts and giant cells, ectatic blood vessels, and reactive periosteal shell of new bone. The difference is in size: osteoid osteoma has a limited growth, and usual size is 1.0 to 1.5 cm, whereas osteoblastoma is greater than 2.0 cm in size.

Answer to question 52: B
In this age, any osseous lesion, even the one having a "benign" appearance, should be considered a **metastasis**, unless proven otherwise.
(**A**) This patient is not in the "metastatic age group," and, in addition, the metastatic lesions usually do not exhibit periosteal reaction. With the features described, the patient most likely has a *primary malignant bone tumor*. (**C**) Although this patient is in the "metastatic age group," the presence of periosteal reaction and a large soft-tissue mass point to the diagnosis of a *primary malignant bone tumor*. (**D**) Punched-out lesions in the skull are classic features of *multiple myeloma*.

(E) In this age, the osteolytic lesion with wide zone of transition and lamellated periosteal reaction may represent *Ewing sarcoma*, *Langerhans cell histiocytosis*, or even *osteomyelitis* but not a metastasis.

Answer to question 53: C

The lateral radiograph of the knee shows a large soft-tissue mass with chondroid calcifications eroding but not invading the posterior cortex of the distal femur and evoking a periosteal reaction. These are the imaging features of **periosteal chondrosarcoma**. The diagnosis is confirmed by histopathologic section showing hyaline cartilage with pleomorphic tumor cells and hyperchromatism of the nuclei consistent with intermediate-grade malignancy. (A) The posterior aspect of the distal femur is a common site of *parosteal osteosarcoma*; however, this tumor presents on radiography as a homogenously sclerotic mass attached to the cortex. (B) *Periosteal chondroma* may exhibit similar radiographic features as periosteal chondrosarcoma; the lesion, however, is much smaller, and the distal femur is not a preferential site, the most common location being the proximal humerus. (D) *Conventional chondrosarcoma* is a medullary lesion, although it may extend into the soft tissues. The tumor under consideration is a surface lesion, without intramedullary involvement. (E) *Tumoral calcinosis* is characterized by the presence of single or multiple periarticular lobulated cystic masses containing chalky material. The masses are painless, usually occur in children and adolescents, and most commonly are formed around the shoulders, hips, and elbow joints, and on the extensile surfaces of the limbs.

Answer to question 54: E

Concerning **clear cell chondrosarcoma**, all of the statements are true.

Answer to question 55: E

The chordoma consists of cord-like arrays and lobules of large polyhedral cells with a vacuolated cytoplasm and vesicular nuclei, referred to as **physaliphorous cells** (from Greek for "bubble bearing").

Answer to question 56: A

In the older patient presenting with back pain, the absence of the pedicle (the "missing pedicle" sign) owing to bone destruction should always be regarded as a **metastasis**, unless proven otherwise. (B) *Congenital absence of the pedicle* is usually diagnosed in much younger age, and the tip-off is the hypertrophy of the contralateral pedicle. The condition is usually asymptomatic. (C) Posterior elements of the vertebra are the common site of an *aneurysmal bone cyst*; the condition, however, occurs in much younger age group, most of the cases diagnosed between ages 5 and 20. In addition, aneurysmal bone cyst usually exhibits expansive imaging features, not present in the case under consideration. (D) Whenever a radiolucent lesion is present in the posterior elements of the vertebra, *osteoblastoma* should be considered in the differential diagnosis; however, similar to the aneurysmal bone cyst, it occurs in much younger age group, majority of the patients being between 10 and 35 years of age. In addition, fluffy densities are usually present within the radiolucent focus. (E) The vertebra is the usual site of *plasmacytoma*; however, unlike the metastatic lesion, the vertebral body not the pedicle is the site of destruction.

Answer to question 57: B

From the given choices, the radiolucent lesion exhibiting **moth-eaten type of bone destruction**, despite lack of a periosteal reaction, most likely represents a malignant bone tumor. (A) *Geographic type of bone destruction* and a *narrow zone of transition* are the hallmarks of a nonaggressive, most likely benign bone lesion. (C) *Soft-tissue mass* may be associated with benign bone lesion, such as an aneurysmal bone cyst, giant cell tumor, or desmoplastic fibroma. It is the *geographic type of bone destruction* that usually (although not always) indicates benignity of the lesion. (D) Again, *geographic type of bone destruction*, *narrow zone of transition*, and uninterrupted, *solid buttress of periosteal reaction* are associated with benign lesions, such as an aneurysmal bone cyst or chondromyxoid fibroma. (E) *Sclerotic lesion with a rough border*, exhibiting *thorny radiations*, is most likely a benign bone island (enostosis). These lesions occasionally demonstrate on skeletal scintigraphy an *increased uptake of radiopharmaceutical tracer* secondary to increased metabolic and osteoblastic activity.

Answer to question 58: C

Although **chordoma** is positive for (A) *S-100 protein*, (B) *cytokeratins*, (D) *carcinoembryonic antigen (CEA)*, and (E) *epithelial membrane antigen (EMA)*, **brachyury**, a protein encoded by *T* gene, has been shown to be the most specific marker for this tumor, rendering specificity above 90%.

Answer to question 59: B

The radiograph shows a mixed radiolucent and sclerotic lesion in the proximal humerus. The proximal part of the lesion shows chondroid calcifications and intact cortex (*arrow*), suggesting a slow-growing tumor. The distal part of the lesion demonstrated more aggressive appearance, osteolytic destruction of medullary portion of bone, and cortical invasion (*open arrow*). These are the imaging features of **dedifferentiated chondrosarcoma**, confirmed on the histopathologic examination. Observe biphasic character of the tumor with low-grade cartilaginous component (*top*) juxtaposed to the noncartilaginous high-grade sarcoma (*bottom and left*), invading the bone trabeculae (*right*). High-grade sarcoma may consist of osteosarcoma, malignant fibrous histiocytoma, fibrosarcoma, rhabdomyosarcoma, or undifferentiated sarcoma. (A) *Mesenchymal chondrosarcoma* histopathologically also exhibits biphasic pattern, which consists of two components: mesenchymal tissue made up of small, round uniform-sized cells with round or ovoid nuclei and well-differentiated cartilaginous matrix containing foci of calcifications and occasionally metaplastic bone. (C) *Undifferentiated pleomorphic sarcoma* is not a biphasic tumor. It is characterized by marked cytologic and nuclear pleomorphism, often with bizarre-appearing giant cells admixed with spindle and histiocyte-like cells. A storiform growth pattern and stromal chronic inflammatory cells are commonly present. (D) *Enchondromatosis* demonstrates completely different imaging and histopathologic features. Although as a component of Ollier disease, the condition may show some aggressive appearance, generally the radiolucent masses of cartilage with foci of calcifications closely resemble solitary enchondromas. Histopathologically, the lesions in enchondromatosis are essentially indistinguishable from those of a solitary enchondromas, although they sometimes tend to be myxoid, more cellular, and may exhibit more cellular atypia. (E) *Chondroblastic osteosarcoma* usually displays a fairly well-differentiated cartilaginous matrix, often with only moderate cytologic signs of malignancy but without the typical lobular pattern of the hyaline cartilage seen in well-differentiated chondrosarcoma. A characteristic feature of this tumor is the indistinct transition from the cartilaginous matrix to osseous matrix, unlike in dedifferentiated chondrosarcoma, where the transition is abrupt.

Answer to question 60: E
Chordoma occurs only at sites in which notochordal remnants are **NOT** normally present. Therefore, although it is a midline lesion of the axial skeleton, it never occurs in the nuclei pulposi.
The statements **A, B, C,** and **D** are all correct.

Answer to question 61: E
The radiograph shows a radiolucent lesion within the medullary portion of the proximal humerus containing various-in-size chondroid calcifications. Observe that the cortex at the site of the lesion is not thickened, there is no evidence of endosteal scalloping and no periosteal reaction. Thickened cortex distal to the lesion represents deltoid tuberosity. The described findings are characteristic features of **enchondroma**. (A) *Medullary bone infarct* also exhibits calcifications and therefore may resemble an enchondroma. The calcifications, however, are coarser and demarcated from the viable bone by serpentine fibro-osseous membrane. (B) Imaging features of *low-grade chondrosarcoma* occasionally can mimic those of *enchondroma*; however, there is focal thickening of the cortex and the presence of deep endosteal scalloping. (C) *Clear cell chondrosarcoma* preferentially affects the articular ends (epiphysis) of long tubular bones. On radiography, the lesion is predominantly lytic, sometimes expansive, commonly with a sclerotic border, and occasionally with central calcifications or ossifications. Endosteal scalloping may be present. The imaging features resemble chondroblastoma. (D) *Chondromyxoid fibroma* is an eccentric lesion, exhibiting narrow zone of transition and geographic type of bone destruction. It commonly is associated with a buttress of solid periosteal reaction. Unlike most of enchondromas, it does not display visible chondroid calcifications.

Answer to question 62: A
Chondromyxoid fibroma DOES NOT exhibit visible chondroid calcifications. The remaining statements are all true.

Answer to question 63: B
The histopathologic section shows in addition to pleomorphic round cells, the characteristic for **Hodgkin lymphoma** binucleate Reed-Sternberg cell with prominent eosinophilic nucleoli. Sclerotic vertebrae are common findings in Hodgkin lymphoma. (A) *Plasmacytoma* exhibits almost invariably osteolytic and not sclerotic features. Moreover, the histopathology shows sheets of atypical plasmacytoid cells. The round nuclei possess a dense, coarse chromatin that has a typical cartwheel-like distribution. (C) *Large B-cell lymphoma* exhibits pleomorphic round cells with well-defined cytoplasmic outline and enlarged cleaved nuclei with prominent nucleoli. The cytoplasm is basophilic. (D) *Langerhans cell histiocytosis* may affect the vertebrae. The characteristic finding is so-called vertebra plana, which represents collapsed of vertebral body secondary to destruction of bone by granulomatous lesion. Histopathology shows agglomerates of more or less densely arranged large rounded cells without cytoplasmic extensions. The characteristic Langerhans cells can be specifically identified in electron microscopy by the presence of racquet-shaped cytoplasmic organelles known as Birbeck granules. (E) *Metastases from thyroid carcinoma* are invariably lytic, not sclerotic. Histopathology may show foci of papillary formation and follicular elements with cells containing clear nuclei with pseudoinclusions.

Answer to question 64: C
Parosteal osteosarcoma is a slow-growing, low-grade tumor that affects only surface of the bone and therefore has the much better prognosis than do the other types of osteosarcomas. It does not produce distant metastases. To the contrary, the other listed lesions, some even benign, may metastasize to the lungs. (A) *Telangiectatic osteosarcoma*, one of the most aggressive types of osteosarcomas, commonly produces lung metastases. (B) *Giant cell tumor*, even a benign variant, also may metastasize to the lungs. According to various reports, about 2% of the patients with this lesion develop pulmonary metastases on average 3 to 4 years after diagnosis. It is of interest, that these metastatic lesions show benign histopathologic features, and some may even regress spontaneously. (D) *Chondroblastoma* is a benign cartilaginous tumor; yet in some instances, it may metastasize to the lungs. These metastases are clinically nonprogressive and may be surgically removed with satisfactory results. (E) *Synovial sarcoma* gives distant metastases including the lungs in high percentage of cases.

Answer to question 65: C

Coronal T1-weighted MR image shows a well-demarcated lesion exhibiting high signal intensity paralleling the signal of subcutaneous fat, with internal focus of low signal intensity. Axial T2-weighted MRI demonstrates that the lesion now becomes of intermediate signal, again paralleling the signal intensity of subcutaneous fat. The focus of low signal intensity (*arrowhead*) represents a calcification. These are the characteristic imaging features of **intraosseous lipoma**. The diagnosis is confirmed on the histopathologic section that shows benign mature lipocytes possessing a large clear cytoplasmic vacuoles that displace the crescent-shaped nuclei to the periphery. There is no evidence of lipoblasts or atypical stellate spindle cells with mitotic figures that are seen in malignant lipomatous tumors. (**A**) *Intramedullary bone infarct* may contain fatty tissue; however, it has characteristic MRI appearance. On T1-weighted images, there is a serpentine band of low signal intensity representing the reactive interface surrounding the central area of bone necrosis; T2-weighted and STIR images demonstrate serpentine low signal line adjacent to a high signal intensity line (so-called double-line sign). (**B**) *Liposarcoma of bone* shows more aggressive imaging features than intraosseous lipoma, and histopathology confirms malignancy demonstrating lipoblasts, atypical stellate, and spindle cells in myxoid stroma, as well as prominent pleomorphism and numerous mitotic figures. (**D**) *Intraosseous ganglion*, most of the time exhibits a sclerotic border, shows no internal calcifications or ossifications, and MRI features of intermediate signal intensity on T1-weighted sequences and high signal on T2 weighting are not consistent with a fatty tumor, but rather with a cystic-like lesion. (**E**) *Langerhans cell histiocytosis* demonstrates no fat signal on any of MRI sequences, and shows characteristic histopathologic features that include aggregates of histiocytic-appearing cells in a mixed inflammatory background with prominent eosinophilia, and Langerhans cells with indistinct cytoplasmic borders and kidney-shaped grooved nuclei.

Answer to question 66: C

Liposarcoma of bone occurs in all age groups, but the majority of the patients are **adults**.
The remaining statements are all true.

Answer to question 67: D

CT section shows a large soft-tissue mass adjacent to the posterior cortex of the distal femur exhibiting ossifications, some well organized, particularly at the periphery (*right side*), some scattered centrally (*left side*) with reverse zoning pattern. The cortex of the bone is not invaded. These imaging features are characteristic of **soft-tissue (extraskeletal) osteosarcoma**. The diagnosis is confirmed by histopathologic section that demonstrates cell-rich malignant tumor with fibrosarcomatous areas and tumor osteoid formation by malignant cells. (**A**) Imaging features of *myositis ossificans* may resemble soft-tissue osteosarcoma, the ossifications, however, instead of being centrally scattered within the mass, are well organized at the periphery of the lesion, creating so-called zonal phenomenon. (**B**) Lesion of *periosteal chondroma*, instead of ossifications, contains chondroid calcifications. In addition, it commonly erodes the adjacent cortex, forming buttress of periosteal reaction. Histopathology shows hyaline cartilage formed by chondrocytes and absence of tumor osteoid. (**C**) *Soft-tissue chondrosarcoma* may mimic soft-tissue osteosarcoma; however, instead of ossifications, it contains calcifications. On histopathologic examination, the tumor is characterized by undifferentiated mesenchymal cells with only rare islands of well-differentiated cartilage and may also exhibit myxoid changes.

Answer to question 68: A

MRI examination shows a classic appearance of **enchondroma**. Coronal T1-weighted MR image of the knee shows a well-defined lobulated lesion in the distal femur exhibiting intermediate-to-low signal intensity. Centrally located foci of low signal represent calcifications. Coronal T2-weighted MRI shows the lesion becomes of high signal, with calcifications remaining of low signal intensity. Histopathologic section confirms the classic features of enchondroma: sparsely cellular tissue and uniform-sized chondrocytes located in rounded lacunae. (**B**) Imaging features of *low-grade chondrosarcoma* may resemble an enchondroma, but cortex is usually focally thickened, and there is evidence of deep endosteal scalloping of the cortex. Histopathology shows cellular pleomorphism and hyperchromatism of the nuclei. (**C**) *Chondromyxoid fibroma* shows slightly more aggressive imaging features, periosteal reaction, and conspicuous lack of calcifications. On histopathologic examination, chondromyxoid fibroma is characterized by large lobulated areas of spindle-shaped or stellate cells distributed within abundant myxoid and chondroid intercellular matrix. (**D**) *Periosteal chondroma* is a surface, not medullary tumor. Histopathology is very similar to enchondroma, although the tumor tissue is more cellular, and some cells may appear atypical. (**E**) *Chondroblastoma* is an epiphyseal lesion, commonly seen in the immature skeleton. MRI shows usually heterogeneous signal of the tumor. Histopathologic features are characteristic, including nodules of fairly mature cartilaginous matrix surrounded by a highly cellular, relatively undifferentiated tissue composed of round and polygonal chondroblast-like cells and giant cells. In addition, the almost pathognomonic fine lattice-like matrix calcifications are present having a spatial arrangement that resembles the hexagonal configuration of chicken wire.

Answer to question 69: E

Giant cells of the osteoclast-like or chondroclast type are usually part of the histopathologic spectrum of **chondroblastoma**. The remaining statements are all true.

Answer to question 70: B

Periosteal chondroma occurs in **children and young adults**, most cases seen in the second and third decades of life. The remaining statements are all true.

Answer to question 71: E
(A) **Telangiectatic osteosarcoma** represents one of the **most aggressive types** of osteosarcomas. It affects males twice as often as females and occurs predominantly during the second and third decades of life. Originally described by Paget in 1854 and subsequently redefined by Gaylord in 1903 as a "malignant bone aneurysm," it was renamed as "hemorrhagic osteosarcoma" by Campanacci in 1971. (B) Most of the tumors arise in the **femur** and **tibia**. (C) **Imaging features of telangiectatic osteosarcoma and aneurysmal bone cyst may overlap**, particularly both lesions may exhibit soft-tissue mass and fluid–fluid levels on MRI. Likewise, the **histopathologic features of both lesions overlap**. In fact, the confusion in diagnosis between telangiectatic osteosarcoma and aneurysmal bone cyst represents one of the most treacherous pitfalls in tumor pathology. The hallmark of telangiectatic osteosarcoma is the presence of anaplastic cells with atypical mitoses forming tumor bone or tumor osteoid, the feature not present in aneurysmal bone cyst. However, some of these tumors exhibit only minimal amount of osteoid production, making it difficult to find it on the biopsy specimens.

Answer to question 72: C
The histopathologic section shows malignant small round and oval cells producing tumor osteoid (*pink material*); therefore, the most likely diagnosis is **small cell osteosarcoma.** Some other malignant and benign lesions may exhibit small round cells, such as Ewing sarcoma, lymphoma, myeloma, mesenchymal chondrosarcoma, metastatic neuroblastoma, or Langerhans cell histiocytosis. Contrary to the small cell osteosarcoma, however, neither of the listed tumors is able to produce tumor osteoid, the hallmark of osteosarcomas. (A) Cells of *osteoblastoma* are able to produce osteoid but not malignant variety. (B) *Fibrous dysplasia* is characterized by metaplastic immature woven bone trabeculae without osteoblasts, haphazardly arranged in the fibrous stroma. (D) *Telangiectatic osteosarcoma* rarely shows tumor osteoid production, and the cells are not small and round, but rather fusiform and spindle. In addition, the giant cells are commonly present in the field of view. (E) *Periosteal osteosarcoma* shows predominantly cartilaginous component, and the tumor cells, particularly at the periphery, are not round but spindled.

Answer to question 73: E
Anteroposterior radiograph of the knee shows a homogeneously sclerotic lesion with small radiating streaks (thorny radiations) in the proximal tibia. CT section shows a high-attenuation lesion with a rough border. These are the characteristic imaging features of a **bone island (enostosis).** Some of the bone islands may show positive radionuclide bone scan due to increased metabolism and osteoblastic activity. The best action is to follow-up the patient with repeat imaging studies in about 6 months. (A) The radiographic and CT features of *bone island* including homogeneity of the lesion and rough border (pseudopodia, thorny radiations, radiating streaks) are diagnostic, and there is no need for additional imaging studies. (B) The lesion definitely does not exhibit imaging features of *osteosarcoma* because there is lack of aggressive findings, and furthermore, osteosarcoma most commonly occurs in children and adolescents. (C) *Metastasis* always should be considered in patients older than 50 years. However, imaging features, particularly the rough border of the lesion and only moderate uptake of the tracer on scintigraphy is more consistent with a bone island. (D) *Osteoma* is a surface and not an intramedullary lesion, so this diagnosis can be assertively excluded.

Answer to question 74: A,B,D,E
The only lesion that should undergo biopsy is the one shown in part (C). The radiograph of the knee shows an eccentric radiolucent lesion with sclerotic border and central calcifications in the lateral aspect of the proximal tibia. The lesion exhibits nonaggressive features including a narrow zone of transition and most likely represents an enchondroma, focus of fibrous dysplasia, nonossifying fibroma, or benign fibrous histiocytoma. The possibility of chondrosarcoma, however, cannot be completely excluded, since the low-grade cartilage tumors may masquerade as benign lesions. **Biopsy of the lesion** is a prudent action. To the contrary, all other lesions under consideration have a very characteristic radiographic appearance, and diagnosis can be made with high degree of accuracy without the biopsy. These conditions belong to the group of so-called don't touch lesions. (A) The radiograph of the left hip shows a large sclerotic lesion in the ilium exhibiting rough border and "thorny radiations" merging with the normal trabeculae of the host bone (*arrow*). Those are the characteristic imaging features of **bone island (enostosis).** The proper action is not to biopsy the lesion but to follow-up the patient with repeat radiologic studies in about 6 months. (B) The radiograph of the femur shows a homogeneously sclerotic lesion abutting the medial cortex with narrow zone of transition. The cortex is normal in thickness, and there is no evidence of a soft-tissue mass. These are the characteristic imaging features of **healed nonossifying fibroma.** No further action is required. (D) An oblique radiograph of the knee in a child (observe the open growth plate) shows a saucer-like defect in the medial cortex of the distal femoral metaphysis at the linea aspera, producing cortical irregularity (*arrow*). This is a classic presentation of benign **periosteal desmoid.** It is a tumor-like proliferation of the periosteum, which has a striking predilection for the posteromedial cortex of the medial femoral condyle. The lesion usually occurs between the ages 12 and 20 years, mainly in boys, and most lesions disappear spontaneously by the end of the second decade. Periosteal desmoid is considered to represent asymptomatic normal variant that does not require biopsy or treatment. (E) A coned-down radiograph of the right ribs shows a large ossific mass in the soft tissues. There is increased density on the periphery of the lesion and more radiolucent center, referred to as zoning phenomenon. In addition, a narrow radiolucent cleft separates the mass from the ribs. These are

the characteristic imaging features of **juxtacortical myositis ossificans**. The zoning phenomenon represents the maturation pattern of the lesion, which is undifferentiated and cellular in the center, and exhibits an increasingly mature ossification toward the periphery. With time, the lesion decreases in size and eventually may disappear completely, or persists as a well-matured ossific focus. It should never be biopsied, although timely repeated imaging studies to document regression of the lesion is a proper action.

Answer to question 75: C

A large number of secondary osteosarcomas arise as a complication of **Paget disease** and characteristically develop in pagetic bone. Most cases of malignant transformation occur in polyostotic Paget disease. Osteosarcoma can develop in any affected bone, although the pelvic bones and femur are the preferential sites of this complication. The other sites commonly affected are the humerus and the tibia. Patients with advanced Paget disease are at greater risk. (**A**) **Osteosarcoma arising in fibrous dysplasia** is a rare event occurring in about 0.5% to 1% of patients with this disorder. In reported cases, the majority of the patients had a polyostotic fibrous dysplasia. The affected sites included craniofacial bones, proximal femur, humerus, and pelvis. (**B**) Radiation therapy for an unrelated previous conditions may also give rise to secondary osteosarcoma. These malignancies account for 3% to 5% of all osteosarcomas, and 50% to 60% of radiation-induced sarcomas. The threshold is approximately 800 to 1,000 cGy, but usually, a dose of at least 3,000 cGy administered within 3 weeks is required to develop this complication. The latent period is between 4 and 42 years, with an average of 11 years. **Postirradiation osteosarcoma** may develop either after radiation therapy for benign bone lesions, such as fibrous dysplasia and giant cell tumor, or after irradiation of malignant conditions such as breast cancer and lymphoma. These tumors may also develop as a result of ingestion and intraosseous accumulation of radioisotopes, as has been described in painters of radium watch dials. (**D**) One of the most common complications of **chronic draining sinus tract of osteomyelitis** is development of squamous cell carcinoma. Less commonly fibrosarcoma and osteosarcoma may develop. In most patients with osteomyelitis, the history of the disease dates to childhood, and sinuses draining for more than 20 years are generally the precursors of malignant neoplasms. (**E**) Secondary **osteosarcoma associated with medullary bone infarcts** is extremely rare complication. More commonly reported malignancies arising in bone infarct are fibrosarcoma, malignant fibrous histiocytoma, and angiosarcoma.

Index

Note: Page numbers in *italics* indicate figures and page numbers followed by t indicate tables.

A

Acidic decalcifiers, 20
Actin, 25
Adamantinoma of long bones
   clinical findings, 334
   definition, 334
   differential diagnosis, 209, 337–339
   epidemiology, 334
   genetics, 337
   gross pathology, 336, *337*
   histopathology, 336–337, *337–339*
   immunohistochemistry, 337
   magnetic resonance imaging, 334
   prognosis, 337
   radiography, 334, *335, 336*
   scintigraphy, 334, *336*
   sites of involvement, 334
   tibia for, 3, *3*
Adult progeria. *See* Werner syndrome
Aneurysmal bone cyst (ABC), 400, 408, 420
   clinical findings, 312
   computed tomography, 314, *318, 319, 322*
   definition, 311–312
   differential diagnosis, 63, 138, 214, 217, 281, 309–311, 321–323, 330
   epidemiology, 312
   genetics, 321
   gross pathology, 314, *326*
   histopathology, 314, 321, *326–328*, 401, 417
   imaging features, 409, 421
   lateral radiograph, 409, 421
   magnetic resonance imaging, 314, *320, 322–325*
   osteoblastoma, 46
   periosteal reaction, 8, *9*
   prognosis, 321
   radiography, 312, *316–318, 320, 322–325*, 400, 416
   at right femur, 3, *5*
   scintigraphy, 312, *319*
   sites of involvement, 312
Aneurysmal-like expansion, *41*
Angiolymphoid hyperplasia, with eosinophilia, 282
Angiomatoid fibrous histiocytoma
   clinical findings, 223
   definition, 223
   epidemiology, 223
   genetics, 225
   gross pathology, 223
   histopathology, 223, 225, *225*
   imaging, 223
   immunohistochemistry, 223, 225
   prognosis, 225
   sites of involvement, 223

Angiosarcoma
   clinical features, 293
   definition, 293
   differential diagnosis, 295
   electron microscopy, 295
   epidemiology, 293
   genetics, 295
   gross pathology, 293, *293*
   histopathology, 293, *294–295*, 295
   imaging, 293
   immunohistochemistry, 295
   prognosis, 295
   radiography, 402, 417
   sites of involvement, 293
Antibodies
   in bone tumor pathology, 26–27
   against hematopoietic and lymphoid cells, and vascular antigens, 25
   against intermediate filaments, 23–25
   against muscle and neuroectodermal antigens, 25–26
Arteriography, 1
Arthritis, inflammatory
   differential diagnosis, 364
   histopathology, 364
   radiography, 364

B

Bacterial infection, Gram stain in, *24*
Benign fibrous histiocytoma
   clinical findings, 189
   definition, 189
   differential diagnosis, 190, 192
   epidemiology, 189
   gross pathology, 189
   histopathology, 189–190, *191, 192*
   immunohistochemistry, 190
   magnetic resonance imaging, 189
   prognosis, 190
   radiography, 189, *190, 191*
   scintigraphy, 189, *191*
   sites of involvement, 189
Benign tumor
   aneurysmal bone cyst, 311–323
   bone-forming lesions
      osteoblastoma, 40–47
      osteoid osteoma, 35–40
      osteoma, 32–35
   cartilage-forming lesions
      chondroblastoma, 124, *129–134*, 134
      chondromyxoid fibroma, 134–138
      enchondroma, 90–97
      enchondromatosis, 97
      Maffucci syndrome, 97
      multiple hereditary osteochondromata, 121, *123–129*

      Ollier disease, 97
      osteochondroma, 114–121
      periosteal chondroma, 99–104, *105–107*
      soft-tissue chondroma, 104
      synovial chondromatosis, 107–113
   fibrous lesions
      benign fibrous histiocytoma, 189–192
      cortical defect/nonossifying fibroma, 181–189
      desmoplastic fibroma, 210–218
      fibrocartilaginous dysplasia, 197–206
      fibrous dysplasia, 194–197
      osteofibrous dysplasia, 206–210
      periosteal desmoid, 192–194
   giant cell reparative granuloma, 323–330
   giant cell tumor, 298–309
   intraosseous lipoma, 330–334
   joints lesions
      juxta-articular myxoma, 366, 368–369
      lipoma arborescens, 364–366
      localized pigmented nodular tenosynovitis, 359–361
      pigmented nodular tenosynovitis, 353–359
      synovial (osteo)chondromatosis, 353
      synovial hemangioma, 362–364
   round cell lesions
      Erdheim-Chester disease, 242–244
      Langerhans cell histiocytosis, 231–240
      Rosai-Dorfman disease, 241–242
   simple bone cyst, 309–311
   vascular lesions
      cystic angiomatosis, 282–284
      epithelioid hemangioma, 282
      glomangioma, 290
      glomangiomatosis, 290
      glomangiomyoma, 290
      glomus tumor, 289
      Gorham disease, 284–285
      intraosseous hemangioma, 273–281
      lymphangioma, 285–289
      lymphangiomatosis, 285–289
      malignant glomus tumor, 290
      symplastic glomus tumor, 290
      synovial hemangioma, 285
Biopsy of lesion, 415, 425
Birbeck granules, 235, *240*, 253
Bizarre parosteal osteochondromatous proliferation (BPOP), 119
Bone abscess
   osteoblastoma, 46
   osteoid osteoma, 40
Bone cyst
   bone destruction and, 6, *7*
   in calcaneus, 3, *5*
   in long bone, 3, *4*

Bone destruction
    geographic, 6, *7*, *66*, 254, *255*, 410, 418, 422
    lesion's growth rate, 6, *7*
    moth-eaten, 6, *7*, 47, 60, 159, *159*, 219, 220, 224, 254, *255*, *258*, *288*, 286, 410, 422
    permeative, 6, 60, 159, *159*, 219, 220, 244, 254, *255*, *258*
    types, *6*, 6–7, *7*
Bone island. See Enostosis
Bone-forming lesions
    benign tumor
        osteoblastoma, 40–47
        osteoid osteoma, 35–40
        osteoma, 32–35
    malignant tumor
        osteosarcomas, 47–78
        secondary osteosarcomas, 78–80
        soft-tissue osteosarcoma, 81–85
Brachyury, 342, 411, 422
Brown tumor of hyperparathyroidism, 240, 268, 284, 309, 393, 396

C

Cafe-au-lait spots, 418
Calcifying enchondroma
    differential diagnosis, 394–395
    histopathology, 395
Camurati-Engelmann disease, 243–244
Cartilage-forming lesions
    benign tumor
        chondroblastoma, 124, *129–134*, 134
        chondromyxoid fibroma, 134–138
        enchondroma, 90–97
        enchondromatosis, 97
        Maffucci syndrome, 97
        multiple hereditary osteochondromata, 121, *123–129*
        Ollier disease, 97
        osteochondroma, 114–121
        periosteal chondroma, 99–104, *105–107*
        soft-tissue chondroma, 104
        synovial chondromatosis, 107–113
    malignant tumor, 138
        clear cell chondrosarcoma, 145–147, 152, *153*
        conventional chondrosarcoma, 139–145, *146–151*
        dedifferentiated chondrosarcoma, 157, 159–165
        mesenchymal chondrosarcoma, 152, 154–157
        myxoid chondrosarcoma, 157
        periosteal chondrosarcoma, 164–169
        secondary chondrosarcomas, 171–175
        soft-tissue chondrosarcoma, 169–171
CD99, 25
Central chondrosarcomas. See Conventional chondrosarcoma
Chondroblastic osteosarcoma
    histopathology, 411, 422–423
    radiography, 411, 422–423
Chondroblastoma, 406, 412, 419–420, 423
    anteroposterior radiograph, 2–3, *3*
    clinical findings, 124
    computed tomography, *130*
    definition, 124
    differential diagnosis, 134, 152
    epidemiology, 124
    genetics, 134
    giant cells of osteoclast-like/chondroclast type, 414, 424
    histopathology, 127, *133–134*, 399, 401, 412–413, 416, 417, 424
    immunohistochemistry, 134
    magnetic resonance imaging, *131, 132*, 412–413, 424
    pathology, 127
    prognosis, 134
    radiography, *129–132*, 399, 400, 416
    sites of involvement, 124
Chondrogenic lesions. See Cartilage-forming lesions
Chondroid matrix, 11, *13*, *14*
Chondroma
    periosteal
        clinical findings, 99
        computed tomography, 99, *106–107*
        definition, 99
        differential diagnosis, 99, 104
        epidemiology, 99
        histopathology, 99, *108*
        magnetic resonance imaging, 99, *107*
        pathology, 99
        prognostic factors, 99
        radiography, 99, *105–107*
        sites of involvement, 99
    soft-tissue, 104, *109*
        differential diagnosis, 361, 374–375
        histopathology, 361
        imaging, 361
Chondromyxoid fibroma, 406, 412, 419, 423
    clinical findings, 135
    definition, 134
    differential diagnosis, 138, 189, 190, 192, 217, 322
    epidemiology, 135
    genetics, 138
    histopathology, 135, *137, 138*, 413–414, 424
    immunophenotype, 138
    at left tibia, 3, *5*
    magnetic resonance imaging, 135, *137*, 413–414, 424
    pathology, 135, 138
    prognostic factors, 138
    radiography, 135, *135, 136*, 406, 411, 420, 423
    sites of involvement, 135
Chondrosarcoma, 138
    classification, *139*
    clear cell (see Clear cell chondrosarcoma)
    conventional
        clinical findings, 139
        computed tomography, 140, *143–145, 148*
        definition, 139
        diagnosis, 406, 419
        differential diagnosis, 143, 145
        epidemiology, 139
        genetics, 143
        histopathology, 140, 143, *150–151*, 410, 422
        magnetic resonance imaging, 140, *146–148*
        pathology, 140, 143
        prognosis, 143
        radiography, 140, *141–142, 144, 146–148*, 410, 411, 422, 423
        scintigraphy, 140, *143*
        sites of involvement, 139
    dedifferentiated
        clinical features, 159
        computed tomography, 159
        definition, 157
        epidemiology, 157
        genetics, 164
        histopathology, 159, *162–165*, 164, 411, 422–423
        magnetic resonance imaging, 159, *160*
        pathology, 159, 164
        prognosis, 164
        radiography, 159, *159, 160*, 411, 422–423
        sites of involvement, 159
    differential diagnosis, 60, 206, 342
    histologic grading, 140t
    low-grade, 97
        histopathology, 413–414, 424
        magnetic resonance imaging, 413–414, 424
    magnetic resonance imaging, 403–404, 418
    mesenchymal, 405, 419
        clinical findings, 154
        definition, 152
        epidemiology, 154
        genetics, 155
        histopathology, 155, *155, 156*, 407, 411, 420, 422–423
        immunohistochemistry, *157*
        magnetic resonance imaging, 154, *154–155*
        pathology, 155
        prognosis, 157
        radiography, 154, *154–155*, 411, 422–423
        sites of involvement, 154
    myxoid, 157
    in pagetic bone, *174, 175*
    periosteal
        clinical findings, 164
        definition, 164
        differential diagnosis, 165
        epidemiology, 164
        histopathology, 165, *168, 169*, 410, 422
        imaging features, 410, 422
        magnetic resonance imaging, *166, 167*
        pathology, 165, 169
        radiography, *165–167*, 410, 422
        scintigraphy, *167*
        sites of involvement, 164
    in primary (osteo) chondromatosis, 175
    radiography, 403–404, 418
    secondary (see Secondary chondrosarcomas)
    soft-tissue, 104
        clinical findings, 169
        computed tomography, 413, 424
        definition, 169
        epidemiology, 169
        genetics, 170
        histopathology, *170*, 377, 413, 424
        immunophenotype, 170
        magnetic resonance imaging, 169, 377
        pathology, 169–170
        prognosis, 170
        radiography, 169, *170*
        scintigraphy, 169
        sites of involvement, 169
Chordoid sarcoma
    definition, 157
    differential diagnosis, 157

epidemiology, 157
pathology, 157
sites of involvement, 157
Chordoma
   clinical findings, 339
   computed tomography, 340, *340*
   definition, 339
   diagnosis, 411, *422*
   differential diagnosis, 342, 344
   epidemiology, 339
   genetics, 342
   gross pathology, 342, *342*
   histopathology, 342, *343*
   immunohistochemistry, 342
   magnetic resonance imaging, 340, *341*
   neoplastic cell, 410, *422*
   prognosis, 342
   radiography, 339–340, *340*
   sites of involvement, 339
Chronic recurrent multifocal osteomyelitis (CRMO), 288–289
CKs. *See* Cytokeratins (CKs)
Clavicle
   gross specimen of, *34*
   osteolytic metastasis in, *385*
   soft-tissue mass, *11*
Clear cell chondrosarcoma
   characteristic features, 405, 410, 419, *422*
   computed tomography, 145, *152*
   definition, 145
   differential diagnosis, 134, 152
   epidemiology, 145
   genetics, 147
   histopathology, 134, 147, *153*
   immunophenotype, 147
   magnetic resonance imaging, 145, *152*
   pathology, 147
   prognosis, 147, 152
   radiography, 145, *152*, 411, *423*
   sites of involvement, 145
Codman triangle, 8, 417
   periosteal reaction, 8, *10*
   radiography, *51*
Computed tomography (CT), 2, 12, 14–17
   aneurysmal bone cyst, 314, *318, 319, 322*
   chondroblastoma, *130*
   chordoma, 340, *340*
   clear cell chondrosarcoma, 145, *152*
   conventional chondrosarcoma, 140, *143–145, 148*
   conventional osteosarcoma, 48, *53*
   cortical metastasis, 382, *386*
   dedifferentiated chondrosarcoma, 159
   desmoplastic fibroma, 210, *216*
   enchondroma, *91*
   enostosis, 414–415, *425*
   Ewing sarcoma, 244, *246*
   fibrous dysplasia, 402–403, *418*
   giant cell tumor, 299, *302, 303*
   glomus tumor, *289*
   hyperparathyroidism, 402–403, *418*
   intraosseous hemangioma, 273, *275, 276*
   intraosseous lipoma, 331, *332*
   Langerhans cell histiocytosis, *237*
   leiomyosarcoma of bone, 344, *344, 345*
   malignant lymphoma, 254, *256–260*
   of Mazabraud syndrome, *205–206*
   of monostotic fibrous dysplasia, *199, 200, 202*
   multiple myeloma, 263, *266*, 402–403, *418*
   multiple osteocartilaginous exostoses, *126, 127, 128*
   myositis ossificans, 413, *424*
   nonossifying fibroma, 182, *185*
   Ollier disease, *102*
   of osteoblastoma, 44, *44*
   osteochondroma, 116, *117*
   of osteofibrous dysplasia, *211–212*
   osteoid osteoma, 35, *38–39*
   osteolytic metastases, *384*, 402–403, *418*
   osteoma, 32, *33*
   of paget osteosarcoma, *80*
   parosteal osteosarcoma, *72*
   periosteal chondroma, 99, *106–107*, 413, *424*
   periosteal desmoid, 192, *193*
   periosteal osteosarcoma, *76*
   of polyostotic fibrous dysplasia, *198, 201*
   sclerotic metastasis, 382, *389*
   sessile osteochondroma, *118*
   soft-tissue chondrosarcoma, 413, *424*
   soft-tissue osteosarcoma, *81*, 413, *424*
   synovial chondromatosis, 109, *110, 111*
   synovial hemangioma, 362, *363*
Congo red stain, 21
Contrast arthrography, 354, *355*
Contrast-enhanced MRI, 14
Conventional chondrosarcoma
   clinical findings, 139
   computed tomography, 140, *143–145, 148*
   definition, 139
   diagnosis, 406, 419
   differential diagnosis, 143, 145
   epidemiology, 139
   genetics, 143
   H&E stain in, *23*
   histopathology, 140, 143, *150–151*, 410, *422*
   magnetic resonance imaging, 140, *146, 147, 148*
   pathology, 140, 143
   prognosis, 143
   radiography, 140, *141–142, 144, 146–148*, 410, 411, *422, 423*
   scintigraphy, 140, *143*
   sites of involvement, 139
Conventional osteosarcoma
   clinical presentation, 47
   complications, 61
   computed tomography, 48, *53*
   definition, 47
   differential diagnosis, 59–61
   epidemiology, 47
   genetics and immunohistochemistry, 58
   gross pathology, 50, *57*
   histopathology, 50, *57–59*, 58
   magnetic resonance imaging, 50, *54–56*, 403–404, *418*
   prognosis, 61
   radiography, 47–48, *49–51*, 403–405, *418, 419*
   scintigraphy, 48, *52–53*
   sites of involvement, 47
Conventional radiography
   benign *vs.* malignant nature, 12
   bone destruction, types, 6, *6–7, 7*
   borders of lesion, 3, *5, 6*
   periosteal reaction, 7–8, *9–10*
   site of lesion, 2–3, *3, 4, 5*
   soft-tissue mass, 11, *11, 12*
   tumor tissue, composition, 11–12, *13, 14*
Cortical desmoid
   clinical findings, 192
   definition, 192
   differential diagnosis, 192–194
   epidemiology, 192
   histopathology, 192, *193*
   imaging, 192, *192, 193*
   prognosis, 192
   sites of involvement, 192
Cortical metastasis
   computed tomography, 382, *386*
   radiography, 382, *385*
Cortical osteoid osteoma, 8, *9*
Cortical thickening, 7
CT. *See* Computed tomography (CT)
Cystic angiomatosis
   clinical findings, 282
   definition, 282
   differential diagnosis, 284
   epidemiology, 282
   gross pathology, 282
   histopathology, 282, *284*
   imaging, 282
   prognosis, 284
   sites of involvement, 282
Cytogenetics, 27–28
Cytokeratins (CKs), 23, *24*
   CK7/CK20 combination, 25, 25t

D

Decalcification, 20–21
Dedifferentiated chondrosarcoma
   clinical features, 159
   computed tomography, 159
   definition, 157
   epidemiology, 157
   genetics, 164
   gross specimen, 159, *160–163*
   H&E stain in, *22*
   histopathology, 159, *162–165*, 164, 411, *422–423*
   magnetic resonance imaging, 159, *160*
   pathology, 159, 164
   prognosis, 164
   radiography, 159, *159, 160*, 411, *422–423*
   sites of involvement, 159
Desmoid tumor of bone
   clinical finding, 210
   definition, 210
   differential diagnosis, 189, 214, 217–218
   epidemiology, 210
   genetics, 214
   gross pathology, 214, *217*
   histopathology, 214, *218*
   imaging, 210
   immunohistochemistry, 214
   prognosis, 214
   radiography, 210, *215–217*
   sites of involvement, 210
Desmoplastic fibroma, 407, *420*
   clinical finding, 210
   definition, 210
   differential diagnosis, 67, 189, 214, 217–218
   epidemiology, 210
   genetics, 214

Desmoplastic fibroma (*Continued*)
   gross pathology, 214, *217*
   histopathology, 214, *218*, 408, 420
   imaging, 210
   immunohistochemistry, 214
   prognosis, 214
   radiography, 210, *215–217*
   sites of involvement, 210
Diaphyseal aclasis, 121, 399, 416
Diffuse osteoporosis, 268, 396
Diffuse-type tenosynovial giant cell tumor.
   See Pigmented villonodular synovitis (PVNS)
Dysplasia epiphysealis hemimelica, 119

E
Electron microscopy (EM), 27
   Erdheim-Chester disease, 243
   Langerhans cell histiocytosis, *27*, 235, *240*
   malignant glomus tumor, 290
Enchondroma, 406, 419
   clinical findings, 91
   complications, 93
   definition, 90
   differential diagnosis, 93, 97, 134, 145, 330, 360, 361
   epidemiology, 90
   genetics, 93
   histopathology, 91, *97, 98*, 413–414, 424
   imaging, 91, 360
   magnetic resonance imaging, 91, *93–96*, 413–414, 424
   malignant transformation
      clinical findings, 171
      epidemiology, 171
      histopathology, 171, *173*
      radiography, *172*
   osteoblastoma, 46
   pathology, 91
   prognosis, 93
   radiography, 91, *91–95*, 402, 411, 418, 423
   right humerus, 3, *4*
   sites of involvement, 90–91
Enchondromatosis, 97
   histopathology, 411, 422–423
   radiography, *97, 99*, 411, 422–423
Enostosis
   computed tomography, 414–415, 425
   histopathology, 393–394
   osteoid osteoma, 40
   radiography, 393, 414–415, 425
Eosinophilic granuloma
   clinical findings, 231, 233
   definition, 231
   differential diagnosis, 236, 240
   electron microscopy, 235
   epidemiology, 231
   immunohistochemistry, 235
   magnetic resonance imaging, 233
   pathology, 233, 235
   radiography, 233
   scintigraphy, 233
Epiphyseal bone abscess, 134
Epithelial component of adamantinoma
   expresses, 400, 416
Epithelial membrane antigen (EMA), 374, *376*
Epithelioid angiosarcoma, *26*

Epithelioid hemangioendothelioma
   clinical findings, 290
   definition, 290
   differential diagnosis, 292–293
   epidemiology, 290
   genetics, 292
   gross pathology, 290
   histopathology, 290, 292, *292*
   imaging, 290
   immunohistochemistry, 292
   prognosis, 292
   sites of involvement, 290
Epithelioid hemangioma
   clinical findings, 282
   definition, 282
   differential diagnosis, 282
   epidemiology, 282
   gross pathology, 282
   histopathology, 282
   imaging, 282
   immunohistochemistry, 282
   prognosis, 282
   sites of involvement, 282
Erdheim-Chester disease
   clinical features, 242
   definition, 242
   differential diagnosis, 243–244, 395
   electron microscopy, 243
   epidemiology, 242
   genetics, 243
   histopathology, 243, *243*
   immunohistochemistry, 243
   magnetic resonance imaging, 242
   pathology, 242–243
   radiography, 242, *242*
   scintigraphy, 242
   sites of involvement, 242
Ewing sarcoma
   bone destruction and, 7, *7*
   clinical features, 244
   computed tomography, 244, *246*
   definition, 244
   differential diagnosis, 59, 65–66, 193, 236, 249, 253, 258
   epidemiology, 244
   in fibula, 3, *5*
   FISH, 28, *28*
   genetics, 249
   histopathology, 245, *251–253*, 399, 407, 416, 420
   immunohistochemistry and, *26*
   magnetic resonance imaging, 244, *247, 248, 250–251*
   Novotny stain in, *24*
   PAS stain in, *24*
   pathology, 245
   periosteal reaction, 8, *10*
   PET, 249–251
   PET-CT, 249–251
   prognosis, 249
   radiography, 244, *244–249*, 399, 402, 416, 417
   scintigraphy, 244
   sites of involvement, 244
Extraskeletal myxoid chondrosarcoma
   clinical findings, 169
   definition, 169

   epidemiology, 169
   genetics, 170
   histopathology, *170*
   immunophenotype, 170
   magnetic resonance imaging, 169
   pathology, 169–170
   prognosis, 170
   radiography, 169, *170*
   scintigraphy, 169
   sites of involvement, 169
Extraskeletal osteosarcoma
   clinical presentation, 81
   definition, 81
   differential diagnosis, 85
   epidemiology, 81
   gross pathology, 81, *84*
   histopathology, 81, *85*
   imaging, 81
   prognosis, 85
   radiography of, *81*
   sites of involvement, 81

F
FCM. *See* Flow cytometry (FCM)
FDG positron emission tomography (FDG PET)
   sclerotic metastasis, 382, *389*
   skeletal metastases, 382, *390, 391–392*
Fibroblastic osteosarcoma
   differential diagnosis, 220
   histopathology, *60*
   radiography, *51*
Fibrocartilaginous dysplasia
   clinical findings, 201
   definition, 197
   differential diagnosis, 201, 206
   epidemiology, 197
   gross pathology, 201
   histopathology, 201
   imaging, 201
   sites of involvement, 201
Fibrocartilaginous mesenchymoma, 206
Fibrohistiocytic lesions
   angiomatoid fibrous histiocytoma, 223–225
   fibrosarcoma, 218–221
   malignant fibrous histiocytoma, 221–223
Fibroma, chondromyxoid
   clinical findings, 135
   definition, 134
   differential diagnosis, 138
   epidemiology, 135
   genetics, 138
   histopathology, 135, *137*, 138
   immunophenotype, 138
   magnetic resonance imaging, 135, *137*
   pathology, 135, 138
   prognostic factors, 138
   radiography, 135, *135, 136*
   sites of involvement, 135
Fibrosarcoma, 408, 421
   clinical findings, 219
   definition, 218
   differential diagnosis, 60, 220–221, 268, 292, 309, 347, 390
   epidemiology, 218
   genetics, 219

gross pathology, 219, *220*
histopathology, 219, *220–221*
imaging, 219
prognosis, 219
sites of involvement, 219
Fibrous cortical defect
   clinical findings, 182
   computed tomography, 182, *185*
   definition, 181
   differential diagnosis, 184, 189, 194
   epidemiology, 182
   gross pathology, 182, *187*
   histopathology, 184, *187–188*
   magnetic resonance imaging, 182, *186*
   prognosis, 184
   radiography, 182, *182–186*
   scintigraphy, 182
   site of involvement, 182
Fibrous dysplasia
   clinical findings, 194
   computed tomography, 402–403, 418
   definition, 194
   differential diagnosis, 67, 138, 197, 338
   epidemiology, 194
   genetics, 197
   gross pathology, 194, *206*
   histopathology, 194, *207, 208*, 403, 408, 414, 418, 420, 425
   imaging, 194
   left tibia, 3, *4*
   osteosarcoma in, 79, 415, 426
   prognosis, 197
   radiography, 408, 420
   sites of involvement, 194
   van Gieson stain in, *23*
Fibrous lesions, benign tumors
   benign fibrous histiocytoma, 189–192
   cortical defect/nonossifying fibroma, 181–189
   desmoplastic fibroma, 210–218
   fibrocartilaginous dysplasia, 197–206
   fibrous dysplasia, 194–197
   osteofibrous dysplasia, 206–210
   periosteal desmoid, 192–194
   with radiographic appearances, 181t
FISH. *See* Fluorescent in situ hybridization (FISH)
^{18}F-labeled 2-fluoro-2-deoxyglucose (^{18}FDG)-PET, 2
Florid reactive periostitis, 77
Flow cytometry (FCM), 27, *27*
Fluorescent in situ hybridization (FISH), 28
   Ewing sarcoma, 28, *28*
Fungal infection, GMS stain in, *24*

G

Gardner syndrome, 399, 416
Gaucher disease, 268, 396
GCRG. *See* Giant cell reparative granuloma (GCRG)
GCT. *See* Giant cell tumor (GCT)
Genetics
   adamantinoma of long bones, 337
   aneurysmal bone cyst, 321
   angiomatoid fibrous histiocytoma, 225
   angiosarcoma, 295
   of bone tumors, 27

   cytogenetics, 27–28
   molecular cytogenetics, 28–29
chondroblastoma, 134
chondromyxoid fibroma, 138
chordoma, 342
clear cell chondrosarcoma, 147
conventional chondrosarcoma, 143
conventional osteosarcoma, 58
dedifferentiated chondrosarcoma, 164
enchondroma, 93
epithelioid hemangioendothelioma, 292
Erdheim-Chester disease, 243
Ewing sarcoma, 249
extraskeletal myxoid chondrosarcoma, 170
fibrosarcoma, 219
fibrous dysplasia, 197
giant cell tumor, 307
intraosseous lipoma, 334
juxta-articular myxoma, 369
leiomyosarcoma of bone, 347
liposarcoma of bone, 348
localized pigmented nodular tenosynovitis, 360
mesenchymal chondrosarcoma, 155
multiple myeloma, 264–265
osteochondroma, 116
osteofibrous dysplasia, 209
osteoid osteoma, 38
pigmented villonodular synovitis, 356
PNET, 249
simple bone cyst, 310
skeletal metastases, 386
synovial (osteo)chondromatosis, 111
synovial sarcoma, 374, *376*
Geode, 134
Giant cell reparative granuloma (GCRG)
   clinical findings, 323
   definition, 323
   differential diagnosis, 330
   epidemiology, 323
   histopathology, 329–330, *330*
   magnetic resonance imaging, 329
   radiography, 329, *329*
   sites of involvement, 323
Giant cell tumor (GCT), 412, 423
   in articular end of long bone, 3, *4*
   clinical findings, 299
   definition, 298
   differential diagnosis, 63–64, 134, 189, 190, 217–218, 220, 223, 309, 322, 330, 390
   epidemiology, 298
   genetics, 307
   gross pathology, 299, *307*
   histopathology, 299, 301, 307, *308, 309*, 390, 401, 404–405, 408, 417, 419, 420
   imaging, 299
   lack of sclerotic border, 401, 417
   matrix mineralization, 407, 420
   prognosis, 307
   radiography, 299, *299–302, 304*, 400, 409, 416, 421
   sites of involvement, 299
   soft-tissue mass, 408, 420
Giant cell tumor of the tendon sheath
   clinical findings, 359
   definition, 359
   differential diagnosis, 360–361, 369

   epidemiology, 359
   genetics, 360
   gross pathology, 360, *360*
   histopathology, 360, *360, 361*
   immunohistochemistry, 360
   magnetic resonance imaging, 359
   prognosis, 360
   radiography, 359, *359*
   sites of involvement, 359
Giant cell–rich osteosarcoma, 400, 416
   clinical presentation, 68
   definition, 68
   epidemiology, 68
   gross pathology, 68, *69*
   histopathology, 68, *70*
   imaging, 68, *68*
   radiography, 405, 419
   sites of involvement, 68
Giemsa stain, 21
   Ewing sarcoma, *251*
   in large B-cell lymphoma, *23*
   multiple myeloma, 267
GLMN gene, 290
Glomangioma, 290
Glomangiomatosis, 290
Glomangiomyoma, 290
Glomus tumor
   clinical findings, 289
   definition, 289
   epidemiology, 289
   histopathology, 289, *289*
   imaging, 289
   sites of involvement, 289
GMS stain. *See* Grocott methenamine silver (GMS) stain
Gomori stain, 21
   in large B-cell lymphoma, *23*
Gorham disease
   clinical finding, 284
   definition, 284
   differential diagnosis, 284–285
   epidemiology, 284
   histopathology, 284, *287*
   imaging, 284
   prognosis, 284
   sites of involvement, 284
Gout
   differential diagnosis, 361, 375
   radiography, 361, 375, *377*
Gram stain, 21
   in bacterial infection, *24*
Grocott methenamine silver (GMS) stain, 21
   in fungal infection, *24*
Gross pathology
   adamantinoma of long bones, 336, *337*
   aneurysmal bone cyst, 314, *326*
   angiomatoid fibrous histiocytoma, 223
   angiosarcoma, 293, *293*
   chondroblastoma, 127
   chordoma, 342, *342*
   clear cell chondrosarcoma, 147
   conventional chondrosarcoma, 140, *149*
   conventional osteosarcoma, 50, *57*
   cystic angiomatosis, 282
   dedifferentiated chondrosarcoma, 159, *160–163*
   desmoplastic fibroma, 214, *217*

Gross pathology (*Continued*)
  enchondroma, 91
  epithelioid hemangioendothelioma, 290
  epithelioid hemangioma, 282
  Erdheim-Chester disease, 243
  Ewing sarcoma, 244
  extraskeletal myxoid chondrosarcoma, 169
  fibrosarcoma, 219, *220*
  fibrous dysplasia, 194, *206*
  giant cell tumor, 299, *307*
  giant cell–rich osteosarcoma, 68, *69*
  high-grade surface osteosarcoma, 77
  intraosseous hemangioma, 276, *280*
  intraosseous lipoma, 331, *333*
  juxta-articular myxoma, 368
  Langerhans cell histiocytosis, 233
  leiomyosarcoma of bone, 344
  lipoma arborescens, 365
  liposarcoma of bone, 347
  localized pigmented nodular tenosynovitis, 360, *360*
  low-grade central osteosarcoma, 67
  lymphangioma, 286
  lymphangiomatosis, 286
  malignant lymphoma, 254
  mesenchymal chondrosarcoma, 155, *155*
  multiple myeloma, 263
  nonossifying fibroma, 182, *187*
  osteoblastoma, 44
  osteochondroma, 116, *119*
  osteoid osteoma, 38, *39*
  osteoma, 32, *34*
  parosteal osteosarcoma, 71, *73*
  periosteal chondroma, 99
  periosteal chondrosarcoma, 165, *168*
  pigmented villonodular synovitis, 354, *356*
  secondary chondrosarcoma, *172*
  simple bone cyst, 310, *315*
  skeletal metastases, 382–383
  soft-tissue chondroma, 104
  soft-tissue osteosarcoma, 81, *84*
  synovial chondromatosis, 109, *113*
  synovial hemangioma, 362
  synovial sarcoma, 369
  telangiectatic osteosarcoma, 61, *63*

H

H&E stain. *See* Hematoxylin and eosin (H&E) stain
Healed nonossifying fibroma, 415, 425
Healing fracture, callus formation of, 405, 419
Hemangioma, 402, 417
Hematoxylin and eosin (H&E) stain, 20, 21
  angiosarcoma, *294*
  cartilage lobules, *97*
  cartilaginous lobules, *97*
  chondroblastic osteosarcoma, *59*
  chondroblastoma, *133*, *134*
  chondromyxoid fibroma, *137*, *138*
  conventional chondrosarcoma, *23*, *150*
  dedifferentiated chondrosarcoma, *22*, *163*
  enchondroma, *98*
  fibrous dysplasi, *207*
  giant cell reparative granuloma, *330*
  hyaline cartilage, *98*
  juxta-articular myxoma, *368*
  Langerhans cell histiocytosis, *238*
  mesenchymal chondrosarcoma, *156*
  multiple myeloma, *267*
  osteoid osteoma, *40*
  pedunculated osteochondroma, *120*
  periosteal chondroma, *108*
  periosteal osteosarcoma, *77*
  pigmented villonodular synovitis, *358*
  pleomorphic intraosseous liposarcoma, *348*
  Rosai-Dorfman disease, *241*
  sessile osteochondroma, *120*
  skeletal metastasis, *395*
  synovial (osteo)chondromatosis, *113*
  telangiectatic osteosarcoma, *64*
Hemophilic arthropathy
  differential diagnosis, 359, 363–364, 366
  histopathology, 359, 364, 366
  magnetic resonance imaging, 366
  radiography, 363
Hereditary multiple diaphyseal sclerosis, 244
Hereditary multiple exostoses, 399, 416
High-grade surface osteosarcoma
  clinical presentation, 77
  definition, 77
  epidemiology, 77
  gross pathology, 77
  histopathology, 78, *79*
  imaging, 77
  radiography, *78*
  sites of involvement, 77
Histopathology
  adamantinoma of long bones, 336–337, *337–339*
  aneurysmal bone cyst, 314, 321, *326–328*, 401, 417
  angiomatoid fibrous histiocytoma, 223, 225, *225*
  benign fibrous histiocytoma, 189–190, *191*, *192*
  brown tumor of hyperparathyroidism, 393, 396
  calcifying enchondroma, 395
  chondroblastic osteosarcoma, 411, 422–423
  chondroblastoma, 127, *133–134*, 399, 401, 412–413, 416, 417, 424
  chondromyxoid fibroma, 135, *137*, *138*, 413–414, 424
  chordoma, 342, *343*
  clear cell chondrosarcoma, 147, *153*
  conventional chondrosarcoma, 140, 143, *150–151*, 410, 422
  conventional osteosarcoma, 50, *57–59*, 58
  cystic angiomatosis, 282, *284*
  dedifferentiated chondrosarcoma, 159, *162–165*, 164, 411, 422–423
  desmoplastic fibroma, 214, *218*, 408, 420
  enchondroma, 91, *97*, *98*, 413–414, 424
  enchondromatosis, 411, 422–423
  enostosis, 393–394
  epithelioid hemangioendothelioma, 290, 292, *292*
  Erdheim-Chester disease, 243, *243*, 395
  Ewing sarcoma, 245, *251–253*, 399, 407, 416, 420
  extraskeletal myxoid chondrosarcoma, 170
  fibrosarcoma, 219, *220–221*, 390, 408, 421
  fibrous dysplasia, 194, *207*, *208*, 403, 408, 414, 418, 420, 425
  Gaucher disease, 396
  giant cell reparative granuloma, 329–330, *330*
  giant cell tumor, 299, 301, 307, *308*, *309*, 390, 401, 404–405, 408, 417, 419, 420
  giant cell–rich osteosarcoma, 68, *70*
  glomus tumor, 289, *289*
  Gorham disease, 284, *287*
  hemophilic arthropathy, 359, 364, 366
  high-grade surface osteosarcoma, 78, *79*
  Hodgkin lymphoma, *262*, 412, 423
  inflammatory arthritis, 364
  intramedullary bone infarction, 412–413, 424
  intraosseous ganglion, 412–413, 424
  intraosseous hemangioma, 276, *281*
  intraosseous lipoma, 331, 334, 412–413, 424
  juxta-articular myxoma, 368, *368*
  Langerhans cell histiocytosis, 233, 235, *238–240*, 396, 407, 412–413, 420, 423, 424
  large B-cell lymphoma, 407, 412, 420, 423
  leiomyosarcoma of bone, 344, *346*
  lipoma arborescens, 359, 363, 365, *368*
  liposarcoma of bone, *347*, 347–348, *348*, 412–413, 424
  localized pigmented nodular tenosynovitis, 360, *360*, *361*
  low-grade central osteosarcoma, 67, *67*
  low-grade chondrosarcoma, 413–414, 424
  lymphangiomatosis, 286, *288*, *288*
  lymphoma, 390, 395
  malignant fibrous histiocytoma, 223, *224–225*
  malignant lymphoma, 254, *260*, *261*, *262*
  mastocytosis, 397
  meniscal cyst, 369
  mesenchymal chondrosarcoma, 155, *155*, *156*, 407, 411, 420, 422–423
  multiple myeloma, 263–264, *267–268*, 396, 407, 420
  myositis ossificans, 375, 413, 424
  myxoid chondrosarcoma, 157, *158*
  nonossifying fibroma, 184, *187–188*, 401, 417
  osteoblastoma, 44, *45–46*, 394, 405, 410, 414, 419, 421, 425
  osteofibrous dysplasia, 208, *213*, 214
  osteoid osteoma, 38, *40*, 405, 410, 419, 421
  osteoma, 32, *34*
  osteopoikilosis, 396
  osteosarcoma, 401, 417
  of paget osteosarcoma, *80*
  parosteal osteosarcoma, 71, *74*, 410, 422
  pedunculated osteochondroma, *120*
  periarticular ganglion, 369
  periosteal chondroma, 99, *108*, 410, 412–413, *413*, 422, 424
  periosteal chondrosarcoma, 165, *168*, *169*, 410, 422
  periosteal desmoid, 192, *193*
  periosteal osteosarcoma, 76, *77*, 414, 425
  pigmented villonodular synovitis, 354, *357*, *358*, 362, 366
  plasmacytoma, 390, 412, 423
  postradiation osteosarcoma, 78
  primitive neuroectodermal tumors, 253
  Rosai-Dorfman disease, 241, *241*
  secondary chondrosarcoma, *173*, *174*

sessile osteochondroma, 120
simple bone cyst, 310, 315–316
skeletal metastases, 383, 393–396
small cell osteosarcoma, 65, 65, 414, 425
soft-tissue chondroma, 104, 109, 361
soft-tissue chondrosarcoma, 170, 377, 413, 424
soft-tissue osteosarcoma, 81, 85, 377, 413, 424
synovial (osteo)chondromatosis, 111, 113, 356, 362, 366, 404, 418
synovial hemangioma, 359, 362, 366, 366
synovial sarcoma, 361, 369, 375, 375–377
telangiectatic osteosarcoma, 61, 63, 63, 64, 414, 425
tumoral calcinosis, 410, 422
undifferentiated pleomorphic sarcoma, 411, 422–423
HMB45, 26
Hodgkin lymphoma
　characteristic for, 423
　histopathology, 254, 262, 412, 423
　increased uptake of radiopharmaceutical tracer, 409, 421
　radiography, 256
Hyperparathyroidism
　brown tumor of, 240, 268, 284, 393, 396
　computed tomography, 402–403, 418

I
IFs. See Intermediate filaments (IFs)
Immunohistochemistry (IHC), 23, 25–26
　adamantinoma of long bones, 337
　angiomatoid fibrous histiocytoma, 223, 225
　antibodies
　　in bone tumor pathology, 26–27
　　against hematopoietic and lymphoid cells, and vascular antigens, 25
　　against intermediate filaments, 23–25
　　against muscle and neuroectodermal antigens, 25–26
　chondroblastoma, 134
　chordoma, 25, 342
　conventional osteosarcoma, 58
　eosinophilic granuloma, 235
　epithelioid hemangioendothelioma, 292
　Erdheim-Chester disease, 243
　Ewing sarcoma, 26
　intraosseous hemangioma, 281
　intraosseous lipoma, 334
　juxta-articular myxoma, 369
　Langerhans cell histiocytosis, 26, 235
　leiomyosarcoma of bone, 344
　liposarcoma of bone, 348
　localized pigmented nodular tenosynovitis, 360
　lymphangiomatosis, 288
　malignant glomus tumor, 290
　malignant lymphoma, 254
　mesenchymal chondrosarcoma, 157
　metastases, 24
　multiple myeloma, 264
　osteofibrous dysplasia, 208
　osteosarcoma, 27
　pigmented villonodular synovitis, 354
　Rosai-Dorfman disease, 241
　round cell lesions, 232t
　skeletal metastases, 386, 394–396

small cell osteosarcoma, 65
synovial sarcoma, 374, 376
Inflammatory arthritis
　differential diagnosis, 364
　histopathology, 364
　radiography, 364
Intermediate filaments (IFs), 23, 25
Intra-articular osteochondroma, 119
Intramedullary bone infarction
　histopathology, 412–413, 424
　magnetic resonance imaging, 412–413, 424
Intraosseous ganglion
　differential diagnosis, 134, 309
　histopathology, 412–413, 424
　lateral radiograph, 409, 421
　magnetic resonance imaging, 412–413, 424
Intraosseous hemangioma
　clinical findings, 273
　computed tomography, 273, 275, 276
　definition, 273
　differential diagnosis, 281
　epidemiology, 273
　gross pathology, 276, 280
　histopathology, 276, 281
　immunohistochemistry, 281
　magnetic resonance angiography, 278, 279
　magnetic resonance imaging, 273, 276–278
　prognosis, 281
　radiography of, 273, 273–275
　scintigraphy, 273
　sites of involvement, 273
Intraosseous lipoma
　clinical findings, 330
　computed tomography, 331, 332
　definition, 330
　differential diagnosis, 334, 348
　epidemiology, 330
　genetics, 334
　gross pathology, 331, 333
　histopathology, 331, 334, 412–413, 424
　immunohistochemistry, 334
　lateral radiograph, 409, 421
　magnetic resonance imaging, 331, 332, 412–413, 424
　prognosis, 334
　radiography, 330–331, 331, 332
　sites of involvement, 330
Intraosseous liposarcoma
　differential diagnosis, 334
　histopathology, 347, 348

J
Jaffe-Campanacci syndrome, 401–402, 405, 417, 419
Joints lesions
　benign tumors
　　juxta-articular myxoma, 366, 368–369
　　lipoma arborescens, 364–366
　　localized pigmented nodular tenosynovitis, 359–361
　　pigmented nodular tenosynovitis, 353–359
　　synovial (osteo)chondromatosis, 353
　　synovial hemangioma, 362–364
　malignant tumors
　　synovial chondrosarcoma, 377
　　synovial sarcoma, 369–377

Juxta-articular myxoma
　clinical findings, 366
　definition, 366
　differential diagnosis, 369
　epidemiology, 366
　genetics, 369
　gross pathology, 368
　histopathology, 368, 368
　immunohistochemistry, 369
　magnetic resonance imaging, 368
　prognosis, 369
　radiography, 368
　sites of involvement, 366
Juxtacortical chondroma. See Periosteal chondroma
Juxtacortical chondrosarcoma. See Periosteal chondrosarcoma
Juxtacortical myositis ossificans, 415, 426
　differential diagnosis, 74–75, 76
Juxtacortical osteoma, 121

K
Kempson-Campanacci lesion. See Osteofibrous dysplasia

L
Langerhans cell histiocytosis (LCH)
　clinical findings, 231, 233
　computed tomography, 237
　definition, 231
　differential diagnosis, 189, 236, 240, 253, 288
　electron microscopy, 235, 240
　epidemiology, 231
　histopathology, 233, 235, 238–240, 396, 407, 412–413, 420, 423, 424
　hole-in-hole appearance, 396
　immunohistochemistry, 235
　magnetic resonance imaging, 233, 235–238, 412–413, 424
　pathology, 233, 235
　periosteal reaction, 8, 9
　prognosis, 235, 236
　radiography, 233, 233–236, 402, 417–418
　scintigraphy, 233, 236
　sites of involvement, 231
Large B-cell lymphoma
　Giemsa stain in, 23
　Gomori stain in, 23
　histopathology, 407, 412, 420, 423
LCH. See Langerhans cell histiocytosis (LCH)
Leiomyosarcoma of bone, 399, 416
　clinical findings, 344
　computed tomography, 344, 344, 345
　definition, 344
　differential diagnosis, 347
　electron microscopy, 344
　epidemiology, 344
　genetics, 347
　gross pathology, 344
　histopathology, 344, 346
　immunohistochemistry, 344
　magnetic resonance imaging, 344, 345
　prognosis, 347
　radiography, 344, 344, 345
　sites of involvement, 344

Lesion
  borders of, 3, 5, 6
  central location, 4
  eccentric location, 5
  matrix, 11–12
  predilection, 3, 4
  site of, 2–3, 3–5
  type of bone destruction, 6, 6–7, 7
Letterer-Siwe disease, 233
Li-Fraumeni syndrome, 399, 416
Lipogranulomatosis, 242–244
Lipoma arborescens, 406, 419
  clinical findings, 365
  definition, 364
  differential diagnosis, 359, 363, 365–366
  epidemiology, 364
  gross pathology, 365
  histopathology, 359, 363, 365, 368
  magnetic resonance imaging, 359, 365, 367–368
  prognosis, 365
  radiography, 363, 365
  sites of involvement, 365
Liposarcoma of bone, 413, 424
  clinical features, 347
  definition, 347
  differential diagnosis, 348
  epidemiology, 347
  genetics, 348
  gross pathology, 347
  histopathology, 347, 347–348, 348, 412–413, 424
  immunohistochemistry, 348
  magnetic resonance imaging, 347, 412–413, 424
  prognosis, 348
  radiography, 347
  sites of involvement, 347
Liposclerosing myxofibrous tumor, 181t, 197
Localized pigmented nodular tenosynovitis
  clinical findings, 359
  definition, 359
  differential diagnosis, 360–361, 369
  epidemiology, 359
  genetics, 360
  gross pathology, 360, 360
  histopathology, 360, 360, 361
  immunohistochemistry, 360
  magnetic resonance imaging, 359
  prognosis, 360
  radiography, 359, 359
  sites of involvement, 359
Low-grade central osteosarcoma
  clinical presentation, 66
  definition, 66
  differential diagnosis, 67
  epidemiology, 66
  genetics, 67
  gross pathology, 67
  histopathology, 67, 67
  imaging, 66–67
  prognosis, 68
  radiography, 66–67
  sites of involvement, 66
Low-grade chondrosarcoma
  differential diagnosis, 97
  histopathology, 413–414, 424
  magnetic resonance imaging, 413–414, 424

Lymphangiography, lymphangiomatosis, 286
Lymphangioma
  clinical findings, 286
  definition, 285
  differential diagnosis, 288–289
  epidemiology, 285
  gross pathology, 286
  histopathology, 286–288
  imaging, 286
  immunohistochemistry, 288
  prognosis, 288
  sites of involvement, 285–286
Lymphangiomatosis
  clinical findings, 286
  definition, 285
  differential diagnosis, 288–289
  epidemiology, 285
  gross pathology, 286
  histopathology, 286, 288, 288
  imaging, 286
  immunohistochemistry, 288
  lymphangiography, 286
  prognosis, 288
  sites of involvement, 285–286
Lymphoma
  differential diagnosis, 243, 347, 390, 395
  malignant
    clinical features, 254
    computed tomography, 254, 256–260
    definition, 254
    differential diagnosis, 258, 263
    epidemiology, 254
    histopathology, 260–262
    immunohistochemistry, 254
    magnetic resonance imaging, 254, 259–260
    pathology, 254
    PET, 259–260
    PET-CT, 259–260
    prognosis, 258
    radiography, 255–260
    scintigraphy, 258
    sites of involvement, 254
    types, 254
Lytic metastases, 221
  in men, 50, 62, 68, 152, 159, 216, 255, 273
  from renal cell carcinoma, 409, 421
  in women, 4, 211, 255, 265, 335, 345, 383, 384, 388, 392

M

Maffucci syndrome, 97, 103, 399, 403, 416, 418
Magnetic resonance angiography, intraosseous hemangioma, 278, 279
Magnetic resonance imaging (MRI), 2, 12, 14–17
  adamantinoma of long bones, 334
  aneurysmal bone cyst, 314, 320, 322–325
  calcifications, 14, 16
  chondroblastoma, 131, 132, 412–413, 424
  chondromyxoid fibroma, 135, 137, 413–414, 424
  chordoma, 340, 341
  clear cell chondrosarcoma, 145, 152
  conventional chondrosarcoma, 140, 146–148
  conventional osteosarcoma, 50, 54–56, 403–404, 418
  cystic angiomatosis, 282

  dedifferentiated chondrosarcoma, 159, 160
  desmoplastic fibroma, 210, 216
  enchondroma, 91, 93–96, 413–414, 424
  epithelioid hemangioendothelioma, 290, 291
  Erdheim-Chester disease, 242
  Ewing sarcoma, 244, 247, 248, 250–251
  fibrosarcoma, 219
  with gadolinium, 14, 16–17
  giant cell reparative granuloma, 329
  giant cell tumor, 14, 16, 299, 303–306
  giant cell–rich osteosarcoma, 14, 17, 68–69
  glomus tumor, 289
  of Gorham disease, 284, 286
  hemophilic arthropathy, 366
  intramedullary bone infarction, 412–413, 424
  intraosseous ganglion, 412–413, 424
  intraosseous hemangioma, 273, 276–279
  intraosseous lipoma, 331, 332, 412–413, 424
  juxta-articular myxoma, 368
  Langerhans cell histiocytosis, 233, 235–238, 412–413, 424
  left proximal humerus, 14, 15
  leiomyosarcoma of bone, 344, 345
  lipoma arborescens, 359, 365, 367–368
  liposarcoma of bone, 347, 412–413, 424
  localized pigmented nodular tenosynovitis, 359
  low-grade chondrosarcoma, 413–414, 424
  of lymphangiomatosis, 286
  malignant fibrous histiocytoma, 221, 222
  malignant lymphoma, 254, 259–260
  Mazabraud syndrome, 205–206, 401–402, 417
  medullary cavity of femur, 14, 16
  melorheostosis, 403–404, 418
  meniscal cyst, 369
  mesenchymal chondrosarcoma, 154, 154–155
  mixed metastases, 392
  of monostotic fibrous dysplasia, 202
  multiple myeloma, 263
  multiple osteocartilaginous exostoses, 127–129
  nonossifying fibroma, 182, 186
  Ollier disease, 102–103
  osteoblastoma, 45
  osteochondroma, 116, 119
  osteofibrous dysplasia, 211–212
  osteoid osteoma, 38, 39
  osteoma, 32
  osteosarcoma, 401–402, 417
  parosteal osteosarcoma, 403–404, 418
  periarticular ganglion, 369
  periosteal chondroma, 99, 107, 412–413, 424
  periosteal chondrosarcoma, 14, 15, 166, 167
  periosteal desmoid, 192
  periosteal osteosarcoma, 76, 403–404, 407, 418, 420
  pigmented villonodular synovitis, 354, 356, 365–366
  plasmacytoma, 266–267
  polyostotic fibrous dysplasia, 203, 204
  proximal humerus, 14, 15, 17
  secondary chondrosarcoma, 173
  sessile osteochondroma, 118
  signal intensity, 14, 15t

simple bone cyst, 310, *313, 314*
skeletal metastases, 382, *391–392, 393*
soft-tissue chondrosarcoma, 377
soft-tissue osteosarcoma, *82–83*, 377
synovial chondromatosis, 109, *112*
synovial hemangioma, 359, 362, *364, 365, 366*
synovial sarcoma, 369, *370–374*
telangiectatic osteosarcoma, *62*
Malignant fibrous histiocytoma
  clinical finding, 221
  complicating medullary bone infarct, *223*
  definition, 221
  differential diagnosis, 59–60, 223
  epidemiology, 221
  genetics, 223
  gross pathology, 221, 223
  histopathology, 223, *224–225*
  imaging, 221
  prognostic factors, 223
  radiography, 221, *221, 222*
  sites of involvement, 221
Malignant glomus tumor, 290
Malignant lymphoma
  clinical features, 254
  computed tomography, 254, *256–260*
  definition, 254
  differential diagnosis, 61, 66, 258, 263
  epidemiology, 254
  histopathology, *260–262*
  immunohistochemistry, 254
  magnetic resonance imaging, 254, *259–260*
  pathology, 254
  PET, *259–260*
  PET-CT, *259–260*
  prognosis, 258
  radiography, *255–260*
  scintigraphy, *258*
  sites of involvement, 254
  types, 254
Malignant transformation
  enchondroma, 171, *172, 173*
  osteochondroma, 171, *172*, 401, 417
  pagetic bone, *174*, 175
  synovial (osteo) chondromatosis, *174*, 175
Malignant tumor
  adamantinoma of long bones, 334–339
  bone-forming lesions
    osteosarcomas, 47–78
    secondary osteosarcomas, 78–80
    soft-tissue osteosarcoma, 81–85
  cartilage-forming lesions, 138
    clear cell chondrosarcoma, 145–147, 152, *153*
    conventional chondrosarcoma, 139–145, *146–151*
    dedifferentiated chondrosarcoma, 157, 159–165
    mesenchymal chondrosarcoma, 152, 154–157
    myxoid chondrosarcoma, 157
    periosteal chondrosarcoma, 164–169
    secondary chondrosarcomas, 171–175
    soft-tissue chondrosarcoma, 169–171
  chordoma, 339–344
  fibrohistiocytic lesions
    angiomatoid fibrous histiocytoma, 223–225

    fibrosarcoma, 218–221
    malignant fibrous histiocytoma, 221–223
  joints lesions
    synovial chondrosarcoma, 377
    synovial sarcoma, 369–377
  leiomyosarcoma of bone, 344–347
  liposarcoma of bone, 347–348
  round cell lesions
    Ewing sarcoma, 244–253
    malignant lymphoma, 254–263
    multiple myeloma, 263–268
  vascular lesions
    angiosarcoma, 293–295
    epithelioid hemangioendothelioma, 290–293
Mastocytosis
  histopathology, 397
  radiography, 396
Mazabraud syndrome
  computed tomography, *205–206*
  magnetic resonance imaging, *205–206*, 401–402, 417
  radiography, *205–206*
McCune-Albright syndrome, 403, 418
Medullary bone infarct, 406, 419
  differential diagnosis, 93, 97, 334
  osteosarcoma with, 415, 426
  radiography, 411, 423
Melan A, 26
Melorheostosis
  magnetic resonance imaging, 403–404, 418
  monostotic form of, 35
  radiography, 403–404, 418
Meniscal cyst
  differential diagnosis, 369
  histopathology, 369
  magnetic resonance imaging, 369
Mesenchymal chondrosarcoma, 405, 419
  clinical findings, 154
  definition, 152
  epidemiology, 154
  genetics, 155
  histopathology, 155, *155, 156*, 407, 411, 420, 422–423
  immunohistochemistry, *157*
  magnetic resonance imaging, 154, *154–155*
  pathology, 155
  prognosis, 157
  radiography, 154, *154–155*, 411, 422–423
  sites of involvement, 154
Metastasis. *See also specific types*
  differential diagnosis, 263, 292–293, 342, 344
  from melanoma, *395*
Metastatic neuroblastoma, 288
Mixed metastases, 382
  magnetic resonance imaging, *392*
  radiography, *388, 392*
Molecular cytogenetics, 28–29
Monostotic fibrous dysplasia, 184, 189, 209, 218, 311
MRI. *See* Magnetic resonance imaging (MRI)
Multicentric osteosarcoma, 397
Multifocal osteoblastic metastases
  mastocytosis, 396–397
  osteopoikilosis, 396
  osteosarcomatosis, 397

Multifocal osteolytic metastases
  brown tumors of hyperparathyroidism, 396
  diffuse osteoporosis, 396
  Gaucher disease, 396
  Langerhans cell histiocytosis, 396
  multiple myeloma, 395–396
Multifocal/multicentric osteosarcoma
  clinical presentation, 69
  definition, 68
  differential diagnosis, 69
  epidemiology, 68
  imaging, 69
  pathology, 69
  prognosis, 69
  sites of involvement, 68
Multiple diaphyseal sclerosis. *See* Ribbing disease
Multiple hereditary osteochondromata, 121
  computed tomography, *126–128*
  magnetic resonance imaging, *127–129*
  radiography, *123–126, 129*
Multiple myeloma, 407, 420
  characteristic features, 403, 418
  clinical features, 263
  computed tomography, 263, *266*, 402–403, 418
  definition, 263
  differential diagnosis, 268, 395–396
  epidemiology, 263
  genetics, 264–265
  histopathology, 263–264, *267–268*, 407, 420
  immunohistochemistry, 264
  magnetic resonance imaging, 263
  prognostic factors, 265
  radiography, 263, *264–266*
  scintigraphy, 263
  sites of involvement, 263
Mutation of p53, 399, 416
Myeloma
  bone destruction and, 6, *7*
  multiple (*see* Multiple myeloma)
MyoD, 25
Myogenin, 25
Myositis ossificans
  computed tomography, 413, 424
  differential diagnosis, 85, 104, 169, 375
  histopathology, 375, 413, 424
  imaging, 375
Myxoid chondrosarcoma
  definition, 157
  differential diagnosis, 157
  epidemiology, 157
  histopathology, *158*
  pathology, 157
  radiography, 157, *158*
  sites of involvement, 157

N

Neurofibromatosis, 403, 418
NF1 gene, 290
Nonossifying fibroma (NOF), 400, 417
  clinical findings, 182
  computed tomography, 182, *185*
  definition, 181
  differential diagnosis, 138, 184, 189, 190, 197, 209, 311, 338
  epidemiology, 182
  gross pathology, 182, *187*
  histopathology, 184, *187–188*, 401, 417

Nonossifying fibroma (NOF) (Continued)
　magnetic resonance imaging, 182, *186*
　prognosis, 184
　radiography, 182, *182–186*, 400, 416
　　at right femur, 3, *5*
　scintigraphy, 182
　site of involvement, 182
Nora lesion, 76–77, 119
Novotny stain, 21
　in Ewing sarcoma, *24*

O

Ollier disease, 97, 403, 418
　computed tomography, *102*
　differential diagnosis, 197, 201
　magnetic resonance imaging, *102–103*
　radiography, *97, 100, 101*
Osteoarthritis, 35, 111
Osteoblastic matrix, 11, *13*
Osteoblastic metastases, 382. *See also* Skeletal metastases
　multifocal
　　mastocytosis, 396–397
　　osteopoikilosis, 396
　　osteosarcomatosis, 397
　radiography, 382, *387*
　solitary
　　calcifying enchondroma, 394–395
　　enostosis, 393–394
　　Erdheim-Chester disease, 395
　　lymphoma, 395
　　osteoblastoma, 394
Osteoblastoma
　clinical findings, 41
　computed tomography, *44*
　definition, 41
　differential diagnosis, 40, 46–47, 190
　epidemiology, 41
　histopathology, *45–46*, 394, 405, 410, 414, 419, 421, 425
　imaging, 41, 44
　magnetic resonance imaging, *45*
　pathology, 44, 46
　prognosis, 46
　radiography, *41–44*, 405, 419
　sites of involvement, 41
Osteocartilaginous exostosis. *See* Osteochondroma
Osteochondroma
　clinical findings, 114
　complications, 119
　　adjacent bone fracture, *121*
　　adjacent bone pressure erosion, *121*
　　bursa exostotica, *122*
　　malignant transformation, *122*
　computed tomography, 116, *117*
　definition, 114
　differential diagnosis, 119, 121
　epidemiology, 114
　features, 403, 418
　genetics, 116
　gross specimen, 116, *119*
　magnetic resonance imaging, 116, *119*
　malignant transformation, 116t, 401, 417
　　clinical findings, 171
　　epidemiology, 171
　　gross specimen, *172*
　　histopathologic findings, 171
　　radiography, *171, 172*
　pathology, 116
　pedunculated (*see* Pedunculated osteochondroma)
　prognosis, 119
　radiography, 114, 116, *117*, 119
　sessile (*see* Sessile osteochondroma)
　sites of involvement, 114
Osteochondromatosis
　synovial, 353
　　clinical findings, 109
　　computed tomography, 109, *110, 111*
　　definition, 107
　　differential diagnosis, 111, 356, 362, 366
　　epidemiology, 107
　　genetics, 111
　　gross pathology, 109, *113*
　　histopathology, 111, *113*, 356, 362, 366
　　magnetic resonance imaging, 109, *112*
　　pathology, 109, 111
　　prognostic factors/complications, 111
　　radiography, 109, *109–112*, 356, 362, 366
　　secondary chondrosarcoma, *173, 174*
　　sites of involvement, 107
Osteofibrous dysplasia, 399, 405, 408, 409, 416, 419, 420, 421
　clinical findings, 208
　definition, 206
　differential diagnosis, 189, 197, 209, 338
　epidemiology, 206, 208
　genetics, 209
　gross pathology, 208
　histopathology, 208, *213, 214*
　imaging, 208
　immunohistochemistry, 208
　prognosis, 209
　radiography of, *210–212*
　sites of involvement, 208
Osteoid osteoma, 399, 416
　clinical findings, 35
　complications, 40
　computed tomography, 35, *38–39*
　definition, 35
　differential diagnosis, 40, 46, 409, 421
　epidemiology, 35
　genetics, 35
　histopathology, 35, *40*, 405, 410, 419, 421
　imaging, 35, *36, 37*
　magnetic resonance imaging, 35, *39*
　pathology, 35
　prognosis, 40
　radiography, 405, 419
　scintigraphy, 35, *37, 38*
　sites of involvement, 35
　ultrasound, 38
Osteolytic metastases. *See also* Skeletal metastases
　computed tomography, *384*, 402–403, 418
　differential diagnosis, 221, 223, 265, 268, 309, 347
　histopathology, 284
　multifocal
　　brown tumors of hyperparathyroidism, 396
　　diffuse osteoporosis, 396
　　Gaucher disease, 396
　　Langerhans cell histiocytosis, 396
　　multiple myeloma, 395–396
　origin, *382*
　radiography, 284, 382, *383–385*
　solitary
　　brown tumor of hyperparathyroidism, 393
　　fibrosarcoma, 390
　　giant cell tumor, 390
　　plasmacytoma, 390
Osteoma
　clinical findings, 32
　definition, 32
　differential diagnosis, 35
　epidemiology, 32
　imaging, 32, *33*
　pathology, 32, *34*
　prognosis, 35
　sites of involvement, 32
Osteomyelitis
　chronic draining sinus tract, 415, 426
　differential diagnosis, 236, 242, 253, 339
　soft-tissue mass in, 11, *11*
Osteopoikilosis, 396
Osteoporosis, *36*, 418
　diffuse, 396
Osteosarcoma, 399, 416
　classification, 48
　conventional
　　clinical presentation, 47
　　complications, 61
　　computed tomography, 48, *53*
　　definition, 47
　　differential diagnosis, 59–61
　　epidemiology, 47
　　genetics, 58
　　gross pathology, 50, *57*
　　histopathology, 50, *57–59*, 58
　　immunohistochemistry, 58
　　magnetic resonance imaging, 50, *54–56*
　　prognosis, 61
　　radiography, 47–48, *49–51*
　　scintigraphy, 48, *52–53*
　　sites of involvement, 47
　differential diagnosis, 47, 143, 193, 249, 253, 258
　in fibrous dysplasia, 415, 426
　giant cell–rich
　　clinical presentation, 68
　　definition, 68
　　epidemiology, 68
　　gross pathology, 68
　　histopathology, 68
　　imaging, 68, *68*
　　sites of involvement, 68
　histologic grading of, 49t
　histopathology, 401, 417
　low-grade central
　　clinical presentation, 66
　　definition, 66
　　differential diagnosis, 67
　　epidemiology, 66
　　genetics, 67
　　gross pathology, 67
　　histopathology, 67, *67*
　　imaging, 66–67
　　prognosis, 68

radiography, 66–67
    sites of involvement, 66
magnetic resonance imaging, 401–402, 417
with medullary bone infarcts, 415, 426
multifocal/multicentric
    clinical presentation, 69
    definition, 68
    differential diagnosis, 69
    epidemiology, 68
    imaging, 69
    pathology, 69
    prognosis, 69
    sites of involvement, 68
periosteal reaction, 8, 10
postirradiation, 415, 426
risk of, 399, 416
small cell
    clinical presentation, 64
    definition, 64
    differential diagnosis, 65–66
    epidemiology, 64
    genetics, 65
    histopathology, 65, 65
    imaging, 64–65
    immunohistochemistry, 65
    prognosis, 66
    sites of involvement, 64
soft-tissue, 11
    histopathology, 377
    magnetic resonance imaging, 377
surface
    high-grade surface osteosarcoma, 77–78
    parosteal osteosarcoma, 69–75
    periosteal osteosarcoma, 75–77
telangiectatic
    clinical presentation, 61
    definition, 61
    differential diagnosis, 63–64
    epidemiology, 61
    genetics, 63
    gross pathology, 61, 63
    histopathology, 61, 63, 63, 64
    imaging, 61
    magnetic resonance imaging, 62
    prognosis, 64
    radiography, 61, 61, 62
    sites of involvement, 61
tumor tissue composition, 11
Osteosarcomatosis, 397

P

Pachydysostosis, 197
Paget disease
    complication, 415, 426
    differential diagnosis, 243–244, 263
    osteolytic phase of, 402–403, 418
Paget osteosarcoma, 79, 416
    computed tomography, 80
    histopathology, 80
Pagetic bone, 426
    chondrosarcoma in, 174, 175
    histopathology, 79, 80
Parosteal lipoma with ossifications, 75
Parosteal myositis ossificans, 35
Parosteal osteoma, 74, 121
Parosteal osteosarcoma, 35, 399, 412, 416, 423
    clinical presentation, 70

definition, 69
differential diagnosis, 71–75, 76, 409, 421
and distal femur, 3, 4
epidemiology, 69
genetics, 71
gross pathology, 71, 73
histopathology, 71, 74, 410, 422
imaging, 70
magnetic resonance imaging, 403–404, 418
prognosis, 75
radiography, 403–404, 410, 418, 422
sites of involvement, 70
PAS stain. See Periodic acid–Schiff (PAS) stain
Pathology
    bone tumors, type, 20, 21t
    decalcification, 20–21
    electron microscopy, 27
    genetics of bone tumors, 27
        cytogenetics, 27–28
        molecular cytogenetics, 28–29
    immunohistochemistry, 23–27
    special stains, 21–23
PCR. See Polymerase chain reaction (PCR)
Pedunculated osteochondroma
    histopathology, 120
    radiography, 114
Periarticular ganglion
    differential diagnosis, 369
    histopathology, 369
    magnetic resonance imaging, 369
Periodic acid–Schiff (PAS) stain, 21
    in Ewing sarcoma, 24
Periosteal chondroma
    in children/young adults, 414, 424
    clinical findings, 99
    computed tomography, 99, 106–107, 413, 424
    definition, 99
    differential diagnosis, 99, 104, 119, 169, 193
    epidemiology, 99
    histopathology, 99, 108, 410, 412–413, 413, 422, 424
    magnetic resonance imaging, 99, 107, 412–413, 424
    pathology, 99
    prognostic factors, 99
    radiography, 99, 105, 106, 107, 410, 422
    sites of involvement, 99
Periosteal chondrosarcoma
    clinical findings, 164
    definition, 164
    differential diagnosis, 76, 165
    epidemiology, 164
    histopathology, 165, 168, 169, 410, 422
    imaging features, 410, 422
    magnetic resonance imaging, 166, 167
    pathology, 165, 169
    radiography, 165–167, 410, 422
    scintigraphy, 167
    sites of involvement, 164
Periosteal desmoid, 415, 425
    clinical findings, 192
    definition, 192
    differential diagnosis, 192–194
    epidemiology, 192
    histopathology, 192, 193
    imaging, 192, 192, 193
    prognosis, 192

sites of involvement, 192
Periosteal osteoblastoma, 104
Periosteal osteosarcoma
    clinical presentation, 75
    definition, 75
    differential diagnosis, 74, 76–77, 165
    epidemiology, 75
    genetics, 76
    gross pathology, 76
    histopathology, 76, 77, 414, 425
    imaging, 75
    magnetic resonance imaging, 403–404, 407, 418, 420
    prognosis, 77
    radiography, 403–404, 418
    sites of involvement, 75
Periosteal reaction, 7–10
    neoplastic and nonneoplastic processes, 8t
    types of, 7, 9–10
PET. See Positron emission tomography (PET)
PET–CT, 18–20
    breast carcinoma, 19, 19–20
    Ewing sarcoma, 249–251
    malignant lymphoma, 259–260
    radiology, 19–20
    sclerotic metastasis, 382, 389
    skeletal metastases, 382, 390–392
    synovial sarcoma, 373–374
PET-MRI, 18–20
Pigmented villonodular synovitis (PVNS)
    clinical findings, 354
    contrast arthrography, 354, 355
    definition, 353
    differential diagnosis, 356, 359, 362, 365–366
    epidemiology, 354
    genetics, 356
    gross pathology, 354, 356
    histopathology, 354, 357, 358, 362, 366
    immunohistochemistry, 354
    magnetic resonance imaging, 354, 356, 365–366
    prognosis, 356
    radiography, 354, 354, 355, 362
    sites of involvement, 354
Plasma cell myeloma. See Multiple myeloma
Plasmacytoma, 409, 421
    differential diagnosis, 220, 223, 265, 268, 293, 309, 342, 390
    histopathology, 412, 423
    magnetic resonance imaging, 266–267
Pleomorphic undifferentiated sarcoma
    clinical finding, 221
    complicating medullary bone infarct, 223
    definition, 221
    differential diagnosis, 223
    epidemiology, 221
    genetics, 223
    gross pathology, 221, 223
    histopathology, 223, 224–225
    imaging, 221
    prognostic factors, 223
    radiography, 221, 221, 222
    sites of involvement, 221
PNET. See Primitive neuroectodermal tumor (PNET)
POEMS syndrome, 263, 403, 407

Polymerase chain reaction (PCR), 29
Polyostotic fibrous dysplasia, 403, 418
    characteristic features, 403, 418
    differential diagnosis, 288–289
    postcontrast MRI, 403, 418
Positron emission tomography (PET), 2, 18–20
    Ewing sarcoma, 249–251
    malignant lymphoma, 259–260
    radiology, 19–20
    of skeletal metastases, 19, *19*, 382
Postirradiation osteosarcoma, 415, 426
Postradiation osteosarcoma
    clinical presentation, 78
    criteria for diagnosis, 78
    definition, 78
    differential diagnosis, 78
    epidemiology, 78
    imaging, 78
    pathology, 78
    prognosis, 78
    sites of involvement, 78
Posttraumatic cyst, 409, 421
Primary (osteo) chondromatosis, chondrosarcoma in, 175
Primitive neuroectodermal tumor (PNET)
    clinical features, 244
    definition, 244
    differential diagnosis, 249, 253
    epidemiology, 244
    histopathology, 245, *253*
    pathology, 245
    prognosis, 249
    sites of involvement, 244
Progressive diaphyseal dysplasia. See Camurati-Engelmann disease
Proximal humerus
    calcified lesion, *92*
    cartilaginous lesion, *106*
    radiolucent lesion, *97, 105*
    resected surgical specimen, *161*
    sessile lesion, *119*
Proximal phalanx
    middle finger, *33, 91*, 417
    osteomyelitis, *11*
    radiolucent lesion, *91*
    saucer-like erosion, *105*
    soft-tissue mass, *170*
Pseudocyst of calcaneus, 334
Pseudotumors of hemophilia
    histopathology, 284
    radiography, 284
PVNS. See Pigmented villonodular synovitis (PVNS)

R

Radiation-induced osteonecrosis, 78
Radiography
    adamantinoma of long bones, 334, *335, 336*
    aneurysmal bone cyst, 312, *316–320, 322–325*, 400, 416
    angiosarcoma, 293, *293*, 402, 417
    benign fibrous histiocytoma, 189, *190, 191*
    chondroblastic osteosarcoma, 411, 422–423
    chondroblastoma, *129–132*, 399, 400, 416
    chondromyxoid fibroma, 135, *135, 136*, 406, 411, 420, 423
    chordoma, 339–340, *340*
    clear cell chondrosarcoma, 145, *152*, 411, 423
    conventional chondrosarcoma, 140, *141–142, 144, 146, 147, 148*, 410, 411, 422, 423
    conventional osteosarcoma, 47–48, *49–51*, 403–404, 405, 418, 419
    cortical metastases, 382, *385*
    cystic angiomatosis, 282, *283*
    dedifferentiated chondrosarcoma, 159, *159, 160*, 411, 422–423
    desmoplastic fibroma, 210, *215–217*
    enchondroma, 91, *91–95*, 402, 411, 418, 423
    enchondromatosis, 97, 99, 411, 422–423
    enostosis, 393, 414–415, 425
    epithelioid hemangioendothelioma, 290, *291*
    Erdheim-Chester disease, 242, *242*
    Ewing sarcoma, 244, *244–249*, 399, 402, 416, 417
    fibrosarcoma, 219, *219*
    fibrous cortical defect, 182, *182*
    fibrous dysplasia, 408, 420
    giant cell reparative granuloma, 329, *329*
    giant cell tumor, 299, *299–302, 304, 305*, 400, 409, 416, 421
    giant cell–rich osteosarcoma, 68–69, 405, 419
    glomus tumor, 289
    Gorham disease, 284, *285*, 286
    gout, 361, 375, 377
    hemangioma, 402, 417
    hemophilic arthropathy, 363
    high-grade surface osteosarcoma, 78
    Hodgkin lymphoma, *256*
    inflammatory arthritis, 364
    of intraosseous hemangioma, 273, *273–275*
    intraosseous lipoma, 330–331, *331, 332*
    juxta-articular myxoma, 368
    Langerhans cell histiocytosis, 233, *233–236*, 402, 417–418
    leiomyosarcoma of bone, 344, *344, 345*
    lipoma arborescens, 363, 365
    liposarcoma of bone, 347
    localized pigmented nodular tenosynovitis, 359, *359*
    low-grade central osteosarcoma, 66–67
    Maffucci syndrome, *103*
    malignant fibrous histiocytoma, 221, *221, 222*
    malignant lymphoma, 255–260
    mastocytosis, 396
    Mazabraud syndrome, 205–206
    medullary bone infarct, 411, 423
    melorheostosis, 403–404, 418
    mesenchymal chondrosarcoma, 154, *154–155*, 411, 422–423
    mixed metastases, 388, *392*
    of monostotic fibrous dysplasia, 195, *196, 199, 202*
    of multicentric osteosarcoma, 70–71
    multiple myeloma, 263, *264, 265, 266*
    multiple osteocartilaginous exostoses, *123–126, 129*
    myxoid chondrosarcoma, 157, *158*
    nonossifying fibroma, 182, *183–186*, 400, 416
    Ollier disease, 97, *100, 101*
    osteoblastic metastases, 382, *387*
    osteoblastoma, *41–44*, 405, 419
    osteochondroma, 114, 116, *117*, 119
    of osteofibrous dysplasia, *210–212*
    osteoid osteoma, 35, *36, 37*, 405, 419
    osteolytic metastases, 382, *383–385*
    osteoma, 32, 33
    osteopoikilosis, 396
    of paget osteosarcoma, *80*
    parosteal osteosarcoma, 72, 403–404, 410, 418, 422
    pedunculated osteochondroma, 114
    periosteal chondroma, 99, *105–107*, 410, 422
    periosteal chondrosarcoma, *165–167*, 410, 422
    periosteal desmoid, 192, *192*, 193
    periosteal osteosarcoma, 75, 403–404, 418
    pigmented villonodular synovitis, 354, *354, 355*, 362
    polyostotic fibrous dysplasia, *197, 198, 201, 203, 204*
    secondary chondrosarcoma, *171–174*
    sessile osteochondroma, *115*, 116
    simple bone cyst, 310, *310–313*, 409, 421
    skeletal lymphangiomatosis, 286, 288
    skeletal metastases, 382
    soft-tissue chondrosarcoma, 170
    soft-tissue osteosarcoma, 81
    synovial (osteo)chondromatosis, 109, *109–112*, 356, 362, 366
    synovial hemangioma, 362, *363*
    synovial sarcoma, 369, *370, 371, 372–374*
    telangiectatic osteosarcoma, 61, *61, 62*
    tumoral calcinosis, 410, 422
    undifferentiated pleomorphic sarcoma, 411, 422–423
Radiology
    computed tomography, 12, 14–17
    conventional radiography
        benign *vs.* malignant nature, 12
        bone destruction, types, 6, *6–7*, 7
        borders of lesion, 3, *5*, 6
        periosteal reaction, 7–8, *9–10*
        site of lesion, 2–3, *3–5*
        soft-tissue mass, 11, *11*, 12
        tumor tissue, composition, 11–12, *13*, 14
    magnetic resonance imaging, 12, 14–17
    PET, PET-CT, and PET-MRI, 01%19–20
    pragmatic analysis, 2
    scintigraphy, 1, 17–19
Radiolucent lesion
    anteroposterior radiograph, *130*
    with chondroid calcifications, *143, 146, 152*
    lateral femoral condyle, *142*
    medial femoral condyle, *132*
    "popcorn"-like calcification, *92*
    proximal humerus, *95, 105*
    proximal phalanx, *91*
    proximal right femur, *141*
    proximal tibia, *136, 142*
Reed-Sternberg cell, 254, *262*, 409, 423
Renal cell carcinoma
    acromial end of left clavicle, *385*
    left hip, *384*
    lytic metastases from, 409, 421
    metastases from, *383*
    right leg, *384*

Revised European-American Lymphoma Classification, 232t
Ribbing disease, 243–244
Rosai-Dorfman disease
    definition, 241
    differential diagnosis, 242
    epidemiology, 241
    histopathology, 241, *241*
    immunohistochemistry, 241
    pathology, 241
    prognosis, 241–242
    scintigraphy, 241
    sites of involvement, 241
Rothmund-Thomson syndrome, 401–402, 417
Round cell lesions
    benign tumor
        Erdheim-Chester disease, 242–244
        Langerhans cell histiocytosis, 231–240
        Rosai-Dorfman disease, 241–242
    histopathologic features, 231t
    immunohistochemistry results, 232t
    malignant tumor
        Ewing sarcoma, 244–253
        malignant lymphoma, 254–263
        multiple myeloma, 263–268
    Revised European-American Lymphoma Classification, 232t

S

S100 protein, 25
Sarcomas. *See also specific types*
    translocation and fusion protein in, 28t, 29
SBC. *See* Simple bone cyst (SBC)
Scintigraphy, 1
    adamantinoma of long bones, 334, *336*
    aneurysmal bone cyst, 312, *319*
    benign fibrous histiocytoma, 189, *191*
    conventional chondrosarcoma, 140, *143*
    conventional osteosarcoma, 48, *52–53*
    enchondroma, 91
    Erdheim-Chester disease, 242
    Ewing sarcoma, 244
    extraskeletal myxoid chondrosarcoma, 169
    fibrous cortical defect, 182
    giant cell tumor, 299, *303*
    of Gorham disease, 284
    Langerhans cell histiocytosis, 233, *236*
    malignant fibrous histiocytoma, 221, *222*
    malignant lymphoma, *258*
    of metastatic disease, 18, *19*
    of monostotic fibrous dysplasia, *199*
    multiple myeloma, 263
    osteoid osteoma, 17, *18*, 35, *37*, *38*
    pathologic process, 19
    periosteal chondrosarcoma, *167*
    polyostotic fibrous dysplasia, *199*
    Rosai-Dorfman disease, 241
    sclerotic metastasis, 382, *389*
    skeletal metastases, 382, *388*, *393*
    synovial sarcoma, 369, *371*
    thallium-201 chloride, 18
Sclerotic metastasis, 382, *389*
    differential diagnosis, 243
Secondary chondrosarcomas
    differential diagnosis, 111
    enchondroma, malignant transformation
        clinical findings, 171
        epidemiology, 171
        histopathology, 171, *173*
        radiography, *172*
    osteochondroma, malignant transformation
        clinical findings, 171
        epidemiology, 171
        gross specimen, *172*
        histopathologic findings, 171
        radiography, *171*, *172*
Secondary osteochondromatosis, 111
Secondary osteosarcomas
    definition, 78
    with fibrous dysplasia, 79
    paget osteosarcoma, 79
    postradiation osteosarcoma, 78–79
Sessile osteochondroma, 35
    computed tomography, *118*
    differential diagnosis, 75, 99
    histopathology, *120*
    magnetic resonance imaging, *118*
    radiography, *115*, *116*, *118*
Shepherd's crook deformity, 403, 418
Simple bone cyst (SBC), 400, 407, 417, 420
    clinical findings, 309
    definition, 309
    differential diagnosis, 217, 310–311, 321, 334
    epidemiology, 309
    genetics, 310
    gross pathology, 310, *315*
    histopathology, 310, *315–316*
    lateral radiograph, 409, 421
    magnetic resonance imaging, 310, *313*, *314*
    no periosteal reaction, 409, 421
    prognosis, 310
    radiography, 310, *310–313*, 409, 421
    sites of involvement, 309
Sinus histiocytosis with massive lymphadenopathy. *See* Rosai-Dorfman disease
Skeletal metastases. *See also* Osteoblastic metastases; Osteolytic metastases
    clinical findings, 382
    definition, 382
    differential diagnosis, 390, 393–397
    epidemiology, 382
    FDG positron emission tomography, 382, *390–392*
    genetics, 386
    gross pathology, 382–383
    histopathology, 383, *393–396*
    immunohistochemistry, 386, *394–396*
    magnetic resonance imaging, 382, *391–393*
    PET, 382
    PET-CT, 382, *390–392*
    radiography, 382
    scintigraphy, 382, *388*, *393*
    sites of involvement, 382
Skeletal scintigraphy, 17–18, 91, 312
Small cell osteosarcoma
    clinical presentation, 64
    definition, 64
    differential diagnosis, 65–66
    epidemiology, 64
    genetics, 65
    histopathology, 65, *65*, 414, 425
    imaging, 64–65
    immunohistochemistry, 65
    prognosis, 66
    sites of involvement, 64
Soft-tissue chondroma
    clinical findings, 104
    differential diagnosis, 104, 361, 374–375
    histopathology, 104, *109*, 361
    imaging, 361
    pathology, 104
    sites of involvement, 104
Soft-tissue chondrosarcoma
    computed tomography, 413, 424
    differential diagnosis, 85, 104
    extraskeletal myxoid chondrosarcoma
        clinical findings, 169
        definition, 169
        epidemiology, 169
        genetics, 170
        immunophenotype, 170
        magnetic resonance imaging, 169
        pathology, 169–170
        prognosis, 170
        radiography, 169
        scintigraphy, 169
        sites of involvement, 169
    histopathology, 377, 413, 424
    magnetic resonance imaging, 377
Soft-tissue mass, 11, *11*, *12*
Soft-tissue osteosarcoma
    clinical presentation, 81
    computed tomography, 413, 424
    definition, 81
    differential diagnosis, 85
    epidemiology, 81
    gross pathology, 81, *84*
    histopathology, 81, *85*, 377, 413, 424
    imaging, 81
    magnetic resonance imaging, 377
    prognosis, 85
    radiography of, *81*
    sites of involvement, 81
Solitary osteoblastic metastasis
    calcifying enchondroma, 394–395
    enostosis, 393–394
    Erdheim-Chester disease, 395
    lymphoma, 395
    osteoblastoma, 394
Solitary osteolytic metastasis
    brown tumor of hyperparathyroidism, 393
    fibrosarcoma, 390
    giant cell tumor, 390
    plasmacytoma, 390
Stress fracture, 40, 409, 421
Surface osteosarcomas
    high-grade surface osteosarcoma
        clinical presentation, 77
        definition, 77
        epidemiology, 77
        gross pathology, 77
        histopathology, 78, *79*
        imaging, 77
        radiography, *78*
        sites of involvement, 77
    parosteal osteosarcoma
        clinical presentation, 70
        definition, 69
        differential diagnosis, 71–75
        epidemiology, 69

Surface osteosarcomas (*Continued*)
    genetics, 71
    gross pathology, 71, *73*
    histopathology, 71, *74*
    imaging, 70
    prognosis, 75
    sites of involvement, 70
  periosteal osteosarcoma
    clinical presentation, 75
    definition, 75
    differential diagnosis, 76–77
    epidemiology, 75
    genetics, 76
    gross pathology, 76
    histopathology, 76, *77*
    imaging, 75
    prognosis, 77
    sites of involvement, 75
  variants of, 71
Symplastic glomus tumor, 290
Synovial (osteo)chondromatosis, 353, 377, 406, 419
  clinical findings, 109
  computed tomography, 109, *110*, *111*
  definition, 107
  differential diagnosis, 111, 356, 362, 366
  epidemiology, 107
  genetics, 111
  gross pathology, 109, *113*
  histopathology, 111, *113*, 356, 362, 366, 404, 418
  magnetic resonance imaging, 109, *112*
  pathology, 109, 111
  prognostic factors/complications, 111
  radiography, 109, *109–112*, 356, 362, 366
  secondary chondrosarcoma, *173*, *174*
  sites of involvement, 107
Synovial hemangioma, 285
  clinical findings, 362
  computed tomography, 362, *363*
  definition, 362
  differential diagnosis, 359, 362–364, 366
  epidemiology, 362
  gross pathology, 362
  histopathology, 359, 362, 366, *366*

  magnetic resonance imaging, 359, 362, *364*, *365*, *366*
  prognosis, 362
  radiography, 362, *363*
  sites of involvement, 362
Synovial sarcoma, 408, 412, 420, 423
  clinical findings, 369
  definition, 369
  differential diagnosis, 85, 104, 361, 374–375, 377
  epidemiology, 369
  genetics, 374, *376*
  gross pathology, 369
  histopathology, 361, 369, 375, *375–377*
  imaging, 361
  immunohistochemistry, 374, *376*
  magnetic resonance imaging, 369, *370–374*
  PET–CT, *373–374*
  prognosis, 374
  radiography, 369, *370–374*
  scintigraphy, 369, *371*
  sites of involvement, 369

T

Telangiectatic osteosarcoma, 400, 412, 417, 423
  clinical presentation, 61
  definition, 61
  differential diagnosis, 63–64, 220, 223, 322–323
  epidemiology, 61
  genetics, 63
  gross pathology, 61, *63*
  histopathology, 61, 63, *63*, *64*, 414, 425
  imaging, 61, 414, 425
  magnetic resonance imaging, *62*
  most aggressive type of osteosarcomas, 414, 425
  prognosis, 64
  radiography, 61, *61*, *62*
  sites of involvement, 61
Touton cells, 235
Trabecular bone
  destruction, 6
  Whole-mount section, *333*
Trevor-Fairbanks disease, 119

Trichrome stain, 21
Tumor tissue, composition, 11–12, *13*, *14*
Tumoral calcinosis
  differential diagnosis, 375
  histopathology, 410, 422
  imaging, 375
  radiography, 410, 422

U

Ultrasound, 1
  osteoid osteoma, 38
Undifferentiated pleomorphic sarcoma
  histopathology, 411, 422–423
  radiography, 411, 422–423

V

van Gieson stain, 21
  in fibrous dysplasia, *23*
Vascular lesions
  benign tumor
    cystic angiomatosis, 282–284
    epithelioid hemangioma, 282
    glomangioma, 290
    glomangiomatosis, 290
    glomangiomyoma, 290
    glomus tumor, 289
    Gorham disease, 284–285
    intraosseous hemangioma, 273–281
    lymphangioma, 285–289
    lymphangiomatosis, 285–289
    malignant glomus tumor, 290
    symplastic glomus tumor, 290
    synovial hemangioma, 285
  malignant tumor
    angiosarcoma, 293–295
    epithelioid hemangioendothelioma, 290–293
Vimentin, 23
von Kossa stain, 21
von Recklinghausen disease of bone, 399, 416

W

Warthin-Starry stain, 21
Werner syndrome, 401–402, 417

RRS1508